Diarrhea: Causes, Diagnosis and Treatment

Diarrhea: Causes, Diagnosis and Treatment

Edited by Emilia Ferguson

hayle medical

New York

Hayle Medical,
750 Third Avenue, 9th Floor,
New York, NY 10017, USA

Visit us on the World Wide Web at:
www.haylemedical.com

ISBN: 978-1-63241-647-6

The publisher's policy is to use permanent paper from mills that operate a sustainable forestry policy. Furthermore, the publisher ensures that the text paper and cover boards used have met acceptable environmental accreditation standards.

Printed in China.

Cataloging-in-Publication Data

Diarrhea : causes, diagnosis and treatment / edited by Emilia Ferguson.
p. cm.
Includes bibliographical references and index.
ISBN 978-1-63241-647-6
1. Diarrhea. 2. Diarrhea--Etiology. 3. Diarrhea--Diagnosis. 4. Diarrhea--Treatment.
I. Ferguson, Emilia.
RC862.D5 D53 2019
616.342 7--dc23

Table of Contents

Preface

This book aims to highlight the current researches and provides a platform to further the scope of innovations in this area. This book is a product of the combined efforts of many researchers and scientists, after going through thorough studies and analysis from different parts of the world. The objective of this book is to provide the readers with the latest information of the field.

Diarrhea is a condition in which a person suffers from loose or liquid bowel movements. The primary cause of diarrhea is an infection in the intestines. The infection may be caused by a bacteria, virus or parasite. It may also be caused by non-infectious health conditions such as lactose intolerance, inflammatory bowel disease, hyperthyroidism, etc. Replacing the loss of fluids and salts through oral rehydration therapy or intravenous rehydration therapy is the most common treatment method. In some chronic cases, antibiotics may also be used to treat diarrhea. This book unravels the recent studies in this medical condition. It aims to elucidate the causes, diagnosis and treatment of the different forms of diarrhea. This book is an essential guide for clinicians, doctors and medical students.

I would like to express my sincere thanks to the authors for their dedicated efforts in the completion of this book. I acknowledge the efforts of the publisher for providing constant support. Lastly, I would like to thank my family for their support in all academic endeavors.

Editor

1

Village-Randomized Clinical Trial of Home Distribution of Zinc for Treatment of Childhood Diarrhea in Rural Western Kenya

Daniel R. Feikin[1]*, Godfrey Bigogo[1,4], Allan Audi[1,4], Sherri L. Pals[2], George Aol[1,4], Charles Mbakaya[4], John Williamson[3], Robert F. Breiman[1], Charles P. Larson[5,6]

1 International Emerging Infections Program, Centers for Disease Control and Prevention Kisumu, Kenya, 2 Division of Global HIV/AIDS, United States Centers for Disease Control and Prevention, Atlanta, Georgia, United States of America, 3 Center for Global Health, United States Centers for Disease Control and Prevention, Atlanta, Georgia, United States of America, 4 Kenya Medical Research Institute, Nairobi, Kenya, 5 International Centre for Diarrhoeal Disease Research, Bangladesh, Dhaka, Bangladesh, 6 Department of Pediatrics, University of British Columbia, Vancouver, Canada

Abstract

Background: Zinc treatment shortens diarrhea episodes and can prevent future episodes. In rural Africa, most children with diarrhea are not brought to health facilities. In a village-randomized trial in rural Kenya, we assessed if zinc treatment might have a community-level preventive effect on diarrhea incidence if available at home versus only at health facilities.

Methods: We randomized 16 Kenyan villages (1,903 eligible children) to receive a 10-day course of zinc and two oral rehydration solution (ORS) sachets every two months at home and 17 villages (2,241 eligible children) to receive ORS at home, but zinc at the health–facility only. Children's caretakers were educated in zinc/ORS use by village workers, both unblinded to intervention arm. We evaluated whether incidence of diarrhea and acute lower respiratory illness (ALRI) reported at biweekly home visits and presenting to clinic were lower in zinc villages, using poisson regression adjusting for baseline disease rates, distance to clinic, and children's age.

Results: There were no differences between village groups in diarrhea incidence either reported at the home or presenting to clinic. In zinc villages (1,440 children analyzed), 61.2% of diarrheal episodes were treated with zinc, compared to 5.4% in comparison villages (1,584 children analyzed, $p<0.0001$). There were no differences in ORS use between zinc (59.6%) and comparison villages (58.8%). Among children with fever or cough without diarrhea, zinc use was low (<0.5%). There was a lower incidence of reported ALRI in zinc villages (adjusted RR 0.68, 95% CI 0.46–0.99), but not presenting at clinic.

Conclusions: In this study, home zinc use to treat diarrhea did not decrease disease rates in the community. However, with proper training, availability of zinc at home could lead to more episodes of pediatric diarrhea being treated with zinc in parts of rural Africa where healthcare utilization is low.

Editor: David Joseph Diemert, The George Washington University Medical Center, United States of America

Funding: Support was provided by The Bill and Melinda Gates Foundation and Centers for Disease Control and Prevention. The funders had no role in study design, data collection and analysis, decision to publish, or preparation of the manuscript.

Competing Interests: The authors have declared that no competing interests exist.

* E-mail: dfeikin@jhsph.edu

Introduction

Diarrhea caused approximately 700,000 deaths in children in 2011, mostly in countries where children are deficient in zinc, an essential trace element for optimal immune response to infections. [1–4] Zinc treatment of a diarrheal episode has been shown to decrease the duration and lessen the severity of that diarrhea episode. [1,5,6] In addition, zinc given for 10–14 days during or shortly after a diarrheal episode has been shown to decrease subsequent diarrhea and acute lower respiratory illness infections over the ensuing few months. [2,7,8] Based on the weight of available evidence, WHO and UNICEF recommend zinc as an adjunct for diarrhea treatment for children in developing countries, and promote zinc use in the recently published integrated Global Action Plan for Pneumonia and Diarrhoea (GAPPD). [6,9].

Scaling up the use of zinc in developing countries has been challenging, due to obstacles of supply, cost, distribution and training. [10,11] Within the public sector, the initial push has been to make zinc available in health-facilities. Yet, many children with diarrhea in developing countries never present to public sector health-facilities, due to constraints of time, distance and cost of transport. [12,13] Distribution of zinc through community health workers (CHWs) has had positive results in several sites in South Asia and Africa. [7,8,14] There are parts of Africa, though, where CHWs do not treat illness in the community. Given the evidence of zinc's prevention of diarrhea and respiratory illness, we investigated whether providing zinc at home for future treatment of diarrhea had a preventative impact at the community level on the reduction of diarrhea incidence. As secondary objectives, we evaluated if availability of zinc in the home had a preventative impact at the community level on the reduction of respiratory disease incidence and would result in more diarrhea episodes being treated with zinc than having zinc available in the clinic only. We used a village-randomized design to facilitate training, distribution, and equity among caretakers within a village.

Methods

The protocol and consent forms were reviewed and approved by the Ethical Review Boards of KEMRI (# 932 and 985) and CDC (# 4566 and 4678). Written informed consent was obtained from children's primary caretakers. The study was registered with ClinicalTrials.gov (#NCT00530829). The protocol for this trial and supporting CONSORT checklist are available as supporting information; see Checklist S1 and Protocol S1.

Surveillance Platform

Population-based infectious disease surveillance (PBIDS) has been ongoing since late 2006 in Asembo, western Kenya. [15] On July 1, 2008, PBIDS included 3,856 children <5 years of age, in 33 villages. Malaria transmission is endemic and occurs year-round. [16] The under-5 mortality ratio was 212 per 1,000 live births in 2008. [17].

The methods for PBIDS have been described. [15,18] In brief, community interviewers visit enrolled households every two weeks to inquire about illnesses, referred to as household morbidity surveillance (HMS). For key symptoms, including cough, fever and diarrhea, participants provide number of days during the past two weeks when they had those symptoms. Health-care seeking, hospital admission, and medication use are also documented. For children <5 years, the mother, or other knowledgeable caretaker, is interviewed. Abbreviated physical exams are done.

In Lwak Hospital, the centrally-located referral facility for PBIDS, medical care is free to PBIDS participants. Patients are examined and diagnosed by clinical officers (similar to physician's assistants). Malaria blood smears are done on all febrile patients. Structured questionnaires record symptoms, vital signs, physical exam findings, diagnosis, and treatment. All children with diarrhea presenting to Lwak Hospital during the study were given zinc, if they were not already taking it for the episode, as standard protocol. We have previously shown that of children in PBIDS with diarrhea who are brought to a clinic, half are brought to Lwak Hospital. [19].

Zinc Study Design

The primary objective was to assess if home zinc availability led to decreased diarrhea incidence in the community. Secondary objectives were if home zinc availability led to decreased respiratory infections in the community, and if more children with diarrhea were treated with zinc when available in the home. For the zinc study, all residents in the 33 PBIDS villages aged 2–59 months of age on December 1, 2007 were identified. Among these, only participants enrolled in PBIDS and found at home after three attempts were eligible for enrollment. Enrollment was rolling until January 2009, whereby children born after the start of the zinc study or who in-migrated were eligible after they reached 2 months of age, whereas children reaching their 5th birthday were excluded. The 33 villages were randomly assigned to receive a 10-day blister pack of 20 mg dispersible zinc-sulfate tablets (Nutriset, France) at home every two months (hereafter referred to as "zinc villages") or to receive no zinc at home, but were told they could obtain it at Lwak Hospital if their child had diarrhea (hereafter referred to as "comparison villages"). All study participants, regardless of village category, presenting to Lwak clinic with diarrhea received a 10-day blister pack of zinc, if they were not already taking it for that episode. Every two months, households of all participants, regardless of study arm, received 2 packets of low-osmolarity ORS. All medicines were given free of charge.

Distribution of home zinc/ORS was done by village reporters, women who lived in the village and had minimal health-related training. Village reporters received a week-long training initially and refresher trainings every 2 months on treatment of diarrhea in children, how and when to use zinc and ORS, when mothers should take their child to the clinic, and were instructed to emphasize that zinc and/or ORS use was not a substitute for taking their child to the clinic. Special emphasis was given in training the village reporters that zinc was to treat only diarrhea, and if a child had other symptoms, such as fever or cough, they might also need an antimalarial or antibiotic at the clinic. [20] At each bi-monthly home visit, the village reporters re-educated mothers on proper use of zinc and ORS. Village reporters, who were unblinded to study arm, delivered zinc and/or OR were every 2 months, regardless of whether the previous supply had been used.

Although part of the MOH essential drug list, zinc was not available in MOH-run health facilities at the start of this study in February 2008. Nor was zinc available in the private sector in rural Kenya at that time. Therefore, zinc was only available to children with diarrhea presenting to Lwak Hospital. By late 2008, zinc had started to become available in MOH-run health facilities in the study area, although stock-outs were frequent.

Participants who had a diarrhea episode reported at the regular bi-weekly HMS visits were visited again seven days later to inquire about ongoing illness, medication use, and any adverse events.

Laboratory

To establish baseline zinc levels in the study area we randomly selected eight children from each of 33 villages, with the intent to enroll the first five who were available and consented for each village, for a goal of 165 children. We measured serum zinc concentrations, using Flame Atomic Absorption Spectrophotometry, at the KEMRI laboratory in Nairobi. Calibration of instruments was done using sera with known concentrations provided by ICDDR-B in Bangladesh. Zinc deficiency in children was considered as a concentration <65 mg/dl. [3,21].

Case Definitions

Case definitions for syndromes for HMS and clinic surveillance are given in Table 1. [15] Definitions for diarrhea, dehydration and ALRI follow WHO's Integrated Management of Childhood Illness guidelines. [22].

Village Randomization

We chose a randomization method that would probabilistically maintain similar numbers of children in each village category, by alternating village assignment, after a random starting assignment, based on an ordered list of villages by population size. Villages were not matched or stratified based on baseline rates of morbidity, mortality or health-seeking patterns. Village randomization was done at KEMRI/CDC after consenting all initial participants in December 2007. Village reporters informed participants of their village group at the time of first home zinc/ORS distribution in January 2008. Mothers from comparison

Table 1. Case definitions for major infectious disease syndromes from clinic and household morbidity surveillance (HMS) in Asembo, western Kenya.

Syndrome	Clinic definition	Household definition
Acute respiratory infection (ARI)	(≥1 symptom): cough, difficulty breathing, chest pain, sore throat, sneezing, ear complaints or runny nose	cough or difficulty breathing
Acute Lower Respiratory Infection (ALRI)	cough or difficulty breathing with one of the following: elevated respiratory rate for age* (non-severe pneumonia;) or IMCI danger sign†, lower chest wall indrawing, stridor, or oxygen saturation <90% (severe/very severe pneumonia)	cough or difficulty breathing and rapid respiration for age* or chest indrawing noted on exam
Diarrhea	≥3 looser than normal stools in a 24 hour period. Severe defined as IMCI danger sign or symptom/sign dehydration‡	≥3 looser than normal stools in a 24 hour period
Acute Febrile Illness (AFI)	documented axillary temperature ≥38.0°C without an obvious cause, defined as cough, difficulty breathing, chest pain, signs of meningitis, or bloody diarrhea (positive malaria smear is not an exclusion)	report of fever, without evidence of another infection defined as cough or difficulty breathing or bloody diarrhea

*Elevated respiratory rate for age based on WHO Integrated Management of Childhood Illness algorithm [14]; <2 months, ≥60 breaths/minute; 2–11 months, ≥50 breaths/minute; 12–59 months, ≥40 breaths/minute.
†IMCI danger signs are maternal report of convulsions, inability to drink or breastfeed, or vomiting everything, or on exam lethargy or unconsciousness [22].
‡IMCI signs/symptoms of dehydration are the following: sunken eyes, slow skin pinch, restless/irritable behavior, drinking eagerly or not at all [22].

villages could not be given zinc by village reporters since their group assignment was by their village of residence; all village reporters were from the villages and knew mothers in their own village.

Data Analysis

We considered the first 2 months (January–February 2008) a pilot study, excluding those months from analysis. Therefore, the study period for analysis was February 2008 to March 2009. We considered the pre-intervention period as October 2006–November 2007, which was when HMS data were available for all villages. Pre-intervention period data were included in analyses to account for baseline differences in disease rates and distance to clinic between village categories. Pre-intervention data on medication use were not available.

Because the population of children in the PBIDS villages was fixed, we calculated what decrease in diarrhea incidence we could detect with a power of 80% or greater at an alpha of 0.05. We estimated the PBIDS population of children 2–59 months old to be approximately 3,000, and assumed a baseline diarrhea incidence of 3.6 episodes per year. Assuming that there would be a 5% decrease in diarrhea rates in the comparison villages during the study period due to zinc use in the clinic, we estimated that we would have the power to detect a difference of 12% in rates between zinc and comparison groups, accounting for correlation of diarrhea events by child using the method described by Rochon. [23].

Baseline characteristics between children in zinc and comparison villages were compared by chi-square or t-test, controlling for clustering at the village level. The percentages of episodes of illness in the zinc and comparison villages that resulted in zinc or other medication use, or care-seeking outside the home, were compared using the F-test in SAS PROC GLIMMIX with village as a random effect to control for clustering; for the analysis of care-seeking we adjusted for seeking care outside the home for similar illness episodes in the pre-intervention period. Rates of illness were compared between children in zinc and comparison villages, both for those resulting in a sick visit to Lwak Hospital and those reported during the biweekly HMS visits. For the HMS, rates were calculated using newly reported episodes divided by the number of total days from which HMS data were available; due to poor recall of symptoms we only calculated rates for the day of the home visit and the three previous days, as we have described before. [15,24] For the clinic, rates were calculated by using the number of clinic visits for a syndrome divided by the person-time of residence in the surveillance area. Children contributed person-time from the date of their enrollment until the end of the study (March 31, 2009), their fifth birthday, or their date of outmigration or death. Rate ratios were calculated between zinc and comparison villages, adjusting for pre-intervention rates of the syndrome in the child's village, distance of the child's compound to Lwak Hospital, and the child's age. For pre-intervention rates, all children in the study villages aged 2–59 months enrolled in morbidity surveillance were used, whereas rates during the intervention period were limited to only those enrolled in the zinc study. Analyses of rates were done using poisson regression with generalized estimating equations to control for correlated observations (PROC GENMOD, SAS version 9.1). A second "per-treatment" analysis was done for clinic visits, where we included only children who took at least one course of zinc (intervention villages) or ORS (comparison villages) during the course of the study. All data analysis was done unblinded to study arm.

Findings

In total, 1,440 children were enrolled in 16 zinc villages and 1,584 in 17 comparison villages (Figure 1). Over 80% of eligible children were enrolled at the outset in both groups; however, for children who were born or in-migrated into the area after the start of the study, only 36–44% were enrolled due to delays in registering children into the surveillance system. Of enrolled children, all were included in the clinic-based analysis, but 17% were excluded from the household-based analysis since no household morbidity data was available for these children during the study period; this was likely due to nobody being at home during biweekly household visits or temporary relocation of residences. During the study period, in the zinc and comparison villages, 96 and 106 children moved out of the study area, 31 and 41 died, and 346 and 431 reached their fifth birthday, respectively.

Zinc and comparison villages were similar in terms of children's age, maternal education, socioeconomic status, and crowding (Table 2). Zinc villages tended to be further from Lwak Hospital than comparison villages (4.7 vs. 3.4 kilometers, $p = 0.07$). At baseline, we collected blood for zinc concentration measurement

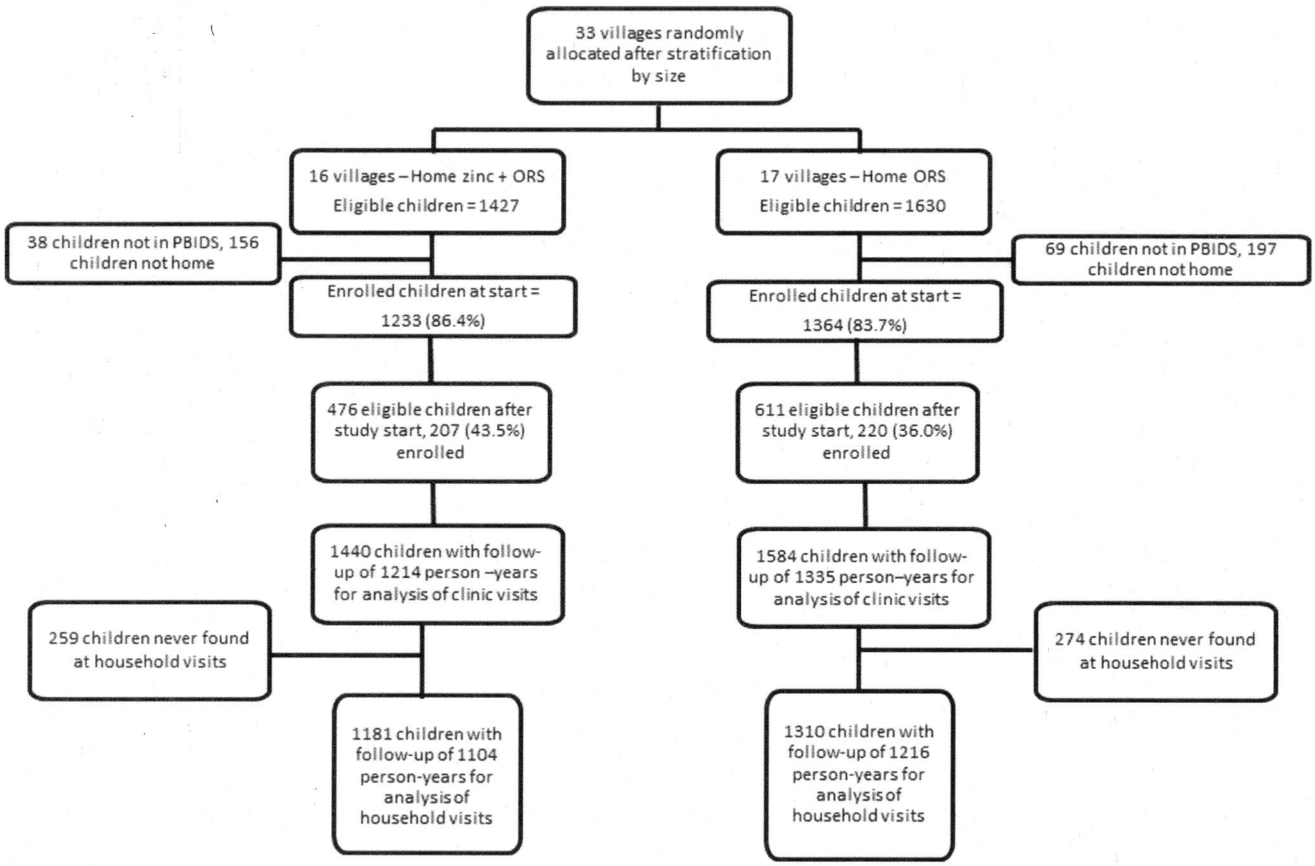

Figure 1. Trial profile. Village randomization and number of children enrolled at the initial enrollment in December 2007 and during the ongoing enrollment during the study period from February 2008–March 2009. Children and person-time contribution given for the analysis of clinic-based surveillance and household morbidity surveillance – see methods. PBIDS = Population-based Infectious Disease Surveillance.

from 151 children who were enrolled and consented. Of these, 135 (89%) blood samples of adequate volume and quality, the median zinc concentration was 72.0 μg/dL (IQR 61–88); 32% of children had low zinc levels (<65 μg/dL). There was no difference between median zinc concentrations of children in the zinc group (72 μg/dL) and comparison group (73.0 μg/dL, $p = 0.87$).

There were 969 7-day follow up visits for diarrheal episodes in zinc villages and 953 in comparison villages. In zinc villages 6.1% of children still had diarrhea versus 5.6% in comparison villages ($p = 0.57$). Among zinc users, the median number of days that zinc had been taken was 8.0 in both village groups. Twenty-one percent of children given zinc had vomited a zinc tablet; 69% of vomiting episodes were limited to the first zinc dose (no difference by village group). The median number of ORS sachets used was 2.0.

Based on self-report of the caretaker at the biweekly HMS visit, in zinc villages 61.2% of all diarrheal episodes were treated with zinc, compared to 5.4% in the comparison villages ($p<0.0001$, Table 3). Similar differences in zinc use were observed for episodes of diarrhea with fever and with cough. There were no differences in ORS use for diarrhea between zinc (59.6%) and comparison villages (58.8%). Diarrheal episodes in zinc villages resulted in less frequent use of antimalarials and antibiotics (Table 3). Children with diarrhea and reported fever in zinc villages (approximately two-thirds of diarrheal episodes) received an antimalarial less frequently (17.8%) than in comparison villages (23.5%, $p = 0.048$). Care-seeking outside the home for diarrhea episodes was similar between village groups. Among children with fever or cough without diarrhea, zinc use was low in both zinc and comparison villages (<0.5%), although care-seeking outside the home was higher in comparison villages for these non-diarrhea syndromes.

Although rates of clinic visitation due to diarrhea were lower in the zinc than comparison villages during the intervention period, this difference was not statistically different after adjustment (Table 4). Similarly, no significant differences were observed between zinc and comparison villages for clinic visits for rates of severe diarrhea, ARI, ALRI, acute febrile illness or malaria parasitemia (Table 4). We found similar results when limiting the clinic-based analysis to only those children who took at least one course of zinc or ORS during the study period (Table 5). There were also no significant differences in the incidence of reported diarrhea, diarrhea with fever, severe diarrhea, ARI, or acute febrile illness at the biweekly household visits (Table 6). However, children in the zinc villages had 32% fewer reported ALRI episodes than in comparison villages (adjusted RR 0.68, 95% CI 0.46–0.99). There were no differences between village groups in hospitalization rates or all-cause mortality (Table 4).

Discussion

We did not observe a community-level impact on diarrhea incidence in home zinc villages despite increased zinc use. There are several potential reasons. First, it is possible that zinc use does not prevent future diarrhea episodes in this setting; most studies on

Table 2. Baseline characteristics for participants in home zinc and comparison villages, western Kenya, February 2008–March 2009.

Characteristic	Home zinc	Comparison	P value*
N	1440	1584	
Age in months (median)	28.2	27.9	0.58
Age categories, n (%)			
2–5 months	202 (14)	246 (16)	0.31
6–11 mo	139 (10)	147 (9)	
12–23 mo	278 (19)	279 (18)	
24–59 mo	821 (57)	912 (58)	
Male, n (%)	732 (51)	772 (49)	0.38
Maternal education beyond primary	291 (20)	322 (20)	0.89
Poorer households†	345 (29)	379 (28)	0.79
Distance from residence to Lwak (median meters)	4728	3351	0.07
# children <5 years in household (median)	2.0	2.0	0.36

*p value controls for cluster design by village.
†Poorer household is defined as the lowest two quintiles using multiple component analysis.

the preventive effect of zinc on diarrhea occurred in South Asia and the epidemiology of diarrhea disease differs in Africa. [2,7,8,25] Second, perhaps not enough children received zinc in the community to precipitate a measureable decrease in community-level incidence. We were not able to enroll as many children as we anticipated, particularly for the household-level morbidity analysis, and so it is possible we were unpowered to detect a difference. We did not, however, see reduced diarrhea rates when restricting the analysis to only children who took zinc. Third, possibly we were unable to detect a real decrease in diarrhea incidence due to limitations in our study design (e.g. baseline differences between village groups), which we were unable to fully adjust for. Moreover, biases in surveillance could have masked an impact on incidence; children given zinc at home might have had reduced health-seeking at clinic because of less perceived need for medication, or caretakers who gave zinc might have been more likely to recall and report diarrheal episodes at the home visits. Although we did not observe a difference in diarrhea rates, we did see marginally less ALRI in the zinc villages reported at the household, but not at the clinic; zinc treatment for diarrhea has been shown to prevent subsequent ALRI in India. [8].

While this study did not provide evidence for a community-level preventative impact of home zinc use, we did show that by providing zinc in the home children with diarrhea were much more likely to receive zinc treatment than when zinc was only available in the health facility. Moreover, having ORS available at home likely resulted in higher uptake of ORS for diarrhea treatment than occurred historically in this area. [9,26,27] In much of rural Africa, such as western Kenya, most children with diarrhea are not taken to health facilities. [12] We have previously shown in our area that only 36% of children with diarrhea seek care at a health facility. [26] Of note, an additional 50% of children sought care at sources besides licensed health facilities, suggesting that making zinc available through drug sellers, community health workers, or private providers could also increase the number of diarrheal episodes treated with zinc.

Our study demonstrated that caretakers of children can be educated to use zinc appropriately at home. In our study, very few caretakers used zinc to treat illnesses without diarrhea. Misuse of zinc has been raised as a concern whereby mothers might substitute one drug, particularly a free one, for other necessary drugs, like antimalarials, which have an extra real or opportunity cost to acquire. [20] Yet, our study did show some potential cautionary information similar to what was shown in a community-based zinc program in Mali in that children with diarrhea with fever tended to be less likely to receive antimalarial medications. [20] Although it is possible that fever could be part of the diarrhea episode, in an endemic malaria area, such as rural western Kenya, all episodes of fever merit either empiric malaria treatment or a reliable diagnostic test to rule out malaria. [28] This speaks to the need for ongoing education of caretakers, or combined home treatment of diarrhea and malaria.

To achieve maximum impact of zinc, we chose to provide zinc to caretakers in the home for several reasons. First, rural western Kenya did not have a well-established system of CHWs at the time of the study, as in other settings in Africa or south Asia. [7,8,20] Second, zinc was not yet available in public or private facilities and was virtually unknown in the community as a treatment for diarrhea. In such a context, we felt that to design a study where zinc was provided to local drug sellers and shops and expect mothers to purchase this new and unknown drug would not result in high levels of zinc usage, even at a minimal price. Third, zinc, along with ORS, is a good candidate for home treatment as it is inexpensive, easy-to-use, and has a low adverse event profile. [5] Mothers already commonly treat children's illnesses at home on their own volition in many parts of Africa. [13,20,26] Although the design we used to deliver zinc and ORS at home is likely not scalable, with the advent of community-based health approaches like in Kenya, alternative strategies, including cost-effectiveness analyses, of delivery of home zinc and ORS to treat diarrhea need to be explored.

Although our study shows safe and proper use of zinc by caretakers at home, alternate approaches to increasing zinc use outside the clinic are possible. Treatment with zinc could be undertaken by community health workers, as in other places. [7,8,10] Moreover, zinc could be made more accessible to caretakers if it was available through non-facility sources of drugs, which in rural Africa could include CHWs through the iCCM strategy [29,30] or drug sellers through local shops and pharmacies, as has been done for effective antimalarial treatment in many parts of Africa. [31].

Table 3. Effect of intervention on drug use and healthcare use for various disease syndromes during the intervention period from household morbidity surveillance (HMS), western Kenya, February 2008–March 2009.

	Home zinc N (%†)	Comparison N (%†)	P value*
All diarrhea (n)	1707	1700	
Zinc	1045 (61.2)	92 (5.4)	<.0001¶
ORS	1018 (59.6)	999 (58.8)	.62
Antimalarial	190 (11.1)	272 (16.0)	.006
Antibiotic	291 (17.1)	383 (22.5)	.018
Sought care†	531 (31.2)	542 (31.9)	.22
Diarrhea+fever (n)	1043	1133	
Zinc	624 (59.8)	72 (6.4)	<.0001
ORS	629 (60.3)	655 (57.8)	.31
Antimalarial	186 (17.8)	266 (23.5)	.048
Antibiotic	253 (24.3)	322 (28.4)	.22
Sought care†	380 (36.5)	412 (36.4)	.26
Diarrhea+cough (n)	701	716	
Zinc	415 (59.2)	45 (6.3)	<.0001
ORS	426 (60.8)	400 (55.9)	.11
Antimalarial	122 (17.4)	150 (21.0)	.28
Antibiotic	192 (27.4)	226 (31.6)	.21
Sought care†	253 (36.1)	255 (35.7)	.61
Fever without diarrhea (n)	6188	6693	
Zinc	13 (0.2)	2 (0.03)	N/A
ORS	25 (0.4)	37 (0.6)	.33
Antimalarial	1510 (24.4)	1701 (25.4)	.81
Antibiotic	1187 (19.2)	1221 (18.2)	.70
Sought care†	2509 (40.6)	3023 (45.3)	.017
Cough without diarrhea (n)	5412	5170	
Zinc	10 (0.2)	1 (0.02)	.039
ORS	12 (0.2)	22 (0.4)	.31
Antimalarial	868 (16.0)	883 (17.1)	.78
Antibiotic	1396 (25.8)	1368 (26.5)	.48
Sought care†	1999 (36.9)	2089 (40.5)	.019

*p-value calculation includes a random effect variable for village, and adjusts for pre-intervention rates of seeking care outside the home by village - F-test in SAS PROC GLIMMIX.
†% given in table is the % of biweekly household visits with illness that resulted in medication use or care-seeking outside the home. Denominator for sought care was slightly lower than for medication use due to some missing data for that variable.
¶For primary outcome, intracluster correlation (ICC) = 0.030.

Our study had several other potential limitations. First, our study was not designed to evaluate the impact of zinc the duration or severity of diarrhea episodes. Because zinc use has been shown to reduce diarrhea duration in multiple settings in several meta-analyses, we expected that in our setting, where approximately one-third of children were zinc-deficient, zinc would be effective in reducing diarrhea duration and did not need to be studied. [1,5,6] Second, zinc was only available for treatment in Lwak Hospital and not other area clinics during most of the study period. Therefore, zinc use was lower than in a setting where all clinics have zinc available. Nonetheless, if we doubled the percentage of diarrhea episodes treated with zinc to account for health-seeking at other area clinics, zinc use would still have been substantially lower (10.8%) among children receiving zinc in the clinics only compared with the children receiving zinc at home (61.2%). [19] Third, because we did not match or stratify villages on incidence of diarrhea or health-seeking at the time of village randomization, there were some baseline differences between village groups. Although we did adjust for baseline rates in our analysis of disease incidence, it is possible that residual confounding due to baseline differences by village group remained. Moreover, we did not have baseline rates of antimicrobial use, so could not adjust for baseline differences in the analysis of the impact of zinc on antimicrobial use, including antimalarials. Fourth, our findings on zinc's impact on prevention might have been biased towards the null by including children younger than six months of age. There is no evidence that zinc use among children <6 months of age shortens duration of diarrhea episodes or prevents subsequent episodes [5,32–34].

Since we undertook this study, the Kenya MOH has fully adopted zinc as part of the essential drug kit available in health facilities. Although we did not show a decrease in community

Table 4. Effect of home zinc on rate of sick visits to Lwak clinic, hospitalization, and mortality, western Kenya, from February 2008–March 2009, controlling for baseline rates of morbidity in home zinc and comparison villages.

	Pre-intervention*		Intervention period†		Adjusted RR‡ (CI 95%)
	Home zinc	Comparison	Home zinc	Comparison	
Person-years observed	2001	2245	1214	1335	
Diarrhea	0.098	0.118	0.146	0.184	1.05 [0.81–1.37]¶
Diarrhea plus reported fever	0.089	0.102	0.138	0.160	1.09 [0.83–1.43]
Diarrhea and malaria	0.025	0.023	0.072	0.090	1.05 [0.74–1.49]
Severe diarrhea	0.040	0.046	0.059	0.059	1.17 [0.79–1.76]
Diarrhea hospitalization	0.027	0.034	0.037	0.051	0.87 [0.56–1.36)
Acute Respiratory Illness	0.406	0.464	0.830	0.904	1.16 [0.98–1.37]
ALRI	0.053	0.065	0.083	0.095	1.06 [0.78–1.45]
ALRI hospitalization	0.035	0.049	0.041	0.055	0.91 [0.59–1.39]
Acute febrile illness	0.030	0.049	0.145	0.162	1.30 [0.99–1.69]
Malaria (Blood smear+)	0.033	0.040	0.530	0.611	1.19 [0.99–1.44]
All-cause hospitalization	0.093	0.126	0.161	0.195	1.06 [0.82–1.38]
Mortality	0.023	0.029	0.024	0.029	0.83 [0.49–1.40]

Intention-to-treat analysis includes all enrolled children. Rates are given as episodes per person-year.
*Pre-intervention period was October 2006 to November 2007.
†While pre-intervention includes all children in the village of appropriate age, the intervention period only includes those enrolled in the home zinc study.
‡Rate ratio is comparing rates between home zinc and comparison groups during the intervention period, adjusted for pre-intervention rates of same syndrome in the child's village, distance of child's compound to Lwak Hospital and child's age.
¶For primary outcome, intracluster correlation (ICC) = 0.027.

incidence of diarrhea when zinc was available in the home, we did show that far more children with diarrhea in rural Kenya, and perhaps most areas of rural Africa, would likely be treated with zinc for diarrhea if zinc were either available in the home or at the community level, rather than in only health facilities. Adequate education, training and monitoring will be essential in adopting

Table 5. Effect of home zinc on rate of sick visits to Lwak clinic, hospitalization, and mortality, western Kenya, from February 2008–March 2009, controlling for baseline rates of morbidity in home zinc and comparison villages.

	Pre-intervention*		Intervention period†		Adjusted RR‡ (CI 95%)
	Home zinc	Comparison	Home zinc	Comparison	
Person-years observed	2001	2245	598	625	
Diarrhea	0.098	0.118	0.22	0.31	0.99 [0.73–1.33]
Diarrhea plus reported fever	0.089	0.102	0.21	0.27	1.02 [0.76–1.39]
Diarrhea and malaria	0.025	0.023	0.10	0.14	0.87 [0.57–1.34]
Severe diarrhea	0.040	0.046	0.10	0.11	1.14 [0.72–1.79]
Diarrhea hospitalization	0.027	0.034	0.06	0.09	0.82 [0.49–1.36)
Acute Respiratory Illness	0.406	0.464	0.86	1.18	0.93 [0.76–1.13]
ALRI	0.053	0.065	0.11	0.15	0.95 [0.65–1.40]
ALRI hospitalization	0.035	0.049	0.06	0.09	0.93 [0.56–1.53]
Acute febrile illness	0.030	0.049	0.16	0.22	1.20 [0.84–1.71]
Malaria (Blood smear+)	0.033	0.040	0.49	0.77	0.89 [0.70–1.12]
All-cause hospitalization	0.093	0.126	0.17	0.29	0.79 [0.57–1.09]
Mortality	0.023	0.029	0.02	0.04	0.69 [0.34–1.41]

Per-treatment analysis includes only children who received at least one course of zinc in home zinc villages and one course of ORS in comparison villages. Rates are given as episodes per person-year.
*Pre-intervention period was October 2006 to November 2007.
†While pre-intervention includes all children in the village of appropriate age, the intervention period only includes those enrolled in the home zinc study who took one course of recommended treatment for diarrhea.
‡Rate ratio is comparing rates between home zinc and comparison groups during the intervention period, adjusted for pre-intervention rates of same syndrome in the child's village, distance of child's compound to Lwak Hospital and child's age.

Table 6. Effect of home zinc on rates of reported morbidity at the household morbidity surveillance (HMS), western Kenya, from February 2008–March 2009, controlling for baseline rates of morbidity in home zinc and comparison villages.

	Pre-intervention*		Intervention†		Adjusted RR‡ (CI 95%)
	Intervention	Comparison	Intervention	Comparison	
Person-years observed	1488	1690	1104	1206	
Diarrhea	2.64	1.69	1.94	1.99	0.96 (0.79–1.15)
Diarrhea plus reported fever	0.94	0.87	1.04	1.10	0.94 (0.81–1.24)
Severe diarrhea	1.90	1.21	1.15	1.32	0.91 (0.73–1.13)
Diarrhea hospitalization (any hospital)	0.04	0.04	0.05	0.06	0.97 (0.42–2.23)
Acute Respiratory Illness	7.32	6.78	7.26	6.83	1.03 (0.95–1.12)
ALRI	0.28	0.24	0.18	0.28	0.68 (0.46–0.99)
Acute febrile illness	10.06	10.13	10.16	10.36	0.99 (0.91–1.07)

Rates are given as episodes per person-year.
*Pre-intervention period was October 2006 to November 2007.
†While pre-intervention includes all children in the village of appropriate age, the intervention period only includes those enrolled in the home zinc study.
‡Rate ratio is comparing rates between home zinc and comparison groups during the intervention period, adjusted for pre-intervention rates of the same syndrome in the child's village, distance of village to Lwak and child's age.

such a strategy. Assuming zinc has the same treatment and preventive impact in rural Africa as elsewhere, greater zinc use would translate into a beneficial public health impact.

Acknowledgments

We thank Rubhana Raqib of the International Centre for Diarrheal Diseases Research, Bangladesh for assistance with laboratory analysis; Allen Hightower for assistance with randomization; and Sonal Patel of the University of Medicine and Dentistry of New Jersey for critical input into the project initiation. This article is published with the approval of the Director of the Kenya Medical Research Institute. The findings and conclusions are those of the authors and do not necessarily represent the views of the Centers for Disease Control and Prevention.

Author Contributions

Conceived and designed the experiments: DRF RFB CPL. Performed the experiments: DRF GB GA CM. Analyzed the data: DRF AA SLP JW. Contributed reagents/materials/analysis tools: CM. Wrote the paper: DRF. Other: Critical review and contribution to written manuscript: GB AA SLP GA CM JW RFB CPL.

References

1. Bhutta ZA, Bird SM, Black RE, Brown KH, Gardner JM, et al. (2000) Therapeutic effects of oral zinc in acute and persistent diarrhea in children in developing countries: pooled analysis of randomized controlled trials. Am J Clin Nutr 72: 1516–1522.
2. Bhutta ZA, Black RE, Brown KH, Gardner JM, Gore S, et al. (1999) Prevention of diarrhea and pneumonia by zinc supplementation in children in developing countries: pooled analysis of randomized controlled trials. Zinc Investigators' Collaborative Group. J Pediatr 135: 689–697.
3. International Zinc Nutrition Consultive Group (2004) Assessment of the risk of zinc deficiency in populations and options for its control. Food Nutr Bull: S91–S204.
4. Walker CL, Rudan I, Liu L, Nair H, Theodoratou E, et al. (2013) Global burden of childhood pneumonia and diarrhoea. Lancet 381: 1405–1416.
5. Lazzerini M, Ronfani L (2012) Oral zinc for treating diarrhoea in children. Cochrane Database Syst Rev 6: CD005436.
6. WHO/UNICEF (2004) Clinical management of acute diarrhoea. Available: http://www.unicef.org/nutrition/files/ENAcute_Diarrhoea_reprint.pdf. Accessed 2012 May 16.
7. Baqui AH, Black RE, El Arifeen S, Yunus M, Chakraborty J, et al. (2002) Effect of zinc supplementation started during diarrhoea on morbidity and mortality in Bangladeshi children: community randomised trial. Bmj 325: 1059.
8. Bhandari N, Mazumder S, Taneja S, Dube B, Agarwal RC, et al. (2008) Effectiveness of zinc supplementation plus oral rehydration salts compared with oral rehydration salts alone as a treatment for acute diarrhea in a primary care setting: a cluster randomized trial. Pediatrics 121: e1279–1285.
9. WHO/UNICEF (2013) Integrated global action plan for the prevention and control of pneumonia and diarrhoea. Geneva. Available: http://www.who.int/maternal_child_adolescent/documents/global_action_plan_pneumonia_diarrhoea/en/. Accessed 2013 May 16.
10. Larson CP, Koehlmoos TP, Sack DA, Scaling Up of Zinc for Young Children Project T (2012) Scaling up zinc treatment of childhood diarrhoea in Bangladesh: theoretical and practical considerations guiding the SUZY Project. Health Policy Plan 27: 102–114.
11. Gill CJ, Young M, Schroder K, Carvajal-Velez L, McNabb M, et al. (2013) Bottlenecks, barriers, and solutions: results from multicountry consultations focused on reduction of childhood pneumonia and diarrhoea deaths. Lancet 381: 1487–1498.
12. Deutscher M, Van Beneden C, Burton D (2012) Putting Surveillance Data into Context: The Role of Health Care Utilization Surveys in Understanding Population Burden of Pneumonia in Developing Countries. J Epidemiology and Public Health in press.
13. Wilson SE, Ouedraogo CT, Prince L, Ouedraogo A, Hess SY, et al. (2012) Caregiver recognition of childhood diarrhea, care seeking behaviors and home treatment practices in rural Burkina Faso: a cross-sectional survey. PLoS One 7: e33273.
14. Winch PJ, Gilroy KE, Doumbia S, Patterson AE, Daou Z, et al. (2006) Prescription and administration of a 14-day regimen of zinc treatment for childhood diarrhea in Mali. Am J Trop Med Hyg 74: 880–883.
15. Feikin DR, Olack B, Bigogo GM, Audi A, Cosmas L, et al. (2011) The burden of common infectious disease syndromes at the clinic and household level from population-based surveillance in rural and urban Kenya. PLoS One 6: e16085.
16. Phillips-Howard PA, Nahlen BL, Wannemuehler KA, Kolczak MS, ter Kuile FO, et al. (2003) Impact of permethrin-treated bed nets on the incidence of sick child visits to peripheral health facilities. Am J Trop Med Hyg 68: 38–43.
17. Hamel MJ, Adazu K, Obor D, Sewe M, Vulule J, et al. (2011) A reversal in reductions of child mortality in western Kenya, 2003–2009. Am J Trop Med Hyg 85: 597–605.
18. Feikin DR, Njenga MK, Bigogo G, Aura B, Aol G, et al. (2013) Viral and bacterial causes of severe acute respiratory illness among children aged less than 5 years in a high malaria prevalence area of western Kenya, 2007–2010. Pediatr Infect Dis J 32: e14–19.

19. Bigogo G, Audi A, Aura B, Aol G, Breiman RF, et al. (2010) Health-seeking patterns among participants of population-based morbidity surveillance in rural western Kenya: implications for calculating disease rates. Int J Infect Dis 14: e967–973.
20. Winch PJ, Gilroy KE, Doumbia S, Patterson AE, Daou Z, et al. (2008) Operational issues and trends associated with the pilot introduction of zinc for childhood diarrhoea in Bougouni district, Mali. J Health Popul Nutr 26: 151–162.
21. Gibson RS, Hess SY, Hotz C, Brown KH (2008) Indicators of zinc status at the population level: a review of the evidence. Br J Nutr 99 Suppl 3: S14–23.
22. WHO (2008) Integrated Management of Childhood Illness. World Health Organization. Available: http://whqlibdoc.who.int/publications/2008/9789241597289_eng.pdf. Accessed 2012 May 16.
23. Rochon J (1998) Application of GEE procedures for sample size calculations in repeated measures experiments. Stat Med 17: 1643–1658.
24. Feikin DR, Audi A, Olack B, Bigogo GM, Polyak C, et al. (2010) Evaluation of the optimal recall period for disease symptoms in home-based morbidity surveillance in rural and urban Kenya. Int J Epidemiol 39: 450–458.
25. Kotloff KL, Nataro JP, Blackwelder WC, Nasrin D, Farag TH, et al (2013) Burden and aetiology of diarrhoeal disease in infants and young children in developing countries (The Global Enterics Multicenter Study): a prospective, case-control study. Lancet. Available: http://dx.doi.org/10.1016/S0140-6736(13)60844-2.
26. Burton DC, Flannery B, Onyango B, Larson C, Alaii J, et al. (2011) Healthcare-seeking behaviour for common infectious disease-related illnesses in rural Kenya: a community-based house-to-house survey. J Health Popul Nutr 29: 61–70.
27. Kenya National Bureau of Statistics (KNBS) and ICF Macro (2010) Kenya Demographic and Health Survey 2008–09. Calverton, Maryland.
28. WHO (2010) Guidelines for the treatment of malaria. In: WHO, editor. 2nd ed. Geneva: WHO. Available: http://whqlibdoc.who.int/publications/2010/9789241547925_eng.pdf. Accessed 2013 May 20.
29. Marsh DR, Hamer DH, Pagnoni F, Peterson S (2012) Introduction to a special supplement: Evidence for the implementation, effects, and impact of the integrated community case management strategy to treat childhood infection. Am J Trop Med Hyg 87: 2–5.
30. George A, Young M, Nefdt R, Basu R, Sylla M, et al. (2012) Community health workers providing government community case management for child survival in sub-saharan Africa: who are they and what are they expected to do? Am J Trop Med Hyg 87: 85–91.
31. Tougher S, Ye Y, Amuasi JH, Kourgueni IA, Thomson R, et al. (2012) Effect of the Affordable Medicines Facility–malaria (AMFm) on the availability, price, and market share of quality-assured artemisinin-based combination therapies in seven countries: a before-and-after analysis of outlet survey data. Lancet 380: 1916–1926.
32. Brooks WA, Santosham M, Roy SK, Faruque AS, Wahed MA, et al. (2005) Efficacy of zinc in young infants with acute watery diarrhea. Am J Clin Nutr 82: 605–610.
33. Fischer Walker CL, Bhutta ZA, Bhandari N, Teka T, Shahid F, et al. (2006) Zinc supplementation for the treatment of diarrhea in infants in Pakistan, India and Ethiopia. J Pediatr Gastroenterol Nutr 43: 357–363.
34. Walker CL, Bhutta ZA, Bhandari N, Teka T, Shahid F, et al. (2007) Zinc during and in convalescence from diarrhea has no demonstrable effect on subsequent morbidity and anthropometric status among infants <6 mo of age. Am J Clin Nutr 85: 887–894.

2

Self-Reported Stomach Upset in Travellers on Cruise-Based and Land-Based Package Holidays

Naomi J. Launders[1,2], Gordon L. Nichols[1,2,5,6*], Rodney Cartwright[3], Joanne Lawrence[4], Jane Jones[4], Christos Hadjichristodoulou[2,5]

1 Gastrointestinal, Emerging and Zoonotic Infections Department, Public Health England, London, United Kingdom, **2** EU Shipsan Trainet Project, Public Health Program, European Agency for Health and Consumers, Luxembourg, Luxembourg, **3** Federation of Tour Operators, London, United Kingdom, **4** Travel and Migrant Health Section, Public Health England, London, United Kingdom, **5** Department of Hygiene and epidemiology, Medical Faculty, University of Thessaly, Larissa, Greece, **6** Norwich Medical School, University of East Anglia, Norwich, United Kingdom

Abstract

Background: International travellers are at a risk of infectious diseases not seen in their home country. Stomach upsets are common in travellers, including on cruise ships. This study compares the incidence of stomach upsets on land- and cruise-based holidays.

Methods: A major British tour operator has administered a Customer Satisfaction Questionnaire (CSQ) to UK resident travellers aged 16 or more on return flights from their holiday abroad over many years. Data extracted from the CSQ was used to measure self-reported stomach upset in returning travellers.

Results: From summer 2000 through winter 2008, 6,863,092 questionnaires were completed; 6.6% were from cruise passengers. A higher percentage of land-based holiday-makers (7.2%) reported stomach upset in comparison to 4.8% of cruise passengers (RR = 1.5, $p<0.0005$). Reported stomach upset on cruises declined over the study period (7.1% in 2000 to 3.1% in 2008, $p<0.0005$). Over 25% of travellers on land-based holidays to Egypt and the Dominican Republic reported stomach upset. In comparison, the highest proportion of stomach upset in cruise ship travellers were reported following cruises departing from Egypt (14.8%) and Turkey (8.8%).

Conclusions: In this large study of self-reported illness both demographic and holiday choice factors were shown to play a part in determining the likelihood of developing stomach upset while abroad. There is a lower cumulative incidence and declining rates of stomach upset in cruise passengers which suggest that the cruise industry has adopted operations (e.g. hygiene standards) that have reduced illness over recent years.

Editor: Martyn Kirk, The Australian National University, Australia

Funding: This study was not formally funded and analysis was performed within the SHIPSAN TRAINET project (EU Project No. 2007206). The funders had no role in study design, data collection and analysis, decision to publish, or preparation of the manuscript.

Competing Interests: All authors work in Public Health Microbiology or Epidemiology. Professor Cartwright has undertaken paid work on behalf of the Travel Industry to investigate outbreaks. Professor Hadjicristodoulou rans an EU funded project called SHIPSAN TRAINET that was involved with passenger ship hygiene and Professor Nichols has also contributed to this project.

* E-mail: gordon.nichols@ecdc.europa.eu

Introduction

Travel by land, air or sea puts the traveller at risk of infectious microorganisms not usually encountered in their home country and brings with it the potential to transport infectious diseases from one area to another [1,2]. Gastrointestinal illness is common in travellers, with one study of package holiday tourists reporting travellers' diarrhoea in 24% of travellers questioned [3]. This may be even higher in those travelling from high to low income countries [4–6]. On cruises, respiratory illness has been shown to be the most common reason for visits to the ship's infirmary, followed by gastrointestinal illness which account for 9–11% of all visits [6,7]. British Tour operators have developed a questionnaire-based means of monitoring stomach upsets in people returning from different countries [8].

Travellers' diarrhoea is generally defined as three or more loose stools in 24 hours, with at least one accompanying symptom (i.e. nausea, vomiting, abdominal cramps, tenesmus, bloody stools or fever), starting during or soon after international travel. Although many episodes of travellers' diarrhoea are self-limiting, prolonged diarrhoea is estimated to occur in 3% of travellers to regions of high risk [9]. As well as causing illness and distress for the traveller, and reducing the enjoyment of foreign holidays, travellers' diarrhoea also impacts on the country of residence. For example it is estimated that 50% of Shigella cases and 20% of Salmonella cases in England, Wales and Northern Ireland are travel-related [10], however, travel history is under-reported. Travel data has also been used to examine disease burden in countries visited [11]. The term stomach upset is undefined and passengers record their response to this depending on their understanding of the term.

Bacterial diseases, such as enterotoxigenic or enteroaggregative *E.* coli [12] and campylobacter [13], are the most common cause of travellers' diarrhoea. However, on cruise ships, norovirus is the most common cause of outbreaks. Although the United States Centres for Disease Control and Prevention Vessel Sanitation Programme (VSP) estimated that the chance of suffering gastrointestinal illness on a seven-day cruise is less than 1% [14], cruise ship outbreaks have been the subject of much media attention, leading to a perception that cruise ship holidays present a high risk of gastroenteritis.

The published literature on stomach upset on passenger ships is limited. There are studies based on investigations by ships doctors [7,15], and the CDC VSP has a gastrointestinal illness surveillance system for cruise ships travelling in US waters. These studies are based on the ships doctor being aware of cases, possibly underestimating the problem. The relative risk for cruise ship passengers compared to those on land-based package holidays has not been investigated.

In this study we examine information from a Questionnaire that is designed for assessing customer satisfaction, but which also asks about illnesses acquired while abroad.

Methods

A major British tour operator regularly administers a Customer Satisfaction Questionnaire (CSQ) to travellers over the age of 16 and resident in the UK, on the return flight of their holiday. The flights targeted for this process are defined by market research needs, and therefore are not random. Passengers were invited to complete a market survey questionnaire that includes a few simple questions about their health on the holiday they are returning from. Data on cruise passengers are predominantly from those who flew to a destination outside the UK to start their cruise. However, from 2005, data were also collected from passengers who had taken a cruise departing from the UK. Data from all questionnaires were entered into a database by a market research company.

The CSQ health data was introduced in the early 1980s as a tool to identify holiday destinations with above average levels of gastrointestinal disturbances among tourists, and tour operators present the results to the authorities responsible for high incidence destinations and encouraged authorities to take remedial actions such as the instigation of food hygiene programmes and the construction of new drinking water and waste water plants. The on-going nature of the CSQs enables the success or otherwise of remedial actions to be assessed, and is an integral part of the Federation of Tour Operators programme to promote improvements in health and safety within destination resorts.

The questionnaire contains questions regarding traveller demographics (age, sex, employment status, occupation), details about their holiday (hotel, resort, region, hotel chain, date of arrival/return, season, length of stay, type of board), customer satisfaction questions, and questions on self-reported illness (stomach upset for >24 hours, sea sickness, colds, sunburn or other illnesses). Definitions for these terms are not provided on the CSQ questionnaire, and are assumed to be common terms understood by the general public. It is assumed that some data will represent questionnaires from the same person travelling on more than one holiday and the analyses are therefore reported as passenger visits rather than populations, and not therefore a cohort.

Cruises were of variable lengths whereas the majority of land based package holidays were predominantly one or two weeks in duration, although some land based holidays were also of variable lengths. The codes used to denote length of stay changed between land, cruise, ski and other types of holiday but there was insufficient information to verify if the coding was correct. It was therefore not feasible to reliably compare land and cruise based holidays by length of stay.

Data from a total of 10,401,470 questionnaires completed during the 12 year period from May 1997 through April 2009 were received from the market research company. Questionnaires completed prior to May 2000 were excluded due to methodological differences, but the relevant questions were unchanged from then. Due to an operational problem (loss of a CSQ file), no data were available for May 2003. The extracted CSQ data was examined as records of foreign visits representing an unspecified percentage of all foreign visits involving a flight. It is understood that some travellers may have completed more than one CSQ if they had travelled on more than one occasion. While use of the surveillance data has been reported previously its limitations are not fully understood [8].

To determine those records related to cruise travel, the hotel names were searched for instances of "cruise" or "CRU". The hotel names were also manually searched and compared with a list of cruise names used by the tour operator. Records were defined as "land-based only", "cruise travel" or "unknown". A total of 1,314 records were rejected as the type of travel could not be determined.

Data were analyzed using SPSS, STATA and Microsoft Excel. Denominator data for the estimated number of holiday visits abroad made by British residents were sourced from the Office for National Statistics International Passenger Survey (IPS) [16]. Data were available per quarter from the IPS. Where data were required for partial quarters an estimate was made assuming the rate of travel was the same throughout that quarter. The season of travel was defined using the date of return, with the summer season defined as May to October and winter season as November through to April of the following year.

Multivariable logistic regression was performed to examine rates of stomach upset with respect to cruise and land travel. All available variables were included in the initial model. Variables which were not significantly associated ($p = 0.05$) with stomach upset in univariate analysis and those with poor response rates (<80%) were removed sequentially, until the best fitting model was generated (backwards regression).

Ethics statement

Data was from voluntarily completed questionnaires. None of the contributers can be identified or contacted.

Results

Customer Satisfaction Questionnaires (CSQs)

A total 6,863,092 CSQs completed from May 2000 (summer 2000) through April 2009 (winter 2008) were accepted for analysis, including 451,387 from cruise passengers (6.6%). Although the participation rate on flights is not known, these records are thought to represent 3.9% of the estimated 174 million package holiday visits abroad made by British residents during that time [16]. Numbers of completed CSQs varied seasonally, with peaks during the summer months for both land-based and cruise-based holiday makers corresponding to the seasonality of trips.

No information was available on the cruise itineraries; however the embarkation port for the majority of cruises was in Spain (62.2%), with 40.2% of all cruises beginning in Majorca, followed by Egypt (13.1%), Greece (13.1%) and the UK (5.8%). Land-based holidays had a larger range of destinations than cruise ship holidays, although the most commonly visited country was also

Table 1. Demographic details of travellers on cruise- and land-based holidays.

	Cruise		Land		
	Count	95% CI	Count	95% CI	p-value†
Number of holiday-makers:	451387		6411705		
Median age group:	55–64		45–54		
Gender: % Men	48.68	48.53–48.83	40.66	40.62–40.7	<0.0005
Social status:					<0.0005
% Unskilled	6.65	6.57–6.73	7.84	7.81–7.86	
% Office/skilled	25.07	24.93–25.2	30.85	30.81–30.89	
% Technical/middle management	9.31	9.22–9.4	10.81	10.78–10.84	
% Professional	20.85	20.72–20.98	16.92	16.89–16.95	
% Student	11.59	11.48–11.69	12.32	12.29–12.34	
% Retired	22.15	22.01–22.28	14.57	14.54–14.59	
% Unemployed	0.84	0.81–0.87	1.21	1.2–1.22	
% House wife/husband	3.55	3.49–3.61	5.48	5.47–5.5	

†Please note that because the sample size is very large and therefore even small effects will appear significant we have chosen P<0.0005 as a cut-off value compared to p values used in other smaller studies (i.e. P<0.01).

Spain (55.6%), followed by Greece (13.4%), Cyprus (7.0%), Portugal (3.3%) and Egypt (2.9%).

The median age group of respondents who had been on cruise-based holidays (55–64 years) was higher than those on land-based holidays (45–54). A higher proportion of cruise passengers were men (48.7%) compared to those on land-based holidays (40.7%). More cruise passengers were retired (22.2% vs. 14.6%), or working as professionals (20.9% vs. 16.9%) than their land-based counterparts (Table 1).

Disease frequencies on land-based versus cruise-based holidays

Of the cruise passengers completing CSQs, 20.9% reported illness, compared to 16.2%, (p<0.05, Risk Ratio (RR) 1.3, CI 1.29–1.3) of those on land-based holidays. However, 10.2% of illness on cruise-based holiday was attributable to seasickness. When seasickness was removed from the analysis, the proportion of respondents reporting illness following cruise ship travel was lower than following land-based holidays (11.7% vs. 16.2%, (p<0.05, RR 0.8, CI 0.79–0.8)). Land-based holiday makers reported a higher proportion of stomach upset, sunburn, fractures and other illnesses than cruise passengers, whereas cruise passengers reported a higher proportion of colds (Table 2). While there were statistically significant differences for these, only stomach upset and sunburn had differences that were large enough to be important.

Determinants of risk for stomach upset

The highest proportions of stomach upset were reported in those under the age of 25, with a steady decline in reporting in travellers over this age. However, for cruise ship passengers 74% of cases were reported in those 45 years of age or over (Figure 1).

A higher proportion of respondents who had been on land-based holidays reported stomach upset than those who had been on cruise-based holidays (7.2% vs. 4.8%; p<0.05, RR 1.5, CI: 1.49–1.54). The proportion of cruise passengers reporting stomach upset decreased over the study period (2000 7.1% (CI 6.9–7.3) vs 2008 3.1% (CI 3.0–3.2)2008 (p<0.05) (Figure 2). The frequency of stomach upset in travellers on land-based holidays increased from 2000 to 2008 (p<0.05). For cruise ship passengers, the reporting of stomach upset peaked during the winter months of each year,

Table 2. Disease frequency in travellers on land- and cruise-based holidays.

Illness*	Land - % ill	Cruise - % ill	Risk Ratio	95% CI	p-value†
Fracture	0.01	0	N/A	N/A	N/A
Cold	2.34	2.45	0.96	0.94–0.98	<0.0005
Sunburn	3.96	1.39	2.85	2.78–2.93	<0.0005
Stomach upset	7.23	4.77	1.51	1.49–1.54	<0.0005
Sea sickness	0.00	10.2	N/A	N/A	N/A
Other	4.32	3.87	1.11	1.1–1.13	<0.0005

*Travellers could report more than one illness. Sea sickness was not reported from land based holidays.
†Please note that because the sample size is very large and therefore even small effects will appear significant we have chosen P<0.0005 as a cut-off value compared to p values used in other smaller studies (i.e. P<0.01). Our judgement is that the differences between land and cruise based are significant for cold, sunburn and stomach upset are significant, but the difference is probably not big enough to be important for colds, whereas it is for sunburn and stomach upset.

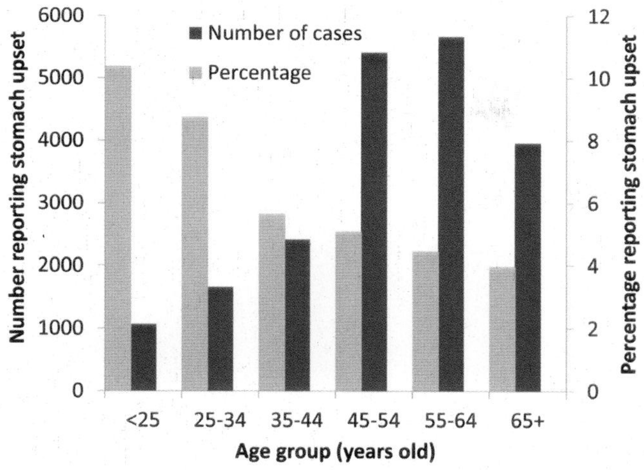

Figure 1. Age distribution of reported stomach upset on cruises.

whereas for travellers on land-based holidays the seasonal pattern was less pronounced (Figure 2).

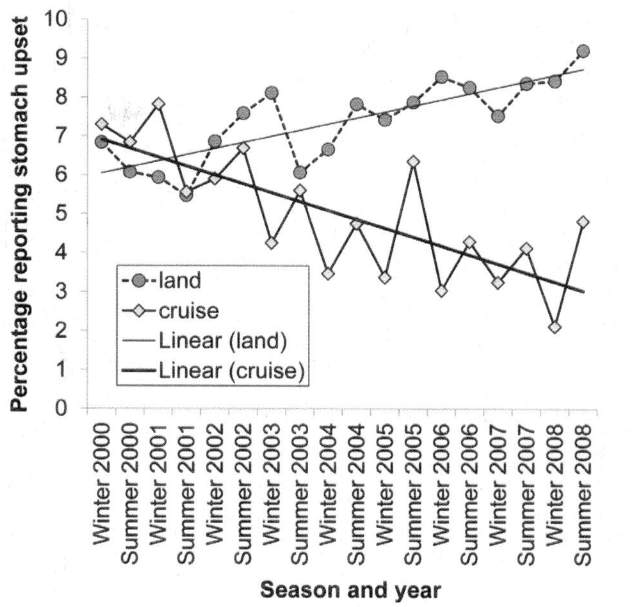

Figure 2. Trends in reports of stomach upset over time. Where S = Summer and W = Winter. Regression line for cruise-related stomach upset per year: $R^2 = 0.8984$; regression line for land-based holiday-related stomach upset: $R^2 = 0.7686$.

Stratification by country

For all countries where CSQs were received for more than 100 cruise passengers, the risk of stomach upset for cruise-based travellers was significantly lower than that for land-based travellers to the same country, with the exception of the United States where no significant difference was seen (Table 3). The largest difference between the proportion of travellers reporting stomach upset on land- and cruise-based holidays was seen in travellers to the Dominican Republic (Land 27.9% vs. Cruise 3.3% ($p<0.05$, RR 8.6, CI 7.59–9.68).

While over 25% of travellers on land-based holidays to Egypt and the Dominican Republic reported stomach upset, in cruise ship passengers the highest proportion of stomach upset was 14.8% in travellers to Egypt, followed by 8.8% in travellers to Turkey (Table 3). Travellers to Greece and Spain reported a low cumulative incidence of stomach upset; however, due to the volume of travellers to these countries, the estimated number of cases in travellers was high. For countries such as Egypt, the opposite was observed, with a relatively high cumulative incidence but low number of cases (Figure 3).

Over the study period, reporting of stomach upset decreased in cruise passengers to both Egypt (31.8% in 2000 vs 13.8% in 2008, $p<0.05$, $r^2 = 0.7903$) and Spain (4.6% in 2000 vs 1.8% in 2008, $p<0.05$, $r^2 = 0.7896$). The reporting of stomach upset in land-based travellers to Spain also decreased, but to a lesser extent (5.9% in 2000 to 4.8% in 2008, $p<0.05$, $r^2 = 0.5266$), whereas no significant decrease was observed in travellers on land-based holidays to Egypt. With the exception of 2001, the incidence of stomach upset in cruises departing from Spain peaked in winter months every year, with 3.3% of all cruise passengers to Spain travelling in the summer seasons reporting stomach upset compared with 3.9% in those travelling during winter ($p<0.05$, RR 0.8, CI 0.8–0.9). For cruises departing from Egypt, 31.8% of passengers reported stomach upset during summer months compared to 9.8% during winter months ($p<0.05$, RR 3.2 CI 3.1–3.4) (Figure 4).

The risk of stomach upset varied greatly within each country. In Spain, for hotels and cruise ships where more than 1,000 CSQs had been completed, 1.7 to 25.3% of travellers to a particular hotel/cruise reported stomach upset (median = 5%), compared with 3.7 to 41.3% for travellers to Egypt (median = 25.1%).

Multivariable analysis

In the multivariable logistic regression model, travellers on land-based holidays were more likely to report stomach upset, and those travelling in the summer months and earlier in the study period were also at increased risk. However, the model was a poor fit for the data (Homer-Lemshow test: $p<0.0005$), suggesting that the risk of stomach upset was not fully explained by these variables.

Discussion

This is a large study of self-reported travel-related stomach upset, but as with any such study, it cannot be assumed that illness directly relates to rates of laboratory diagnosed infection, and in addition some misclassifications may have occurred. For travellers on cruise-based holidays, travellers may have misclassified stomach upset (including norovirus infection) and sea-sickness. However, sea sickness is generally short lived, and therefore the time aspect of the definition of stomach upset (>24 hours) should remove some of this misclassification. Because stomach upset is a colloquial term suggesting nausea and epigastric pain there is a question of whether people will report diarrhoea and vomiting as an upset stomach. The view we took was that amongst people in the UK returning from holiday the box would most likely be ticked for upset stomach in most passengers who had experienced diarrhoea and/or vomiting. There could also be misclassification through stomach upset recorded by passengers including dyspepsia in addition to diarrhoea and vomiting. There is no record of the percentage of passengers completing the survey, and because CSQ completion was voluntary there could be biases related to who completes such forms. The CSQ data will probably under-ascertain illness because many people will only develop symptoms after the return flight. However, despite these caveats and limitations previous evidence suggests that the analysis of this

Table 3. Incidence of stomach upset on land- and cruise-based holidays to countries for which >100 CSQs were received from cruise passengers.

	Land	Cruise	Risk Ratio	95% CI	p-value†
Country[a]	No. of cases (%)[c]	No. of cases (%)[c]			
Turkey	16048 (13.3)	33 (8.8)	1.50	1.08–2.08	0.0116
Spain	197641 (5.5)	9790 (3.5)	1.59	1.56–1.62	<0.0005
Greece	42880 (5.0)	1522 (2.6)	1.94	1.85–2.04	<0.0005
Cyprus	20385 (4.6)	140 (3.2)	1.41	1.2–1.67	<0.0005
Portugal	9240 (4.4)	126 (3.2)	1.35	1.14–1.61	0.0006
UK Cruise[b]	N/A	436 (1.7)			
Egypt	49352 (26.6)	8759 (14.8)	1.80	1.76–1.84	<0.0005
United States	2328 (4.2)	17 (3.7)	1.13	0.71–1.81	0.5986
Dominican Republic	38436 (27.9)	252 (3.3)	8.57	7.59–9.68	<0.0005
Barbados	609 (5.4)	181 (4.0)	1.37	1.16–1.61	<0.0005
Thailand	436 (12.7)	287 (6.6)	1.93	1.68–2.23	<0.0005

[a]: Country of cruise departure for cruises, country of holiday stay for land-based holidays. It is expected that most cruises will stop at many ports and allow shore trips, so the departure country may not reflect the exposure risks on the cruise.
[b]: UK cruise data only available from 2005 onwards.
[c]: Cases of stomach upset (and as a % of total passenger trips.
†Please note that because the sample size is very large and therefore even small effects will appear significant we have chosen $P<0.0005$ as a cut-off value compared to p values used in other smaller studies (i.e. $P<0.01$).

data is useful and informative [8] and the CSQ data provide records of over six million questionnaires completed by individual travellers over a nine-year period. An additional area that may cause inaccuracy is that cruise holidays may be shorter than land-based holidays. While it would have been nice to estimate the incidence of stomach upset per day of the holiday the data did not allow this to be done in a way that accurately reflected risk.

Our study found lower levels of stomach upset in package holiday travellers (7.2%) than previously reported (25.7%) [3][4][5]. Unlike our study these considered a broader range of traveller and we think that it is difficult to directly compare our results to these studies. This large retrospective study provides an interesting comparison of self-reported illness on cruise- and land-based holidays, and highlights the utility of alternative datasets in epidemiology. In this study, both demographic factors and holiday choice factors were shown to play a part in determining the likelihood of developing stomach upset while abroad. The finding that destination is the main determinant of illness reinforces the message that to improve traveller's health, the sanitation and health within destination countries must be improved. Further elucidation of the risk factors for acquiring a travel-related illness will allow travel health practitioners to tailor their advice for each

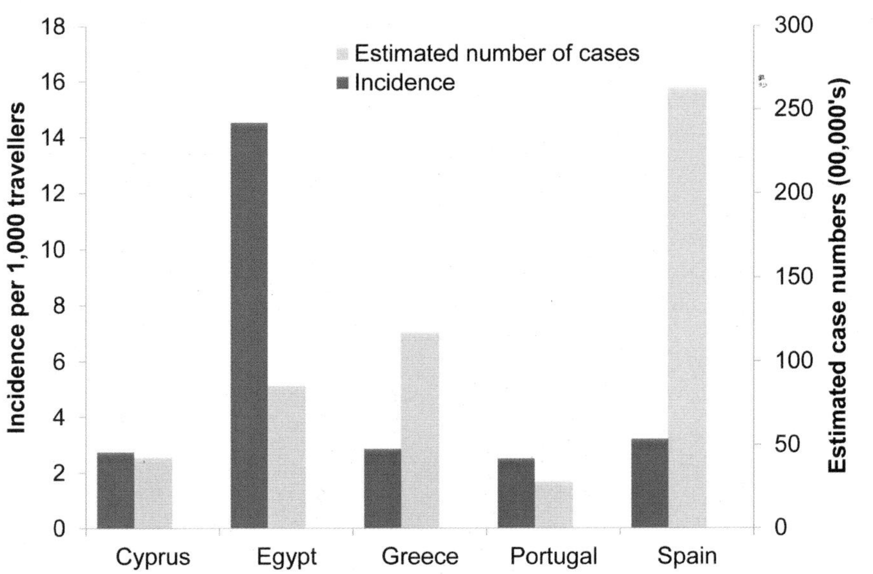

Figure 3. Incidence and estimated number of cases of stomach upset in travellers (both cruise- and land-based) in the period from Jan 2001 to Dec 2008.

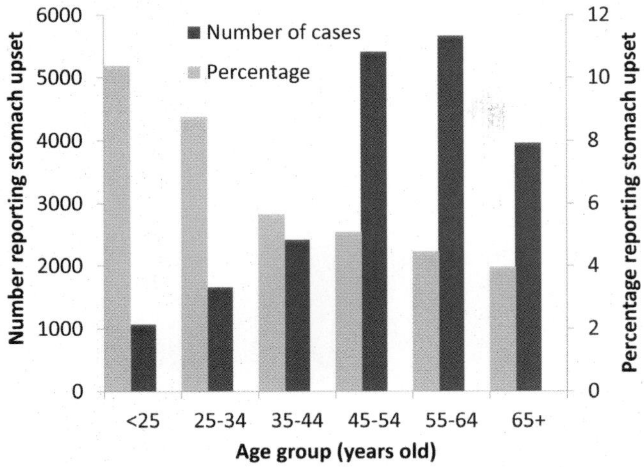

Figure 4. Seasonal distribution of prevalence of reported stomach upset in cruise passengers on cruises departing Spain and Egypt. S = Summer and W = Winter.

traveller, and for travellers to make informed choices about their holiday destinations. The lower incidence and declining rates of stomach upset in cruise ship passengers over the nine years study period suggest that cruise industry measures to improve hygiene have reduced self-reported stomach upset, although the data does not indicate what these changes are.

Cruise ships passengers are seen as at high risk for gastrointestinal illness, in part due to the media interest in large norovirus outbreaks. Successful surveillance and reporting systems such as that run by the Centers for Disease Control Vessel Sanitation Program [17,18] may also alter the perception of risk, providing a better surveillance mechanism than for many land-based locations. Although outbreaks on cruise ships with high attack rates have been reported [19,20], this study suggests the proportion of travellers reporting stomach upset is lower in cruise ship passengers than for those on land-based package holidays when sea sickness is excluded.

As with other studies [8,10,21,22], our study showed an increased risk of stomach upset when travelling outside of Europe and North America. The level of public health infrastructure, including access to clean drinking water and adequate sewage facilities, will affect the risk of stomach upset for travellers to that country [8], particularly for land-based travellers who are more exposed to a country's infrastructure. Cruise passengers staying on land as part of their holiday or participating in on-shore excursions in countries with poor public health infrastructure are also at risk, as are passengers of cruise ships which are using food and water purchased in such countries. As well as the risks posed by poor public health infrastructure, the risk of stomach upset is also dependent on the hygiene levels of individual resorts, hotels and cruises, as shown in the high variability in stomach upset rates between resorts or cruises in an individual country. This is particularly true in the package holiday market, where travellers may consume the majority of their meals in the hotel or on the cruise.

Our study has shown that the rates of self-reported stomach upset on cruise ships show strong seasonality. The different seasonal patterns in Egypt and Spain may be due to a predominance of different aetiological agents on the two types of cruises. The majority of reported outbreaks on large cruise ships in high income countries are due to norovirus [23,24]. Incidence of norovirus peaks in winter months and may account for the winter peaks in reports of stomach upsets in passengers departing from Spain. In contrast, reported stomach upset in passengers departing from Egypt peaked in the summer. Most of the cruises departing from Egypt were smaller river cruises, perhaps lessening the propensity for large norovirus outbreaks and presenting more frequent opportunities to go ashore. The high summer temperatures may have increased the likelihood of bacterial contamination of food or water either on board or ashore.

The decreasing trend observed in stomach upset reported on cruise ships is encouraging. Over the past ten years great effort has been made by cruise ship lines, Port Health Authorities and inspectorate organisations to improve the hygiene standards on ships. The cruise lines have sound business reasons for their continued interest in reducing the incidence of gastrointestinal illness on their ships. Furthermore, the US Vessel Sanitation Program inspection and scoring system has provided a strong incentive for ships travelling to the United States to maintain the highest hygiene standards. In September 2010, the European project for ship sanitation training network (SHIPSAN TRAINET) published the European Manual for Hygiene Standards and Communicable Disease Surveillance on Passenger Ships, and a ship inspection programme has been piloted [25]. It is hoped that with the strong collaboration of cruise lines, Port Health Authorities and national, trans-national and international organisations the incidence of infectious diseases, including gastroenteritis, will continue to fall from the current levels which are still higher than passengers would expect.

In this study it was not possible to produce a well fitted multivariable model to examine stomach upset. This is likely due to the limited information collected on the CSQs and the complex interplay of factors determining a person's risk of travel-related stomach upset. Behaviour choices, such as the types of meals consumed and how stringently hygiene advice is followed, have previously been shown to have an influence on the risk of travellers becoming ill while abroad on both land [3,26] and cruise holidays [19,27], and this level of detail was not available on the CSQs. Furthermore, for cruise ship travel, no details of the itinerary were available, so the start point of the cruise has been used for analysis of destinations. Finally, no information was available regarding whether cruise passengers stayed in land-based accommodation in the country of cruise departure prior to boarding the ship.

The systematic collection of CSQ data over many years has been instrumental in some major public health improvements in many holiday countries. It may be useful for the Travel Industry to discuss the methods for collection and use of this data with Public Health England to examine ways of improving the health benefits.

Acknowledgments

The authors would like to thank George Kafatos (Health Protection Agency) for his input in the statistical analysis of data, and the market research company and British tour operator for the provision of these data. This study was performed in collaboration with SHIPSAN TRAINET (EU Project No. 2007206). Thanks to Jan Semenza for comments on the draft manuscript.

Author Contributions

Conceived and designed the experiments: GN NL RC JL CH JJ. Performed the experiments: NL GN RC. Analyzed the data: NL GN RC JL JJ. Wrote the paper: NL GN JL RC CH JJ.

References

1. Mouchtouri VA, Nichols G, Al GR (2010) State of the art: public health and passenger ships. Int Marit Health 61: 53–98.
2. Soto SM (2009) Human migration and infectious diseases. Clin Microbiol Infect 15 Suppl 1: 26–28.
3. Evans MR, Shickle D, Morgan MZ (2001) Travel illness in British package holiday tourists: prospective cohort study. J Infect 43: 140–147.
4. Pitzurra R, Steffen R, Tschopp A, Mutsch M (2010) Diarrhoea in a large prospective cohort of European travellers to resource-limited destinations. BMC Infect Dis 10: 231.
5. Redman CA, Maclennan A, Wilson E, Walker E (2006) Diarrhea and respiratory symptoms among travelers to Asia, Africa, and South and Central America from Scotland. J Travel Med 13: 203–211.
6. Steffen R, Tornieporth N, Clemens SA, Chatterjee S, Cavalcanti AM, et al. (2004) Epidemiology of travelers' diarrhea: details of a global survey. J Travel Med 11: 231–237.
7. Peake DE, Gray CL, Ludwig MR, Hill CD (1999) Descriptive epidemiology of injury and illness among cruise ship passengers. Ann Emerg Med 33: 67–72.
8. Cartwright RY (2003) Food and waterborne infections associated with package holidays. J Appl Microbiol 94 Suppl: 12S–24S.
9. Schultsz C, van den EJ, Cobelens F, Vervoort T, van Gompel A, et al. (2000) Diarrheagenic Escherichia coli and acute and persistent diarrhea in returned travelers. J Clin Microbiol 38: 3550–3554.
10. Health Protection Agency (2010) Foreign travel associated illness: a focus on travellers' diarrhoea, 2010 report.
11. de Jong B (2006) The comparative burden of salmonellosis in the European Union member states, associated and candidate countries.
12. Shah N, DuPont HL, Ramsey DJ (2009) Global etiology of travelers' diarrhea: systematic review from 1973 to the present. Am J Trop Med Hyg 80: 609–614.
13. DuPont HL (2009) Systematic review: the epidemiology and clinical features of travellers' diarrhoea. Aliment Pharmacol Ther 30: 187–196.
14. Cramer EH, Blanton CJ, Blanton LH, Vaughan GH Jr, Bopp CA, et al. (2006) Epidemiology of gastroenteritis on cruise ships, 2001–2004. Am J Prev Med 30: 252–257.
15. Tomaszewski R, Nahorski WL (2008) Interpopulation study of medical attendance aboard a cruise ship. Int Marit Health 59: 61–68.
16. Office for National Statistics (2010) International Passenger Survey, Travel Trends. 2000–2009.
17. Centers for Disease Control and Prevention (2005) Vessel Sanitation Program Operations Manual 2005.
18. Cramer EH, Blanton CJ, Otto C (2008) Shipshape: sanitation inspections on cruise ships, 1990–2005, Vessel Sanitation Program, Centers for Disease Control and Prevention. J Environ Health 70: 15–21.
19. Chimonas MA, Vaughan GH, Andre Z, Ames JT, Tarling GA, et al. (2008) Passenger behaviors associated with norovirus infection on board a cruise ship–Alaska, May to June 2004. J Travel Med 15: 177–183.
20. Verhoef L, Depoortere E, Boxman I, Duizer E, van Duynhoven Y, et al. (2008) Emergence of new norovirus variants on spring cruise ships and prediction of winter epidemics. Emerg Infect Dis 14: 238–243.
21. Greenwood Z, Black J, Weld L, O'Brien D, Leder K, et al. (2008) Gastrointestinal infection among international travelers globally. J Travel Med 15: 221–228.
22. Northey G, Evans MR, Sarvotham TS, Thomas DR, Howard TJ (2007) Sentinel surveillance for travellers' diarrhoea in primary care. BMC Infect Dis 7: 126.
23. Centers for Disease Control and Prevention (2011) Outbreak updates for international cruise ships.
24. World Health Organization (2001) Compendium of foodborne and waterborne disease and legionnaires disease associated with ships, 1970–2000.
25. EU Shipsan Trainet Project. (2012) European Manual for Hygiene Standards and Communicable Disease Surveillance on Passenger Ships. European Commission.
26. Swaminathan A, Torresi J, Schlagenhauf P, Thursky K, Wilder-Smith A, et al. (2009) A global study of pathogens and host risk factors associated with infectious gastrointestinal disease in returned international travellers. J Infect 59: 19–27.
27. Neri AJ, Cramer EH, Vaughan GH, Vinje J, Mainzer HM (2008) Passenger behaviors during norovirus outbreaks on cruise ships. J Travel Med 15: 172–176.

3

Diversity of Rotavirus Strains Causing Diarrhea in <5 Years Old Chinese Children

Yue Li[1¶], Song-Mei Wang[2¶], Shan-Shan Zhen[1¶], Ying Chen[1], Wei Deng[3], Paul E. Kilgore[4], Xuan-Yi Wang[1]*

1 Key Laboratory Medical Molecular Virology, MoE/MoH, and the Institutes of Biomedical Sciences, Shanghai Medical College, Fudan University, Shanghai, People's Republic of China, **2** Training Center of Medical Experiments, Shanghai Medical College, Fudan University, Shanghai, People's Republic of China, **3** Department of Health Statistics & Social Medicine, School of Public Health, Shanghai Medical College, Fudan University, Shanghai, People's Republic of China, **4** Eugene Applebaum College of Pharmacy and Health Sciences, Wayne State University, Detroit, United States of America

Abstract

Background: We conducted a systematic review of the diversity and fluctuation of group A rotavirus strains circulating in China.

Methods and Findings: Studies of rotavirus-based diarrhea among children less than 5 years, published in English or Chinese between 1994 and 2012, were searched in PubMed, SinoMed, and CNKI and reviewed by applying standardized algorithms. The temporal and spatial trends of genotyping and serotyping were analyzed using a random-effects model. Ninety-three studies met the inclusion/exclusion criteria and were included in the meta-analysis. Overall, 22,112 and 10,660 rotavirus samples had been examined for G and P types, respectively. The most common G types were G1 (39·5%), G3 (35·6%), G2 (1·3%), and G9 (0·1%). Among P types, P[8] (54·6%) was the predominant type, followed by P[4] (11·1%) and P6 (0·1%). The most common G-P combinations were G3P[8] (32·1%) and G1P[8] (24·5%), followed by G2P[6] (13·2%) and G2P[4] (10·1%). Before 2000, serotype G1 was the predominant strain and accounted for 74·3% of all rotavirus infections; however, since 2000, G3 (45·2%) has been the predominant strain. Rotavirus P types showed little variation over the study period.

Conclusion: Despite the variation of serotypes observed in China, the G1, G2, G3, and G4 serotypes accounted for most rotavirus strains in recent decades. These results suggest that Chinese children will be adequately protected with currently available or forthcoming rotavirus vaccines.

Editor: Yury E Khudyakov, Centers for Disease Control and Prevention, United States of America

Funding: The authors have no support or funding to report.

Competing Interests: The authors have declared that no competing interests exist.

* E-mail: xywang@shmu.edu.cn

¶ Yue Li, Song-Mei Wang, Shan-Shan Zhen are Co-first authors.

Introduction

Acute gastroenteritis is a leading cause of childhood illness in China [1,2]. Rotavirus is the pathogen most commonly identified as causing severe gastroenteritis in children less than 5 years old. In China, published data show that rotavirus-associated hospitalizations account for 32% to 50% of all hospitalizations for diarrhea among infants and children <5 years of age [3–8]. Beside of the current rotavirus vaccine (ie, the Lanzhou lamb rotavirus vaccine, LLR), which was developed and licensed in China in 2000, Two reassortant vaccines are being developed in China, one of which is based on the UK-bovine reassortant rotavirus vaccine originally developed at the National Institutes of Health (USA). To successfully develop and introduce a rotavirus vaccine in China, a full picture on the distribution of rotavirus G and P types is needed.

Methods

Search strategy

We identified studies of diarrhea caused by rotavirus among children less than 5 years old in mainland China, published before June, 2012, using standardized search algorithms for systematic reviews [9]. Scientific articles published in English or Chinese were identified using PubMed (United States), SinoMed (Chinese Bio-Medical Literature Service System, China), and CNKI (National Knowledge Infrastructure, China) databases. Standardized medical subject heading (MeSH) term "rotavirus" and free word "China" were used to search each database.

Definitions

To facilitate identification of reports, a suspected case of rotavirus diarrhea was defined as a child less than 5 years old who was admitted for treatment of diarrhea to a healthcare facility. A confirmed case of rotavirus diarrhea was defined as a child for whom rotavirus infection was proven by means of an enzyme immunoassay performed on fecal specimens.

Review strategy

Endnote® (version X, Thomson Reuters, Inc., Philadelphia, PA) bibliographic software was used to create an electronic library of citations identified in the database searches. PubMed searches were performed using Endnote®, and duplicate records were

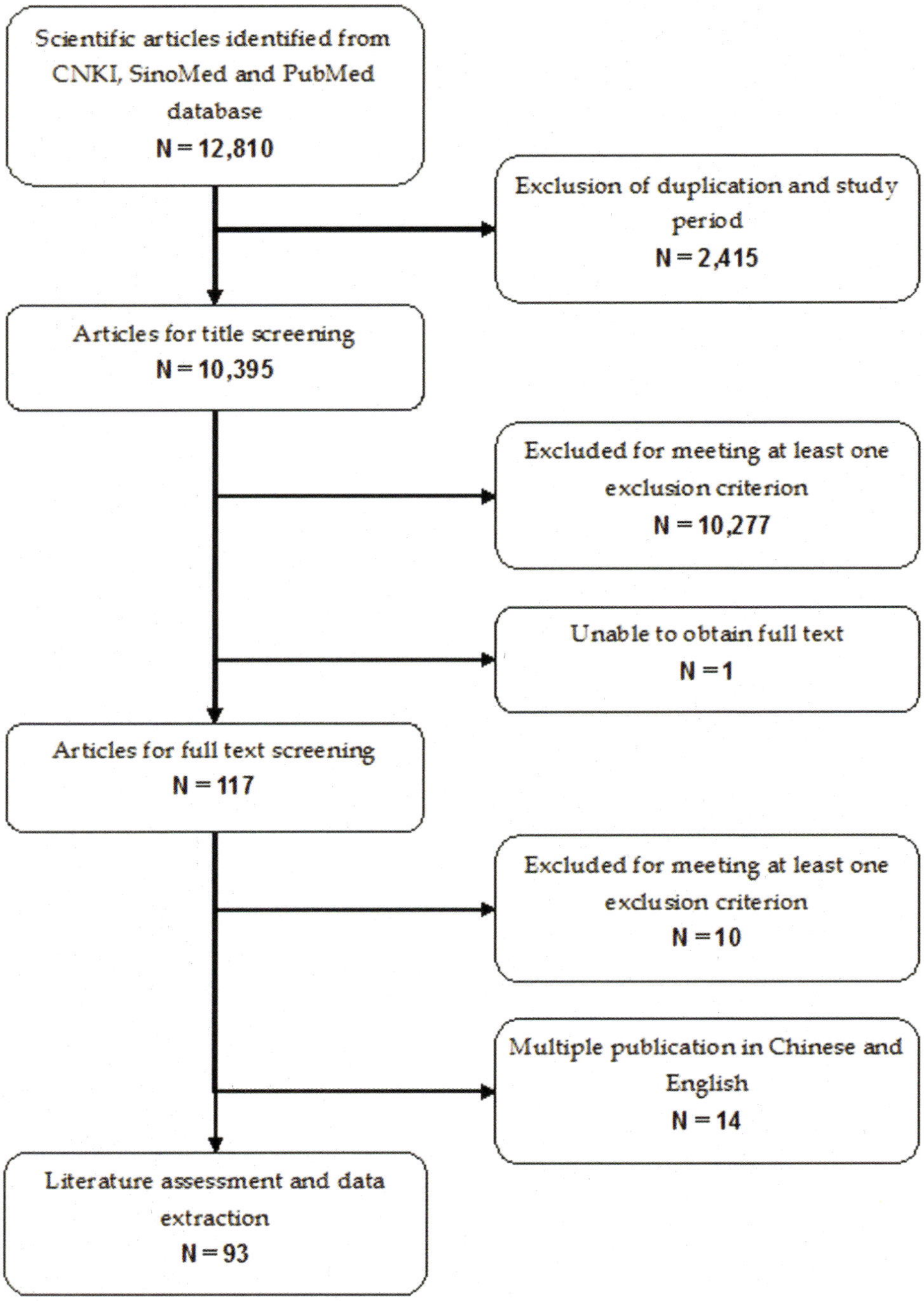

Figure 1. Eligibility of studies for inclusion in this systematic review. The initial search identified 12,810 rotavirus-related citations from CNKI, SinoMed, and PubMed. A total of 93 studies that met the inclusion and exclusion criteria were included in the pooled analysis.

deleted. Each study was assigned a unique identification code to enable tracking of reviews and analysis after title/abstract screening. Two independent reviewers were trained to perform the title/abstract screening and thereafter full text screening. Disagreements were resolved by consensus between the two reviewers and the corresponding author. For each article that met the inclusion criteria we used a structured questionnaire to appraise its quality based on study design, sources of specimens, study scope, case definitions, and diagnostic methods. To identify differences in homogeneity among the articles, each question was assigned a score, with zero being the lowest and five being the highest. Mean points per question were calculated for each article. Articles with ≥3·0 points/question were considered moderate/high quality. A structured questionnaire was used for data extraction, and the EpiData program (version 3·1) was used for data entry.

A pilot study was conducted to refine the questionnaire for quality assessment, and inclusion/exclusion criteria. The principles of Transparent Reporting of Systematic Reviews and Meta-Analysis (PRISMA) were implemented throughout the study.

Study inclusion and exclusion criteria

All studies published before June, 2012, in English or Chinese languages, obtained from the sources defined above, were

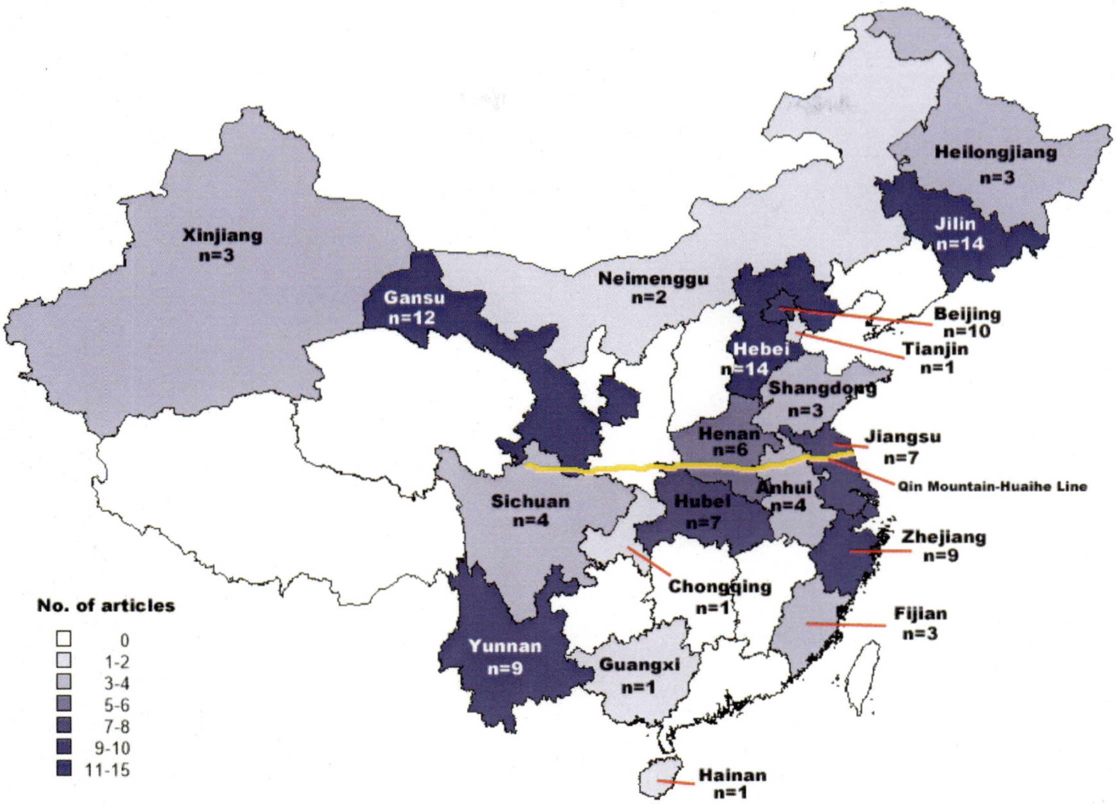

Figure 2. Distribution of included articles by province. The 93 studies included in the pooled analysis came from 22 provinces.

considered for inclusion. To be included, published reports possessed the following characteristics: 1) the study population was composed exclusively of children less than 5 years old living in mainland China; 2) group A rotavirus strains were reported as the etiologic agent; 3) results reported data on rotavirus G and P types; and 4) the strains used for G and P typing numbered at least 50. Reports were excluded from final analysis if their content was limited to a description of diagnostic methods, traditional medical therapies, case reports, health education, or policy analysis or if they focused solely on reporting community outbreaks and nosocomial cases, as these data could bias the distribution of serotypes or genotypes found in annual endemic transmission.

Analytical strategy and statistical analysis

The temporal and spatial distributions of rotavirus G and P types were analyzed to describe changes over time and by region within China. Differences among studies in the use of an enzyme immunoassay (EIA) or polymerase chain reaction (PCR)-based test for rotavirus were considered when appraising study quality, but test results using either method were pooled for the meta-analysis. To study temporal variations in rotavirus strain types, the extracted data were grouped by the year the study was published, namely 1994–1999, and 2000–2012, considering the implementation of LLR vaccine in 2000 in China. The Qinling Mountain-Huaihe River line, which is commonly recognized as the north-south dividing line of mainland China [10], was applied to define the geographic regions, namely South (subtropical zone) and North (warm temperate zone).

Before the original data were synthesized, homogeneity across studies was tested by use of the Q statistic ($P<0{\cdot}10$)[11]. If substantial heterogeneity existed, the random-effects model was used; otherwise, the fixed-effects model is preferred to summarize the pooled percentage, as well as 95% confidence intervals [12]. In order to detect potential bias introduced by the heterogeneous quality of publications, the pooled percentages from all studies and high-quality articles (mean score per question $\geq 3{\cdot}0$) were calculated and compared. If there was significant difference, outputs derived from high-quality articles would be presented. All analyses were performed using STATA version 10·0 (Stata Corp, College Station, Texas, USA). Statistical significance was assessed using $P<0{\cdot}05$.

Ethics

This study was reviewed and approved by the Institutes of Biomedical Sciences Institutional Review Board, Fudan University.

Results

Overview of studies

The initial search identified 12,810 rotavirus-related citations from CNKI, SinoMed, and PubMed. After first excluding duplicate records, 10,277 and 10 studies were excluded after review of title/abstract and full text information, respectively (**Figure 1**). A total of 93 studies (83 Chinese articles and 10 English articles) that met the inclusion and exclusion criteria were included in the pooled analysis. Of these, 24 (25·8%) studies were appraised as moderate/high quality, with a mean score $\geq 3{\cdot}0$ per question. Approximately 70% of specimens were collected from inpatients treated in city- or county-level hospitals. The majority of studies were conducted in eastern provinces of China (n = 51, 54·8%). Other studies were identified from central (n = 33, 35·5%) and western provinces (n = 27, 29·0%) (**Figure 2**). Regarding the G- and P-typing, most studies (>90%) tested only for common G

Table 1. Characteristics of all studies included in the meta-analysis (n = 93).

Characteristic	Studies (n)	%
Journal		
International English	10	10·8
Domestic Chinese core	43	46·2
Domestic Chinese non-core	40	43·0
Study region*		
Eastern	51	54·8
Central	33	35·5
Western	27	29·0
Source of specimens		
Outpatient	7	7·5
Inpatient	65	69·9
Both	21	22·6
Study scope		
Nation	10	10·8
Province	17	18·2
City/county	66	71·0
Typing confirmed by sequencing		
Yes	8	8·6
No	85	91·4
Case inclusion criteria		
Presented	40	43·0
Not presented	53	57·0
Diagnostic method for RV infection		
ELISA^	77	82·8
PAGE$	16	17·2
Mean score after quality assessment		
<2·5	28	30·1
2·5 -	41	44·1
3·0-	16	17·2
≥3·5	8	8·6

^: Abbreviations: ELISA = enzyme-linked immunosorbent assay;
$: Abbreviations: PAGE = polyacrylamide gel electrophoresis.
*: Since several studies reported data from different regions, the total percentage exceeds 100%.

and P types, namely G1–G4, G9 as well as P[4], P[6], P[8], P[9], and P[10]. Out of 93 studies included in final analysis, only 8 studies (8·6%) reported rotavirus G and P types identified by nucleic acid sequencing (**Table 1**).

During the data analysis, heterogeneity was found in most of the analytical indicates; therefore, the random-effects model was applied throughout the analysis. When the outputs derived from all articles versus those from high-quality articles were compared, there was no difference in the temporal and spatial trends of rotavirus strain diversity; however, the magnitude of percentage showed slight inconsistencies. Thus, only analyses using all publications are presented hereafter.

Diversity of rotavirus strains by region and by year

Overall, 22,112 and 10,660 rotavirus samples were examined for G and P types, respectively, from the 93 studies. In the past 19 years (1994–2012), the most common G types were G1 (39·5%), G3 (35·6%), and G2 (1·3%), followed by G9 (0·1%), but not G4 (<0·01%). For the P type, P[8] (54·6%) was predominant, followed by P[4] (11·1%) and P6 (0·1%) (**Tables 2 and 3**). The most common G-P combinations were G3P[8] (32·1%) and G1P[8] (24·5%), followed by G2P[6] (13·2%) and G2P[4] (10·1%) (**Table 4**).

To determine the temporal trends of rotavirus strain distribution, we divided the time span at the year 2000, because before 2000, genotype G1 was the predominant strain and accounted for 74·3% of rotavirus infections, followed by G2 (6·1%) and G3 (4·7%). However after 2000, G3 (45·2%) became the predominant strain, followed by G1 (21·3%). Notably, G9 (0·2%), which was first identified in Yunnan province in 1998, increased in the most recent period (**Table 2**). In comparison, P types remained consistent across time periods. P[8] was always the predominant strain followed by P[4]. These top two strains were responsible for around 60% of rotavirus infection in each time period (**Table 3**).

There was good agreement on the spatial trends of rotavirus strain distribution between the North and the South of China. Similar to the trends countrywide, G3 replaced G1 and became the most prevalent strain in both regions. A slight difference was that more G9 strains were identified in the North after 2000 (**Table 2**). No differences in the distribution of P types was found by region (**Table 3**).

Among the less-common strains, G5, G8, P[9], and P[10] were notable. G5 emerged in 2003 in Hebei province. G8 mixed with G1 was first reported in Guanzhou city in 1994 and thereafter was identified in Beijing, Wuhan, Hunan, and Gansu provinces and reached a prevalence of 2% in some instances. Besides P[8], P[4], and P[6], P[9] and P[10] were relatively common strains during each time period. Comparatively, P[9] strains were identified more frequently in the South, and P[10] strains were more frequent in the North (**Table S1**).

Discussion

In the most recent global systematic review, human serotypes G1, G2, G3, G4, and G9 were responsible for ~90% of rotavirus infection among children less than 5 years of age [13]. A similar distribution of G types, as well as the temporal trends of rotavirus infection in China was obtained from our comprehensive systematic review, which covered studies over a 19-year time span. The prevalence of the G1 serotype, which accounted for > 70% of rotavirus infection before 2000, decreased to ~20% after 2000. In contrast, the number of identified G3 strains increased from 4·7% to 45·2% during the same period, and G9 emerged and reached a zenith of 19·2% in 2005 in the Xinjiang Autonomous Region [14]. Regardless of the fluctuation of G and P types overall, serotypes G1, G2, and G3 accounted for ~80% of circulating strains in China, while the genotypes P[8] and P[4] were predominant consistently during that time period and represented ~70% of rotavirus infections.

Currently it is not clear whether serotype-specific immunity plays an important role in protection against rotaviral gastroenteritis. However, the monovalent serotype G6 vaccine RIT 4237 was highly effective in locations where G1 was the predominant serotype, though homotypic immunity was found to be no more significant than heterotypic immunity in a multicenter study of RRV-TV in the USA. This results indicated the development of vaccine candidates should be based on human-animal reassortants containing the common serotype of human strains [15]. Two vaccine candidates have been developed in China. One, developed by Lanzhou Vaccine Institute, is a human-ovine reassortant

Table 2. Distribution of common G types among children <5 years old with rotaviral diarrhea in China, 1994–2012.

Classification (number of studies)	Pooled percentage of G types among children with rotaviral diarrhea % (95% CI)					
	G1	G2	G3	G4	G9	G untyped
By Year (Countrywide)						
Before 2000 (n = 17)	74·3(71·6–77·1)	6·1(5·1–7·1)	4·7(3·8–5·6)	0·0(0·0–0·1)	0·0	0·4(0·1–0·7)
After 2000 (n = 81)	21·3(20·4–22·3)	0·9(0·8–1·1)	45·2(40·5–49·8)	0·0(0·0–0·1)	0·2(0·1–0·2)	10·9(9·8–11·9)
Overall (n = 93)	39·5(34·7–44·3)	1·3(1·1–1·5)	35·6(31·0–40·3)	0·0(0·0–0·1)	0·1(0·0–0·1)	6·7(6·1–7·3)
By region and year						
North						
Before 2000 (n = 12)	70·0(66·3–73·8)	6·6(5·2–7·9)	33·2(30·3–36·2)	0·0(0·0–0·1)	0·0(0·0–0·1)	0·5(0·1–0·9)
After 2000 (n = 41)	20·0(18·8–21·3)	1·2(0·9–1·5)	43·0(37·4–48·6)	0·0(0·0–0·1)	0·3(0·2–0·4)	10·2(8·8–11·5)
Overall (n = 49)	34·6(32·9–36·2)	1·7(1·4–2·0)	33·2(30·3–36·2)	0·0(0·0–0·1)	0·1(0·0–0·2)	6·1(5·3–6·8)
South						
Before 2000 (n = 8)	79·3(72·5–86·2)	6·8(4·8–8·9)	1·5(0·8–2·3)	0·0(−0·1–0·2)	0·0(0·0–0·1)	0·3(0–0·5)
After 2000 (n = 42)	24·2(22·5–26·0)	0·6(0·4–0·8)	47·6(37·4–57·9)	0·1(0·0–0·1)	0·1(0·0–0·2)	11·9(10·0–13·8)
Overall (n = 49)	39·9(29·3–45·5)	0·9(0·7–1·2)	37·4(29·3–45·5)	0·1(0·0–0·1)	0·1(0·0–0·1)	7·7(6·7–8·8)

vaccine containing human G2, G3, G4, and ovine P[12]. This human-ovine reassortant vaccine is being tested for efficacy in a large-scale phase III trial that recruited 12,000 infants less than 6 months old. Another candidate, which expresses human virus VP7 from serotypes G1, G2, G3, G4, G8, and G9, and VP4 (P[5]) from a bovine strain, is being developed by the Wuhan Vaccine Institute and is ready to enter clinical trials. With regard to serotype distribution, all those vaccine candidates could provide satisfactory protection of Chinese children, due to the broad coverage of prevalent serotypes in China.

Globally, a remarkable increase in the number of G8 strains in the African region was observed in recent year compared to the review article published in 1998 [13,16], along with its identification in European countries [17], South Korea [18], India [19], Australia [20], and Asian countries. Although it is currently an unusual strain in China, since its emergence in Guangzhou city in 1994 [21], it has been identified in several provinces in the North and the South and even reached a prevalence of 2% over the past two decades [22–25]. Because G8 is presently circulating through China, it would make sense to add G8 in the construction of new vaccines. Despite the concern that might arise regarding the potential of G8 spreading, a study of RotaTaq demonstrated low incidence and low concentration of shedding when it was administered to infants [26–28]. These findings suggest that the vaccine strain is much less well adapted to growth at the infant intestinal mucosal surface, thus horizontal transmission among infants would be unlikely. Besides serotype, genotype might also play an important role in protection. Unfortunately, however, neither vaccine candidate included the most prevalent human virus VP4 (P[8]), which might render it less efficacious.

Table 3. Distribution of common P types among children <5 years old with rotaviral diarrhea in China, 1994–2012.

Classification (number of studies)	Pooled percentage of P types among children with rotaviral diarrhea % (95% CI)			
	P4	P6	P8	P untypable
By Year(Countrywide)				
Before 2000 (n = 7)	8·2(6·4–10·1)	0·3(0·1–0·7)	49·9(36·6–66·2)	7·6(5·2–10·0)
After 2000 (n = 55)	8·7(8·0–9·5)	0·0(0·0–0·1)	55·3(48·5–62·1)	20·9(18·8–23·1)
Overall (n = 61)	11·1(10·2–12·0)	0·1(0·0–0·2)	54·6(48·7–60·6)	18·3(16·5–20·1)
By region and year				
North				
Before 2000 (n = 5)	17·2(10·2–24·2)	0·1(0·2–0·4)	53·1(29·0–77·2)	7·1(4·2–10·0)
After 2000 (n = 29)	7·4(6·4–8·3)	0·1(0·0–0·1)	56·4(48·4–64·3)	22·7(19·2–26·2)
Overall (n = 33)	7·3(6·5–8·1)	0·1(0·0–0·1)	55·4(42·7–68·1)	19·1(16·6–21·7)
South				
Before 2000 (n = 4)	6·6(4·0–9·3)	9·7(4·3–15·1)	42·9(34·1–51·7)	9·7(4·2–15·2)
After 2000 (n = 27)	11·3(10·0–12·7)	0·0(0·0–0·0)	53·2(37·0–69·3)	19·8(16·6–23·1)
Overall (n = 31)	0·6(0·4–0·8)	0·0(0·0–0·0)	51·4(37·52–65·3)	18·0(15·2–20·9)

Table 4. Distribution of common G-P combinations among children <5 years old with rotaviral diarrhea in China, 1994–2012.

G-P combination	Pooled percentage of G-P types %(95% CI) [number of studies]		
	North	South	Countrywide
G1P4	2·7(1·9–3·8)[9]	9·7(5·5–13·9)[11]	5·1(3·5–6·7)[20]
G1P8	28·5(19·0–38·1)[12]	21·6(15·9–27·2)[18]	24·5(19·9–29·2)[30]
G2P4	10·6(6·8–14·3)[13]	9·9(5·8–14·0)[10]	10·1(7·7–12·5)[22]
G2P6	13·2(3·5–22·8)[1]	-[0]	13·2(3·5–22·8)[1]
G3P4	5·2(3·0–7·4)[14]	6·6(4·3–8·9)[12]	5·7(4·2–7·2)[26]
G3P8	35·1(24·8–45·5)[14]	29·0(19·0–39·0)[17]	32·1(25·0–39·2)[31]

There are several limitations with our systematic review. First, not all studies aimed to identify the full spectrum of G and P types. Most studies focused on the common G and P types, namely G1–G4, and P[4], P[6], P[8], P[9], and P[10]. The unusual G and P types, such as G8 and G12 probably were misclassified or untypable, and thus we did not get full insight into the rotavirus strains circulating in mainland China. Notably, the prevalence of G and P untypable strains increased after 2000. Second, although the diversity of circulating rotavirus strains is very broad across the country, the virulence of each strain might not be equal. Unfortunately, we were not able to associate the severity of illness with the genotype of the corresponding strains, due to a paucity of data. Finally, differences between EIA- and PCR-based serotyping and genotyping might introduce heterogeneity and bias the accuracy of magnitude, rather than the trends.

In summary, continuing national epidemiological surveillance studies of the circulating strains of rotavirus will be vital to promoting future vaccine successes and to interpreting vaccine failures.

Author Contributions

Conceived and designed the experiments: PEK XYW. Performed the experiments: YL SMW SSZ YC. Analyzed the data: YL SMW WD XYW. Wrote the paper: PEK XYW.

References

1. Wang XY, Du L, Von Seidlein L, Xu ZY, Zhang YL, et al. (2005) Occurrence of shigellosis in the young an elderly in rural China: results of a 12-months population-based surveillance study. Am J Trop Med Hyg in press.
2. Yu WL (1989) Survey on the prevention and treatment of diarrhoea in part of regions, China. Zhong Hua Liu Xing Bing Xue Za Zhi 10: 257–260.
3. Fang ZY, Wang B, Kilgore PE, Bresee JS, Zhang LJ, et al. (2005) Sentinel hospital surveillance for rotavirus diarrhea in the People's Republic of China, August 2001 - July 2003. J Infect Dis 192: s94–99.
4. Sun LW, Tong ZL, Li LH, Zhang J, Chen Q, et al. (2003) Surveillance finding on rotavirus in Changchun children's hospital during July 1998-June 2001. Zhong Hua Liu Xing Bing Xue Za Zhi 24: 1010–1012.
5. Tong ZL, Ma L, Zhang J, Hou AC, Zheng LS, et al. (2003) Epidemiological study of rotavirus diarrhea in Beijing, China - a hospital-based surveillance from 1998–2001. Zhong Hua Liu Xing Bing Xue Za Zhi 24: 1100–1103.
6. Wang XY, Riewpaiboon A, von Seidlein L, Chen XB, Kilgore PE, et al. (2009) The potential cost-effectiveness of a rotavirus immunization program in rural China. Clin Infect Dis 49: 1202–1210.
7. Wang XY, Xu ZY, von Seidlein L, Zhang YL, Zhao SJ, et al. (2005) Incidence of diarrhea caused by rotavirus infections in rural Zhengding, China: prospective, population-based surveillance. J Infect Dis 192: s100–105.
8. Orenstein EW, Fang ZY, Xu J, Liu C, Shen K, et al. (2007) The epidemiology and burden of rotavirus in China: a review of the literature from 1983 to 2005. Vaccine 25: 406–413.
9. Stroup DF, Berlin JA, Morton SC, Olkin I, Williamson GD, et al. (2000) Meta-analysis of observational studies in epidemiology: a proposal for reporting. JAMA 283: 2008–2012.
10. Editorial Office (2002) Encyclopedia of China. Beijing: Encyclopedia of China Publishing House.
11. Cochran WG (1954) The combination of estimates from different experiments. Biometrics 10: 101–129.
12. DerSimonian R, Laird N (1986) Meta-analysis in clinical trials. Control Clin Trials 7: 177–188.
13. Bányai K, László B, Duque J, Steele AD, Nelson EA, et al. (2012) Systematic review of regional and temporal trends in global rotavirus strain diversity in the pre rotavirus vaccine era: insights for understanding the impact of rotavirus vaccination programs. Vaccine 30: A122–130.
14. Yang XL, Matthijnssens J, Sun H, Muhamaiti J, Zhang B, et al. (2008) Temporal changes of rotavirus strain distribution in a city in the northwest of China, 1996-2005. Int J Infect Dis 12: e11–17.
15. Cunliffe NA, Bresee JS, Hart CA (2002) Rotavirus vaccines: development, current issues and future prospects. J Infect Dis 45: 1–9.
16. Cunliffe NA, Kilgore PE, Bresee JS, Steele AD, Luo N, et al. (1998) Epidemiology of rotavirus diarrhoea in Africa: a review to assess the need for rotavirus immunization. Bull World Health Organ 76: 525–537.
17. Iturriza-Gómara M, Dallman T, Bányai K, Böttiger B, Buesa J, et al. (2011) Rotavirus genotypes co-circulating in Europe between 2006 and 2009 as determined by EuroRotaNet, a pan-European collaborative strain surveillance network. Epidemiol Infect 139: 895–909.
18. Le VP, Kim JY, Cho SL, Nam SW, Lim I, et al. (2008) Detection of unusual rotavirus genotypes G8P[8] and G12P[6] in South Korea. J Med Virol 80: 175–182.
19. Miles MG, Lewis KD, Kang G, Parashar UD, Steele AD (2012) A systematic review of rotavirus strain diversity in India, Bangladesh, and Pakistan. Vaccine 30: A131–139.
20. Kirkwood CD, Cannan D, Boniface K, Bishop RF, Barnes GL, et al. (2008) Australian Rotavirus Surveillance Program annual report, 2007/08. Commun Dis Intell Q Rep 32: 425–429.
21. Chang RX, Pan RF, Zhu B, Zhang Y, Xiao W, et al. (2002) Genotypes of VP4 and VP7 of rotaviruses identified from infants and young children with diarrhea in Guangzhou City. Zhong Hua Er Ke Za Zhi 40: 405–408.
22. Li JH, Zhou SF, Liu YZ, Deng ZH, Huang W, et al. (2012) Etiological Study on Viral Diarrhea Among Infants and Young Children in Surveillance Hospitals of Hunan Province from 2009 to 2010. Shi Yong Yu Fang Yi Xue 19: 337–341.
23. Qiao H, Nilsson M, Abreu ER, Hedlund KO, Johansen K, et al. (1999) Viral diarrhea in children in Beijing, China. J Med Virol 57: 390–396.
24. Tang SW, Wang B, Li Y, Yang JH, Ye LX, et al. (2004) VP7 genotype of group A rotavirus isolated from children with diarrhea in Wuhan. Hua Zhong Yi Xue Za Zhi 28: 73–74.
25. Wei KF, Yang JJ, Liu XF, Liu JD, Chen JH, et al. (2010) Analysis of children rotavirus diarrhea in Lanzhou in 2009. Zhong Guo Wei Sheng Jian Yan Za Zhi 20: 2025–2028.
26. Clark HF, Borian FE, Modesto K, Plotkin SA (1990) Serotype 1 reassortant of bovine rotavirus WC3, strain WI79-9, induces a polytypic antibody response in infants. Vaccine 8: 327–332.
27. Clark HF, Offit PA, Ellis RW, Eiden JJ, Krah D, et al. (1996) The development of multivalent bovine rotavirus (strain WC3) reassortant vaccine for infants. J Infect Dis 174: S73–80.
28. Treanor JJ, Clark HF, Pichichero M, Christy C, Gouvea V, et al. (1995) Evaluation of the protective efficacy of a serotype 1 bovine-human rotavirus reassortant vaccine in infants. Pediatr Infect Dis J 14: 301–307.

4

Enteric Pathogens in Stored Drinking Water and on Caregiver's Hands in Tanzanian Households with and without Reported Cases of Child Diarrhea

Mia Catharine Mattioli[1], Alexandria B. Boehm[1], Jennifer Davis[1,2], Angela R. Harris[1], Mwifadhi Mrisho[3], Amy J. Pickering[1,2*]

1 Environmental and Water Studies, Department of Civil and Environmental Engineering, Stanford University, Stanford, California, United States of America, **2** Woods Institute for the Environment, Stanford University, Stanford, California, United States of America, **3** Ifakara Health Institute, Bagamoyo Research and Training Unit, Bagamoyo, Tanzania

Abstract

Background: Diarrhea is one of the leading causes of mortality in young children. Diarrheal pathogens are transmitted via the fecal-oral route, and for children the majority of this transmission is thought to occur within the home. However, very few studies have documented enteric pathogens within households of low-income countries.

Methods and Findings: The presence of molecular markers for three enteric viruses (enterovirus, adenovirus, and rotavirus), seven *Escherichia coli* virulence genes (ECVG), and human-specific *Bacteroidales* was assessed in hand rinses and household stored drinking water in Bagamoyo, Tanzania. Using a matched case-control study design, we examined the relationship between contamination of hands and water with these markers and child diarrhea. We found that the presence of ECVG in household stored water was associated with a significant decrease in the odds of a child within the home having diarrhea (OR = 0.51; 95% confidence interval 0.27–0.93). We also evaluated water management and hygiene behaviors. Recent hand contact with water or food was positively associated with detection of enteric pathogen markers on hands, as was relatively lower volumes of water reportedly used for daily hand washing. Enteropathogen markers in stored drinking water were more likely found among households in which the markers were also detected on hands, as well as in households with unimproved water supply and sanitation infrastructure.

Conclusions: The prevalence of enteric pathogen genes and the human-specific *Bacteroidales* fecal marker in stored water and on hands suggests extensive environmental contamination within homes both with and without reported child diarrhea. Better stored water quality among households with diarrhea indicates caregivers with sick children may be more likely to ensure safe drinking water in the home. Interventions to increase the quantity of water available for hand washing, and to improve food hygiene, may reduce exposure to enteric pathogens in the domestic environment.

Editor: Lionel G. Filion, University of Ottawa, Canada

Funding: This study was supported by the National Science Foundation (SES-0827384) and by the Stanford University Shah Research Fellowship. The funders had no role in study design, data collection and analysis, decision to publish, or preparation of the manuscript.

Competing Interests: The authors have declared that no competing interests exist.

* E-mail: amyjanel@stanford.edu

Introduction

Over 6.5 million children died in 2012 before reaching their fifth birthday [1]. Globally, almost 10% of these deaths are attributed to diarrhea, and the highest rates of child mortality occur in sub-Saharan Africa [1]. The east African country of Tanzania is a nation that continues to struggle with the burden of childhood diarrhea. In 2010, diarrheal diseases were responsible for almost 9% of all deaths of Tanzanian children under the age of five, just behind malaria (11%) and pneumonia (15%) [2]. Diarrhea-causing pathogens are transmitted via the fecal-oral route and, in low-income countries like Tanzania, it has been suggested that up to 88% of all child diarrhea cases can be attributed to inadequate sanitation, unsafe water, and/or insufficient hygiene [3]. The large diarrheal burden in Tanzania is consistent with the fact that only half of the Tanzanian population has access to improved drinking water sources, and only 10% has access to improved sanitation [4].

Fecal contamination is traditionally monitored using fecal indicator bacteria (FIB) characteristic of animal and human feces (*e.g., Escherichia coli*, enterococci, and fecal coliforms). The concentration of these organisms is regularly used to evaluate health risk associated with different exposure pathways, such as recreational water use and drinking water [5]. For young children, exposure to feces is thought to occur primarily within the home [6], and previous research in low-income countries has documented high levels of FIB in household stored drinking water [7–9] and on hands of mothers [10–13].

Several studies have investigated the behavioral determinants of FIB levels in stored water and on hands in order to identify the most promising household-level interventions for preventing childhood diarrhea. Safe storage containers and point-of-use (POU) treatments have been found to significantly reduce FIB contamination of household stored drinking water [14,15]. Other studies investigating hand contamination found that increasing the frequency of hand washing with soap reduces FIB contamination on hands, whereas some household chores increase hand contamination [16,17].

Several studies have found associations between FIB on hands and/or in stored drinking water and diarrheal illness in children [18–20]. For example, one study in the Philippines found that children drinking water with high levels of *E. coli* had significantly higher rates of diarrhea than those drinking less contaminated water [19], and a recent study in Tanzania found FIB contamination on hands to be significantly associated with diarrheal illness among household members [17]. However, other research suggests that FIB are inadequate indicators of the health risks associated with fecal contamination in the home [21–23]. For example, in Ecuador Levy *et al.* found childhood diarrhea to be associated with levels of *E. coli* in drinking water, but not with the concentration of enterococci or somatic coliphage [24]. Similarly, a meta-analysis by Gundry *et al.* was unable to determine any clear relationship between FIB levels in household drinking water and incidence of child diarrhea [22].

One possible reason for the equivocal findings regarding the relationship between FIB and child diarrhea is that FIB are present in both human and non-human animal feces [5]. In addition, FIB have historically been used to assess water quality in countries with temperate climates. They have subsequently been found to occur naturally and even proliferate in water [25,26], soil [27–29], and sands [30], particularly in tropical environments [31,32]. As such, FIB in water and on hands are often not strongly associated with the presence of human enteric pathogens [33–36], and there is very limited research on the association between indicators and pathogens in South America, Asia, and Africa [37]. In particular, viruses such as human enterovirus, adenoviruses, and rotavirus show limited association with FIB [33,37–43]. Given the low infectious dose of these viruses, as well as their significant contribution to child diarrhea globally, the limited utility of FIB to indicate viral presence in water and on hands is of particular concern [44,45].

For these reasons, in low-income countries with widespread fecal contamination, FIB are likely not adequate indicators for understanding the relationship between water management and hygiene behaviors and diarrheal illness among young children. Molecular fecal markers such as human-specific *Bacteroidales* that are unique to human fecal sources [46], as well as molecular markers of enteric pathogens, may be better indicators of contamination. In turn, such indicators may be more useful for identifying behavioral interventions that can prevent childhood diarrhea. However, few studies have reported the prevalence of enteric pathogens or human-specific fecal contamination in the household environment of low-income countries [16,33,47].

In a recent study conducted in Bagamoyo, Tanzania, Mattioli *et al.* analyzed source water, stored drinking water, and hand rinse samples from 93 households for molecular markers of enteric viruses and *E. coli* virulence genes [33]. The authors found a significant association between viral markers on hands and in stored drinking water, as well as between *E. coli* virulence genes in stored and source waters. FIB were found not to be good predictors of viral markers in water or on hands, although turbidity was associated with viral markers on hands. However, Mattioli *et al.* did not examine the association between microbial contamination and either child health or water management and hygiene behaviors among sampled households.

The present study builds on Mattioli *et al.* [33] by using data collected from 223 households in Bagamoyo, Tanzania to investigate whether the presence of enteropathogen and human-specific *Bacteroidales* genes in water and on hands is associated with reported cases of child diarrhea. Of the 223 households, 213 households are distinct from those described previously [33]. In addition, we combine the microbial data collected uniquely for this study with data from the 93 households described in Mattioli *et al.* [33] in order to evaluate the association of water management and hygiene behaviors with enteropathogen and human-specific *Bacteroidales* genes in stored drinking water and hand rinse samples.

Methods

Setting

The study was conducted in Bagamoyo, Tanzania (06°28′S, 38°55′E), approximately 70 km north of Dar es Salaam. Households–defined as groups of people that sleep and eat together in a dwelling on a regular basis–that included at least one child under five years of age were enrolled in the study. The data used in the present study were collected from a subset of 1219 households surveyed during the baseline phase of a household water and hygiene behavioral intervention trial from March-May 2010 [33].

Data Collection

In each participating household, a hand rinse sample was taken from the respondent (adult female caregiver). Hand rinse sampling involves the participant placing her hands, one at a time, into a sterile sample bag containing 350 ml of sterile distilled water, a sampling method used successfully in a number of previous studies [13,16,17,33]. A sample of stored water that was intended for drinking and cooking was also collected from each household. Enumerators documented whether or not the water storage container was covered, then asked each respondent to extract water in the manner she usually would, pouring it into a 1.63 liter sterile sample bag (VWR, Radnor, PA). Enumerators noted whether the respondent's hand touched the water during extraction, as well as the extraction method used (*e.g.*, decanting, filling a cup or bowl). Enumerators inquired whether and how the water had been treated, and for how long the water had been stored prior to sampling. Finally, respondents were asked to identify the water source from which the stored water had been collected. Water samples were tested for chlorine using a dip chlorine strip (Hach Co., Loveland, CO); because chlorine was never detected, there was no need to add sodium thiosulfate to neutralize residual.

Along with water and hand rinse samples, enumerators conducted interviews with the female caretaker of the youngest child in the household. Information was collected regarding household water management and hygiene behaviors, water supply and sanitation services, household socioeconomic and demographic characteristics, and illness status of household members. Tanzanian enumerators participated in a 4-week training that included instruction on survey content and administration, electronic data collection, and sterile sampling technique. The survey instrument underwent multiple iterations and pre-tests.

Ethics Statement

Participants were informed in the local language (Kiswahili) of all study procedures and the time required for participation. Written informed consent was obtained from the mother or primary female adult caretaker of the under-five children in the household. When younger caregivers were interviewed (15–17), an adult household member was present. The Tanzanian Commission for Science and Technology, the Tanzanian National Institute for Medical Research (NIMRI) Ethics Sub-Committee, the Ifakara Health Institute Institutional Review Board (IRB), and Stanford University's IRB (IRB Protocol #17971) approved the consent procedures and study protocol.

Laboratory Analysis

All water and hand rinse samples were stored in a cooler on ice and transported to a local laboratory for microbial analysis by membrane filtration within six hours of collection. The turbidity of the water and hand rinse samples was measured using a LaMotte 2020e Turbidity Meter (LaMotte Company, Chestertown, MD). The fecal indicator bacteria, *E. coli* and enterococci, were enumerated following USEPA Methods 1604 and 1600, respectively [48,49]. $MgCl_2$ was added to the water and hand rinse filters to facilitate capture of viral particles [50], and the samples were subsequently passed through a 0.45 μm-pore size membrane filter as outlined in Mattioli *et al.* [33]. The filters were then treated with RNAlater (Qiagen, Germantown, MD) to stabilize RNA/DNA [51] and stored at −80°C. *E. coli* membrane filters with *E. coli* biomass (from EPA method 1604) were removed from agar after counting and were treated with RNAlater and stored at −80°C. Filters were stored for up to 5 months at −80°C until being transported back to Stanford University (Stanford, CA, USA) for molecular processing. Details on field and lab blanks, turbidity measurements, filtration volumes, culture assay detection limits, and sample transport were previously described by Mattioli *et al.* [33].

The presence or absence of the nucleic acids from three enteric viruses (enterovirus, adenovirus, and rotavirus), the human-specific *Bacteroidales* marker, as well as seven *E. coli* virulence genes was measured in all samples. These pathogens were chosen for analysis because rotavirus, pathogenic *E. coli*, and *Shigella* spp. are believed to be major viral and bacterial etiologies of childhood diarrhea [52,53]; in addition, enteroviruses and adenoviruses are recognized as important etiological agents of gastroenteritis for children in the developing world [45,54].

Presence of *E. coli* virulence genes in preserved *E. coli* biomass was determined using multiplex polymerase chain reactions (PCR) [33]. This method determines the presence of diarrheagenic *E. coli* virulence genes that are commonly found in *Shigella* spp., as well as five different pathotypes of *E. coli* including enteroinvasive *E. coli* (EIEC), enteropathogenic *E. coli* (EPEC), enteroaggregative *E. coli* (EAEC), enterotoxigenic *E. coli* (ETEC), and enterohemorragic *E. coli* (EHEC) [47]. These virulence genes include *stx1* and *stx2* (present in EHEC), *eaeA* (present in EHEC and EPEC), *STIb* and *LTI* (present in ETEC), *ipaH* (present in EIEC and *Shigella* spp.), and *aggR* (present in EAEC) [55].

The three enteric viruses (enterovirus [56], rotavirus [57], and adenovirus [58]) and the human-specific *Bacteroidales* fecal marker (BacHum) [59] were detected using end-point PCR (BacHum) or reverse transcriptase-PCR (viruses) with a hydrolysis probe. Details on nucleic acid extraction, molecular detection assays, assay detection limits, and inhibition analyses can be found in Mattioli *et al.* [33].

Statistical Analysis

Data were analyzed using SAS Enterprise Guide version 4.3 (SAS Institute Inc., Cary, NC). The term 'enteric virus' is defined as the presence or absence of at least one of the three enteric viruses measured. The acronym ECVG is defined as the presence or absence of at least one of the seven *E. coli* virulence genes measured, and the term BacHum is defined as the presence or absence of the human-specific *Bacteroidales* fecal marker. Results are considered statistically significant at a level of $p \leq 0.05$.

A matched case-control study design was used to evaluate the relationship between cases of diarrhea in children under five and the presence of molecular markers of enteric pathogens on hands of mothers and in household stored water. Out of the 1219 households surveyed in the larger household water and hygiene behavioral intervention trial, the total number of children classified as sick with GI illness was 113 (among 112 unique households). These children served as our 'cases' in the case-control study. A case of gastrointestinal illness (GI) was defined as a child having three or more loose/watery stools per 24 hour period, blood in the stool, and/or vomiting using a two-day recall period. Reported GI illness was thus nearly contemporaneous with the sampling and interview. Healthy children (no reported symptoms) in the same household as a GI case were excluded from being controls. Children presenting with non-GI symptoms (*e.g.*, coughing, congestion) and their siblings were also excluded from being controls.

Cases were matched to controls post sample collection by one-to-one propensity score matching (PSM) with no replacement using STATA (version 11; Stata Corporation, College Station, TX) [60]. PSM was employed to reduce the chance of bias resulting from systematic differences between cases and controls and to improve effect estimation efficiency [61]. The following variables were included in the model to generate the propensity scores for matching: child age; the number of families in the housing unit; the number of times mother reported washing hands with soap the day prior to interview; whether the household was located in an urban or rural community; whether the mother reported that the youngest child uses a latrine regularly; whether the household has an on-plot water source; if the child's palms were observed to have visible dirt; whether the mother works outside the home; the number of liters of water collected *per capita* per day; and whether the household's main drinking water source type was a borewell or tap. An equal number of children (among 111 unique households) were selected by PSM as matched controls.

Conditional logistic regression was used to calculate matched odds ratios (OR) representing the association between childhood diarrhea and the presence of contamination on the primary caregiver's hands and in the household's stored drinking water (case-control analysis). Exact p-values and confidence intervals (CI) were calculated. As a robustness check and to control for potential confounders in the case-control analysis, bivariate analyses of household demographics and water, sanitation, and hygiene behaviors/characteristics between case and control households were performed. The bivariate analyses showed which factors were independently associated with child case status. The student's T-test was used to compare mean values between case and control households. Pooled variances were used unless the Equality of Variances Folded F-Statistic was significant ($p<0.05$), in which case a Satterthwaite Test of unequal variance was used. The chi-square test was used to test for differences in proportions of binary variables between case and control households; when $N <5$ a Fisher's exact test was used. An ANOVA test was used to evaluate differences in proportions between case and control households for categorical variables, and the Wilcoxon-Mann-Whitney Test was used for non-parametric comparisons for non-normally distributed continuous variables. Variables with a p-value ≤ 0.20 in the bivariate analysis were included in a multivariate logistic regression model of diarrhea. Model reduction was performed by backwards selection until all remaining variables were found to be significant ($p \leq 0.05$). Adjusted odds ratios (AOR) and 95% confidence intervals were calculated using conditional logistic regression, adjusting for those variables independently associated with diarrhea [62]. The possibility of overmatching with PSM was also assessed and is described in the Supporting Information (SI).

Multivariate logistic regression was used to model the presence of contamination (separate models were estimated for ECVG, enteric virus, and BacHum) on hands and in household stored water as a function of hand hygiene and water management behaviors, respectively. Each separate model included data from 306 unique households. Two hundred twenty-three of these households were part of the case-control analysis presented above. The additional 83 households were drawn from the dataset published by Mattioli *et al.* [33].

The hand hygiene behaviors examined in the model of hand contamination include reported liters *per capita* per day used for hand washing; whether the respondent reported washing her hands with soap within one hour prior to having her hand rinse taken; and the respondent's reported activity immediately prior to having the hand rinse sample taken (*i.e.,* washing clothes, dishes, or child; hand washing; food preparation/eating/serving; or other activity such as gardening/farming and sweeping; *versus* sitting).

The water management behaviors examined in the model of stored drinking water contamination include whether the respondent reported actively treating her stored water (*i.e.,* boiling, chlorinating, filtering, or solar water disinfection); the reported length of time the sampled water had been stored in the home; whether the observed extraction method of stored water for sampling by the respondent was "risky" (*i.e.,* dipping a short-handled cup, mug, or bowl); whether the stored drinking water was reportedly collected from an improved source; the average reported amount of time that household members spend fetching water per day; and whether the bacterial or viral gene(s) being modeled was present in the respondent's hand rinse sample. The models also include control variables for the presence of an infant in the household, household monthly expenditure *per capita*, and whether the household uses a facility with improved sanitation infrastructure. Other control variables considered but that did not contribute significantly to any of the models include whether the household used a private or shared latrine; the number of children under five in the household; whether the primary caregiver worked outside of the home, and whether the primary caregiver was able to read and write.

For the purposes of this manuscript, improved sanitation infrastructure is defined as a toilet or latrine with a cement slab, septic tank, or flush tank into a piped sewer system or pit latrine. This definition differs from the WHO/UNICEF Joint Monitoring program definition [63] in which only privately owned sanitation facilities are considered improved. This definition allowed us to examine for the effects of private versus shared sanitation and improved versus unimproved sanitation infrastructure separately in our models.

Results

Matched Case-control Analysis

Among the 113 children classified as sick with GI illness within the 48 hours prior to interview, 80 children were reported to have 3 or more loose/watery stools per 24 hour period, 6 were reported to have blood in the stool, and 53 were reported to have vomited. Variables used in the PSM method, as well as household demographics and water, sanitation, and hygiene characteristics stratified by case *versus* control status are presented in Table S1.

At least one of the three enteric viruses measured was found on 21% of mother's hands (47/222) and in 3% of stored water samples (7/216). Rotavirus was the most frequently detected virus both on hands (10%) and in stored water (2%). Enterovirus was detected in 8% of hand samples, but was never detected in household stored water; adenovirus was detected in 5% of hand rinse samples and in 1% of stored water samples. BacHum was found in 39% of hand rinse samples (86/222) and in 14% of stored water samples (30/216).

More than half (59%) of all households in the study had at least one *E. coli* virulence gene (ECVG) detected in their stored water, and 41% of respondents had ECVG detected on their hands. The presence of individual virulence genes among all water and hand rinse samples processed for the case-control analysis is reported in Table S2. Across case and control households, the mean *E. coli* and enterococci concentration in household stored water was 1.5 (SD 1.0) and 0.5 (SD 0.6) log CFU/100 ml (N = 219), respectively. The mean *E. coli* and enterococci concentration in hand rinse samples was 2.5 (SD 1.0) and 2.7 (SD 1.0) log CFU/2 hands (N = 223), respectively. The concentration of FIB on hands and in stored drinking water stratified by case status can be found in Table S2. There was no significant difference between case and control households in the concentration of *E. coli* or enterococci found on mother's hands or in stored drinking.

Table 1 presents the prevalence of molecular markers of enteric viruses and ECVG in household stored water and hand rinse samples, stratified by case and control households, as well as the odds ratios from the matched case-control analysis. The presence of ECVG in a household's stored water was associated with a 2-fold *decrease* in the odds of at least one child under five years of age in the household reporting symptoms of diarrhea (OR = 0.51 [95% CI 0.27–0.93]; $p = 0.03$). Similarly, the presence of the *E. coli* virulence gene, Lt1, on the primary caregiver's hands (suggesting the presence of the *E. coli* pathotype enterotoxigenic *E. coli* (ETEC) [55]) was also associated with a significant decrease in the odds of a child in the household having diarrhea (OR = 0.25 [95% CI 0.05, 0.93]; $p = 0.04$).

There were no significant associations between virus detection in water or hand rinses and diarrhea case status in children. The presence of each enteric virus on hands and in stored water was consistently associated with increased odds of a child in the household having diarrhea (Table 1), although none achieved statistical significance. The presence of at least one enteropathogen molecular marker (enteric virus or ECVG) on hands or in water was also not significantly associated with diarrhea.

The presence of BacHum in either stored water or hand rinse samples was not associated with the odds of a child having diarrhea at the time of visit. Similarly, the presence of FIB (*E. coli* or enterococci) on hands or in stored water was not associated with cases of diarrhea. Higher concentrations of FIB in stored water (categorical variable: 1 to <11, 11 to 100, or >100 CFU/100 mL, Table 1) were also not associated with the odds of a child having diarrhea.

Case and control households were found to be similar with respect to the variables used in the PSM (Table S1, all $p > 0.05$). Cases and controls had no statistically different characteristics (all $p > 0.05$), with one exception: a larger percentage of control households had their stored drinking water covered (98% *versus* 89%, $p < 0.01$). The results of the bivariate analyses performed as a robustness check and to control for other potential confounders in the case-control analysis can be found in the SI (Results S1 and Table S1). The revised odds ratios after adjusting for the variables

Table 1. Prevalence of *E. coli* virulence genes (ECVG), enteric virus genes, human-specific *Bacteroidales* genes, and FIB detected in household stored drinking water and hand rinse samples of respondents with at least one child younger than five years old that were either sick with diarrhea (cases) versus matched healthy children under five years of age (controls).

	HANDS						STORED WATER					
	Case (%)	Control (%)	OR	95% CI[c]		P	Case (%)	Control (%)	OR	95% CI[c]		P
ECVG [a]	40.0	44.1	0.86	0.48	1.53	0.68	52.7	67.9	0.51	0.27	0.93	0.03[†]
ipaH	20.0	31.5	0.50	0.24	1.01	0.05	23.2	33.9	0.58	0.31	1.07	0.09
aggR	13.6	15.3	0.92	0.39	2.19	1.00	21.4	32.1	0.54	0.26	1.07	0.08
Lt1	4.5	13.5	0.25	0.05	0.93	0.04[†]	11.6	17.0	0.71	0.31	1.57	0.46
STIb	0.0	0.9	1.00*	0.00	19.00	1.00	1.8	1.8	1.00	0.07	13.80	1.00
eaeA	4.5	5.4	0.83	0.20	3.28	1.00	17.0	15.2	1.15	0.51	2.64	0.85
stx1	9.1	17.1	0.53	0.22	1.19	0.14	20.5	30.4	0.54	0.26	1.07	0.08
stx2	0.0	0.9	1.00*	0.00	19.00	1.00	0.0	2.7	0.26*	0.00	1.71	0.25
Enteric Virus [b]	24.8	17.0	1.69	0.82	3.66	0.18	4.6	1.8	2.50	0.41	26.25	0.45
Rotavirus	12.4	8.0	1.56	0.63	4.07	0.40	3.7	0.0	5.29*	0.90	∞	0.13
Adenovirus	6.2	4.5	1.50	0.36	7.23	0.75	0.9	1.8	0.50	0.01	9.61	1.00
Enterovirus	8.8	6.3	1.60	0.46	6.22	0.58	0.0	0.0				
At least 1 enteric virus or ECVG	55.8	54.0	1.12	0.63	1.97	0.79	54.0	66.4	0.59	0.32	1.08	0.09
Human *Bacteroidales*	33.6	43.8	0.64	0.35	1.13	0.13	11.1	16.2	0.67	0.27	1.59	0.42
Escherichia coli[¥]	81.4	74.3	1.44	0.76	2.80	0.29	81.4	87.6	0.63	0.28	1.37	0.28
1 to <11 CFU/100 mL							13.3	20.4	0.48	0.16	1.39	0.21
11 to 100 CFU/100 mL							31.9	33.6	0.70	0.25	1.85	0.57
>100 CFU/100 mL							36.3	33.6	0.79	0.29	2.04	0.75
Enterococcus[¥]	84.1	87.6	0.71	0.28	1.73	0.54	79.6	89.4	0.48	0.20	1.06	0.07
1 to <11 CFU/100 mL							18.6	15.9	0.60	0.20	1.75	0.43
11 to 100 CFU/100 mL							31.0	38.1	0.47	0.19	1.10	0.09
>100 CFU/100 mL							30.1	35.4	0.46	0.17	1.16	0.11

The study consisted of 112 unique case households (containing 113 case children) and 111 unique households with only healthy children (containing 113 matched, control children).
[a]At least one of the seven pathogenic *E. coli* virulence genes (ECVG) measured present.
[b]At least one of the three enteric viruses measured (rotavirus, adenovirus, enterovirus) present.
[c]CI, confidence interval.
[¥]Presence/Absence of CFU per 2 hands; Presence/Absence or within specified range of CFU/100 mL stored drinking water with 0 CFU/100 mL as the reference group.
*Indicates a median unbiased estimate.
[†]Statistically significant ($p \leq 0.05$).

significantly associated with case status are presented in Table S3. Since there were no substantive differences between the adjusted case-control analyses and the unadjusted analyses, the case-control results were considered robust. The incorporation of numerous matching variables in the PSM model may have overmatched households, causing the case-control effect estimates to be biased downward [61,64,65]. Therefore, the potential effect of overmatching on our results was assessed. The results of the overmatching analysis (see SI and Tables S4, S5, S6, and S7) show that matching case and control children on several control variables did not affect the results.

Behavioral Determinants of Enteric Pathogen and Fecal Markers

We modeled ECVG, enteric virus, and BacHum presence in hand rinse samples and household stored water as a function of hygiene and water management behaviors. Household socioeconomic and demographic characteristics, as well as water supply, sanitation, and hygiene practices of all 306 households used in the models can be found in Table S8. Among the households modeled, twenty-five percent of households included an infant (<1 yr) present at the time of visit, with an average of 1.3 (SD 0.5) children under the age of five. The age of the primary caregivers in our study ranged from 16 to 68 years (median 25 yr). Households reported spending an average of $17 US (SD $9) per month per person. Only 15% of households had an on-plot water source, but 85% reported using an improved source as their main source of drinking water according to the WHO/UNICEF Joint Monitoring program definition [63] (*e.g.*, tap, borewell, or rainwater). A minority of households (16%) reported to have treated their stored water. At the time of sampling, mean storage time was 33 hours (SD 29), and 94% of stored water containers were observed to be covered. Thirty-eight percent of households had access to a sanitation facility with improved sanitation infrastructure, and 51% percent of households reported having a private sanitation facility.

The models of ECVG, enteric virus, and BacHum presence in hand rinse samples and household stored water are presented in Tables 2 and 3, respectively. We found a limited number of significant determinants of hand contamination. The liters *per capita* used per day for hand washing (natural-log transformed) was the only statistically significant explanatory hygiene behavior in the model of enteric virus presence on hands ($p<0.01$). Results indicate that doubling the quantity of water used *per capita* per day for hand washing was associated with a 2-fold decrease in the odds of a respondent having an enteric virus on her hands. In the model of ECVG presence on hands, the odds of detecting ECVG was approximately three times greater for those respondents who reported handling food or washing (both $p<0.01$) prior to sampling versus those reporting sitting. No hand hygiene behaviors were significant in the model of BacHum. It is important to note that our model explains only a small portion of the variation in microbial prevalence on hands, highlighting the unexplained variability in hand contamination within these communities.

Contamination of stored water was associated with several water management variables. Stored drinking water collected from an improved source was associated with a 2.7-fold reduction in the odds of detecting ECVG contamination ($p = 0.02$) and a 5.6-fold decrease in the odds of detecting BacHum ($p<0.01$). Conversely, the odds of enteric virus and BacHum being present in a household's stored water was 32.7 and 3.6 times greater for households where enteric viruses or BacHum were also present on the hands of the respondent (both $p<0.01$). Also, the use of a facility with improved sanitation infrastructure was associated with a 1.7-fold decrease in the odds of detecting ECVG in the household's stored drinking water ($p = 0.04$).

Discussion

The overall prevalence of enteropathogen genes and the human-specific *Bacteroidales* molecular marker in stored drinking water and hand rinse samples analyzed for this study (Table S2) was similar to that found in Bagamoyo, Tanzania by Mattioli *et al.* [33]. Other studies in Tanzania have also documented ECVG, enteric virus, and *Bacteroidales* molecular markers in soil, on household surfaces, on produce, and on hands in Tanzania [16,47].

Unexpectedly, our study found that the presence of ECVG in stored water and on hands was associated with decreased odds of a child under the age of five having reported diarrhea–indicating a higher prevalence of ECVG among control households. One possible explanation for the observed negative association between ECVG presence and diarrhea is that an episode of child diarrhea in the household might have triggered efforts by the primary caregiver to improve stored drinking water quality, such as treatment or collection from an improved source. A greater percentage of respondents caring for children with diarrhea reported boiling their stored drinking water (16%) than those in control households (9%), although the difference did not reach statistical significance ($p = 0.1$). Notably, a prior study in Tanzania also found microbial water quality to be cleaner among households with child diarrhea [17].

Asymptomatic pathogen shedding among healthy control children could help explain the absence of association between the pathogens detected in the household environment and child diarrhea. A recent study to identify the etiology of child diarrhea in Tanzania found that 52% of healthy controls were infected with an enteric pathogen [53]. Asymptomatic shedding could be the result of subclinical infections, persistent shedding after illness symptoms have subsided, ingestion of pathogens below an infectious dose, or immunity developed by those children living in households with persistent pathogen contamination [66–69].

Several reported water management and hygiene behaviors were found to be significantly associated with molecular indicators of pathogen contamination in the household. For example, modeling the presence of enteric virus marker on hands suggests that the volume of water used for hand washing may be important in reducing enteric virus transmission. Currently, the World Health Organization does not recommend a minimum volume of water per person per day specifically for hand washing, with the assumption that this volume is dependent on level of service and water fetching distance [70]. Households in our study reported using an average of 1.8 L (SD = 1.3) per person per day for hand washing and had an average of 5.4 people (SD = 2.3) per household (Table S8). Therefore, for a household in our study to reduce their risk of viral hand contamination by 2-fold, each household would have to access an average of 19.3 extra L of water (3.6 L per person) per day for hand washing. This would be roughly equivalent to a household collecting one extra 20-L jerry can of water per day.

Respondents reporting activities involving washing soiled household items (such as clothes or dishes), and those who reported handling food immediately prior to sampling, were more likely to have ECVG detected on their hands. This may suggest, as proposed by others [71], that water used for washing might serve as a transport mechanism for bacterial pathogens within the home. Previous studies found Tanzanian fresh market produce to be contaminated with ECVG [47] and have detected increased levels of FIB on hands after handling produce or preparing food [16]. This may imply that bacterial pathogens could also be transferred from produce to hands and would explain the association between ECVG on hands and recent food handling observed in this study.

Stored drinking water collected from households using improved water sources was less likely to be contaminated with ECVG and BacHum. This result adds nuance to published evidence of significant post-supply FIB contamination of stored water, particularly stored water collected from improved sources [8,14,72,73]. Together this suggests that while stored water may become re-contaminated with FIB after collection, improvements to water sources may still provide safer water at the point-of-use by preventing bacterial pathogens and human feces from entering drinking water prior to collection. Households with improved sanitation infrastructure also had reduced odds of ECVG detection in their stored water, suggesting that, like water sources, improvements to sanitation infrastructure (*e.g.*, the addition of a concrete slab, septic tank, or flush tank) may reduce the risk of pathogenic bacteria entering the household's stored drinking water.

Stored water collected from the household of a respondent with BacHum detected on her hands was more likely to be contaminated with BacHum, implying that hands may be a source of human fecal contamination in stored drinking water. However, due to the cross-sectional study design, we cannot confirm the directionality of contamination. Interestingly, reported water treatment, storage time, use of a "risky" extraction method, and water fetching time were not found to be associated with markers of pathogen or human fecal presence in stored water. This result stands in contrast to other research which found higher FIB levels in drinking water of households that performed risky extraction methods [14] and lower FIB levels in households that actively treated stored water [15] or were served by on-site water sources [74]. However the results are consistent with previous research in Tanzania identifying fecal contamination on hands as the strongest predictor of fecal contamination levels in stored water [17]. Thus, the effects of safe water management behaviors may be offset or muted by contamination from hand contact.

Viral marker prevalence may have been too low in this study to detect significant associations with diarrhea or water management

Table 2. Binary logistic regression model of *E. coli* virulence genes (ECVG), enteric virus genes, and human-specific *Bacteroidales* genes presence in hand rinse samples as a function of hygiene behaviors.

	HANDS																	
	ECVG, N = 256*						**Enteric Virus, N = 258***						**Human-Specific *Bacteroidales*, N = 258***					
	pseudo $R^2 = 0.09$, Max-rescaled $R^2 = 0.12$						pseudo $R^2 = 0.06$, Max-Rescaled $R^2 = 0.10$						pseudo $R^2 = 0.03$, Max-Rescaled $R^2 = 0.04$					
	Likelihood Ratio: $\chi2 = 24.31$, $p<0.01$						Likelihood Ratio: $\chi^2 = 16.60$, $p = 0.06$						Likelihood Ratio: $\chi^2 = 6.93$, $p = 0.64$					
Variable	**ß**	**SE**	**P**	**OR**	**95% CI**		**ß**	**SE**	**P**	**OR**	**95% CI**		**ß**	**SE**	**P**	**OR**	**95% CI**	
Intercept	−0.87	0.33	0.01				−1.43	0.37	0.00				−0.57	0.32	0.07			
Liters per capita per day used for hand washing[a]	−0.01	0.27	0.98	0.99	0.59	1.68	−1.00	0.34	0.00[†]	0.37	0.19	0.72	−0.15	0.26	0.56	0.86	0.51	1.43
Respondent washed hands within 1 h prior to sampling[b]	−0.08	0.30	0.77	0.92	0.51	1.64	−0.67	0.38	0.08	0.51	0.24	1.09	−0.13	0.29	0.66	0.88	0.50	1.56
Washing (clothes, dishes, hands, child) vs. Sitting[b, c]	1.04	0.41	0.01[†]	2.84	1.28	6.32	−0.22	0.56	0.69	0.80	0.27	2.39	0.05	0.41	0.91	1.05	0.47	2.34
Hand Washing vs. Sitting[b, c]	0.90	1.43	0.53	2.46	0.15	40.77	1.41	1.44	0.32	4.12	0.25	68.73	−13.76	894.20	0.99	<0.01	<0.01	>999.9
Food Preparation vs. Sitting[b, c]	1.23	0.34	0.00[†]	3.41	1.74	6.69	0.10	0.41	0.81	1.11	0.49	2.48	0.55	0.33	0.10	1.73	0.90	3.34
Other vs. Sitting[b, c]	−0.25	0.57	0.66	0.78	0.25	2.39	0.31	0.58	0.59	1.37	0.44	4.24	−0.38	0.56	0.49	0.68	0.23	2.04
Use of facility with improved sanitation infrastructure[b]	−0.30	0.29	0.30	0.74	0.43	1.30	0.16	0.34	0.64	1.17	0.60	2.26	0.29	0.28	0.30	1.34	0.78	2.30
Infant (<1 yr) present in household[b]	0.49	0.30	0.11	1.63	0.90	2.96	−0.27	0.37	0.47	0.77	0.37	1.58	−0.14	0.30	0.63	0.87	0.48	1.56
Regular monthly expenditures per person per 1000 TZS[d]	0.06	0.10	0.53	1.06	0.88	1.28	0.22	0.11	0.04	1.24	1.01	1.53	0.01	0.09	0.95	1.01	0.84	1.20

[a]Ln-transformed.
[b]Binary variables with values of 0 and 1.
[c]Refers to the reported activity prior to the respondent having their hand rinse sample taken.
[d]TZS Tanzanian Shillings.
*N <306 because sample was lost or survey response not collected.
[†]Statistically significant ($p \leq 0.05$).

Table 3. Binary logistic regression model of *E. coli* virulence genes (ECVG), enteric virus genes, and human-specific *Bacteroidales* gene presence in household stored water as a function of water management behaviors.

	STORED WATER																	
	ECVG, N = 276*						**Enteric Virus, N = 267***						**Human-Specific *Bacteroidales*, N = 267***					
	pseudo $R^2 = 0.06$, Max-Rescaled $R^2 = 0.09$						pseudo $R^2 = 0.11$, Max-Rescaled $R^2 = 0.45$						pseudo $R^2 = 0.13$ Max-Rescaled $R^2 = 0.24$					
	Likelihood Ratio: $\chi^2 = 17.83$, $p = 0.04$						Likelihood Ratio: $\chi^2 = 32.17$, $p<0.01$						Likelihood Ratio: $\chi^2 = 35.57$ $p<0.01$					
Variable	**ß**	**SE**	**P**	**OR**	**95% CI**		**ß**	**SE**	**P**	**OR**	**95% CI**		**ß**	**SE**	**P**	**OR**	**95% CI**	
Intercept	1.34	0.89	0.13				−25.02	418.8	0.95				−3.89	1.38	0.00			
Stored water reportedly treated[b, c]	−0.11	0.37	0.77	0.90	0.43	1.87	0.40	1.29	0.76	1.49	0.12	18.76	0.02	0.60	0.98	1.02	0.32	3.26
Time water stored in household (h)[a]	0.09	0.11	0.45	1.09	0.87	1.37	−0.41	0.36	0.25	0.66	0.33	1.34	0.47	0.25	0.06	1.60	0.99	2.60
Observed extraction method of stored water was risky[b, d]	−0.04	0.38	0.92	0.96	0.46	2.03	12.16	285.8	0.97	1.90×10^6	<0.01	>999.9	−0.17	0.56	0.77	0.85	0.28	2.56
Stored water reportedly collected from improved source[b, e]	−1.01	0.41	0.01[†]	0.36	0.16	0.82	11.01	306.1	0.97	6.02×10^4	<0.01	>999.9	−1.69	0.45	0.00[†]	0.18	0.08	0.45
Water Fetching Time Per Day (min)[a]	0.03	0.15	0.87	1.03	0.77	1.37	−0.15	0.42	0.72	0.86	0.38	1.96	0.37	0.25	0.14	1.44	0.89	2.35
Modeled contamination present on hands of primary caregiver[b]	0.26	0.26	0.33	1.30	0.77	2.17	3.49	1.11	0.00[†]	32.7	3.68	290.42	1.28	0.43	0.00[†]	3.60	1.55	8.38
Use of facility with improved sanitation infrastructure[b]	−0.55	0.27	0.04[†]	0.58	0.34	0.98	−0.70	0.87	0.42	0.50	0.09	2.75	0.41	0.44	0.35	1.51	0.64	3.59
Infant (<1 yr) present in household[b]	−0.07	0.30	0.80	0.93	0.52	1.66	−11.96	243.5	0.96	0.00	<0.01	>999.9	−0.35	0.52	0.50	0.71	0.25	1.96
Regular monthly expenditures per person per 1000 TZS[f]	−0.08	0.09	0.37	0.92	0.77	1.10	−0.42	0.35	0.23	0.66	0.33	1.30	−0.05	0.14	0.75	0.95	0.72	1.26

[a]Ln-transformed.
[b]Binary variables with values of 0 and 1.
[c]Boiling, chlorinating, filtering, or SODIS (versus no treatment including settling).
[d]Cup, mug, or bowl (versus pouring, long handled dipper, or spigot).
[e]Borewell, rainwater, or tap (versus shallow well, cart/tanker, surface water, or vendor).
[f]TZS Tanzanian Shillings.
*N <306 because sample was lost or survey response not collected.
[†]Statistically significant (p≤0.05).

behaviors given our sample size. Also, the lower limit of detection of the viral assays ranged from 10^0 to 10^2 genomic units per 100 ml stored water or per two hands. Thus, health relevant concentrations below our detection limit could have been present but been undetected in our study [75]. Despite these limitations, viral prevalence trended toward an increase in the odds of a child having diarrhea in the household, and therefore should be prioritized for further research. Our findings suggest that research focused on child exposure to enteric pathogens in the household environment should include rotavirus, as it was the most prevalent virus found in both hand rinses and stored water of sample households. Rotavirus was also recently reported to be one of the most important etiological agents of childhood diarrhea in a multi-country, prospective case-control study [76].

The results presented herein should be interpreted in consideration of several study limitations. The cross-sectional design precludes determining the direction of effect between child diarrhea, behaviors, and exposure. Also, previous research has shown that microbial contamination of hands and drinking water can vary significantly over time [14,16], and our cross sectional study design does not allow us to consider this variability. In addition, only nucleic acids of enteric pathogens were detected in this study; our methods do not characterize the infectivity or viability of the pathogens targeted. Diarrhea and many of the water management and hygiene behaviors used in our models were self-reported by the respondent; self-reported data has been found to introduce inaccuracy and bias into estimates of behavior [77]. Finally, we were unable to measure all potential enteric pathogens (*e.g.*, protozoa) [76] in this study, and it is possible that these unmeasured pathogens may have had a positive association with diarrhea.

Few studies have looked at enteric pathogen and human fecal molecular markers in household environments of low-income communities [16,33,47]; this study contributes new knowledge by examining the association between hygiene and water management behaviors and the presence of these markers. The identification of behaviors associated with molecular markers of enteric pathogens and human fecal contamination on hands and in water in Bagamoyo can be used to inform the development of more efficacious interventions aimed at reducing the burden of childhood diarrhea in other low-income communities. For example, our work suggests that increasing the quantity of water available for hand washing may reduce enteric virus transmission from hands. In addition, improvements in food hygiene practices and sanitation infrastructure may help alleviate pathogenic *E. coli* contamination within the home, while improved source water may prevent human fecal and pathogenic *E. coli* contamination of a household's stored drinking water. To our knowledge, this is the first study to examine the association between child diarrhea and molecular markers of enteric pathogens in household stored water and hand rinses. Our results warrant further investigation into why stored drinking water was less frequently contaminated with bacterial pathogens in households with sick children. In combination, our analyses highlight the need to better understand the relative contribution and interdependence of household exposure routes to the burden of child diarrhea.

Supporting Information

Table S1 Child-level descriptive statistics from the case-control analysis. The table includes variables used in the PSM, as well as household (HH) demographics, and water, sanitation, and hygiene characteristics by case and control status.

Table S2 ECVG, enteric virus gene, Human *Bacteroidales* gene, and FIB (*Escherichia coli* and *Enterococcus*) prevalence for households in the case-control study.

Table S3 Adjusted, matched case-control analysis results.

Table S4 Unmatched household case-control analysis results using original controls.

Table S5 Unmatched household case-control analysis results using additional controls.

Table S6 Prevalence (%) of ECVG, enteric virus genes, and Human *Bacteroidales* genes in additional control households. The additional households, along with the original (case-control analysis) control households, were used in the robustness checks.

Table S7 Robustness checks logistic regression results. These results were used to evaluate whether the propensity score is significantly associated with pathogen presence in the original (case-control analysis) control households.

Table S8 Household-level descriptive statistics from the water management and hygiene behavior models. Household-level demographics, and water, sanitation, and hygiene characteristics of the households used in the logistic regression model of contamination as a function of water management and hygiene behaviors.

Methods S1 Detailed description of methods used for the overmatching analysis.

Results S1 Results of robustness checks and overmatching analysis.

Acknowledgments

The authors acknowledge Rebecca Gilsdorf, Michael Harris, Debbie Lee, Emily Viau, and Maggie Montgomery for their support in the field and the laboratory. We acknowledge our collaborators Salim Abdulla and Omar Juma at the Ifakara Health Institute in Bagamoyo, Tanzania. This project would not have been possible without the Tanzanian lab and field teams and participating households.

Author Contributions

Conceived and designed the experiments: MCM ABB JD ARH MM AJP. Performed the experiments: MCM ARH AJP. Analyzed the data: MCM AJP. Contributed reagents/materials/analysis tools: ABB JD MM. Wrote the paper: MCM ABB JD ARH MM AJP.

References

1. Walker CL, Rudan I, Liu L, Nair H, Theodoratou E, et al. (2013) Global burden of childhood pneumonia and diarrhoea. Lancet 381: 1405–1416.
2. Liu L, Johnson HL, Cousens S, Perin J, Scott S, et al. (2012) Global, regional, and national causes of child mortality: an updated systematic analysis for 2010 with time trends since 2000. Lancet 379: 2151–2161.
3. Prüss-Üstün A, Bos R, Gore F, Bartram J (2008) Safer water, better health: costs, benefits and sustainability of interventions to protect and promote health. Geneva: World Health Organization.
4. Organization WH, UNICeF (2012) Progress on sanitation and drinking water: 2012 update. Geneva: World Health Organization.
5. Dufour AP, Ballentine P (1986) Ambient Water Quality Criteria for Bacteria-1986 (Bacteriological ambient water quality criteria for marine and fresh recreational waters). Washington, DC: U.S. Environmental Protection Agency.
6. Cairncross AM (1990) Health Impacts in Developing Countries: New Evidence and New Prospects. Water and Environment Journal 4: 571–575.
7. Trevett AF, Carter RC, Tyrrel SF (2005) The importance of domestic water quality management in the context of faecal-oral disease transmission. J Water Health 3: 259–270.
8. Wright J, Gundry S, Conroy R (2004) Household drinking water in developing countries: a systematic review of microbiological contamination between source and point-of-use. Trop Med Int Health 9: 106–117.
9. Jensen PK, Ensink JH, Jayasinghe G, van der Hoek W, Cairncross S, et al. (2002) Domestic transmission routes of pathogens: the problem of in-house contamination of drinking water during storage in developing countries. Trop Med Int Health 7: 604–609.
10. Luby SP, Agboatwalla M, Raza A, Sobel J, Mintz ED, et al. (2001) Microbiologic effectiveness of hand washing with soap in an urban squatter settlement, Karachi, Pakistan. Epidemiol Infect 127: 237–244.
11. Luby SP, Agboatwalla M, Billhimer W, Hoekstra RM (2007) Field trial of a low cost method to evaluate hand cleanliness. Trop Med Int Health 12: 765–771.
12. Pinfold JV (1990) Faecal contamination of water and fingertip-rinses as a method for evaluating the effect of low-cost water supply and sanitation activities on faeco-oral disease transmission. II. A hygiene intervention study in rural north-east Thailand. Epidemiol Infect 105: 377–389.
13. Davis J, Pickering AJ, Rogers K, Mamuya S, Boehm AB (2011) The effects of informational interventions on household water management, hygiene behaviors, stored drinking water quality, and hand contamination in peri-urban Tanzania. Am J Trop Med Hyg 84: 184–191.
14. Levy K, Nelson KL, Hubbard A, Eisenberg JN (2008) Following the water: a controlled study of drinking water storage in northern coastal Ecuador. Environ Health Perspect 116: 1533–1540.
15. Sobsey MD, Stauber CE, Casanova LM, Brown JM, Elliott MA (2008) Point of use household drinking water filtration: A practical, effective solution for providing sustained access to safe drinking water in the developing world. Environ Sci Technol 42: 4261–4267.
16. Pickering AJ, Julian TR, Mamuya S, Boehm AB, Davis J (2011) Bacterial hand contamination among Tanzanian mothers varies temporally and following household activities. Trop Med Int Health 16: 233–239.
17. Pickering AJ, Davis J, Walters SP, Horak HM, Keymer DP, et al. (2010) Hands, water, and health: fecal contamination in Tanzanian communities with improved, non-networked water supplies. Environ Sci Technol 44: 3267–3272.
18. Brown JM, Proum S, Sobsey MD (2008) *Escherichia coli* in household drinking water and diarrheal disease risk: evidence from Cambodia. Water Sci Technol 58: 757–763.
19. Moe CL, Sobsey MD, Samsa GP, Mesolo V (1991) Bacterial indicators of risk of diarrhoeal disease from drinking-water in the Philippines. Bull World Health Organ 69: 305–317.
20. VanDerslice J, Briscoe J (1995) Environmental interventions in developing countries: interactions and their implications. Am J Epidemiol 141: 135–144.
21. Jensen PK, Jayasinghe G, van der Hoek W, Cairncross S, Dalsgaard A (2004) Is there an association between bacteriological drinking water quality and childhood diarrhoea in developing countries? Trop Med Int Health 9: 1210–1215.
22. Gundry S, Wright J, Conroy R (2004) A systematic review of the health outcomes related to household water quality in developing countries. J Water Health 2: 1–13.
23. Khush RS, Arnold BF, Srikanth P, Sudharsanam S, Ramaswamy P, et al. (2013) H2S as an indicator of water supply vulnerability and health risk in low-resource settings: a prospective cohort study. Am J Trop Med Hyg 89: 251–259.
24. Levy K, Nelson KL, Hubbard A, Eisenberg JN (2012) Rethinking indicators of microbial drinking water quality for health studies in tropical developing countries: case study in northern coastal Ecuador. Am J Trop Med Hyg 86: 499–507.
25. Power ML, Littlefield-Wyer J, Gordon DM, Veal DA, Slade MB (2005) Phenotypic and genotypic characterization of encapsulated *Escherichia coli* isolated from blooms in two Australian lakes. Environ Microbiol 7: 631–640.
26. Viau EJ, Goodwin KD, Yamahara KM, Layton BA, Sassoubre LM, et al. (2011) Bacterial pathogens in Hawaiian coastal streams–associations with fecal indicators, land cover, and water quality. Water Res 45: 3279–3290.
27. Byappanahalli MN, Whitman RL, Shively DA, Sadowsky MJ, Ishii S (2006) Population structure, persistence, and seasonality of autochthonous *Escherichia coli* in temperate, coastal forest soil from a Great Lakes watershed. Environ Microbiol 8: 504–513.
28. Anderson KL, Whitlock JE, Harwood VJ (2005) Persistence and differential survival of fecal indicator bacteria in subtropical waters and sediments. Appl Environ Microbiol 71: 3041–3048.
29. Byappanahalli MN, Fujioka RS (1998) Evidence that tropical soil environment can support the growth of Escherichia coli. Water Science and Technology 38: 171–174.
30. Yamahara KM, Walters SP, Boehm AB (2009) Growth of enterococci in unaltered, unseeded beach sands subjected to tidal wetting. Appl Environ Microbiol 75: 1517–1524.
31. Fujioka RS, Tenno K, Kansako S (1988) Naturally occurring fecal coliforms and fecal streptococci in Hawaii's freshwater streams. Toxicity Assessment 3: 613–630.
32. Ferguson AS, Mailloux BJ, Ahmed KM, van Geen A, McKay LD, et al. (2011) Hand-pumps as reservoirs for microbial contamination of well water. J Water Health 9: 708–717.
33. Mattioli MC, Pickering AJ, Gilsdorf RJ, Davis J, Boehm AB (2013) Hands and water as vectors of diarrheal pathogens in Bagamoyo, Tanzania. Environ Sci Technol 47: 355–363.
34. Lemarchand K, Lebaron P (2003) Occurrence of *Salmonella* spp. and *Cryptosporidium* spp. in a French coastal watershed: relationship with fecal indicators. FEMS Microbiol Lett 218: 203–209.
35. Horman A, Rimhanen-Finne R, Maunula L, von Bonsdorff CH, Torvela N, et al. (2004) *Campylobacter* spp., *Giardia* spp., *Cryptosporidium* spp., noroviruses, and indicator organisms in surface water in southwestern Finland, 2000–2001. Appl Environ Microbiol 70: 87–95.
36. Bonadonna L, Briancesco R, Ottaviani M, Veschetti E (2002) Occurrence of Cryptosporidium oocysts in sewage effluents and correlation with microbial, chemical and physical water variables. Environ Monit Assess 75: 241–252.
37. Wu J, Long SC, Das D, Dorner SM (2011) Are microbial indicators and pathogens correlated? A statistical analysis of 40 years of research. J Water Health 9: 265–278.
38. Jiang S, Noble R, Chu W (2001) Human adenoviruses and coliphages in urban runoff-impacted coastal waters of Southern California. Appl Environ Microbiol 67: 179–184.
39. Noble RT, Fuhrman JA (2001) Enteroviruses detected by reverse transcriptase polymerase chain reaction from the coastal waters of Santa Monica Bay, California: low correlation to bacterial indicator levels. Hydrobiologia 460: 175–184.
40. Harwood VJ, Levine AD, Scott TM, Chivukula V, Lukasik J, et al. (2005) Validity of the indicator organism paradigm for pathogen reduction in reclaimed water and public health protection. Appl Environ Microbiol 71: 3163–3170.
41. Pusch D, Oh DY, Wolf S, Dumke R, Schroter-Bobsin U, et al. (2005) Detection of enteric viruses and bacterial indicators in German environmental waters. Arch Virol 150: 929–947.
42. Baggi F, Demarta A, Peduzzi R (2001) Persistence of viral pathogens and bacteriophages during sewage treatment: lack of correlation with indicator bacteria. Res Microbiol 152: 743–751.
43. Ferguson AS, Layton AC, Mailloux BJ, Culligan PJ, Williams DE, et al. (2012) Comparison of fecal indicators with pathogenic bacteria and rotavirus in groundwater. Sci Total Environ 431: 314–322.
44. Fong TT, Lipp EK (2005) Enteric viruses of humans and animals in aquatic environments: health risks, detection, and potential water quality assessment tools. Microbiol Mol Biol Rev 69: 357–371.
45. Ramani S, Kang G (2009) Viruses causing childhood diarrhoea in the developing world. Curr Opin Infect Dis 22: 477–482.
46. Bernhard AE, Field KG (2000) A PCR assay To discriminate human and ruminant feces on the basis of host differences in Bacteroides-Prevotella genes encoding 16S rRNA. Appl Environ Microbiol 66: 4571–4574.
47. Pickering AJ, Julian TR, Marks SJ, Mattioli MC, Boehm AB, et al. (2012) Fecal contamination and diarrheal pathogens on surfaces and in soils among Tanzanian households with and without improved sanitation. Environ Sci Technol.
48. USEPA (2002) Method 1604: Total coliforms and *Escherichia coli* in water by membrane filtration using a simultaneous detection technique (MI Medium). Washington, D.C.: United States Environmental Protection Agency, Office of Water.
49. USEPA (2009) Method 1600: Enterococci in water by membrane filtration using membrane-Enterococcus Indoxyl-D-Glucoside Agar (mEI). Washington, D.C.: United States Environmental Protection Agency, Office of Water.
50. Victoria M, Guimaraes F, Fumian T, Ferreira F, Vieira C, et al. (2009) Evaluation of an adsorption-elution method for detection of astrovirus and norovirus in environmental waters. J Virol Methods 156: 73–76.
51. Keating DT, Malizia AP, Sadlier D, Hurson C, Wood AE, et al. (2008) Lung tissue storage: optimizing conditions for future use in molecular research. Exp Lung Res 34: 455–466.
52. Ashbolt NJ (2004) Microbial contamination of drinking water and disease outcomes in developing regions. Toxicology 198: 229–238.
53. Gascon J, Vargas M, Schellenberg D, Urassa H, Casals C, et al. (2000) Diarrhea in children under 5 years of age from Ifakara, Tanzania: a case-control study. J Clin Microbiol 38: 4459–4462.

54. Silva PA, Stark K, Mockenhaupt FP, Reither K, Weitzel T, et al. (2008) Molecular characterization of enteric viral agents from children in northern region of Ghana. J Med Virol 80: 1790–1798.
55. Kaper JB, Nataro JP, Mobley HL (2004) Pathogenic *Escherichia coli*. Nat Rev Microbiol 2: 123–140.
56. Walters SP, Yamahara KM, Boehm AB (2009) Persistence of nucleic acid markers of health-relevant organisms in seawater microcosms: implications for their use in assessing risk in recreational waters. Water Res 43: 4929–4939.
57. Jothikumar N, Kang G, Hill VR (2009) Broadly reactive TaqMan assay for real-time RT-PCR detection of rotavirus in clinical and environmental samples. JIN2@cdc.gov. J Virol Methods 155: 126–131.
58. Jothikumar N, Cromeans TL, Hill VR, Lu X, Sobsey MD, et al. (2005) Quantitative real-time PCR assays for detection of human adenoviruses and identification of serotypes 40 and 41. Appl Environ Microbiol 71: 3131–3136.
59. Kildare BJ, Leutenegger CM, McSwain BS, Bambic DG, Rajal VB, et al. (2007) 16S rRNA-based assays for quantitative detection of universal, human-, cow-, and dog-specific fecal *Bacteroidales*: a Bayesian approach. Water Res 41: 3701–3715.
60. Dehejia RH, Wahba S (2002) Propensity score-matching methods for nonexperimental causal studies. Review of Economics and statistics 84: 151–161.
61. Wacholder S, Silverman DT, McLaughlin JK, Mandel JS (1992) Selection of controls in case-control studies. III. Design options. Am J Epidemiol 135: 1042–1050.
62. Howard CM, Handzel T, Hill VR, Grytdal SP, Blanton C, et al. (2010) Novel risk factors associated with hepatitis E virus infection in a large outbreak in northern Uganda: results from a case-control study and environmental analysis. Am J Trop Med Hyg 83: 1170–1173.
63. WHO-UNICEF (2012) Progress on Drinking Water and Sanitation: 2012 Update. Geneva: World Health Organization.
64. Day NE, Byar DP, Green SB (1980) Overadjustment in case-control studies. Am J Epidemiol 112: 696–706.
65. Breslow NE, Day NE, Cancer IAfRo (1980) Statistical methods in cancer research. vol. 1: The analysis of case-control studies.
66. Levine MM, Robins-Browne RM (2012) Factors that explain excretion of enteric pathogens by persons without diarrhea. Clinical infectious diseases : an official publication of the Infectious Diseases Society of America 55 Suppl 4: S303–311.
67. VanDerslice J, Briscoe J (1993) All coliforms are not created equal: A comparison of the effects of water source and in-house water contamination on infantile diarrheal disease. Water Resources Research 29: 1983–1995.
68. Black RE, Merson MH, Rowe B, Taylor PR, Alim AA, et al. (1981) Enterotoxigenic *Escherichia coli* diarrhoea: acquired immunity and transmission in an endemic area. Bulletin of the World Health Organization 59: 263.
69. Valentiner-Branth P, Steinsland H, Fischer TK, Perch M, Scheutz F, et al. (2003) Cohort study of Guinean children: incidence, pathogenicity, conferred protection, and attributable risk for enteropathogens during the first 2 years of life. J Clin Microbiol 41: 4238–4245.
70. Howard G, Bartram J (2003) Domestic water quantity, service level, and health. Geneva: World Health Organization.
71. Thompson J (2001) Drawers of Water II: 30 years of change in domestic water use & environmental health in east Africa. Summary. Iied.
72. Kremer M, Leino J, Miguel E, Zwane AP (2011) Spring cleaning: Rural water impacts, valuation, and property rights institutions*. The Quarterly Journal of Economics 126: 145–205.
73. Gasana J, Morin J, Ndikuyeze A, Kamoso P (2002) Impact of water supply and sanitation on diarrheal morbidity among young children in the socioeconomic and cultural context of Rwanda (Africa). Environ Res 90: 76–88.
74. Brown J, Hien VT, McMahan L, Jenkins MW, Thie L, et al. (2012) Relative benefits of on-plot water supply over other 'improved' sources in rural Vietnam. Trop Med Int Health 18: 65–74.
75. Haas CN, Rose JB, Gerba C, Regli S (1993) Risk assessment of virus in drinking water. Risk Anal 13: 545–552.
76. Kotloff KL, Nataro JP, Blackwelder WC, Nasrin D, Farag TH, et al. (2013) Burden and aetiology of diarrhoeal disease in infants and young children in developing countries (the Global Enteric Multicenter Study, GEMS): a prospective, case-control study. The Lancet.
77. Curtis V, Cousens S, Mertens T, Traore E, Kanki B, et al. (1993) Structured observations of hygiene behaviours in Burkina Faso: validity, variability, and utility. Bull World Health Organ 71: 23–32.

5

Levofloxacin-Based First-Line Therapy versus Standard First-Line Therapy for *Helicobacter pylori* Eradication: Meta-Analysis of Randomized Controlled Trials

Musthafa Chalikandy Peedikayil[1]*, Fahad Ibrahim AlSohaibani[1], Abdullah Hamad Alkhenizan[2]

1 Department of Medicine, King Faisal Specialist Hospital & Research Center, Riyadh, Kingdom of Saudi Arabia, **2** Department of Family Medicine & Polyclinics, King Faisal Specialist Hospital & Research Center, Riyadh, Kingdom of Saudi Arabia

Abstract

Background: First-line levofloxacin-based treatments eradicate *Helicobacter pylori* with varying success. We examined the efficacy and safety of first-line levofloxacin-based treatment in comparison to standard first-line therapy for *H pylori* eradication.

Materials and Methods: We searched literature databases from Medline, EMBASE, and the Cochrane Register of Randomized Controlled Trials through March 2013 for randomized controlled trials comparing first-line levofloxacin and standard therapy. We included randomized controlled trials conducted only on naïve *H pylori* infected patients in adults. A systematic review was conducted. Meta-analysis was performed with Review Manager 5.2. Treatment effect was determined by relative risk with a random or fixed model by the Mantel-Haenszel method.

Results: Seven trials were identified with 888 patients receiving 7 days of first-line levofloxacin and 894 treated with standard therapy (Amoxicillin, Clarithromycin and proton pump inhibitor) for 7 days. The overall crude eradication rate in the Levofloxacin group was 79.05% versus 81.4% in the standard group (risk ratio 0.97; 95% CI; 0.93, 1.02). The overall dropout was 46 (5.2%) in the levofloxacin group and 52 (5.8%) for standard therapy. The dizziness was more common among group who took Levofloxacin based treatment and taste disturbance was more common among group who took standard therapy. Meta-analysis of overall adverse events were similar between the two groups with a relative risk of 1.06 (95% CI 0.72, 1.57).

Conclusion: *Helicobacter pylori* eradication with 7 days of Levofloxacin-based first line therapy was safe and equal compared to 7 days of standard first-line therapy.

Editor: Antony Bayer, Cardiff University, United Kingdom

Funding: The authors have no funding or support to report.

Competing Interests: The authors have declared that no competing interests exist.

* E-mail: musthafacpdr@gmail.com

Introduction

Helicobacter pylori infection is one of the most common chronic human bacterial infections. The consequences of infection are chronic gastritis, gastric and duodenal ulcers, gastric cancer, and primary gastric lymphoma of mucosa-associated lymphoid tissue type (MALT lymphoma) [1]. Eradication of *H pylori* may cure dyspepsia [2], peptic ulcer disease, and MALT lymphoma [3].

Various consensus groups, including the group at the Maastricht consensus meeting [2], recommended a triple-therapy regimen containing a proton pump inhibitor (PPI), clarithromycin, and either amoxicillin or metronidazole as first-line treatment for the eradication of *H pylori* [2]. However, recent reports indicate that these regimens achieve only about a 70% eradication rate [4–5]. The most important cause for the reduced success of standard triple therapy is the increasing rate of *H pylori* clarithromycin/metronidazole resistance [6].

There have not been any new drugs recently developed to treat *H pylori*. Thus, many investigators have examined various combinations of antibiotics or sequential therapies to improve the eradication rate. Many studies have investigated levofloxacin-based regimens as second-line treatments, including meta-analyses [7]. The 2012 Maastricht consensus guideline recommends the levofloxacin-PPI containing regimen for patients who have failed standard first-line treatment [2]. Many studies have examined levofloxacin-PPI as a first-line therapy for eradication of *H pylori* infection [8–10]. However, the eradication rates achieved with first-line levofloxacin-based treatments are not uniform. Some reports show improved efficacy with levofloxacin-based regimens in comparison to standard first-line therapy, whereas others have found equivalent or poorer responses [9,11–12].

Conclusive data regarding the role of levofloxacin-based first-line therapy for *H pylori* eradication does not currently exist. A meta-analysis may provide meaningful answers to this question. Thus, a systematic review and meta-analysis was conducted. First objective was to do a meta-analysis of data from all of the available randomized, controlled trials that compared 7 days of Levoflox-

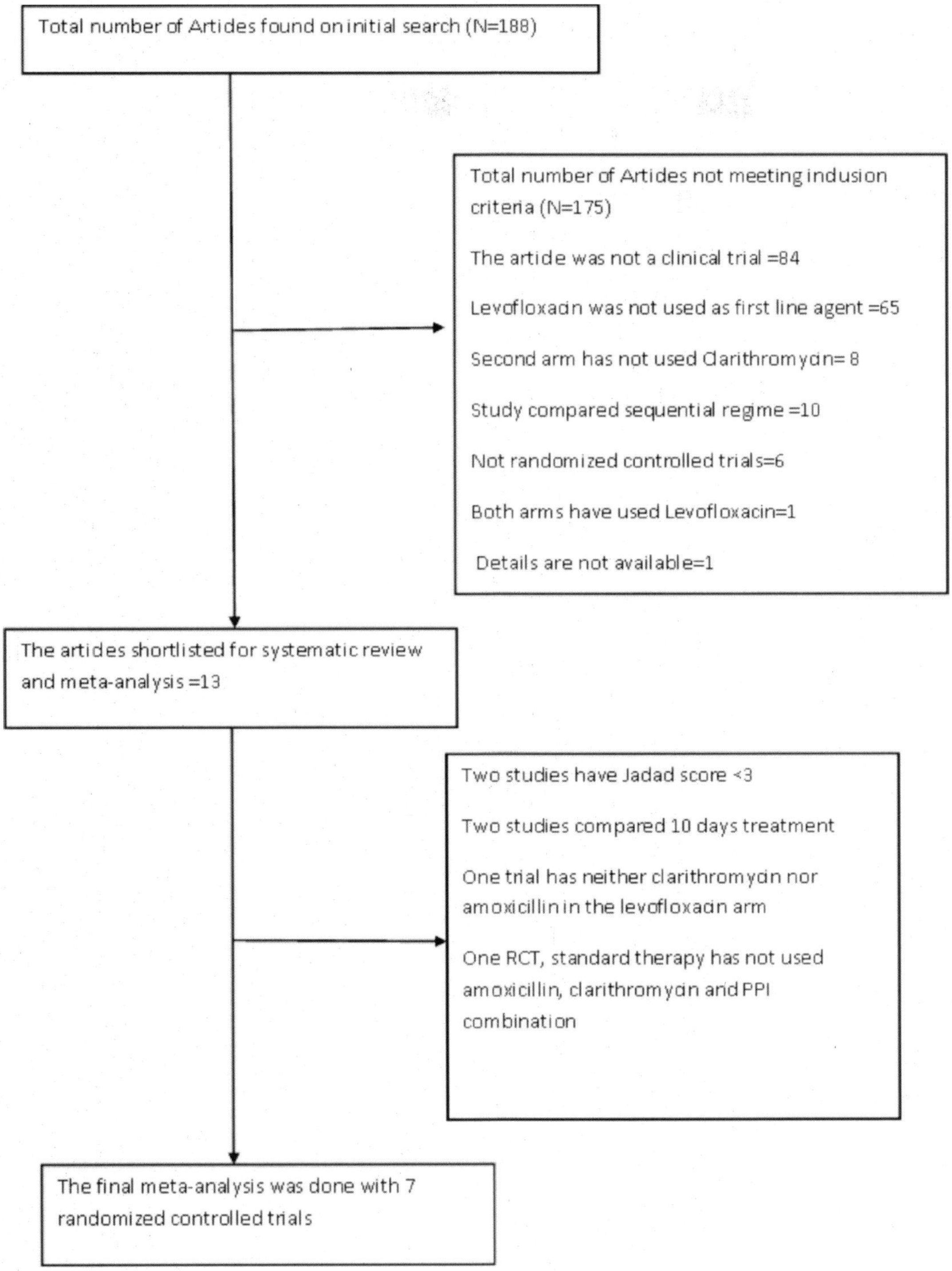

Figure 1. Flow chart showing study selection.

acin based treatment to 7 days of Amoxicillin, Clarithromycin and PPI as first line treatment for *H pylori* eradication. The second objective was to perform a meta-analysis of adverse effects of levofloxacin-based first-line therapy versus standard first-line therapy.

Materials and Methods

Selection of studies

A particular trial was included in the meta-analysis if it satisfied following. (1) The study must have been a randomized, controlled trial. (2) The presence of *H pylori* infection before and after treatment must be confirmed by one or more diagnostic methods.

Table 1. Quality assessment of selected studies.

Author	Randomization	Concealment of allocation	Blinding	Adequacy of blinding	Drop out described	Jadad score
Assem M	Yes	Yes	Open label	N D	Yes	3
Chen LW	Yes	Yes	Open label	N D	Yes	3
Choi KH	Yes	Yes	Double Blind	Adequate	Yes	5
Hung IF	Yes	Yes	Open label	N D	Yes	3
Iacopini F	Yes	Yes	Open label	N D	Yes	3
Liou JM	Yes	Yes	N D	N D	Yes	3
Nista EC	Yes	Yes	Open label	N D	Yes	3

ND = Not described.

(3) The subjects must have been at least 18 years old. (4) The patients were naïve to *H pylori* eradication treatment. (5) One group was treated with standard first-line therapy containing a minimum of two antibiotics and one PPI (amoxicillin, clarithromycin, with a PPI). (6) The levofloxacin-based treatment group was treated with a minimum of two antibiotics, including levofloxacin, and one PPI. Randomized, controlled trials (RCTs) with more than two treatment groups were selected if two of the treatment groups satisfied the inclusion and exclusion criteria. Studies or articles were excluded if sequential therapy was the only treatment regimen, levofloxacin was included in all of the treatment groups, studies included known antibiotic susceptibility tests, manuscripts were review articles, *H pylori* eradication therapy was provided for treatment failures, or if data were incomplete.

Literature search

Medline, EMBASE, and the Cochrane Register of Randomized Controlled Trials were searched for relevant studies. In addition, a manual search was performed on the references of relevant published articles. The literature search was performed without any restrictions on language. The Medline search was performed with the keywords levofloxacin and *Helicobacter pylori* and included articles from 1956–March 2013. The Cochrane library was searched for articles with the keywords levofloxacin, *Helicobacter pylori*, and randomization. Each title and abstract was read, and potential articles were recorded on a short list. All of the articles on the short list were downloaded or purchased. EndNote version X3 (Thomson Reuters) was used at various stages for collecting, storing, and finding duplicate references. Duplicates were identified and removed.

Data extraction

Each researcher independently collected data in a predefined data extraction form. Any difference of opinion between researchers was resolved to reach a consensus. The following data were collected from each paper: year of publication, institution, study design, quality of the study, tests performed to confirm the diagnosis and eradication, gender, age, medications in each arm, drop outs, and adverse events. Additional data regarding medications were collected and included the drug name, dose, frequency of treatment, and duration of treatment. Eradication rates expressed in the trials as intention to treat analysis were used.

Quality assessment

Each investigator independently assessed the quality of the studies by using the Jadad-Score. This score was entered into the predefined data extraction form. The following quality indicators were assessed: randomization (generation of allocation sequence), allocation of concealment, blinding, description of dropouts, and description of loss of follow-up. The maximum score was five. A higher score represented a higher quality paper. In this meta-analysis, studies with scores of three and above were included in the final meta-analysis.

Statistical analysis

Data were independently extracted by the same reviewer and cross-checked. Discrepancies were resolved by discussion. Data synthesis was performed with the Cochrane Statistics package RevMan version 5.2. Relative risk (RR) and risk difference (RD) with 95% confidence intervals (CI) were reported. If there was a statistically significant RR, then the number needed to treat (NNT) was calculated. Heterogeneity was tested by the I^2 statistics method. A value greater than 50% indicated substantial heterogeneity. Potential causes of heterogeneous treatment effects were explored by pre-specified subgroup analysis. If statistically significant heterogeneity existed between studies, the weighted estimate of the typical treatment effect across trials (relative risk) was calculated with the random effects model to ensure robust results.

Results

Description of selected studies

The literature search was performed with predefined keywords through different search engines as described in the methods section. Our initial search revealed a total of 188 articles. Each abstract was reviewed to find suitable RCTs that satisfied the inclusion and exclusion criteria. Figure 1 shows the flow diagram of the process by which articles were selected. Finally, 13 RCTs met our predefined inclusion and exclusion criteria and were qualified for the meta-analysis [8–9,11–21]. From 13 RCTs, two of them [16,20] were excluded because of their Jadad score was <3, three of them [8,11,14], compared 10 days of levofloxacin based regimen to 10 days of standard therapy, and the study by Zullo et al [21] was excluded because the standard arm was unique and contained 7 days of Clarithromycin, Tinidazole, Bovine Lactoferrin and Rabeprazole. The quality of each RCT was based on the Jadad score (Table 1).

Several articles reporting results for levofloxacin-based first-line therapy for *H pylori* eradication were excluded. The RCTs by Cammarota et al. and Di Caro et al. were excluded, because all of the treatment groups included levofloxacin [22,23]. The RCT by Antos et al. was excluded, because the study included patients with

Table 2. Details of treatment effects, common adverse events, and drop outs for studies included in the meta-analysis.

Author	Medications	Duration of Rx (N)	Eradication (N)	Recruitment (N)	Eradication rate ITT (%)	Drop out (N)	Adverse events (N)	Adverse events	NNT	Relative risk reduction (95% CI)
Assem M [13] LEVO arm	AMOX 1 gm. BID; LEVO 500 mg BID; ESOM 20 mg BID.	7	127	150	84.7	4	120	Nausea, Diarrhea, Taste disturbance		
Assem M [13] STD Arm	AMOX 1 gm BID; CLAR 500 mg BID; ESOM 200 mg BID	7	118	150	78.6	5	132	Nausea, Diarrhea, Taste disturbance	16.7	7.1 (−3.5 to 16)
Chen LW [15] LEVO arm	CLAR 500 mg QD; LEVO 500 mg QD; ESO 40 mg QD	7	71	90	78.9	5	8	Taste disturbance		
Chen LW [15] STD arm	AMOX 1 gm BID; CLAR 500 mg BID; ESO 40 mg BID.	7	74	99	74.8	13	12	Taste disturbance, Skin rash	24.1	5.2 (−10.8 to 19)
Choi KH [17] LEVO arm	AMOX 1 gm BID; LEVO 200 mg BID; OMEP 20 mg BID.	7	64	98	65.3	11	72	Diarrhea, anorexia, nausea		
Choi KH [17] STD arm	AMOX 1 gm BID; CLAR 500 mg BID; OMEP 20 mg BID	7	77	99	77.8	9	111	Diarrhea, anorexia, nausea, taste disturbance	−8	−19 (−42 to 0.4)
Hung IF [9] LEVO arm	AMOX 1 gm BID; LEVO 500 mg QD; ESOM 20 BID.	7	128	150	85.3	0	31	Dizziness, diarrhea		
Hung IF [9] STD arm	AMOX 1 gm BID; CLAR 500 mg BID; ESOM 20 mg BID.	7	139	150	92.7	0	43	Diarrhea, taste disturbance	−13.6	−8.6 (−17.7 to −0.2)
Iacopini F [12] LEVO arm	AZIT 500 mg QD; LEVO 500 mg QD; ESOM 20 mg QD.	7	54	83	65	6	11	Taste disturbance, diarrhea		
Iacopini F [12] STD arm	AMOX 1 gm BID; CLAR 500 mg BID; ESOM 20 mg BID.	7	53	81	65	11	35	Taste disturbance, nausea, diarrhea	−2.68	−0.6 (−25.7 to 20)
Liou JM [18] LEVO arm	AMOX 1 gm BID; LEVO 750 mg QD; LANS 30 mg BID.	7	161	217	74.2	16	163	Diarrhea, dizziness, taste disturbance		
Liou JM [18] STD arm	AMOX 1 gm BID; CLAR 500 mg BID; LANS 30 mg BID.	7	180	215	83.7	9	128	Diarrhea, taste disturbance,	−10.5	−12.8 (−24.5 to −2.3)
Nista EC [19] LEVO arm	CLAR 500 mg BID; LEVO 500 mg QD; ESOM 20 mg BID.	7	87	100	87	4	51	Taste disturbance		
Nista EC [19] STD arm	AMOX 1 gm BID; CLAR 500 mg BID; ESOM 20 mg BID.	7	75	100	75	5	38	Diarrhea	8.3	13.8 (1.2 to 25)

Abbreviations
AMOX = Amoxicillin; LEVO = Levofloxacin; ESOM = Esomeprazole; CLAR = Clarithromycin; OMEP = Omeprazole; LANS = Lansoprazole; AZIT = Azithromycin.
Rx = treatment; BID = twice daily; QD = once daily; N = number; NNT = number needed to treat; ITT = intention to treat; LEVO arm = levofloxacin arm; STD arm = standard arm.
gm = gram; mg = milligram.

Study or Subgroup	Levofloxacin based triple Events	Levofloxacin based triple Total	Clarithromycin based trip Events	Clarithromycin based trip Total	Weight	Risk Ratio M-H, Fixed, 95% CI
Assem M 2010	136	150	118	150	16.3%	1.15 [1.05, 1.27]
Chen LW 2010	71	90	74	99	9.7%	1.06 [0.90, 1.23]
Choi KH 2011	64	98	77	99	10.6%	0.84 [0.70, 1.00]
Hung IF 2009	129	150	139	150	19.2%	0.93 [0.86, 1.00]
Iacopini F 2005	54	83	53	81	7.4%	0.99 [0.80, 1.24]
Liou JM 2010	161	217	180	215	24.9%	0.89 [0.80, 0.98]
Nista EC 2006	87	100	87	100	12.0%	1.00 [0.90, 1.11]
Total (95% CI)		**888**		**894**	**100.0%**	**0.97 [0.93, 1.02]**
Total events	702		728			

Heterogeneity: $Chi^2 = 20.35$, df = 6 (P = 0.002); $I^2 = 71\%$
Test for overall effect: Z = 1.28 (P = 0.20)

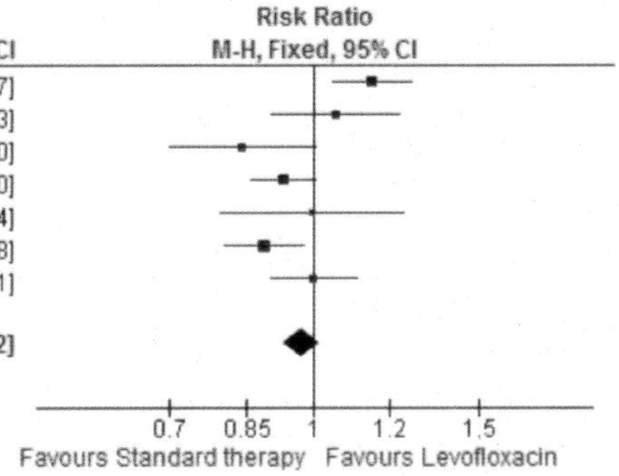

Figure 2. Forest plot showing the treatment effect of 7 randomized controlled trials. The crude eradication rate was similar between Levofloxacin based first line treatment and standard first line treatment for the eradication of *H pylori*.

one or more previous treatment failures [24]. The study by Schrauwen et al. was excluded, because it was not a randomized, controlled trial, and both groups were treated with levofloxacin. Finally, the study by Castro-Fernandez et al. was excluded, because the study was not a randomized, controlled trial [25].

The cumulative number of *H pylori*-infected patients enrolled in the 7 studies included in our meta-analysis was 1782, which included 888 who received levofloxacin-based first-line therapy and 894 treated with standard first-line therapy. The selected studies were from different countries. Two of the selected RCTs were from Italy; two studies were from Taiwan, one each from Hong King, Korea and one from Middle East (Saudi Arabia and Egypt).

All of the patients were older than 18 years. Further, none of the patients had received prior treatment for *H pylori* infection. All of the RCTs confirmed the diagnosis of *H pylori* infection by upper endoscopy with gastric biopsy and histology except for one study, which confirmed the diagnosis by Urea breath test. All researchers have confirmed Eradication of *H pylori* infection a urea breath test.

Five of the 7 RCTs included the combination of levofloxacin, amoxicillin, and a PPI as first-line therapy (levofloxacin arm) and two RCTs included levofloxacin, clarithromycin, and a PPI. All seven RCTs included standard therapy with amoxicillin, clarithromycin, and a PPI. Four studies had two treatment arms and other three RCTs had 3 treatment arms. Table 2 describes treatment effects, common adverse events, and drop outs of seven trials which are included in the meta-analysis.

Meta-analysis of seven trail's crude eradication rate was 79.05% versus 81.4% in the standard group and 79.5% in the levofloxacin-based first-line therapy. The difference in the crude eradication was not statistically significant with a relative risk of risk ratio of 0.97; 95% CI; 0.93, 1.02. Figure 2 shows the Forest plot of meta-analysis of 7 RCTs.

The heterogeneity of treatment effects in the meta-analysis was significant. Statistical analysis indicated that the I^2 statistics for the heterogeneity of the meta-analysis of seven RCTs were 71%.

The overall dropout was 46 (5.2%) in the levofloxacin group and 52 (5.8%) for standard therapy. The dizziness was more common among group who took Levofloxacin based treatment, and taste disturbance was more common among group who took standard therapy. Meta-analysis of overall adverse events were similar between the two groups with a relative risk of 1.06 (95% CI 0.72, 1.57). Figure 3 shows the Forest plot for the results of meta-analysis side effect with both treatment regimens.

The funnel plot (figure 4) of all seven included studies showed a symmetric pattern suggested that there are no publication biases.

Discussion

The most significant finding of this meta-analysis was that levofloxacin-based first-line therapy and standard therapy for previously untreated *H pylori*-infected patients achieved equivalent

Study or Subgroup	Levofloxacin Events	Levofloxacin Total	Standard Events	Standard Total	Weight	Risk Ratio M-H, Random, 95% CI
Abdominal Pain	26	888	33	894	10.4%	0.79 [0.48, 1.31]
Bloating	20	888	18	894	9.4%	1.12 [0.60, 2.10]
Constipation	9	888	12	894	7.8%	0.76 [0.32, 1.78]
Diarrhea	95	888	129	894	11.9%	0.74 [0.58, 0.95]
Dizziness	129	888	37	894	11.4%	3.51 [2.46, 5.00]
Headache	38	888	37	894	10.8%	1.03 [0.66, 1.61]
Nausea	75	888	73	894	11.6%	1.03 [0.76, 1.41]
Skin Problem	15	888	17	894	9.0%	0.89 [0.45, 1.77]
Taste Disturbance	68	888	119	894	11.8%	0.58 [0.43, 0.76]
Vomiting	10	888	4	894	6.0%	2.52 [0.79, 8.00]
Total (95% CI)		**8880**		**8940**	**100.0%**	**1.06 [0.72, 1.57]**
Total events	485		479			

Heterogeneity: $Tau^2 = 0.32$; $Chi^2 = 73.01$, df = 9 (P < 0.00001); $I^2 = 88\%$
Test for overall effect: Z = 0.29 (P = 0.77)

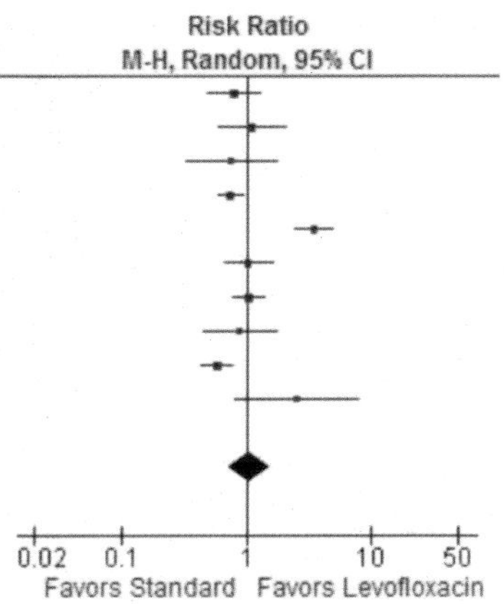

Figure 3. The Forest plot showing meta-analysis of common side-effects related to levofloxacin-based first line therapy, and standard first-line therapy. Overall side effects were equal for both levofloxacin and standard treatment.

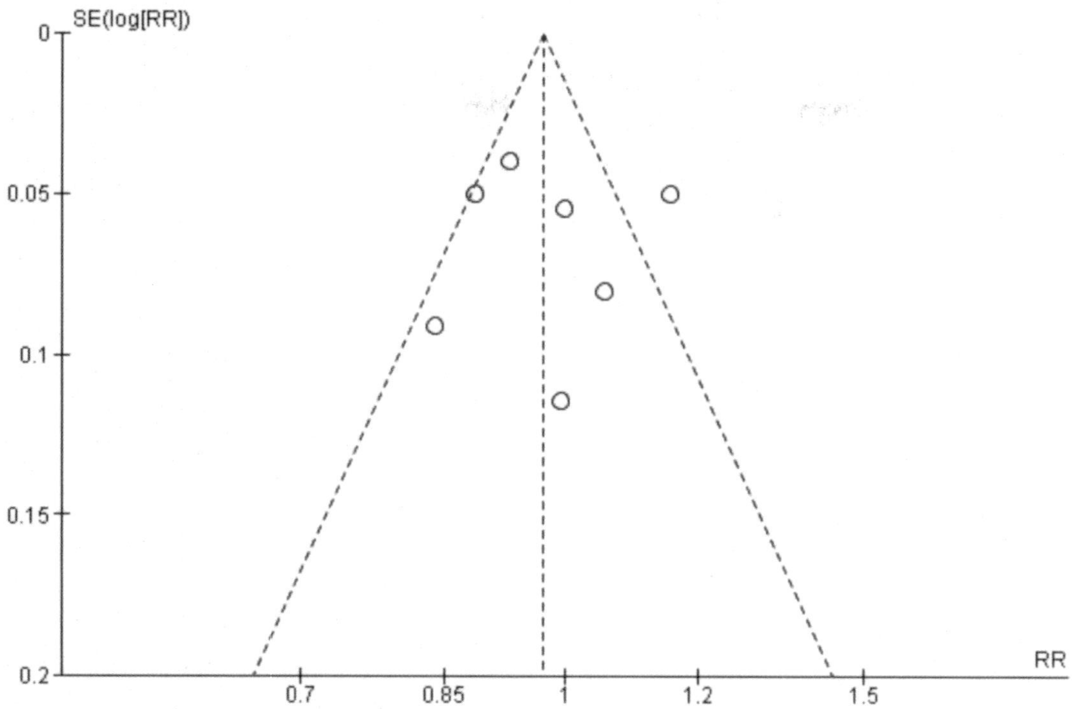

Figure 4. Funnel plot of included studies showing symmetrical distribution, and no publication bias.

outcomes. The overall eradication rates of the seven RCTs were 79.05% for levofloxacin-based regimens and 81.4% for standard therapy. The overall adverse events were similar between these two regimens.

Significant heterogeneity was observed in our meta-analysis. The obvious reasons for high heterogeneity were not evident. The main difference in the studies was in the study population. Otherwise duration of the treatment and medications used in the levofloxacin based first line therapy and standard therapy was more or less similar.

Since the year 2000, many investigators have published individual studies examining treatment of *H. pylori* with levofloxacin-based first-line therapy. The current meta-analysis included only randomized, controlled trials with predefined inclusion and exclusion criteria. Hence, we were forced to exclude many excellent studies from our meta-analysis. The *H. pylori* eradication rates in the excluded studies ranged from 75% to 96% with levofloxacin-based first-line therapy [22–23,25–26]. The results of these individual studies support the concept that the efficacy and safety of levofloxacin-based first-line therapy is equivalent to standard first-line therapy.

Prior to this meta-analysis, another meta-analysis was performed, in which Zhang et al [27] compared levofloxacin-based first-line therapy to standard therapy. The previous meta-analysis found that a PPI and levofloxacin-based triple therapy was more effective than standard triple therapy with a lower rate of adverse events compared to standard triple therapy. That article was published in the Chinese language in 2009, and only the abstract was available in the English language. Therefore, the details of the RCTs that were included in that meta-analysis were not available to us.

The recently updated guidelines by the Maastricht IV/Florence Consensus Report [2], the American College of Gastroenterology Guideline on the management of *H pylori* [28], and Second Asia–Pacific Consensus Guidelines for *H pylori* infection [29] recommend levofloxacin-based triple therapy as a second-line treatment for *H pylori* infections. Two meta-analyses support these recommendations. The levofloxacin-PPI-based regimen was successful in 81% of patients with previous eradication failures compared to 70% of patients who responded to quadruple therapy [30]. The second meta-analysis reviewed the levofloxacin-based triple salvage therapy (levofloxacin+amoxicillin+PPI), which was found to be superior to bismuth-based quadruple salvage therapy [31].

Should we recommend levofloxacin-based regimens as first-line therapies for *H pylori* eradication? Our current meta-analysis suggests that levofloxacin-based first-line treatment is as effective as standard therapy for *H pylori* eradication, and the adverse events and dropout rates are also equal. Noticeably, the overall eradication rates for *H pylori* with both levofloxacin-based regimens and standard therapy were around 80%.

The second reason for not recommending levofloxacin-based therapy as a first-line treatment modality for *H pylori* infection is the increasing incidence of levofloxacin-resistant *H pylori* strains from different parts of the world, especially countries in which quinolone consumption is high. Levofloxacin-resistant *H pylori* has been reported in the range of non-existent in Malaysia to 30.3% in China [32–33]. Levofloxacin resistance has been reported to be 11.7% [95% CI 6.5–20.3%)] in Ireland with much higher rates of resistance in subjects older than 45 years (19.1%) in comparison to those younger than 45 years (2.6%) [34]. *H pylori* resistance to levofloxacin was 5% in Poland and 5.3% in Iran [6,35]. An Italian study by Zullo et al. reported a levofloxacin resistance rate of 19.1% with higher resistance rates in older patients compared to younger patients (28.4% vs. 14.4%, $P = 0.048$) [36]. In Taiwan, the prevalence of levofloxacin resistance in *H pylori* isolates has increased from 3.2% in isolates collected before 2004 to 16.3% in isolates collected after 2004 [37].

Various studies indicate that resistance will reduce the efficacy of levofloxacin-based regimens in the eradication of *H pylori.* In Italy, the eradication rate decreased significantly from 75% in levofloxacin-susceptible patients to 33.3% in patients with levofloxacin-resistant strains [38]. A study from the U.S.A. suggests that levofloxacin resistance may be associated with prior quinolone exposure during the past 10 years [39].

There are some suggestions that levofloxacin-based first-line therapy may be used in areas where clarithromycin resistance is higher than 20%, along with levofloxacin resistance is below 10%. For patients who are allergic to penicillin, instead of Metronidazole-containing regimens, the levofloxacin based regime can be used as a first line therapy [40–41]. However, these regimens have not yet been compared in the first-line setting. Thus, further studies are needed to test this concept.

Although there are a few limitations to this meta-analysis, such as heterogeneity, there are numerous strengths. Levofloxacin-based first-line therapy has been included in clinical practice since the year 2000. However, a thorough meta-analysis investigating the role of levofloxacin in the eradication of *H pylori* has been lacking. Our meta-analysis was successful in identifying all of the important randomized, controlled trials with strict criteria and provided clear answers to various questions. To our knowledge, no other meta-analysis comparing first-line levofloxacin-based therapy to first-line standard therapy has been published in the English language.

Conclusions

This meta-analysis suggests that levofloxacin-based first-line therapy and standard therapy have equivalent efficacy and safety profiles for eradication of *H pylori*. There is not sufficient evidence to support replacement of the current standard first-line therapy with levofloxacin-based first-line therapy. Levofloxacin-based first-line therapy may be a valuable alternative for patients with penicillin allergies and in areas in which quinolone resistance is very low and clarithromycin resistance is very high. Each country should determine the prevalence of antibiotic resistance within their community before introducing new treatment regimens for *H pylori*.

Acknowledgments

Bioscience writers and Mrs Rehna Ruksana Musthafa for editing the manuscript. **Ethics:** Ethics committee of our institute has approved the research proposal. The systematic review and meta-analysis was conducted as per guidelines from the clinical guidelines by the Cochrane Collaboration, and followed by PRISMA systematic review guidelines and PRISMA checklist and flow diagrams.

Author Contributions

Conceived and designed the experiments: MCP. Performed the experiments: MCP. Analyzed the data: MCP FAS AHA. Wrote the paper: MCP.

References

1. Correa P (1997) Helicobacter pylori as a pathogen and carcinogen. J Physiol Pharmacol 48 Suppl 4:19–24.
2. Malfertheiner P, Megraud F, O'Morain CA, Atherton J, Axon ATR, et al (2012) Management of Helicobacter pylori infection–the Maastricht IV/Florence Consensus Report. Gut 61:646–64.
3. Bayerdorffer E, Neubauer A, Rudolph B, Thiede C, Lehn N, et al (1995) Regression of primary gastric lymphoma of mucosa-associated lymphoid tissue type after cure of Helicobacter pylori infection. MALT Lymphoma Study Group. Lancet 345:1591–4.
4. Jafri NS, Hornung CA, Howden CW (2008) Meta-analysis: sequential therapy appears superior to standard therapy for Helicobacter pylori infection in patients naive to treatment. Ann Intern Med 148:923–31.
5. Malfertheiner P, Megraud F, O'Morain C, Bazzoli F, El-Omar E, et al (1997) Current European concepts in the management of Helicobacter pylori infection–the Maastricht Consensus Report. The European Helicobacter Pylori Study Group (EHPSG). Eur J Gastroenterol Hepatol 9:1–2.
6. Karczewska E, Wojtas-Bonior I, Sito E, Zwolinska-Wcislo M, Budak A (2011) Primary and secondary clarithromycin, metronidazole, amoxicillin and levofloxacin resistance to Helicobacter pylori in southern Poland. Pharmacol Rep 63:799–807.
7. Li Y, Huang X, Yao L, Shi R, Zhang G (2010) Advantages of Moxifloxacin and Levofloxacin-based triple therapy for second-line treatments of persistent Helicobacter pylori infection: a meta analysis. Wien Klin Wochenschr 122:413–22.
8. Cuadrado-Lavin A, Salcines-Caviedes JR, Carrascosa MF, Dierssen-Sotos T, Cobo M, et al (2012) Levofloxacin versus clarithromycin in a 10 day triple therapy regimen for first-line Helicobacter pylori eradication: a single-blind randomized clinical trial. J Antimicrob Chemother 67:2254–9.
9. Hung IF, Chan P, Leung S, Chan FS, Hsu A, et al (2009) Clarithromycin-amoxycillin-containing triple therapy: a valid empirical first-line treatment for Helicobacter pylori eradication in Hong Kong? Helicobacter 14:505–11.
10. Molina-Infante J, Gisbert JP (2011) Levofloxacin in first-line eradication regimens for Helicobacter pylori: better test antibiotic susceptibility before treating. Gut 60:1605; author reply -6.
11. Molina-Infante J, Perez-Gallardo B, Fernandez-Bermejo M, Hernandez-Alonso M, Vinagre G, et al (2010) Clinical trial: clarithromycin vs. levofloxacin in first-line triple and sequential regimens for Helicobacter pylori eradication. Aliment Pharmacol Ther 31:1077–84.
12. Iacopini F, Crispino P, Paoluzi OA, Consolazio A, Pica R, et al (2005) One-week once-daily triple therapy with esomeprazole, levofloxacin and azithromycin compared to a standard therapy for Helicobacter pylori eradication. Dig Liver Dis 37:571–6.
13. Assem M, El Azab G, Rasheed MA, Abdelfatah M, Shastery M (2010) Efficacy and safety of Levofloxacin, Clarithromycin and Esomeprazol as first line triple therapy for Helicobacter pylori eradication in Middle East. Prospective, randomized, blind, comparative, multicenter study. Eur J Intern Med 21:310–4.
14. Basu PP, Rayapudi K, Pacana T, Shah NJ, Krishnaswamy N, et al (2011) A randomized study comparing levofloxacin, omeprazole, nitazoxanide, and doxycycline versus triple therapy for the eradication of Helicobacter pylori. Am J Gastroenterol 106:1970–5.
15. Chen LW, Chien RN, Chang JJ, Fang KM, Chang LC (2010) Comparison of the once-daily levofloxacin-containing triple therapy with the twice-daily standard triple therapy for first-line Helicobacter pylori eradication: a prospective randomised study. Int J Clin Pract 64:1530–4.
16. Cheng H, Hu FL, Zhang GX, Shi RH, Du YQ, et al (2010) [Levofloxacin-based triple therapy for first-line Helicobacter pylori eradication treatment: a multi-central, randomized, controlled clinical study]. Zhonghua Yi Xue Za Zhi 90:79–82.
17. Choi KH, Chung WC, Lee KM, Paik CN, Kim EJ, et al (2011) Efficacy of levofloxacin and rifaximin based quadruple therapy in Helicobacter pylori associated gastroduodenal disease: a double-blind, randomized controlled trial. J Korean Med Sci 26:785–90.
18. Liou JM, Lin JT, Chang CY, Chen MJ, Cheng TY, et al (2010) Levofloxacin-based and clarithromycin-based triple therapies as first-line and second-line treatments for Helicobacter pylori infection: a randomised comparative trial with crossover design. Gut 59:572–8.
19. Nista EC, Candelli M, Zocco MA, et al (2006) Levofloxacin-based triple therapy in first-line treatment for Helicobacter pylori eradication. Am J Gastroenterol 101:1985–90.
20. Rispo A, Di Girolamo E, Cozzolino A, Bozzi R, Morante A, et al (2007) Levofloxacin in first-line treatment of Helicobacter pylori infection. Helicobacter 12:364–5.
21. Zullo A, De Francesco V, Scaccianoce G, Manes G, Efrati C, et al (2007) Helicobacter pylori eradication with either quadruple regimen with lactoferrin or levofloxacin-based triple therapy: a multicentre study. Dig Liver Dis 39:806–10.
22. Cammarota G, Cianci R, Cannizzaro O, Cuoco L, Pirozzi G, et al (2000) Efficacy of two one-week rabeprazole/levofloxacin-based triple therapies for Helicobacter pylori infection. Aliment Pharmacol Ther 14:1339–43.
23. Di Caro S, Zocco MA, Cremonini F, et al (2002) Levofloxacin based regimens for the eradication of Helicobacter pylori. Eur J Gastroenterol Hepatol 14:1309–12.
24. Antos D, Schneider-Brachert W, Bastlein E, et al (2006) 7-day triple therapy of Helicobacter pylori infection with levofloxacin, amoxicillin, and high-dose esomeprazole in patients with known antimicrobial sensitivity. Helicobacter 11:39–45.
25. Castro-Fernandez M, Lamas E, Perez-Pastor A, et al (2009) Efficacy of triple therapy with a proton pump inhibitor, levofloxacin, and amoxicillin as first-line

treatment to eradicate Helicobacter pylori. Rev Esp Enferm Dig 101:395–8, 9–402.
26. Schrauwen RW, Janssen MJ, de Boer WA (2009) Seven-day PPI-triple therapy with levofloxacin is very effective for Helicobacter pylori eradication. Neth J Med 67:96–101.
27. Zhang ZF, Zhao G, Liu LN (2008) [Effectiveness and safety of proton pump inhibitor and levofloxacin based first-line triple therapy in the eradication of Helicobacter pylori: a meta-analysis]. Zhonghua Yi Xue Za Zhi 88:2722–5.
28. Chey WD, Wong BC (2007) American College of Gastroenterology guideline on the management of Helicobacter pylori infection. Am J Gastroenterol 102:1808–25.
29. Fock KM, Katelaris P, Sugano K, Ang TL, Hunt R, et al (2009) Second Asia-Pacific Consensus Guidelines for Helicobacter pylori infection. J Gastroenterol Hepatol 24:1587–600.
30. Gisbert JP, Morena F (2006) Systematic review and meta-analysis: levofloxacin-based rescue regimens after Helicobacter pylori treatment failure. Aliment Pharmacol Ther 23:35–44.
31. Saad RJ, Schoenfeld P, Kim HM, Chey WD (2006) Levofloxacin-based triple therapy versus bismuth-based quadruple therapy for persistent Helicobacter pylori infection: a meta-analysis. Am J Gastroenterol 101:488–96.
32. Goh KL, Navaratnam P (2011) High Helicobacter pylori resistance to metronidazole but zero or low resistance to clarithromycin, levofloxacin, and other antibiotics in Malaysia. Helicobacter 16:241–5.
33. Liao J, Zheng Q, Liang X, Zhang W, Sun Q, et al (2013) Effect of Fluoroquinolone Resistance on 14-day Levofloxacin Triple and Triple Plus Bismuth Quadruple Therapy. Helicobacter 18(5):373–7.
34. O'Connor A, Taneike I, Nami A, Fitzgerald N, Ryan B, et al (2013) Helicobacter pylori resistance rates for levofloxacin, tetracycline and rifabutin among Irish isolates at a reference centre. Ir J Med Sci 182(4):693–5.
35. Talebi Bezmin Abadi A, Ghasemzadeh A, Taghvaei T, Mobarez AM (2012) Primary resistance of Helicobacter pylori to levofloxacin and moxifloxacine in Iran. Intern Emerg Med 7:447–52.
36. Zullo A, Perna F, Hassan C, Ricci C, Saracino I, et al (2007) Primary antibiotic resistance in Helicobacter pylori strains isolated in northern and central Italy. Aliment Pharmacol Ther 25:1429–34.
37. Chang WL, Sheu BS, Cheng HC, Yang YJ, Yang HB, et al (2009) Resistance to metronidazole, clarithromycin and levofloxacin of Helicobacter pylori before and after clarithromycin-based therapy in Taiwan. J Gastroenterol Hepatol 24:1230–5.
38. Perna F, Zullo A, Ricci C, Hassan C, Morini S, et al (2007) Levofloxacin-based triple therapy for Helicobacter pylori re-treatment: role of bacterial resistance. Dig Liver Dis 39:1001–5.
39. Carothers JJ, Bruce MG, Hennessy TW, et al (2007) The relationship between previous fluoroquinolone use and levofloxacin resistance in Helicobacter pylori infection. Clin Infect Dis 44:e5–8.
40. Gisbert JP, Pajares R, Pajares JM (2007) Evolution of Helicobacter pylori therapy from a meta-analytical perspective. Helicobacter 12 Suppl 2:50–8.
41. Gisbert JP, Perez-Aisa A, Castro-Fernandez M, Barrio J, Rodrigo L, et al (2010) Helicobacter pylori first-line treatment and rescue option containing levofloxacin in patients allergic to penicillin. Dig Liver Dis 42:287–90.

6

Anti-Allergic Role of Cholinergic Neuronal Pathway via α7 Nicotinic ACh Receptors on Mucosal Mast Cells in a Murine Food Allergy Model

Takeshi Yamamoto[1], Toshihisa Kodama[1], Jaemin Lee[1], Naho Utsunomiya[1], Shusaku Hayashi[1], Hiroshi Sakamoto[2], Hirofumi Kuramoto[3], Makoto Kadowaki[1]*

1 Division of Gastrointestinal Pathophysiology, Institute of Natural Medicine, University of Toyama, Toyama, Toyama, Japan, **2** Department of Physical Therapy, Health Science University, Fujikawaguchiko, Yamanashi, Japan, **3** Department of Applied Biology, Kyoto Institute of Technology, Kyoto, Kyoto, Japan

Abstract

The prevalence of food allergy (FA) has increased in developed countries over the past few decades. However, no effective drug therapies are currently available. Therefore, we investigated cholinergic anti-inflammatory pathway as a regulatory system to ameliorate disrupted mucosal immune homeostasis in the gut based on the pathophysiological elucidation of mucosal mast cells (MMCs) in a murine FA model. BALB/c mice sensitized with ovalbumin received repeated oral ovalbumin for the development of FA. FA mice developed severe allergic diarrhea and exhibited enhanced type 2 helper T (Th2) cell immune responses in both systemic immunity and mucosal immunity, along with MMCs hyperplasia in the colon. MMCs were localized primarily in the strategic position of the mucosal epithelium. Furthermore, the allergic symptoms did not develop in p85α disrupted phosphoinositide-3 kinase-deficient mice that lacked mast cells in the gut. Vagal stimulation by 2-deoxy-D-glucose and drug treatment with nicotinic ACh receptor (nAChR) agonists (nicotine and α7 nAChR agonist GTS-21) alleviated the allergic symptoms in the FA mice. Nicotine treatment suppressed MMCs hyperplasia, enhanced MPO and upregulated mRNA expression of Th1 and Th2 cytokines in the FA mice colon. MMCs, which are negatively regulated by α7 nAChRs, were often located in close proximity to cholinergic CGRP-immunoreactive nerve fibers in the FA mice colon. The present results reveal that the cholinergic neuroimmune interaction via α7 nAChRs on MMCs is largely involved in maintaining intestinal immune homeostasis and can be a target for a new therapy against mucosal immune diseases with homeostatic disturbances such as FA.

Editor: Kenji Hashimoto, Chiba University Center for Forensic Mental Health, Japan

Funding: This research was supported by a Grant-in-Aid for Scientific Research from the Ministry of Education, Culture, Sports, Science and Technology of Japan (http://www.jsps.go.jp/j-grantsinaid/index.html) to T. Yamamoto (No. 25460891) and M. Kadowaki (No. 24590879). The funders had no role in study design, data collection and analysis, decision to publish, or preparation of the manuscript.

Competing Interests: The authors have declared that no competing interests exist.

* E-mail: makotok@inm.u-toyama.ac.jp

Introduction

Food allergy (FA) is an abnormal immunologic reaction to food proteins, and its prevalence has increased in developed countries over the past few decades. However, the pathogenic mechanisms underlying FA are not fully understood, and no effective drug therapies are yet available. The only way to avoid allergic reactions to food is to avoid the foods that trigger these responses [1].

It is well known that type 2 helper T (Th2) cell-biased immune responses are responsible for allergic diseases. There is a growing body of work that has examined the interaction between T cells and mast cells and how these relationships might alter immunity to foreign antigens [2]. Th2 cell-associated cytokines, such as IL-4, IL-5, IL-9 and IL-13, are involved in B cell class switching to IgE and in the differentiation and maturation of mast cells and Th2 cells [3,4,5].

In the pathological Th2 cell-biased immunological environment, mast cells are usually positioned close to the external environment to respond to the pathogens, and mast cells play a central role as an effector cell and a conductor cell in the pathogenesis of various allergic diseases [5,6]. The activation of mast cells results in the release of various inflammatory mediators, such as proteases, eicosanoids, biogenic amines, cytokines and chemokines [2]. Despite their strategic location in the mucosa of the intestinal microenvironment, the role of mast cells in FA has not been well investigated.

We previously demonstrated that the number of mucosal mast cells (MMCs) is greatly increased in the colonic mucosa of ovalbumin (OVA)-induced FA mice [7]. Mast cells are classified as MMCs or connective tissue mast cells (CTMCs). Considerable evidence has demonstrated that MMCs are morphologically, biochemically and functionally distinct from CTMCs [2]. CTMCs reside in connective tissues, such as the skin, whereas MMC progenitors migrate to intestinal or bronchial mucosal tissues, where MMCs are able to mature following antigen exposure. CTMCs contain high concentrations of histamine in their granules and mainly contribute to allergic symptoms, such as congestion, itch, urticaria and anaphylaxis, whereas MMCs contain low concentrations of histamine [8]. Consequently, anti-histamine agents have no effect on FA. Furthermore, CTMC stabilizers (e.g., tranilast, ketotifen, and cromolyn) are frequently used for the treatment of various allergic disorders, while these stabilizers fail to exert therapeutic effects on FA, which is supported by our finding that these stabilizers are not able to suppress MMC activation [9].

Recent advances in neuroscience and immunology have revealed a bidirectional interaction between the nervous and immune systems. Therefore, the function of the intestine may be modulated by neuro-immune interactions, but this interaction is not fully understood. Mast cells are ubiquitous in the body, and these cells are often found in close proximity to nerve fibers in various tissues, including the lamina propria of the intestine [3,4,10,11]. Mast cells and nerves are assumed to communicate bilaterally to modulate neuro-physiological effects and mast cell functions [12], which suggests that the neuro-immune interaction may be involved in the pathology of allergic diseases.

Until now, findings on the cholinergic regulation of immune responses have been accumulated in various inflammatory experimental models [13,14,15,16], while there has been little information obtained on the cholinergic control in allergic models, especially in FA models. We have already shown that nicotine exerts an inhibitory effect on antigen-induced degranulation in mucosal-type murine bone marrow-derived mast cells (mBMMCs) through α7 nicotinic ACh receptors (nAChRs), which is reversed by the α7 nAChR antagonist methyllycaconitine [17].

Therefore, an elucidation of the cholinergic regulatory pathway has provided new concepts in understanding and treating FA.

Materials and Methods

Ethics statement

This study was carried out in strict accordance with the recommendations in the Guide for the Care and Use of Laboratory Animals of the National Institutes of Health. The Animal Experiment Committee at the University of Toyama approved all of the animal care procedures and experiments (authorization no. S-2009 INM-9).

Animals

Male BALB/c mice, C57BL/6 mice and BALB/c nude (nu/nu) mice (5 weeks old) were purchased from Japan SLC (Shizuoka, Japan). BALB/c background p85α subunit-disrupted class Ia phosphoinositide-3 kinase (PI3K)-deficient ($PI3K^{-/-}$) mice were gifted from Drs. Shigeo Koyasu (Keio University, Tokyo, Japan) and Takashi Kadowaki (the University of Tokyo, Tokyo, Japan). All mice were housed in the experimental animal facility at the University of Toyama and were provided free access to food and water.

Induction of food allergy

The murine model of FA was initiated as described previously.8 Briefly, male BALB/c mice (5 weeks old) were sensitized twice at 2-week intervals using an intraperitoneal injection of 50 µg OVA (fraction V; Sigma-Aldrich, St. Louis, MO) in the presence of 1.3 mg/100 µl aluminium hydroxide gel adjuvant (Sigma-Aldrich). Two weeks after systemic priming, the mice received repeated oral administrations of 50 mg/0.3 ml OVA every other day. Diarrhea resulting from FA was assessed by visual monitoring for up to 1 hour following oral challenge. Profuse liquid stool was detected as allergic diarrhea, and the diarrhea-presenting mice were considered to be FA mice.

For the pharmacological evaluation of an activation of nicotinic AChRs (nAChRs) in the FA model, a non-selective nAChR agonist nicotine (Sigma-Aldrich) or a selective α7 nAChR agonist GTS-21 (10 mg/kg, Taiho, Tokushima, Japan) was subcutaneously administered to mice 1 hour before the oral OVA challenges. A central vagal stimulant 2-deoxy-D-glucose (2-DG, 200 mg/kg, Sigma-Aldrich) was intraperitoneally administered 30 minutes before OVA challenges. Furthermore, hexamethonium (C6, 100 mg/kg, Sigma-Aldrich) as a non-selective nAChR antagonist was intraperitoneally administered 30 minutes before 2-DG administration. A CTMC stabilizer disodium cromoglycate (cromolyn, 100 mg/g, Sigma-Aldrich), a CTMC and MMC stabilizer doxantrazole (10 mg/kg, Sigma-Aldrich) or an anti-inflammatory drug prednisolone (10 mg/kg, Sigma-Aldrich) was administered 1 hour before OVA challenges.

One hour after the 6th oral OVA challenge, the proximal colon and spleen were used for morphological and biological analyses, and plasma was for measurement of OVA-specific IgE and mouse mast cell protease (mMCP)-1 (a marker of mouse MMCs) levels. Plasma OVA-specific IgE level was measured using an ELISA kit (DS Pharma Biomedical, Osaka, Japan). Plasma mMCP-1 level was measured using an ELISA kit (Moredun Scientific). These measurements were performed according to the manufacturers' instructions.

Measurement of myeloperoxidase activity

One hour after the 6th oral OVA challenge, the entire colon of each mouse was excised. Each colon was weighed and cut into small pieces. The colon was homogenized on ice in 1 ml of 0.5% hexadecyltrimethylammonium bromide in 50 mM potassium phosphate buffer (pH 6.0) using a Polytron homogenizer (Kinematica, Littau, Switzerland) and fortified with an additional quantity of the same buffer to 100 mg of the colon in 1 ml. The homogenate was frozen and thawed three times and then was vortex-mixed. The suspension was centrifuged at 15,000×*g* for 20 minutes at 4°C. Myeloperoxidase (MPO) activity of the resulting supernatant was measured. The supernatant (100 µl) was vortex-mixed with 2.87 ml of 0.5 mM *o*-dianisidine in 50 mM potassium phosphate buffer (pH 6.0) and 30 µl of 0.05% hydrogen peroxide. The mixture was measured spectrophotometrically at 460 nm for 4 minutes of incubation. MPO activity is expressed as units per wet weight of the colon in grams (gwwt).

Expression of cytokine mRNA

One hour after the 6th oral OVA challenge, 2 cm of the proximal colon and spleen were excised. Total RNA was extracted from the tissues using Sepasol Super (Nacalai Tesque, Kyoto, Japan) according to the manufacturer's instructions. Reverse transcription was performed using the Exscript RT reagent kit (Takara Bio, Ohtsu, Japan) and random primers, followed by real-time PCR. Real-time PCR amplification of IL-4, IL-5, IFN-γ and GAPDH was performed using SYBR Premix Ex Taq (Takara Bio). The following primer pairs were used:

IL-4, forward 5′-GGTCTCAACCCCCAGCTAGT-3′ and reverse 5′-GCCGATGATCTCTCTCAAGTGAT-3′;

IL-5, forward 5′-GAAGTGTGGCGAGGAGAGAC-3′ and reverse 5′-GCACAGTTTTGTGGGGTTTT-3′;

IFN-γ, forward 5′-CGGCACAGTCATTGAAAGCCTA-3′ and reverse 5′-GTTGCTGATGGCCTGATTGTC-3′;

GAPDH, forward 5′-TGACCACAGTCCATGCCATC-3′ and reverse 5′-GACGGACACATTGGGGGTAG-3′.

The PCR reaction conditions consisted of 10 seconds at 95°C followed by 40 cycles of 5 seconds at 95°C and 20 seconds at 63°C. Target mRNA levels were normalized to those of GAPDH as an internal control in each sample. The results are expressed as the ratio relative to the naïve group average.

Morphological analysis

One hour after the 6th oral OVA challenge, the proximal colon was excised. The proximal colon was fixed with 4% paraformaldehyde (w/v) in 0.1 M sodium phosphate buffer (PB; pH 7.3) and immersed for 12–18 hours at 4°C. The tissue was washed with 0.01 M phosphate-buffered saline (PBS; pH 7.3), cryoprotected with 30% sucrose in 0.01 M PBS and embedded in OCT compound. Frozen sections (25 μm) were cut at −20°C using a cryostat microtome (Leica Microsystems, Nussloch, Germany). The sections were soaked for 12–18 hours in 0.01 M PBS containing 0.3% Triton X-100 to increase permeability, and they were then exposed to normal donkey serum (1:10; Jackson Immunoresearch Laboratories, West Grove, PA) for 30 minutes to reduce the nonspecific binding of antisera and washed in 0.01 M PBS. The sections were exposed to each primary antibody for 12–18 hours, washed with 0.01 M PBS and incubated with the appropriate secondary antibody for 2 hours. All incubations were performed at room temperature. The following primary antibodies were used: goat anti-choline acetyltransferase (ChAT) (1:200; Chemicon, Temecula, CA), sheep anti-mouse mast cell protease (mMCP)-1 (1:5,000; Moredun Scientific, Midlothian, UK) and rabbit anti- CGRP (1:10,000; Chemicon). Cy3-conjugated donkey anti-sheep IgG (1:200; Jackson Immunoresearch Laboratories, West Grove, PA) and Alexa 488-conjugated donkey anti-rabbit IgG (1:200; Jackson Immunoresearch Laboratories) were used as secondary antibodies. The preparations were examined using a fluorescence microscope (IX71 system; Olympus, Tokyo, Japan) with a U-MWIG3 filter set (Olympus) and photographed using an Olympus digital camera (DP70; Olympus). The preparations were also observed using confocal laser-scanning microscopy (LSM700; Carl Zeiss, Oberkochen, Germany) to examine the proximity between mMCP-1-positive cells and CGRP-immunoreactive (IR) nerve fibers in the colonic mucosa of the FA mice. Stacks of confocal sections were three-dimensionally reconstructed and observed using Imaris software (Bitplane, Zurich, Switzerland). Surface rendering of each channel was performed in an optimal intensity threshold setting. The intensity threshold setting was optimized by visual comparison between the original and the three-dimensional rendered result.

Furthermore, a segment of the proximal colon was opened along the mesenteric border and fixed with 4% paraformaldehyde. The whole-mount preparation of longitudinal muscle with adherent enteric plexus was dissected from the proximal colon, and the aforementioned immunohistochemical procedures were performed to examine the ChAT and CGRP immunoreactivities in nerve cell bodies of the enteric neurons.

Sections (1 μm thick) of the fixed colon embedded in LR white resin (Sigma-Aldrich) were stained with 1% toluidine blue and observed with light microscopy for the analysis of mast cells.

The brightness and contrast of the images were modified using Adobe Photoshop Elements 2.0 (Adobe Systems, San Jose, CA).

Electron microscopy

For electron microscopy, the FA mice were perfusion-fixed with 2% paraformaldehyde and 2.5% glutaraldehyde in 0.1 M PB and the proximal colon was removed. The colon was transversely sectioned into 0.5–1.0 mm thick sections with a razor blade. The sections were post-fixed for 1 hour by 1% OsO_4 in 0.1 M PB, dehydrated in graded ethanol and embedded in EPON 812 (Shell Chemical, Houston, Tex). Ultrathin sections were cut using an LKB 2088-V ultramicrotome (LKB, Bromma, Sweden). The ultrathin sections were collected on copper grids, stained with lead citrate and uranyl acetate and examined with an electron microscope (H-7500, Hitachi, Tokyo, Japan).

Statistical analysis

The data are expressed as the means ±SE. The statistical comparisons were performed using Student's unpaired *t*-test, the chi-squared test and one-way repeated measures ANOVA followed by Tukey's HSD. A significant difference was defined as $P<0.05$.

Results

Induction of food allergy in mice

Repeated oral OVA challenges to systemically OVA primed mice produced FA associated with allergic diarrhea in Th2-prone BALB/c mice (FA mice, $n=5$–7), but not in Th1-prone C57BL/6 mice ($n=8$) (Figure 1A). The occurrence of allergic diarrhea reached about 80.0% after the 6th OVA challenge. However, repeated OVA challenges without systemic OVA priming did not induce allergic diarrhea in BALB/c mice ($n=5$) (Figure 1A).

The plasma level of OVA-specific IgE was elevated after the systemic OVA priming, and subsequent repeated oral OVA challenges caused a remarkable elevation of the OVA-specific IgE level (naïve mice 0.0±0.0 μg/ml, OVA primed mice

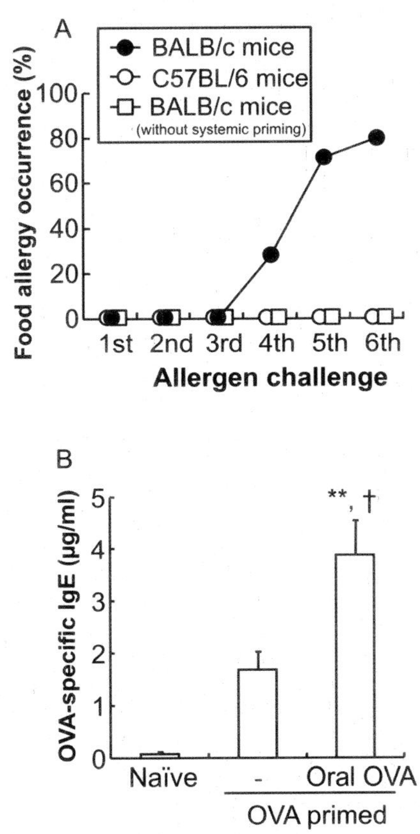

Figure 1. Induction of Th2-mediated food allergy. The allergic responses were induced by two instances of systemic OVA priming and repeated oral OVA (50 mg) challenges. *A*: Systemically primed BALB/c mice (closed circle) and C57BL/6 mice (open circle) and non-systemically primed BALB/c mice (open square) were subjected to food allergy (FA)-inducing oral OVA challenges ($n=5$–8 mice per group). *B*: The level of OVA-specific IgE in the plasma of naïve mice, systemically primed mice, and systemically primed and repeated oral OVA challenged mice is shown. The level of OVA-specific IgE in the plasma was determined using an ELISA kit. Data are expressed as means ±SE. $^{**}P<0.01$ vs. naïve mice. $^{\dagger}P<0.05$ vs. systemically primed mice ($n=5$ mice per group).

1.7±0.2 μg/ml, oral OVA challenged OVA primed mice 3.8±0.7 μg/ml; **$P<0.01$ vs. naïve mice, †$P<0.05$ vs. OVA primed mice; $n=5$ mice per group) (Figure 1B).

Systemic and mucosal immune responses in food allergy mice

The expression of Th1 and Th2 cytokine mRNA was measured using real-time PCR. In systemic immunity (spleen, Figure 2A), mRNA levels of Th2 cytokines (IL-4 and IL-5) were significantly increased in the FA mice (IL-4: naïve mice 1.0±0.2, FA mice 3.7±0.8, *$P<0.05$ vs. naïve mice; IL-5: naïve mice 1.0±0.4, FA mice 3.2±0.9, *$P<0.05$ vs. naïve mice; $n=5$–6 mice per group), whereas the Th1 cytokine (IFN-γ) mRNA level was significantly decreased in the FA mice (naïve mice 1.0±0.1, FA mice 0.5±0.1; **$P<0.01$ vs. naïve mice; $n=6$ mice per group). On the other hand, in mucosal immunity (proximal colon, Figure 2B), Th2 cytokine (IL-4 and IL-5) mRNA levels were significantly increased in the FA mice (IL-4: naïve mice 1.0±0.7, FA mice 2.9±0.6, *$P<$ 0.05 vs. naïve mice; IL-5: naïve mice 1.0±0.2, FA mice 11.3±1.4, **$P<0.01$ vs. naïve mice; $n=4$ mice per group), and the Th1 cytokine (IFN-γ) mRNA level exhibited a tendency to be increased in the FA mice (naïve mice 1.0±0.3, FA mice 2.4±0.8; $n=5$–8 mice per group).

Mucosal mast cell hyperplasia in the colon of food allergy mice

We investigated mucosal mast cells in the proximal colon by immunohistochemistry. As shown in Figure 3A, very few MMCs (mMCP-1-positive cells) were scattered in the lamina propria and submucosal layer of the mice colon two weeks after twice systemic OVA priming. The distribution of MMCs was similar to that in the proximal colon of the vehicle-treated control mice. MMCs began to occur in the mucosal epithelium of the primed mice proximal colon two days after the second oral OVA administration, and the number of MMCs was dramatically elevated in the mucosal epithelium of the primed mice colon in proportion to the OVA challenge time. MMCs were localized primarily in the mucosal epithelium of the upper half of the crypts throughout the primed mice colon two days after the fifth oral OVA administration.

To investigate the degranulation of mucosal mast cells, we measured the concentration of plasma mMCP-1 by ELISA (Figure 3B). There was no detectable plasma mMCP-1 in naïve mice. In contrast, the repeated OVA challenges resulted in a dramatic increase in the plasma mMCP-1 level (naïve mice 0.0±0.0 μg/ml, FA mice 29.0±8.0 μg/ml; **$P<0.01$ vs. naïve mice; $n=5$ mice per group).

Involvement of T cell in the development of food allergy in mice

In the FA mouse model, we used BALB/c nude mice that lack functional T cells due to their thymus deficiency. The nude mice did not exhibit any sign of allergic responses following exposure to

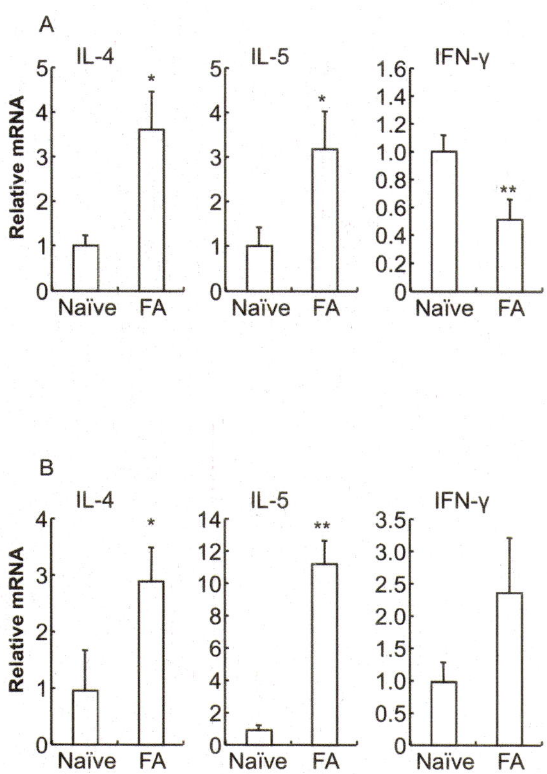

Figure 2. Induction of predominant Th2 cytokine responses in food allergy mice. IL-4, IL-5 and IFN-γ cytokine mRNA expression in the spleen (*A*) and proximal colon (*B*) from naïve mice and FA mice were measured by real-time PCR. Relative mRNA levels of cytokines were normalized to GAPDH expression. Data are expressed as means ±SE. *$P<0.05$, **$P<0.01$ vs. naïve mice ($n=4$–8 mice per group).

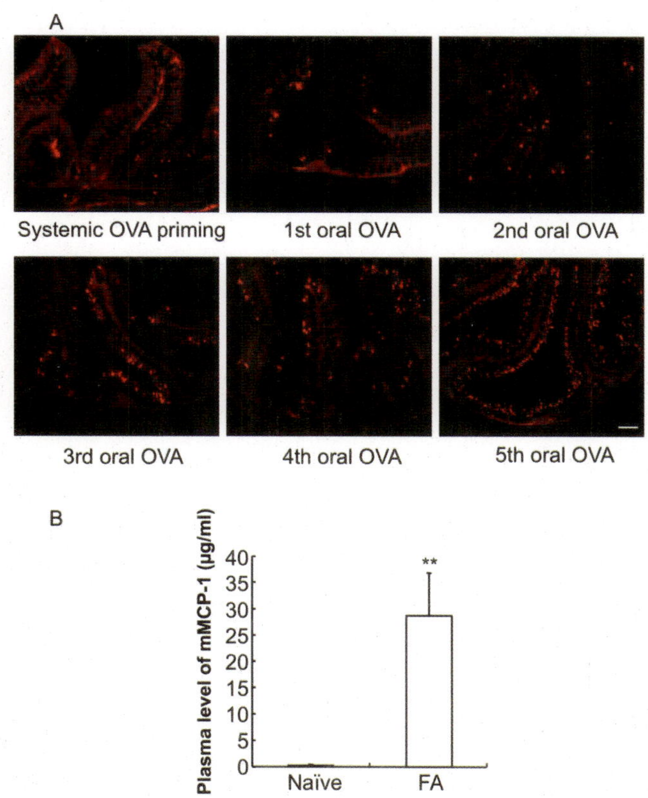

Figure 3. Mucosal mast cell hyperplasia and degranulation in the colon of food allergy mice. *A*: The proximal colons of systemically OVA primed mice and oral OVA-challenged mice after each oral OVA challenge were stained with anti-mouse mast cell protease-1 (mMCP-1) antibodies. Scale bar represents 200 μm. *B*: The concentration of mMCP-1 in the plasma of naïve mice and FA mice is shown. The concentration of mMCP-1 in the plasma was determined using an ELISA kit. Data are expressed as means ±SE. **$P<0.01$ vs. naïve mice ($n=5$ mice per group).

repeated oral allergen challenges (Figure 4A, $n = 5$ mice per group) and that OVA-specific IgE and mMCP-1 were not detected in the plasma of nude naïve mice and nude FA mice (Figure 4B: $^{**}P<0.01$ vs. wild-type (WT) naïve mice, $^{††}P<0.01$ vs. WT FA mice: $n = 3–5$ mice per group; Figure 4C: $^{*}P<0.05$ vs. WT naïve mice, $^{††}P<0.01$ vs. WT FA mice: $n = 3–5$ mice per group). Furthermore, no increase of mucosal mast cells was observed in the mucosal layer of the proximal colons of nude FA mice as compared to those of WT mice in the FA model (Figure 4D).

Characteristics of mast cells in the colon of food allergy mice

Mast cells were observed in the proximal colon of the FA mice and contained many granules intensely stained with toluidine blue (Figure 5A). Only a few mast cells were observed in the lamina propria. These mast cells contained numerous granules in the cytoplasm, most of which exhibited reddish violet metachromasia with toluidine blue (Figure 5B), indicating that these mast cells exhibit properties of CTMCs because in rodents, CTMC granules stain purple, and MMC granules stain blue with toluidine blue [18]. However, a few granules in these mast cells in the lamina propria were nonmetachromatic and were larger than metachromatic granules (Figure 5B; arrows).

Many MMCs were observed in the mucosal epithelium, and the majority of MMC granules were larger (Figure 5C) and were spherical or polymorphic in shape (Figure 5C; arrows). In addition, these MMC granules, which exhibited nonmetachromasia, were strongly stained with toluidine blue, but some were weakly stained.

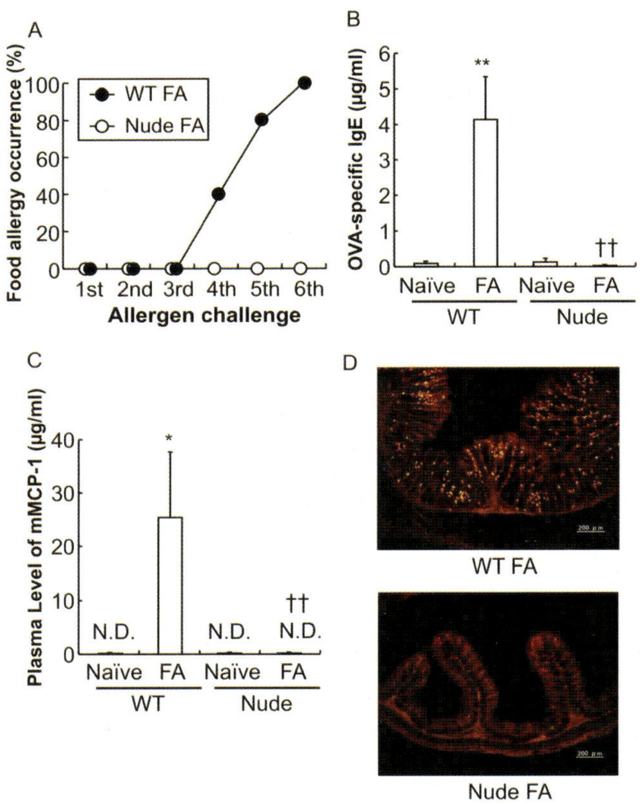

Figure 4. Induction of food allergy in athymic nude mice. *A*: The occurrence of allergic diarrhea in wild-type (WT) FA mice and nude FA mice after each oral OVA challenge is shown (n = 5 mice per group). *B*: The level of OVA-specific IgE in the plasma of WT naïve mice, WT FA mice, nude naïve mice and nude FA mice is shown. The level of OVA-specific IgE in the plasma was determined using an ELISA kit. $^{**}P<0.01$ vs. WT naïve mice, $^{††}P<0.01$ vs. WT FA mice ($n = 3–5$ mice per group). *C*: The level of mMCP-1 in the plasma of WT naïve mice, WT FA mice, nude naïve mice and nude FA mice is shown. The level of mMCP-1 in the plasma was determined using an ELISA kit. $^{*}P<0.05$ vs. WT naïve mice, $^{††}P<0.01$ vs. WT FA mice ($n = 3–5$ mice per group). *D*: The proximal colon of WT FA mice and nude FA mice after the 6th oral OVA challenge was stained with anti-mMCP-1 antibodies. Scale bars represent 200 µm.

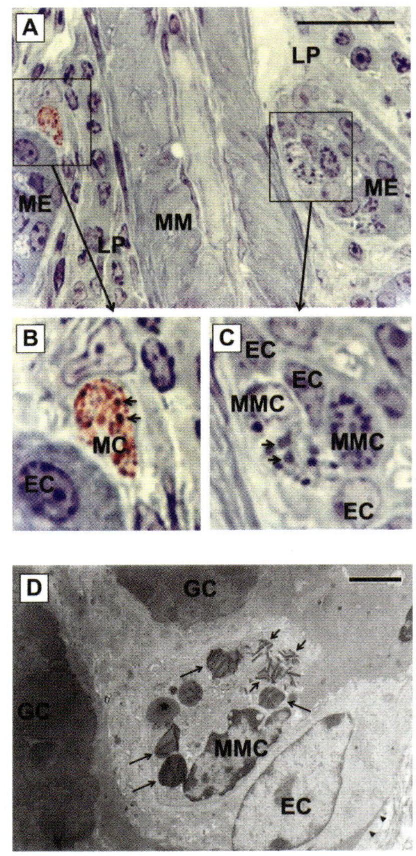

Figure 5. Morphology of mast cells in the colon of food allergy mice. Sections (1 µm thick) of the fixed colon embedded in resin were stained with 1% toluidine blue and were observed with light microscopy for the analysis of mast cells. *A*: On the left hand side of the picture, a mast cell (surrounded by a square) with metachromatic granules was observed in the lamina propria. On the other side, two mast cells (surrounded with another square) with nonmetachromatic granules were localized in the mucosal epithelium. ME: mucosal epithelium, LP: lamina propria, MM: muscularis mucosa. Scale bar represents 50 µm. *B*: An image of higher magnification of the mast cell in the lamina propria. Most of granules of the mast cell exhibited metachromasia, but a few granules (arrows) were nonmetachromatic. MC: mast cell, EC: epithelial cell. *C*: An image of higher magnification of mucosal mast cells (MMCs) in the mucosal epithelium. The granules in MMCs did not exhibit metachromasia and some of the granules were polymorphic in shape (arrows). MMC: mucosal mast cell. *D*: Electron microscopic analysis of mucosal mast cells in the proximal colon of food allergy mice. A variety of morphologies of granules was seen in a MMC: one (asterisk) showed amorphous inner structure, some (long arrows) showed crystals with amorphous matrix and others (short arrows) seemed to be occupied by the crystalline structure. Arrowheads indicate basement membrane. GC: goblet cell. Scale bar represents 4 µm.

Ultrastructural characteristics of mucosal mast cells in food allergy mice

MMCs in the mucosal epithelium of the FA mice proximal colon have been examined with the electron microscope (Figure 5D). Many MMCs were observed within the mucosal epithelium, and they were characterized by the presence of peculiar large granules (0.5–2.5 μm) in the cytoplasm. MMCs had specific granules of varying size, shape and electron-density. Many of the granules (Figure 5D, long arrows) contained crystalline inclusions with cylindrical shape and had irregular contours and showed polymorphic shapes. Other granules seemed to be occupied by crystalline structures (Figure 5D, short arrows). Some of the granules had relatively homogeneous matrix with round or oval contours without the crystalline inclusion (Figure 5D, asterisk).

Critical involvement of mast cells in the pathogenesis of food allergy in mice

Mice that specifically lack only mast cells have not been reported/generated; two mouse strains, WBB6F1/J-Kit^{W}/Kit^{W-v} and C57BL/6-Kit^{W-sh}/Kit^{W-sh} are profoundly deficient in mast cells. These mice are most frequently used to analyze the *in vivo* functions of mast cells, but we could not employ these strains to examine the role of mast cells in the induction of FA because the genetic background of these mice is not BALB/c and these mice have other phenotypic abnormalities, such as gastric ulcer and intestinal motility disorder.

Therefore, in this study, we employed $PI3K^{-/-}$ mice with a BALB/c genetic background that exhibit a selective loss of gastrointestinal mast cells [19]. As a result, $PI3K^{-/-}$ mice failed to develop allergic diarrhea ($PI3K^{-/-}$ FA mice) (Figure 6A, $n = 5$ mice per group). As shown in Figure 6B, immunohistochemical staining with the mMCP-1 antibody revealed that MMCs were dramatically increased in the proximal colon of WT FA mice, whereas only a few mast cells were observed in the mucosal layer of $PI3K^{-/-}$ FA mice. Plasma mMCP-1 was almost undetectable in $PI3K^{-/-}$ naïve mice and $PI3K^{-/-}$ FA mice (Figure 6C: $^{**}P<0.01$ vs. WT naïve mice, $^{\dagger\dagger}P<0.01$ vs. WT FA mice; $n = 3$–5 mice per group).

Furthermore, in systemic immunity (spleen, Figure 6D), mRNA levels of Th2 cytokines (IL-4 and IL-5) were increased in $PI3K^{-/-}$ FA mice as compared to $PI3K^{-/-}$ naïve mice (IL-4: $^{*}P<0.05$ vs. WT naïve mice, $^{**}P<0.01$ vs. $PI3K^{-/-}$ naïve mice; IL-5: $^{**}P<0.01$ vs. WT naïve mice; $n = 4$–7 mice per group), which is similar to those in WT FA mice. On the other hand, in mucosal immunity (proximal colon, Figure 6E, lower expression of mRNA for Th2 cytokines was found in $PI3K^{-/-}$ FA mice as compared to WT FA mice (IL-4: $^{*}P<0.05$ vs. WT naïve mice, $^{\dagger\dagger}P<0.01$ vs. WT FA mice; IL-5: $^{*}P<0.05$ vs. WT naïve mice; $n = 4$–7 mice per group).

Effect of mast cell stabilizers on the induction of food allergy in mice

The critical involvement of MMCs in the pathogenesis of FA was pharmacologically investigated in the FA model. The subcutaneous administration of a CTMC and MMC dual stabilizer doxantrazole (10 mg/kg) completely prevented the allergic responses following exposure to repeated oral allergen challenges, whereas the oral treatment with cromolyn (100 mg/kg), a CTMC stabilizer failed to suppress these responses (Figure 7: $^{**}P<0.01$ vs. FA mice; $n = 10$–15 mice per group). In addition, mice treated with an anti-inflammatory drug prednisolone (10 mg/kg) did not exhibit any sign of allergic diarrhea in the FA model.

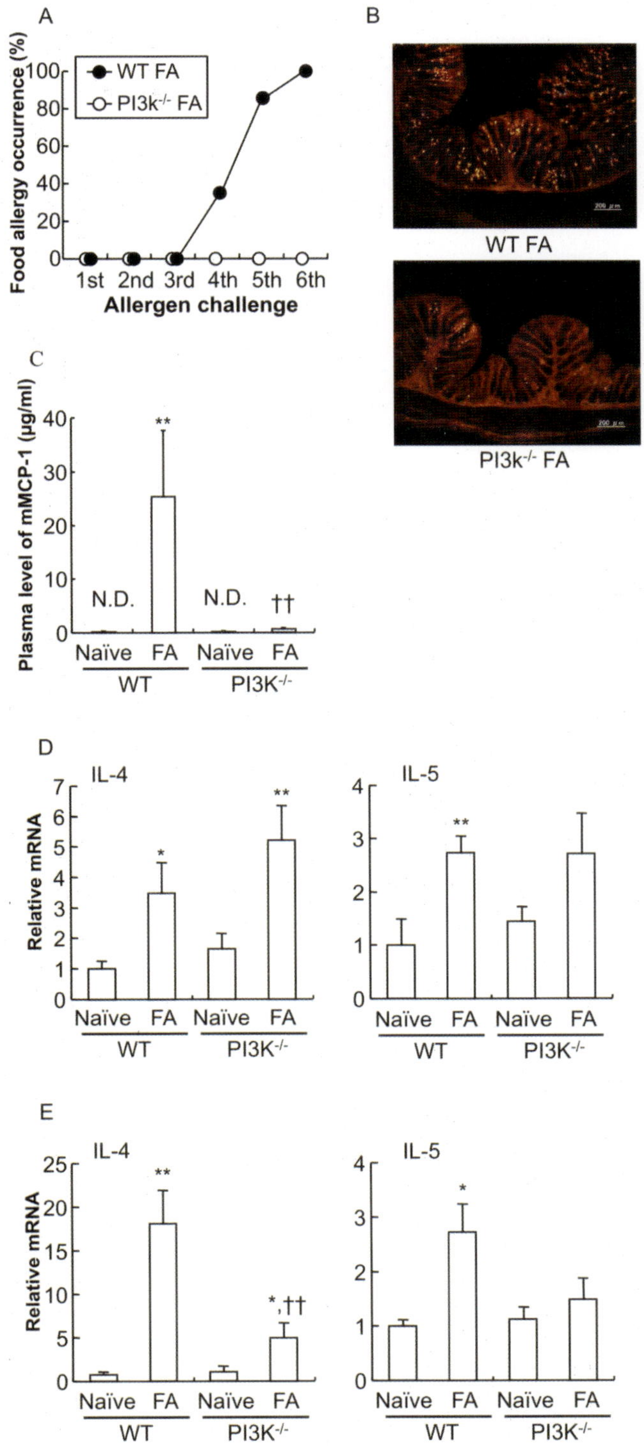

Figure 6. Induction of food allergy in PI3K-deficient mice. $PI3K^{-/-}$ mice as a gastrointestinal mast cell-deficient murine model were subjected to FA-inducing oral OVA challenges. *A*: The occurrence of allergic diarrhea in WT mice (WT FA mice) and $PI3K^{-/-}$ mice ($PI3K^{-/-}$ FA mice) after each oral OVA challenge is shown ($n = 5$ mice per group). *B*: The proximal colon of FA-induced $PI3K^{-/-}$ mice after oral OVA challenge was stained with anti- mMCP-1 antibodies. Scale bars represent 200 μm. *C*: The level of mMCP-1 in the plasma of $PI3K^{-/-}$ naïve mice and $PI3K^{-/-}$ FA mice is shown. The level of mMCP-1 in the plasma was determined using an ELISA kit. Data are expressed as means ±SE. $^{**}P<0.01$ vs. WT naïve mice, $^{\dagger\dagger}P<0.01$ vs. WT FA mice ($n = 3$–5 mice per group). IL-4 and IL-5 cytokine mRNA expression in the spleen (*D*) and proximal colon (*E*) from WT naïve mice, WT FA mice, $PI3K^{-/-}$

naïve mice and PI3K$^{-/-}$ FA mice were measured by real-time PCR. Relative mRNA levels of cytokines were normalized to GAPDH expression. *$P<0.05$, **$P<0.01$ vs. each naïve mice, ††$P<0.01$ vs. WT FA mice ($n=4$–7 mice per group).

Cholinergic anti-inflammatory pathway in food allergy mice

To investigate whether vagal activity influences the development of FA, we examined the effect of 2-deoxy-D-glucose (2-DG), a central vagal stimulant on the FA model. Intraperitoneal injection of 2-DG (200 mg/kg) significantly ameliorated allergic diarrhea. After the 6th OVA challenge, the occurrence of allergic diarrhea was significantly decreased from 100.0% to 54.5% (Figure 8A: *$P<0.05$ vs. vehicle, $n=11$–18 mice per group). The therapeutic effect of 2-DG was significantly blocked by the subcutaneous injection of the non-selective nAChR antagonist hexamethonium (C6) at 32 mg/kg (Figure 8A: †$P<0.05$ vs. 2-DG, $n=11$ mice per group).

We next examined the therapeutic effect of nAChR activation on the development of FA. The subcutaneous injection of nicotine attenuated the induction of allergic diarrhea at 1 and 3.2 mg/kg (Figure 8B: *$P<0.05$, **$P<0.01$ vs. FA mice, $n=10$–74 mice per group). The selective α7 nAChR agonist GTS-21 was used to determine whether α7 nAChR mediated the therapeutic effect of nicotine. The subcutaneous injection of GTS-21 (10 mg/kg) resulted in a significant suppression of allergic diarrhea (Figure 8C: *$P<0.05$, **$P<0.01$ vs. FA mice, $n=23$–40 mice per group).

Effect of nicotine treatment on the systemic and mucosal immune responses in food allergy mice

The number of MMCs that was dramatically increased in the proximal colon of the FA mice was significantly decreased in that of nicotine-treated FA mice (Figure 9A).

MPO activity in the colon of the FA mice was significantly increased approximately 2.5-fold compared to that in the naïve mice colon, and the subcutaneous injection of nicotine significantly suppressed the increment of MPO activity in the FA mice (Figure 9B: naïve mice 534.8±56.5 units/gwwt, FA mice 1285.7±123.5 units/gwwt, nicotine-treated FA mice 740.5±138.4 units/gwwt; *$P<0.05$ vs. naïve mice, †$P<0.05$ vs. FA mice; $n=3$–10 mice per group).

In contrast, the plasma level of OVA-specific IgE remained unchanged in nicotine-treated FA mice compared to the FA mice (Figure 9C: naïve mice 0.1±0.0 μg/ml, FA mice 3.8±0.7 μg/ml, nicotine-treated FA mice 4.3±0.4 μg/ml; **$P<0.01$ vs. naïve mice; $n=5$ mice per group).

To investigate the effects of nicotine treatment on the cytokine profile in the FA mice, cytokine mRNA expression was detected by real-time PCR. In systemic immunity (spleen), the upregulated Th2 cytokine (IL-4 and IL-5) mRNA expression observed in the FA mice was not significantly changed by nicotine treatment (Figure 9D: $n=6$ mice per group), which is almost consistent with no effect of nicotine on the enhanced plasma OVA-specific IgE level in the FA mice (Figure 9C). In contrast, the downregulated Th1 cytokine (IFN-γ) mRNA expression observed in the FA mice was significantly increased in nicotine-treated FA mice (Figure 9D: *$P<0.01$ vs. FA mice, $n=6$ mice per group). On the other hand, in mucosal immunity (proximal colon), the upregulated mRNA expression of both Th1 (IFN-γ) and Th2 (IL-4 and IL-5) cytokines was significantly suppressed in nicotine-treated FA mice (Figure 9E: *$P<0.05$, **$P<0.01$ vs. FA mice, $n=3$–6 mice per group).

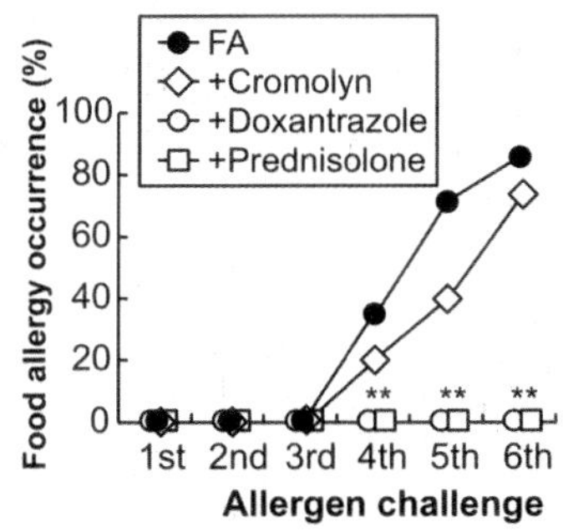

Figure 7. Effect of mast cell stabilizers on the induction of food allergy in mice. The occurrence of allergic diarrhea in FA mice (closed circle) and cromolyn-treated mice (open diamond) after each oral OVA challenge is shown ($n=14$–15 mice per group). In addition, mice treated with the subcutaneous administration of doxantrazole (open circle, 10 mg/kg) or the oral administration of prednisolone (open square, 10 mg/kg) did not exhibit any sign of allergic responses in the FA model. **$P<0.01$ vs. FA mice ($n=10$ mice per each group).

Morphological analysis of mucosal mast cell–cholinergic nerve interactions in the colon of food allergy mice

We have demonstrated that α7 nAChRs are expressed in mBMMCs and that the stimulation of α7 nAChRs can negatively regulate the activation of mBMMCs [17]. Therefore, we investigated the morphological interaction of MMCs and cholinergic nerve fibers in the lamina propria of the FA mouse proximal colon. It was difficult to investigate the morphological interaction of MMCs and cholinergic nerve fibers using two-dimensional images with fine-resolution in the colon. Therefore, digital images acquired by confocal laser-scanning microscopy were three-dimensionally reconstructed and observed using Imaris software (Figure 10A). The majority of mMCP-1-positive MMCs (green) were located in close vicinity of the CGRP-IR cholinergic nerve fibers (red) in the FA mouse proximal colon (Figure 10B, C, D: arrows). Furthermore, we verified that CGRP-IR neurons (Figure 10E: arrows) exhibited ChAT immunoreactivities in the myenteric and submucosal neurons of the mouse enteric nervous system.

Discussion

In this study, we provide evidence that MMCs are primarily responsible for the pathology of the FA model and that the cholinergic neuro-immune interaction via α7 nAChRs on MMCs play a crucial role in controlling pathological immune activation to restore the homeostasis in the intestine.

The neuro-immune interaction can be targeted for the design of novel therapeutic agents for the treatment of intestinal immune diseases.

Our murine FA model exhibited various features of type 1 hypersensitive allergic reactions, such as allergic diarrhea within 1 hour after oral antigen exposure, antigen-specific IgE hyperproduction and MMC hyperplasia and degranulation. In addition, Th1-prone C57BL/6 mice did not develop the allergic diarrhea.

Taken together, these data suggest that enhanced Th2-mediated immune responses are responsible for the pathology of our murine FA model.

In the mRNA analysis of cytokines, the FA mice exhibited Th2-biased immune responses in systemic immunity. On the other hand, in mucosal immunity, Th2 immune responses were significantly enhanced, whereas Th1 immune responses were not decreased, but rather increased, indicating that there is a

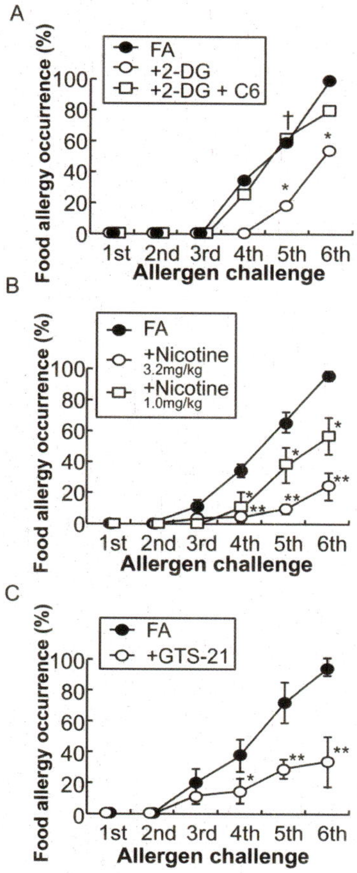

Figure 8. Cholinergic control of food allergy in mice. *A*: The occurrence of allergic diarrhea in FA mice (closed circle), 2-deoxy-d-glucose (2-DG)-treated mice (open circle) and hexamethonium (C6)-treated mice prior to 2-DG administration (open square) after each oral OVA challenge is shown. $^*P<0.05$ vs. FA mice. †$P<0.05$ vs. 2-DG mice ($n=11$–18 mice per group). *B*: The occurrence of allergic diarrhea in FA mice (closed circle) and nicotine-treated mice (3.2 mg/kg; open circle, 1.0 mg/kg; open square, and 0.32 mg/kg; open diamond) after each oral OVA challenge is shown. $^*P<0.05$, $^{**}P<0.01$ vs. FA mice ($n=10$–74 mice per group). *C*: The occurrence of allergic diarrhea in FA mice (closed circle) and GTS-21-treated mice (open circle) after each oral OVA challenge is shown. $^*P<0.05$, $^{**}P<0.01$ vs. FA mice ($n=23$–40 mice per group).

difference between the systemic immune responses and the mucosal immune responses in the FA mice. Furthermore, these enhanced Th2 responses were almost consistent with those observed in other murine OVA-induced FA models, but Th1 responses in the mucosal immunity were different from those in the other models [20,21]. Kweon et al. observed increased IFN-γ production in the spleen and no IFN-γ production in the colon using ELISA in another murine FA model with allergic diarrhea [21], and Brandt et al. reported no change of IFN-γ mRNA expression in the jejunum of their FA mice with allergic diarrhea [20]. These discrepancies may be due to differences in immunization protocols, cytokine measurement methods and tissue segments. Thus, our murine FA model is characterized by the activation of not only Th2 but also Th1 immune responses in the mucosal immunity of the FA mice colon [7].

Furthermore, to determine whether T cells have a pathological role in the development of FA, we examined whether food allergic diarrhea was induced in nude mice that lack functional T cells due

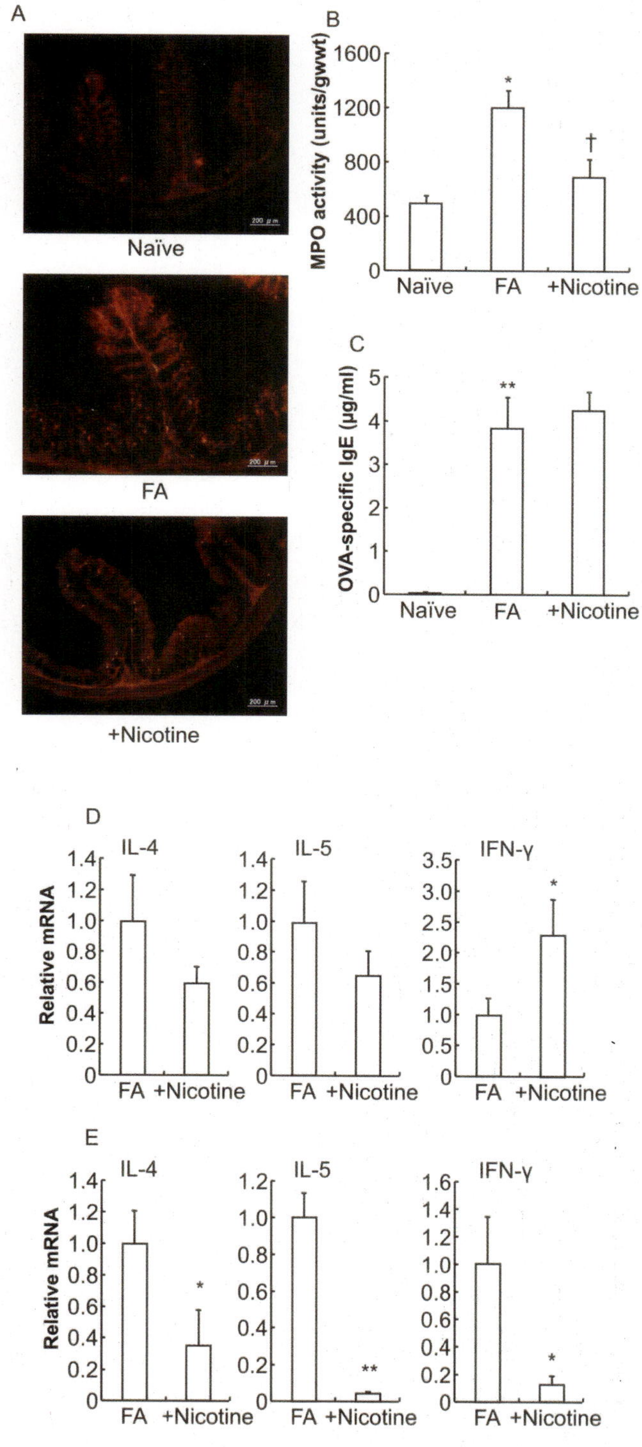

Figure 9. Effect of nicotine on the pathology of food allergy in mice. *A*: The proximal colons of naïve mice, FA mice, and mice treated with the subcutaneous administration of nicotine were stained with mMCP-1 antibodies. Scale bars represent 200 μm. *B*: MPO activity was measured in the colon of naïve mice, FA mice and nicotine-treated FA mice. $^*P<0.01$ vs. naïve mice. †$P<0.05$ vs. FA mice ($n=3$–10 mice per group). *C*: The level of OVA-specific IgE in the plasma of naïve mice, FA mice and nicotine-treated FA mice is shown. The level of OVA-specific IgE in the plasma was determined using an ELISA kit. $^{**}P<0.01$ vs. naïve mice ($n=5$ mice per group). IL-4, IL-5 and IFN-γ cytokine mRNA expression in the spleen (*D*) and proximal colon (*E*) from FA mice and nicotine-treated FA mice were measured by real-time PCR. Relative mRNA levels of cytokines were normalized to GAPDH expression. $^*P<0.05$, $^{**}P<0.01$ vs. FA mice ($n=3$–6 mice per group).

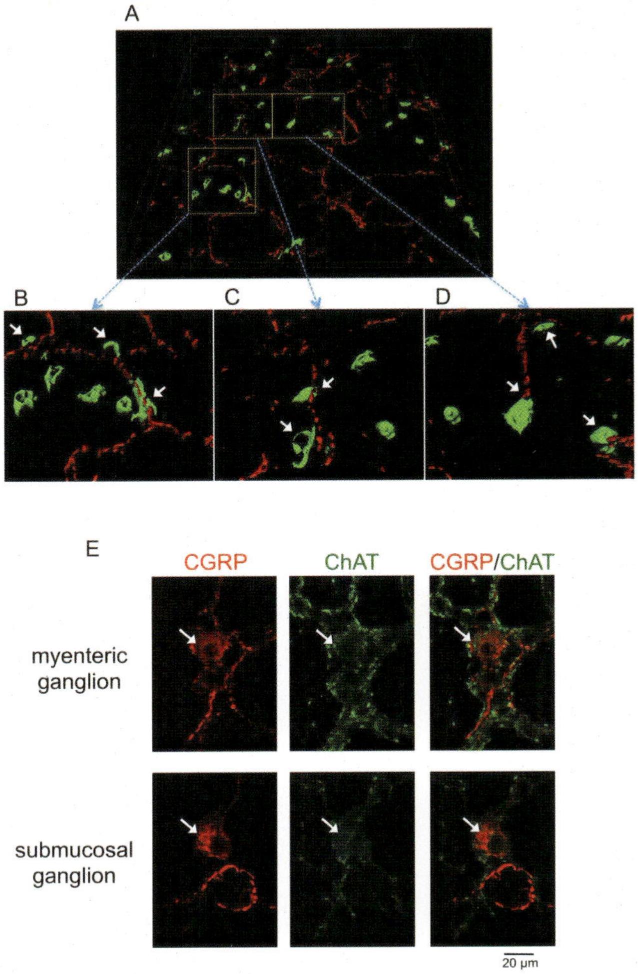

Figure 10. Spatial relationship of mucosal mast cells and cholinergic nerve fibers in the FA mouse colon. *A*: Three-dimensional reconstruction of the confocal images reveals the morphological interaction of mMCP-1-positive MMCs (green) and cholinergic CGRP- immunoreactive nerve fibers (red). Major grid space represents 20 μm. *B–D*: High-magnification images of three boxed regions in (*A*). *E*: CGRP- immunoreactive neurons (arrows) exhibited ChAT immunoreactivities in the myenteric and submucosal ganglion of the mouse enteric nervous system. Scale bar represents 20 μm.

to their thymus deficiency. We found that nude mice failed to exhibit allergic responses in the FA mouse model and that increased OVA-specific IgE and mMCP-1 levels in the plasma and mastocytosis in the mucosa of the proximal colon were not detected in nude naïve mice and nude FA mice. In addition, in this study, OVA-challenged mice without systemic priming failed to exhibit allergic diarrhea. Thus, these results indicate that the T-cell-mediated immune responses in the systemic immunity are essentially required for the development of the allergic responses in our FA model.

This study revealed that mMCP-1 immunoreactive MMCs increased in the mucosal epithelium of the FA mice colon, which is similar to previous reports on the appearance of mast cells in the jejunal mucosa of oral allergen–induced diarrhea mice [20] and parasite-infected mice [22,23]. Thus, these findings suggest that MMCs are localized in the strategic position to enhance a rapid expulsion of food antigens or parasites from the gut by bioactive products released from MMCs.

The toluidine blue staining revealed a difference between mast cells in the lamina propria and MMCs in the mucosal epithelium of the FA mice colon. Most of the granules of mast cells in the lamina propria, but not MMCs exhibited metachromasia presumably caused by sulfate radicals of proteoglycan such as heparin, suggesting that the difference results from chemical properties of substances contained in the granules of mast cells and that the granules of MMCs in the mucosal epithelium have depleted the reactive substances.

In the previous studies with mMCP-1-deficient mice in the parasite infection model, the light microscopic analysis reveals that MMCs in the jejunal mucosa of the deficient mice have smaller, less intensely toluidine blue-positive granules than those in WT mice and that the granules of MMCs in the deficient mice are uniformly round, whereas those in WT mice are irregularly shaped [23]. Furthermore, previous ultrastructural analysis demonstrates that crystalline inclusions with a cylindrical shape abundantly exist in the irregularly shaped granules of MMCs in the jejunal mucosa of the murine parasite infection model [23], which is consistent with the present findings using the electron microscopy in the granules of MMCs in the mucosal epithelium of the FA mice colon. However, in the mMCP-1 deficient mice, the shapes of MMC granules are regular and oval, and no crystalline structures are observed within the granules in the parasite infection model [23]. Taken all together, it is suggested that the disappearance of matrix constituents such as chondroitin sulfate in the granules of mast cells may be related to the formation of crystalline structures of chymases such as mMCP-1.

The PI3K family is involved in signal transduction that regulates cell proliferation, survival and differentiation. In particular, PI3K is involved in many functions of immune cells [24], and in mast cells, the activation of class Ia PI3K is required in the downstream signaling cascades initiated by the stimulation of high-affinity IgE receptor FcεRI. $PI3K^{-/-}$ mice are observed to be deficient in gastrointestinal mast cells but still have abundant dermal mast cells [19], indicating that the p85α subunit of PI3K is required for the development of gastrointestinal mast cells, but not dermal mast cells.

$PI3K^{-/-}$ mice failed to develop FA in our FA model, which were attributed to a deficiency of mast cells in the intestine, because: 1) mast cells can promote T-cell migration by producing chemokines [25,26], 2) mast cell products can promote dendritic cells to acquire a Th2 cell-inducing phenotype [2,27], and 3) mast cells themselves can produce Th2 cytokines, such as IL-4, 5 and 13 [2,25].

Furthermore, despite our finding that nicotine treatment atteuated allergic diarrhea in the FA mouse model, nicotine had no effect on the enhanced plasma IgE level.

Thus, these data suggest that the pathogenesis of FA is mainly attributed to mast cell hyperplasia in the intestine, but not antigen-specific IgE hyperproduction. Taken all together, our results indicate that MMCs critically contribute to the development of FA through orchestrating Th2 immune responses in the mucosal immunity of the FA mice.

The cross-talk between the autonomic nervous system and immune system is becoming increasingly elucidated to be of great importance for the maintenance of immune homeostasis. Several lines of evidence indicate that parasympathetic vagus nerve, through release of acetylcholine, plays a counter-regulatory role to restore immune homeostasis in diverse inflammatory disease models, such as ischemia-reperfusion injury [28], pancreatitis [29], peritonitis [30], DSS-induced colitis [31] and postoperative ileus [32,33]. The anti-inflammatory properties of the vagus nerve in these mouse models are primarily attributed to the suppression of macrophage activation that leads to the induction of inflammation through the release of the central inflammatory mediator TNF-α. Recently, it has become clear that nAChRs are expressed in various immune cells [14,32] as well as macrophages [34]. However, it still remains unclear whether the stimulation of nAChRs on these immune cells ameliorates diverse inflammatory diseases. In particular, it is worth noting that it is unknown whether cholinergic activation via nAChRs serves as an anti-inflammatory pathway in Th2-related diseases, especially allergic diseases.

In this FA study, vagal stimulation with 2-DG ameliorated the development of FA, which was reversed by the nAChR antagonist C6, indicating that vagus nerves exhibit anti-allergic properties via nAChRs. The therapeutic potential of the cholinergic agonist nicotine in inflammatory diseases has recently been demonstrated. In fact, nicotine has been shown to suppress inflammatory responses in various clinical studies, animal models and in vitro studies [12,35,36,37]. Notably, in a randomized double-blind study, nicotine patches in combination with conventional therapy have ameliorated ulcerative colitis, in which Th2-mediated phenomena tend to predominate, as compared to placebo patches and conventional therapy; however, nicotine patch treatment has caused adverse side effects, such as nausea, dizziness, headache and addiction due to non-selectivity of nicotine for subtypes of nAChRs [38].

In this study, nicotine treatment significantly ameliorated FA, mainly due to the suppression of upregulated mucosal immune responses via α7 nAChRs on immune cells. Therefore, the therapeutic effects of nicotine and GTS-21 on the FA model raise the possibility that a strategy for drug discovery against FA by targeting α7 nAChRs could potentially have therapeutic benefits.

Moreover, we have demonstrated that mBMMCs express α7 nAChRs and that their activation exerts inhibitory effects on antigen-IgE-mediated degranulation in mBMMCs [17]. In addition, our results in this study reveal that MMCs can orchestrate the allergic and inflammatory responses in the mucosal immune environment of the FA mice colon. Therefore, it is suggested that nicotine treatment suppresses the activation of MMCs through α7 nAChRs on MMCs, thereby reducing the number of MMCs and the plasma mMPC-1 level, which results in the significant amelioration of FA.

Furthermore, to examine whether the cholinergic anti-allergic pathway is a hard-wired connection between the immune and nervous systems closely interacting to regulate FA, we undertook morphological analysis in the mucosa of the FA mouse colon. Previous reports and this study demonstrate that in the mouse enteric nervous system, CGRP is exclusively contained in intrinsic primary afferent neurons that are immunoreactive for choline acetyltransferase [39,40], indicating that CGRP-IR neurons contain ACh as a neurotransmitter in the mouse colon. Our morphological findings of the close proximity between MMCs and CGRP-IR cholinergic nerve fibers in the colonic mucosa of the FA mice imply that the neural cholinergic regulation of immune responses occurs via nAChRs on immune cells, which is consistent with previous reports [14,32]. Collectively, it is suggested that cholinergic nerve fibers closely communicate with MMCs to regulate mast cell functions in the FA mice colon.

Further investigation of this cholinergic counter-regulatory nerve-immune interactions in the intestine will provide new insights to elucidate FA. In addition, new strategies for drug discovery that target the hard-wired connection via α7 nAChRs can lead to novel drug therapies against diverse intestinal immune diseases.

Author Contributions

Conceived and designed the experiments: MK. Performed the experiments: TY TK JL NU SH HS HK MK. Analyzed the data: JL TY. Contributed reagents/materials/analysis tools: TY JL HS HK. Wrote the paper: MK JL TY.

References

1. Sicherer SH, Sampson HA (2010) Food allergy. J Allergy Clin Immunol 125: S116–125.
2. Abraham SN, St John AL (2010) Mast cell-orchestrated immunity to pathogens. Nat Rev Immunol 10: 440–452.
3. Eigenmann PA, Frossard CP (2003) The T lymphocyte in food-allergy disorders. Curr Opin Allergy Clin Immunol 3: 199–203.
4. MacDonald TT, Di Sabatino A (2009) The immunologic basis for gastrointestinal food allergy. Curr Opin Gastroenterol 25: 521–526.
5. Paul WE, Zhu J (2010) How are T(H)2-type immune responses initiated and amplified? Nat Rev Immunol 10: 225–235.
6. Dawicki W, Marshall JS (2007) New and emerging roles for mast cells in host defence. Curr Opin Immunol 19: 31–38.
7. Yamamoto T, Fujiwara K, Yoshida M, Kageyama-Yahara N, Kuramoto H, et al. (2009) Therapeutic effect of kakkonto in a mouse model of food allergy with gastrointestinal symptoms. Int Arch Allergy Immunol 148: 175–185.
8. Metcalfe DD, Baram D, Mekori YA (1997) Mast cells. Physiol Rev 77: 1033–1079.
9. Kageyama-Yahara N, Suehiro Y, Maeda F, Kageyama S, Fukuoka J, et al. (2010) Pentagalloylglucose down-regulates mast cell surface FcepsilonRI expression in vitro and in vivo. FEBS Lett 584: 111–118.
10. Bienenstock J, Goetzl EJ, Blennerhassett MG (2003) Autonomic neuroimmunology. London: CRC Press. 392 p.
11. van Diest SA, Stanisor OI, Boeckxstaens GE, de Jonge WJ, van den Wijngaard RM (2012) Relevance of mast cell-nerve interactions in intestinal nociception. Biochim Biophys Acta 1822: 74–84.
12. Bauer O, Razin E (2000) Mast Cell-Nerve Interactions. News Physiol Sci 15: 213–218.
13. de Jonge WJ, Ulloa L (2007) The alpha7 nicotinic acetylcholine receptor as a pharmacological target for inflammation. Br J Pharmacol 151: 915–929.
14. Rosas-Ballina M, Tracey KJ (2009) Cholinergic control of inflammation. J Intern Med 265: 663–679.
15. Tracey KJ (2009) Reflex control of immunity. Nat Rev Immunol 9: 418–428.
16. van Der Zanden EP, Boeckxstaens GE, de Jonge WJ (2009) The vagus nerve as a modulator of intestinal inflammation. Neurogastroenterol Motil 21: 6–17.
17. Kageyama-Yahara N, Suehiro Y, Yamamoto T, Kadowaki M (2008) IgE-induced degranulation of mucosal mast cells is negatively regulated via nicotinic acetylcholine receptors. Biochem Biophys Res Commun 377: 321–325.
18. Miller HR, Walshaw R (1972) Immune reactions in mucous membranes. IV. Histochemistry of intestinal mast cells during helminth expulsion in the rat. Am J Pathol 69: 195–208.
19. Fukao T, Yamada T, Tanabe M, Terauchi Y, Ota T, et al. (2002) Selective loss of gastrointestinal mast cells and impaired immunity in PI3K-deficient mice. Nat Immunol 3: 295–304.
20. Brandt EB, Strait RT, Hershko D, Wang Q, Muntel EE, et al. (2003) Mast cells are required for experimental oral allergen-induced diarrhea. J Clin Invest 112: 1666–1677.
21. Kweon MN, Yamamoto M, Kajiki M, Takahashi I, Kiyono H (2000) Systemically derived large intestinal CD4(+) Th2 cells play a central role in STAT6-mediated allergic diarrhea. J Clin Invest 106: 199–206.
22. Friend DS, Ghildyal N, Austen KF, Gurish MF, Matsumoto R, et al. (1996) Mast cells that reside at different locations in the jejunum of mice infected with Trichinella spiralis exhibit sequential changes in their granule ultrastructure and chymase phenotype. J Cell Biol 135: 279–290.

23. Wastling JM, Knight P, Ure J, Wright S, Thornton EM, et al. (1998) Histochemical and ultrastructural modification of mucosal mast cell granules in parasitized mice lacking the beta-chymase, mouse mast cell protease-1. Am J Pathol 153: 491–504.
24. Koyasu S (2003) The role of PI3K in immune cells. Nat Immunol 4: 313–319.
25. Galli SJ, Nakae S, Tsai M (2005) Mast cells in the development of adaptive immune responses. Nat Immunol 6: 135–142.
26. Nakajima T, Inagaki N, Tanaka H, Tanaka A, Yoshikawa M, et al. (2002) Marked increase in CC chemokine gene expression in both human and mouse mast cell transcriptomes following Fcepsilon receptor I cross-linking: an interspecies comparison. Blood 100: 3861–3868.
27. Mazzoni A, Siraganian RP, Leifer CA, Segal DM (2006) Dendritic cell modulation by mast cells controls the Th1/Th2 balance in responding T cells. J Immunol 177: 3577–3581.
28. Bernik TR, Friedman SG, Ochani M, DiRaimo R, Ulloa L, et al. (2002) Pharmacological stimulation of the cholinergic antiinflammatory pathway. J Exp Med 195: 781–788.
29. van Westerloo DJ, Giebelen IA, Florquin S, Bruno MJ, Larosa GJ, et al. (2006) The vagus nerve and nicotinic receptors modulate experimental pancreatitis severity in mice. Gastroenterology 130: 1822–1830.
30. van Westerloo DJ, Giebelen IA, Florquin S, Daalhuisen J, Bruno MJ, et al. (2005) The cholinergic anti-inflammatory pathway regulates the host response during septic peritonitis. J Infect Dis 191: 2138–2148.
31. Ghia JE, Blennerhassett P, Kumar-Ondiveeran H, Verdu EF, Collins SM (2006) The vagus nerve: a tonic inhibitory influence associated with inflammatory bowel disease in a murine model. Gastroenterology 131: 1122–1130.
32. Dhawan S, Cailotto C, Harthoorn LF, de Jonge WJ (2012) Cholinergic signalling in gut immunity. Life Sci 91: 1038–1042.
33. The FO, Boeckxstaens GE, Snoek SA, Cash JL, Bennink R, et al. (2007) Activation of the cholinergic anti-inflammatory pathway ameliorates postoperative ileus in mice. Gastroenterology 133: 1219–1228.
34. Wang H, Yu M, Ochani M, Amella CA, Tanovic M, et al. (2003) Nicotinic acetylcholine receptor alpha7 subunit is an essential regulator of inflammation. Nature 421: 384–388.
35. Andersson U, Tracey KJ (2012) Reflex principles of immunological homeostasis. Annu Rev Immunol 30: 313–335.
36. Lakhan SE, Kirchgessner A (2011) Anti-inflammatory effects of nicotine in obesity and ulcerative colitis. J Transl Med 9: 129.
37. Yoshikawa H, Kurokawa M, Ozaki N, Nara K, Atou K, et al. (2006) Nicotine inhibits the production of proinflammatory mediators in human monocytes by suppression of I-kappaB phosphorylation and nuclear factor-kappaB transcriptional activity through nicotinic acetylcholine receptor alpha7. Clin Exp Immunol 146: 116–123.
38. Pullan RD, Rhodes J, Ganesh S, Mani V, Morris JS, et al. (1994) Transdermal nicotine for active ulcerative colitis. N Engl J Med 330: 811–815.
39. Furness JB, Robbins HL, Xiao J, Stebbing MJ, Nurgali K (2004) Projections and chemistry of Dogiel type II neurons in the mouse colon. Cell Tissue Res 317: 1–12.
40. Qu ZD, Thacker M, Castelucci P, Bagyanszki M, Epstein ML, et al. (2008) Immunohistochemical analysis of neuron types in the mouse small intestine. Cell Tissue Res 334: 147–161.

7

An Investigation of the Diversity of Strains of Enteroaggregative *Escherichia coli* Isolated from Cases Associated with a Large Multi-Pathogen Foodborne Outbreak in the UK

Timothy J. Dallman[1], Marie A. Chattaway[1], Lauren A. Cowley[1], Michel Doumith[2], Rediat Tewolde[3], David J. Wooldridge[4], Anthony Underwood[3], Derren Ready[5], John Wain[6], Kirsty Foster[7], Kathie A. Grant[1], Claire Jenkins[1]*

1 Gastrointestinial Bacteria Reference Unit, Public Health England, London, United Kingdom, **2** Antimicrobial Resistance and Healthcare Associated Infections Reference Unit, Public Health England, London, United Kingdom, **3** Applied Laboratory and Bio- Informatics Unit, Public Health England, London, United Kingdom, **4** Department for Bio-analysis and Horizon Technologies, Next Generation Sequencing, Public Health England, London, United Kingdom, **5** Public Health Laboratory London, Barts & The London Hospital Trust, London, United Kingdom, **6** Innovation Centre, University of East Anglia, Norwich, United Kingdom, **7** North East Public Health England Centre, Newcastle upon Tyne, United Kingdom

Abstract

Following a large outbreak of foodborne gastrointestinal (GI) disease, a multiplex PCR approach was used retrospectively to investigate faecal specimens from 88 of the 413 reported cases. Gene targets from a range of bacterial GI pathogens were detected, including *Salmonella* species, *Shigella* species and Shiga toxin-producing *Escherichia coli*, with the majority (75%) of faecal specimens being PCR positive for *aggR* associated with the Enteroaggregative *E. coli* (EAEC) group. The 20 isolates of EAEC recovered from the outbreak specimens exhibited a range of serotypes, the most frequent being O104:H4 and O131:H27. None of the EAEC isolates had the Shiga toxin (stx) genes. Multilocus sequence typing and single nucleotide polymorphism analysis of the core genome confirmed the diverse phylogeny of the strains. The analysis also revealed a close phylogenetic relationship between the EAEC O104:H4 strains in this outbreak and the strain of *E. coli* O104:H4 associated with a large outbreak of haemolytic ureamic syndrome in Germany in 2011. Further analysis of the EAEC plasmids, encoding the key enteroaggregative virulence genes, showed diversity with respect to FIB/FII type, gene content and genomic architecture. Known EAEC virulence genes, such as *aggR, aat* and *aap,* were present in all but one of the strains. A variety of fimbrial genes were observed, including genes encoding all five known fimbrial types, AAF/1 to AAF/V. The AAI operon was present in its entirety in 15 of the EAEC strains, absent in three and present, but incomplete, in two isolates. EAEC is known to be a diverse pathotype and this study demonstrates that a high level of diversity in strains recovered from cases associated with a single outbreak. Although the EAEC in this study did not carry the *stx* genes, this outbreak provides further evidence of the pathogenic potential of the EAEC O104:H4 serotype.

Editor: Axel Cloeckaert, Institut National de la Recherche Agronomique, France

Funding: These authors have no support or funding to report.

Competing Interests: The authors have declared that no competing interests exist.

* E-mail: claire.jenkins@phe.gov.uk

Introduction

The Enteroaggregative *Escherichia coli* (EAEC) group is a large, diverse group of diarrhoeagenic *E. coli* originally defined by their adherence to HEp-2 cells in a stacked brick formation [1]. Generally, EAEC are detected and identified using PCR targeting EAEC associated virulence genes that are predominately plasmid encoded, including a regulator of multiple plasmid virulence factors (*aggR*), the anti-aggregation transporter gene (*aat*) and the gene encoding dispersin (*aap*) [2–4]. AggR also activates the expression of the chromosomal *aai* genes encoding a Type VI Secretion System (T6SS) [5].

Virulence gene content associated with EAEC is highly variable between different strains, as illustrated in studies aimed at genotyping EAEC from a variety of clinical sources, healthy control groups and outbreaks [6–9]. In these studies, strains show inconsistent presence and concordance of EAEC virulence genes by PCR in specimens from symptomatic and asymptomatic cases. These data suggest that the full genetic component of this phenotype is not yet fully understood and, although most of these genes are found on the aggregative virulence plasmid, their inheritability is complex.

Early research on EAEC linked these strains to persistent diarrhoea in children in developing countries but EAEC have since been shown to be a significant cause of acute diarrhoea and important in the aetiology of intestinal infections in industrialized countries [10]. Two independent, large, prospective studies of diarrhoea aetiology conducted in the UK (1993–1996) and USA (2002–2004) reported a similar EAEC prevalence in patients with diarrhoea: 4.6% (160/3506) and 4.5% (37/823) in the UK and

Table 1. Phenotypic and genotypic characteristic of the 20 strains of EAEC isolated from faecal specimens linked to the outbreak.

Isolate Number	Isolate ID	Serotype	MLST	Plasmid type	Fimbrial type	Antibiotic resistance profile (ESBL *)
1	216/13	O104:H4	678	FIB_25 FII_48	I	AMP/SUL/STR/TET/TMP/NAL
2	218/13	O104:H4	678	FIB_25 FII_48	I	AMP/SUL/STR/TET/TMP/NAL
3	1062/13	O104:H4	678	FIB_25 FII_48	I	AMP/SUL/STR/TET/TMP/NAL
4	1063/13	O104:H4	678	FIB_25 FII_48	I	AMP/SUL/STR/TET/TMP/NAL
5	1070/13	O104:H4	678	FIB_25 FII_48	I	AMP/SUL/STR/TET/TMP/NAL
6	0219/13	O131:H27	10	FIB_5 FII_17	I	AMP/SUL/STR/TET/TMP/NAL
7	0220/13	O131:H27	10	FIB_5 FII_17	I	AMP/SUL/STR/TET/TMP/NAL
8	1071/13	O131:H27	10	FIB_5 FII_17	I	AMP/SUL/STR/TET/TMP/NAL
9	1072/13	O131:H27	10	FIB_5 FII_17	I	AMP/SUL/STR/TET/TMP/NAL
10	1073/13	O131:H27	10	FIB_5 FII_17	I	AMP/SUL/STR/TET/TMP/NAL
11	1074/13	O131:H27	10	FIB_5 FII_17	I	AMP/SUL/STR/TET/TMP/NAL
12	0215/13	O20:H19	278	FIB_5 FII_17	IV	AMP/SUL/TMP/CAZ/CTX/CPR/CEF *
13	0221/13	O20:H19	278	FIB_5 FII_17	IV	AMP/SUL/TMP/CAZ/CTX/CPR/CEF *
14	0222/13	O19a:H30	38	FIB_33 FII_1	III	AMP/SUL/STR/TMP/NAL/CAZ/CTX/CEF
15	1061/13	O55:H19	10	FIB_33 FII_1	III	AMP/SUL/STR/TEM/NAL
16	1065/13	O63:H12	1664	FIB_33 FII_1	III	AMP/SUL/STR/TET/TMP/NAL/CIP/CAZ/CTX/CEF
17	0214/13	O?:H19	746	FII	III	NAL
18	0217/13	O33:H16	295	FII_9	II	AMP/CHL/STR/TET/TMP/NAL
19	1064/13	O?:H21	227	FII_9	II	AMP/SUL/STR/TET/TMP/NAL/CAZ/CTX/CPR/CEF *
20	1060/13	O111:H4	226	repB	-	AMP/CHL/COL/TET/NAL

Key: AMP Ampicillin; CAZ ceftazidime; CTX Cefataxime; CEF Ceftiofur; CPR cefpirome; NAL nalidixic acid; STR Streptomycin; SUL Sulphonamide; TET tetracycline; TMP Trimethoprim.

US studies, respectively, and 1.7% in control subjects from both studies [11,12]. Clinical symptoms include watery diarrhoea, often with mucus, low grade fever, abdominal pain, nausea and vomiting [10].

Several EAEC foodborne outbreaks of gastroenteritis have been documented, notably in Japan, the UK and Italy [13–15]. Recently, a strain of enteroaggregative Shiga toxin-producing *E. coli* O104:H4 was identified as the cause of a foodborne outbreak of bloody diarrhoea and haemolytic ureamic syndrome (HUS) in Germany and France [16–20]. Case-control, cohort and trace back studies implicated fenugreek sprouts from Egypt as the source of the infection [21]. Detailed and timely microbiological outbreak investigations were followed by whole genome sequencing of strains of *E. coli* O104:H4 by various international groups [17,19,22–23].

In March 2013, a large outbreak of GI disease occurred in the North East of England and cases were linked to a food festival. Four hundred and thirteen cases reported illness including symptoms of persistent diarrhoea and abdominal pain immediately following the event, and a total of 592 cases were identified following an on-line questionnaire. One hundred and ten specimens were submitted to the regional Public Health England and local hospital laboratories. Using traditional culture methods, *Salmonella enterica* serotype Agona was isolated from 25 cases and 4 further cases had other *Salmonella* species. Cohort and trace back studies implicated a contaminated, fresh curry leaves from Pakistan as the source of the infection.

The low number of cases testing positive for *Salmonella* species raised the suspicion that this was a multi-pathogen outbreak and further testing using a pan pathogen PCR was requested by the Outbreak Control Team. Subsequently, strains of EAEC harbouring *aggR* were isolated from PCR positive faecal specimens. The aim of this study was to use whole genome sequencing to explore the genomic diversity of the 20 strains of EAEC harbouring *aggR* by determining their phylogenetic relationship, plasmid type and virulence gene content and to assess the likely contribution of each strain type to the reported symptoms of GI disease.

Material and Methods

Microbiology

Retrospectively, 88 faecal specimens from cases associated with the outbreak were tested for the presence of other bacterial GI pathogens using a multiplex GI pathogens PCR [24]. Although the faecal specimens had been stored for over 10 weeks at 4°C, an attempt was made to isolate the pathogens detected by the multiplex PCR by testing individual colonies for the *stx*, *ipaH* and *aggR* target genes, associated with Shiga toxin-producing *Escherichia coli* (STEC), *Shigella* species and EAEC respectively. For faecal specimens positive for *aggR*, 20 colonies were picked from bacterial growth on MacConkey or Sorbitol MacConkey agar plates and retested using the same PCR. Those colonies harbouring the *aggR* genes were identified biochemically as *E. coli* and serotyped using antisera raised in rabbits to the *E. coli* somatic O antigens.

Library preparation and whole genome sequencing

DNA was extracted for sequencing using the Wizard kit (Promega UK). Paired-end libraries were generated using the Illumina Nextera XT sample preparation kit. Automated

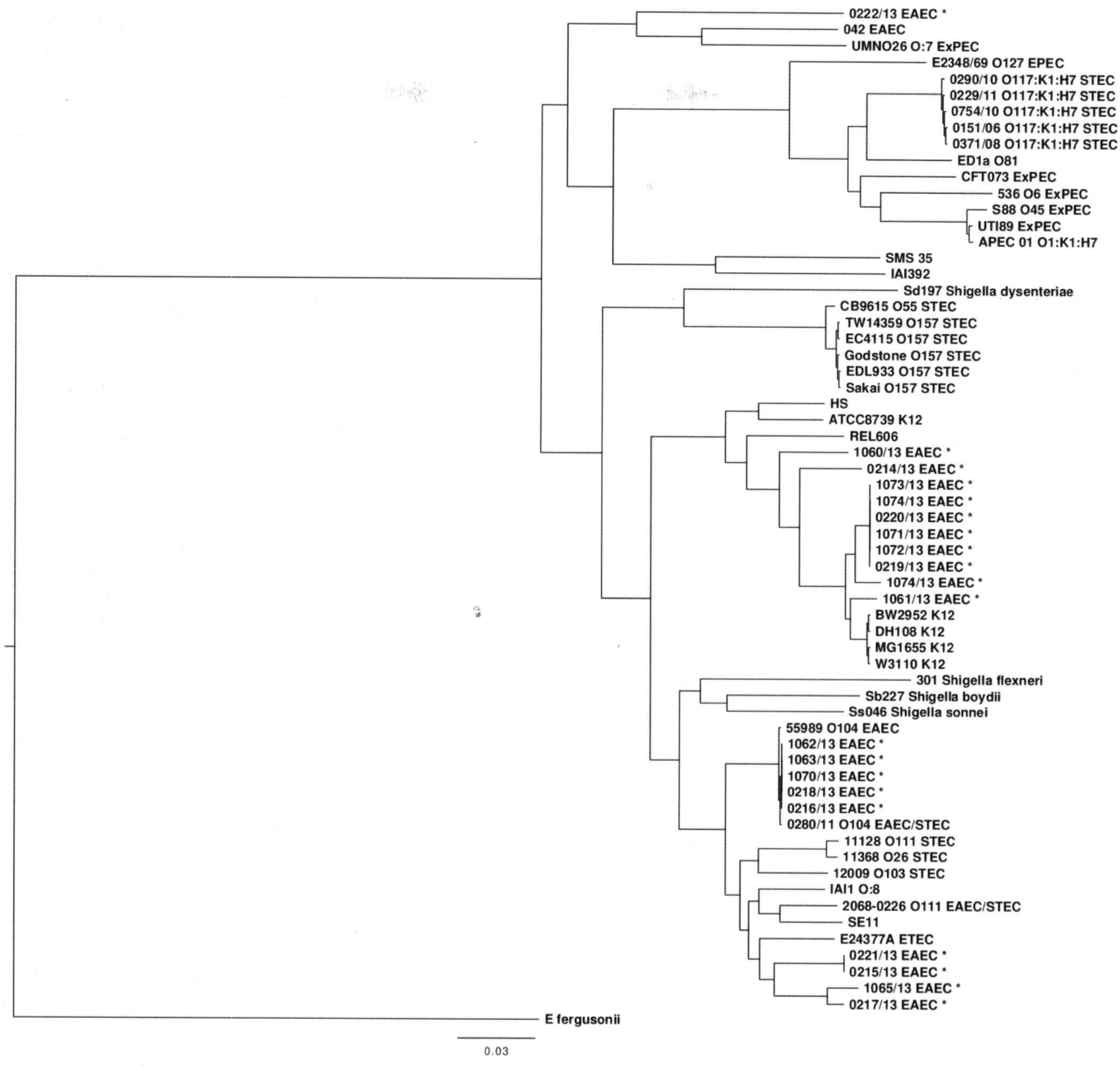

Figure 1. Whole genome chromosomal phylogeny of strains of *E. coli* and *Shigella* spp using previously published sequences and showing the 20 strains of EAEC isolates during this outbreak (highlighted in red). EAEC Enteroaggregative *E. coli*; EHEC Enterohaemorrhagic *E. coli*; ExPEC Extraintestinal Pathogenic *E. Coli*; EPEC Enteropathogenic *E. coli*; ETEC Enterotoxigenic *E. coli*.

platforms were used for sample preparation, library generation and quality checks. Assessment of fragment sizes was performed on the Perkin Elmer Labchip GX after fragmentation and clean-up. After normalisation, samples were pooled by hand and library quantification was performed using the KAPA library quantification kit for Illumina sequencing, on an ABI Viia7. Libraries were diluted to 15 pM and denatured at 96°C on a heat block for 2 minutes before being placed on ice for 5 minutes. Denatured libraries were spiked with 5% phiX and loaded on a Rapid flowcell by the Illumina cBot instrument. Paired-end sequencing was performed on the Illumina HiSeq 2500 instrument running HCS 2.0.10.0 using the TruSeq Rapid SBS kit (200 cycle) and TruSeq Paired-end rapid cluster kit. The following cycle parameters were used for sequencing: Read 1: 101, Index read 1: 8, Index read 2: 8 and Read 2: 101. RTA version 1.17.21.3 was used for generation of base call files.

Spades version 2.5.1 [25] was used to produce *de novo* assemblies of the sequenced paired-end fastq file. The number of contigs produced ranged from 221 to 552 per sample with N50s from 48338 to 192731 nucleotides.

Phylogenetic analysis

Illumina reads were mapped to the reference EAEC strain 55989 using BWA-SW [26]. The Sequence Alignment Map output from BWA was sorted and indexed to produce a Binary Alignment Map (BAM) using Samtools [27]. GATK2 [28] was

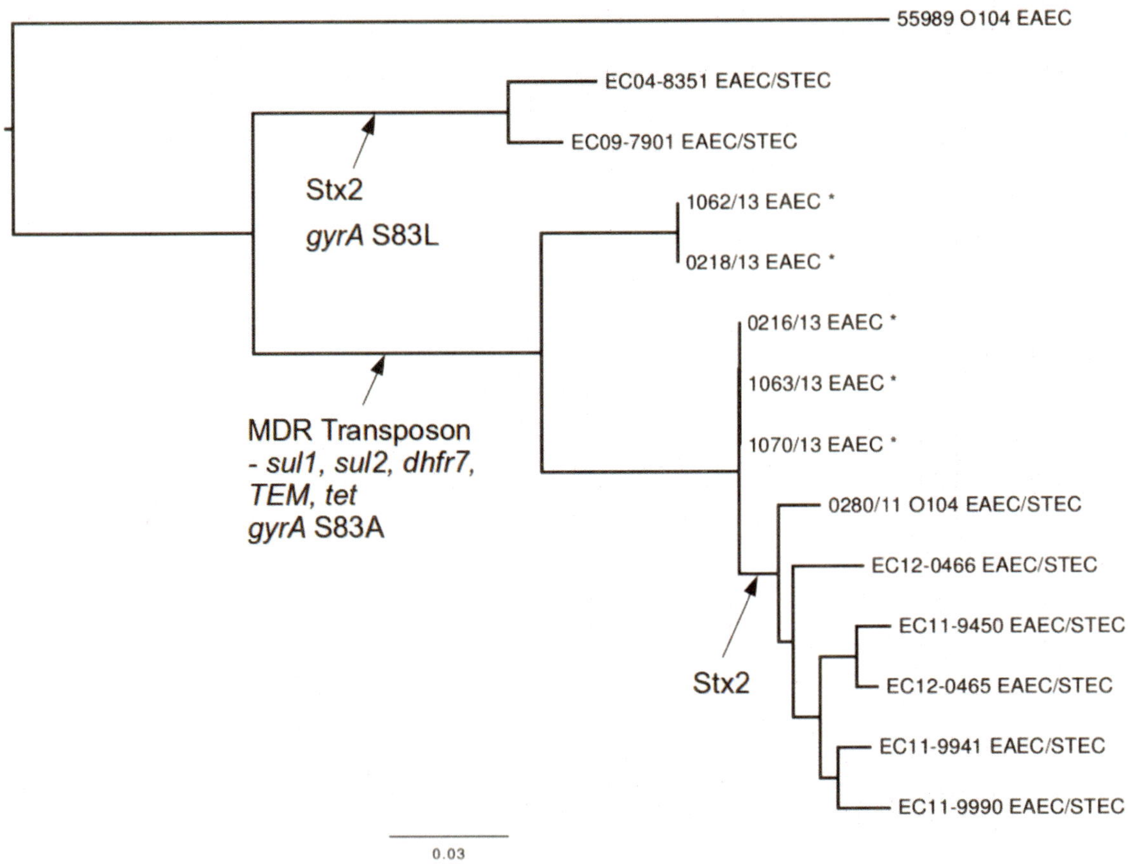

Figure 2. Chromosomal phylogeny of sequenced EAEC ST687 (strains including five strains isolated during this study marked *) represented as a maximum-likelihood tree. Previously published genome sequences included 280/11 isolated from a case linked to the outbreak in Germany in 2011 and 55989 isolated in the late 1990s in the Central African Republic. Other strains were previously described in Grad *at al.* 2013.

used to create a Variant Call Format (VCF) file from each of the BAMs, which were further parsed to extract only single nucleotide polymorphism (SNP) positions which were of high quality in all genomes (MQ>30, DP>10, 128 GQ>30, Variant Ratio >0.9). Pseudosequences of polymorphic positions were used to create approximate maximum likelihood trees using FastTree [29] under the General time reversible (GTR) model of nucleotide evolution.

Multilocus sequence typing (MLST)

MLST types were identified by mapping the reads against all *E. coli* allele variants held in the Achtman MLST database (www.mlst.ucc.ie/mlst/dbs/Ecoli) using a modification of the SRST software [30].

Plasmid FIB/FII typing

Plasmid incompatibility groups were determined using the specific sequences for plasmid replicon types defined by Carattoli *et al.* 2005 [31]. These sequences were searched for using blastn against the assembled genomes. Retrieved IncF and IncI replicon sequences were extracted *in silico* and further characterised to sequence type level according to the new scheme described in the plasmid MLST database (pMLST: www.pubmlst.or/plasmid/)

BRIG analysis

Assembled genomes were loaded into BRIG as concentric rings [32] and compared against the pAA reference genome using blastn. pAA annotations from genbank file were added in the final ring.

Mapping of known EAEC virulence genes

Illumina reads were mapped to a panel of putative EAEC virulence factors (*aggR, aatA, aatB, aatC, aatP, aap, SepA, IDI* and *aaiC*) using BWA-SW [26]. The number of reads that mapped to each position was calculated using Samtools mpileup [27]. The aggregative fimbrial adhesion type was determined based on mapping to each of the five variable fimbrial subunits AAF/I to AAFV (*aggA, aafA, agg3a, hdaA, aaf5a*) [33–37].

Determination of the presence or absence of AAI operon T6SS components using BLAST

AAI operon T6SS coding genes were extracted from the reference strain 55989 genbank file (http://www.ncbi.nlm.nih.gov/nuccore/NC_011748.1) and made into a BLAST database. Each of the assembled genomes was queried against the database using blastn to recover whether it had significant hits for each component of the AAI.

Data Submission

The short read sequence data has been deposited in the NCBI Short Read Archive under the BioProject PRJNA245029

Table 2. Number of mapped reads to the EAEC virulence genes in each outbreak isolate.

Isolate Number	Isolate ID	Serotype	AggR	aatA	aap	sepA	IDI	aaiC
1	216/13	O104:H4	1001	759	752	387	631	1780
2	218/13	O104:H4	1752	1783	874	443	1278	2213
3	1062/13	O104:H4	1932	1593	1525	805	1360	2195
4	1063/13	O104:H4	1483	1145	1133	733	1056	1165
5	1070/13	O104:H4	1554	1345	866	434	897	3219
6	0219/13	O131:H27	1799	799	540	128	591	2335
7	0220/13	O131:H27	1792	739	563	172	584	2683
8	1071/13	O131:H27	3501	1705	1054	347	1123	2228
9	1072/13	O131:H27	5185	2300	1607	366	1472	5146
10	1073/13	O131:H27	3337	1599	973	273	999	1879
11	1074/13	O131:H27	5160	2455	1357	378	1566	1943
12	0215/13	O20:H19	1826	1545	831	271	781	1841
13	0221/13	O20:H19	757	615	366	136	264	1390
14	0222/13	O19a:H30	685	568	493	118	393	**0**
15	1061/13	O55:H19	1813	1859	1206	355	1127	1598
16	1065/13	O63:H12	2339	2313	1448	383	1558	**2**
17	0214/13	O?:H19	2380	1963	1901	**32**	1533	**270**
18	0217/13	O33:H16	794	620	716	**10**	827	2842
19	1064/13	O?:H21	3008	3045	2159	**1**	2291	**0**
20	1060/13	O111:H4	**0**	**0**	**0**	**0**	**0**	**193**

Where the average coverage is less than 10% across the length of the gene the cell in the table is highlighted in bold.

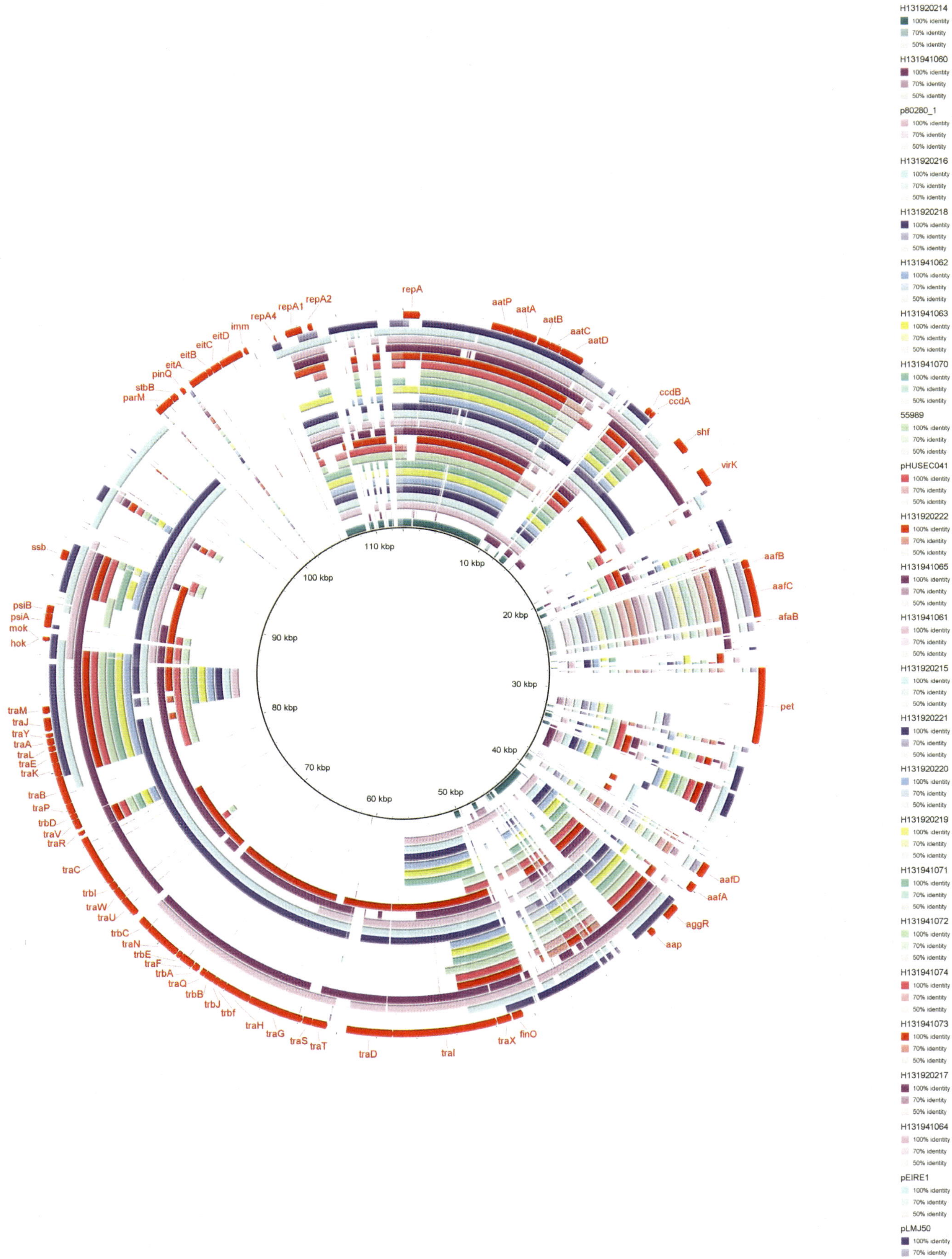
repA
aatP
aatA
aatB
aatC
aatD
ccdB
ccdA
shf
virK
aafB
aafC
afaB
pet
aafD
aafA
aggR
aap
finO
traX
traI
traD
traT
traS
traG
traH
trbf
trbJ
trbB
traQ
trbA
traF
trbE
traN
trbC
traU
traW
trbI
traC
traR
traV
trbD
traP
traB
traK
traE
traL
traA
traY
traJ
traM
hok
mok
psiA
psiB
ssb
parM
stbB
pinQ
eitA
eitB
eitC
eitD
imm
repA4
repA1
repA2
110 kbp
10 kbp
20 kbp
30 kbp
40 kbp
50 kbp
60 kbp
70 kbp
80 kbp
90 kbp
100 kbp
H131920214
100% identity
70% identity
50% identity
H131941060
100% identity
70% identity
50% identity
p80280_1
100% identity
70% identity
50% identity
H131920216
100% identity
70% identity
50% identity
H131920218
100% identity
70% identity
50% identity
H131941062
100% identity
70% identity
50% identity
H131941063
100% identity
70% identity
50% identity
H131941070
100% identity
70% identity
50% identity
55989
100% identity
70% identity
50% identity
pHUSEC041
100% identity
70% identity
50% identity
H131920222
100% identity
70% identity
50% identity
H131941065
100% identity
70% identity
50% identity
H131941061
100% identity
70% identity
50% identity
H131920215
100% identity
70% identity
50% identity
H131920221
100% identity
70% identity
50% identity
H131920220
100% identity
70% identity
50% identity
H131920219
100% identity
70% identity
50% identity
H131941071
100% identity
70% identity
50% identity
H131941072
100% identity
70% identity
50% identity
H131941074
100% identity
70% identity
50% identity
H131941073
100% identity
70% identity
50% identity
H131920217
100% identity
70% identity
50% identity
H131941064
100% identity
70% identity
50% identity
pEIRE1
100% identity
70% identity
50% identity
pLMJ50
100% identity
70% identity
50% identity

Figure 3. Assembled genomes displayed as concentric rings using BRIG and BLASTed against pAA genbank file as a reference. Coloured bars represent regions of homology. The darker shades represent a high percentage similarity, lighter shades represent lower levels of similarity and the absence of colour signifies absence of the gene.

Results

Detection of multiple GI pathogens by PCR

Retrospectively, 88 specimens from cases associated with the outbreak were tested for the presence of other bacterial GI pathogens using a multiplex GI pathogens PCR [24]. A variety of bacterial GI pathogens were detected by PCR from 88 of the stored faecal specimens from cases associated with the outbreak including *Salmonella* (3 cases), STEC (5 cases) and *Shigella* (29 cases). The *aggR* gene was identified in 65 (75%) specimens. Twenty strains of EAEC harbouring *aggR* were isolated from the 65 PCR positive faecal specimens. No STEC or *Shigella* species were isolated.

Phylogeny of EAEC isolated from the cases associated with the outbreak

Ten different serotypes and nine MLSTs were identified among the EAEC isolated from the outbreak cases (Table 1). The most commonly observed serotypes were O131:H27 (6), O104:H4 (5) and O20:H19 (2), and the most frequently identified STs, corresponding with these serotypes, were ST10, ST678 and ST278 respectively.

SNP analysis confirmed that the strains were phylogenetically diverse between serotypes (Figure 1). Strains belonging to the same serotype clustered on the same branch of the tree, however, even within the same serotype, isolates were phylogenetically distinct. Figure 2 shows a phylogeny based on 3115 core SNPs of 14 strains of *E. coli* O104:H4 and illustrates the relationship between the EAEC O104:H4 strains in this study with sporadic strains of *E. coli* O104:H4 and the strain associated with the *E. coli* O104:H4 outbreak in Germany in 2011 [22,23]. Although none of the EAEC O104:H4 isolates in this study had the *stx* gene they share a common ancestor with the German outbreak strain 280/11 and the sporadic *stx* harboring enteroaggregative strains characterised by Grad *et al* (23). All five strains of *E. coli* O104:H4 isolated during this study share the MDR genomic island conferring resistance to ampicillin, the sulphonamides, streptomycin and tetracycline, and the S83A gyrA mutation in common with German outbreak strain and the closely related EAEC/STEC sporadic isolates from France. The EAEC O104:H4 strains isolated in this study are phylogenetically integrated with strains of EAEC/STEC suggesting either multiple gain or gain then loss of the *stx* phage within the O104:H4 serotype.

None of the EAEC O104:H4 isolates in this study had the *stx* gene or carried the extended spectrum beta lactamase (ESBL) plasmid characteristic of the 280/11 strain, although three other strains isolated during this study were identified phenotypically and genotypically as being ESBL-producers (Table 1).

Replicon types of the EAEC plasmids encoding the key enteroaggregative virulence genes (pEAEC)

Multiple replicon types were observed with multiple combinations of FII and FIB proteins, with all but three plasmids having both the FIB and FII replicon types (Table1). Plasmids of type FIB5_FII17 were carried by strains belonging to two serotypes, O131:H27 and O20:H19. The plasmid type FIB25_FII48 harboured by the strains of EAEC O104:H4 was the same FIB/FII type described in the strains of *E. coli* O104:H4 linked to the 2011 German outbreak (Table 1).

pEAEC encoded virulence genes and genomic architecture

Several plasmid encoded genes associated with EAEC have been described in previous studies. These include the transcriptional activator *aggR*, the anti-aggregation transporter locus *aat*, the anti-aggregative dispersin protein *aap* (2–4), the aggregative adherence fimbriae (AAF) (30–34), the serine protease autotransporter toxin *SepA* [38] and the recently described putative isopentenyl isomerase (IDI) enzymes [39]. Table 2 shows the number of reads that mapped to these targets in each outbreak isolate. All of the strains, apart from *E. coli* O111:H4 designated 1060/13, had sequence reads that mapped to *aggR, aat, aap* and the putative IDI enzymes. This isolate originally tested positive with the *aggR* PCR subsequently tested negative following storage on Dorset Egg medium at room temperature. It is likely that this isolate lost the EAEC plasmid during storage. The serine protease *sepA* was present in 16 of the 20 EAEC strains isolated from the cases associated with the outbreak. Whilst the pEAEC virulence gene complement was conserved, the genomic context in terms of flanking IS elements was highly variable across the different plasmids (Figure 3).

Five types of pEAEC associated AAF have been described [33–37] and all five fimbriae types were identified in the strains analysed during this study. Strains of EAEC belonging to serotypes O104:H4 and O131:H27 had AAF/I fimbriae, as seen in the aggregative plasmid of *E. coli* O104:H4 linked to the 2011 German outbreak. Those strains belonging to serotype O20:H19 had the Type IV fimbriae (HdaA) [36]. AAF/II, AAF/III and AAF/V fimbriae were detected in five strains belonging to five different serotypes but three harbouring the same plasmid type, FIB33_FII1 (Table 2).

AAI operon encoding the putative T6SS

A 117 kb pathogenicity island, first described in the chromosome of EAEC 042, has been implicated as an EAEC pathogenicity factor. Twenty-five contiguous genes (*aaiA–Y*) in this island were previously shown to be transcriptionally activated by the plasmid encoded AggR protein and encoded for a T6SS [5]. In the EAEC strains isolated from the outbreak cases described in this study, the AAI operon was present in its entirety in the strains belonging to serotypes O104:H4, O131:H27, O20:H19 and O55:H19, whilst the island was absent in the strains belonging to the serotypes O19a:H30, O?:H21 and O63:H12 (Figure 3). Table 3 shows the distribution of the putative T6SS genes, *aaiA* to *aaiN*, in the outbreak strains. In the EAEC strains designated 1060/13 and 0214/13 (serotypes O111:H4 and O?:H19 respectively), a contig with 84% identity to the AAI operon and no homology to the NCBI non-redundant database was identified. In the EAEC O?:H19 isolate this homologue to *aai* was co-located on a contig with a plasmid addiction system suggestive of a non-chromosomal location in these strains.

Discussion

Historically, outbreaks have been associated with strains of a single pathogen exhibiting similar, if not identical, phenotypic and genotypic characteristics. However, the multiplex PCR approach to detection of GI pathogens directly from faecal specimens has provided good evidence that many individual cases of diarrhoea

Table 3. The distribution of the putative T6SS genes *aaiA* to *aaiN* in the outbreak strains.

Serotypes									
Gene	**O104:H4**	**O33:H27**	**O20:H19**	**O55:H19**	**O111:H4**	**O?:H19**	**O19a:H30**	**O63:H12**	**O?:H21**
aaiA	X	X	X	X	X	X			
aaiB	X	X	X	X	X	X			
aaiC	X	X	X	X					
aaiD	X	X	X	X	X	X			
aaiE	X	X	X	X	X	X			
aaiF	X	X	X	X	X	X			
aaiG	X	X	X	X	X	X			
aaiH	X	X	X	X					
aaiI	X	X	X	X					
aaiJ	X	X	X	X	X	X			
aaiK	X	X	X	X	X	X			
aaiL	X	X	X	X	X	X			
aaiM	X	X	X	X	X	X			
aaiN	X	X	X	X	X	X			

X indicates the genes was present on the genome.

and outbreaks of GI disease are associated with multiple pathogens [40–41]. Although there was clear microbiology evidence that established GI pathogens, such as *Salmonella* and *Shigella* species, played a significant part, the symptoms described by the cases and the presence of *aggR* in 75% of the specimens retrospectively tested by PCR, suggested that certain serotypes of the EAEC isolated, contributed to the GI disease associated with this outbreak. However, the variety of EAEC serotypes identified in the 20 strains isolated presented a complex picture.

Initially, it was suggested that the variation in serotype in the outbreak strains was masking a closer phylogenetic relationship. However, the phylogenetic tree created by comparing SNPs in the core genome showed that, although strains of the same serotype were relatively closely related, those of different serotypes were diverse. EAEC belong to several lineages with different evolutionary histories demonstrating independent acquisition of the plasmids encoding EAEC virulence genes [42]. Conversely, strains with a recent common ancestor, e.g. those that share an MLST sequence type, may have different pathotypes [43]. For example, *E. coli* O104:H4 ST678 has been shown to be STEC and EAEC [19]. The pathotype distribution is explained with multiple loss/gain events of pathogenicity elements.

Although strains of EAEC have been shown to harbour a wide diversity of plasmids that encode the enteroaggregative phenotype even in conserved chromosomal backgrounds [19], it was considered possible that similar plasmids would be found in the different strains of EAEC linked to this outbreak, given their spatial and temporal association. However, analysis of the plasmid genomes showed that they demonstrated a high level of variation in replicon type, gene content and genomic architecture. Some plasmid similarity was seen within strains of the same MLST and serotype but wide diversity was observed between different MLST and serotypes. The interspersing of different plasmids in the phylogeny suggests that the aggregative phenotype (specifically the presence of *aggR, aat* and *aap*) has been acquired by several different replicons of F-plasmids on multiple occasions. This level of strain and plasmid diversity has not previously been identified in isolates of EAEC from the same outbreak, although EAEC outbreaks involving more than one serotype and variation in pEAEC have been described previously [14,44]

Generally, *aggR, aat* and *aap* were conserved between strains of EAEC linked to this outbreak but a variety of fimbrial genes were identified. The presence of AAF is required for mediating the aggregative adherence seen in EAEC. To date five non-homologous AAF fimbiral structural proteins have been described and a representative of each was identified in strains belonging to this outbreak.

aaiA-P comprise a T6SS apparatus for *aaiC* and was the first example of a conserved chromosomal aggregative genotype whose expression is under the control of a conserved plasmid encoded pathogenicity factor *AggR* [5]. In this study, five isolates all harbouring *aggR* and *aat*, had a missing or an incomplete AAI operon. This raises a question regarding the pathogenic potential of the *aggR*-positive but AAI operon deficient strains, in relation to those *aggR*-positive strains with complete AAI cassettes. Previous prevalence studies detecting the *aaiA* show its presence in between 26 and 44% of phenotypic aggregative *E. coli* [45,46]. Animal models for investigating EAEC virulence have been described previously [47] and further virulence studies are required. Interestingly, two strains (EAEC O111:H4 and O?:H19) had incomplete AAI operons encoding a T6SS. These regions were homologous to those found in serotypes O104:H4, O131:H27, O20:H19 and O55:H19 but with a different *aaiC* component. In addition, there was some evidence that it may be plasmid-encoded.

It was suggested that certain strains of EAEC may have been carried asymptomatically by the cases before the outbreak occurred. Hwoever, it was not possible to compare the serotypes isolates following the outbreak with the serotypes of strains of EAEC currently circulating in England as there are very little data on domestically acquired strains of EAEC. Surveillance data indicates that the majority of strains of EAEC isolate in England are from cases of travellers' diarrhoea [12,50].

One hypothesis is that not all the strains of EAEC associated with this outbreak had the same level of pathogenicity and that only certain EAEC serotypes isolated contributed to the symptoms described. For example, a complete AAI operon may increase the pathogenic potential of strains of *E. coli* harbouring the pEAEC. Other studies have suggested that strains harbouring different fimbrial types maybe more pathogenic that others. Nüesch-Inderbinen *et al.* (2013) [48] showed a statistically significant association of the agg3C gene with the asymptomatic state. The presence of AAF/I and AAF/II have been associated with symptomatic cases [6,49].

Importantly, although colonies of EAEC O104:H4 were isolated from only five outbreak cases, all faecal specimens were retrospectively tested by PCR for the presence of the O104 O-antigen gene (*wzx*O104) [51]. The PCR detected *wzx*O104 in faecal specimens from 36 cases. The EAEC serotype O104:H4, with and without *stx2*, has been previously identified as a cause of GI disease. Furthermore, although the EAEC O104:H4 in this study did not carry the *stx* genes, this outbreak provides further evidence of the pathogenic potential of this EAEC serotype. EAEC is known to be a diverse pathotype and this study demonstrates this diversity can be seen within a single outbreak.

Acknowledgments

We would like to acknowledge Jennifer Collins and Michelle Payne at Newcastle PHE Regional Laboratory for their microbiological expertise. We would also like to thank Martin Day for producing the antibiotic resistance data. We are grateful to Dr Rohini Manuel and colleagues at Public Health Laboratory London for supporting the use of the GI multiplex PCR for outbreak investigations.

Author Contributions

Conceived and designed the experiments: TD LC MD RT AU KF KG CJ. Performed the experiments: TD MC LC DW DR KF CJ. Analyzed the data: TD LC CJ. Contributed reagents/materials/analysis tools: TD LC MD JW DR KF. Wrote the paper: TD KF KG CJ.

References

1. Nataro JP, Kaper JB, Robins-Browne R, Prado V, Vial P, et al. (1987) Patterns of adherence of diarrheagenic *Escherichia coli* to HEp-2 cells. Pediatr Infect Dis J 6: 829–31.
2. Nataro JP, Yikang D, Yingkang D, Walker K (1994) AggR, a transcriptional activator of aggregative adherence fimbria I expression in enteroaggregative *Escherichia coli*. J Bacteriol 176: 4691–9
3. Sheikh J, Czeczulin JR, Harrington S, Hicks S, Henderson IR, et al. (2002) A novel dispersin protein in enteroaggregative *Escherichia coli*. J Clin Invest 110: 1329–37.
4. Nishi J, Sheikh J, Mizuguchi K, Luisi B, Burland V, et al. (2003) The export of coat protein from enteroaggregative *Escherichia coli* by a specific ATP-binding cassette transporter system. J Biol Chem 278: 45680–9.
5. Dudley EG, Thomson NR, Parkhill J, Morin NP, Nataro JP (2006) Proteomic and microarray characterization of the AggR regulon identifies a pheU

pathogenicity island in enteroaggregative *Escherichia coli*. Mol Microbiol 61: 1267–82.
6. Jenkins C, Chart H, Willshaw GA, Cheasty T, Tompkins DS (2007) Association of putative pathogenicity genes with adherence characteristics and fimbrial genotypes in typical enteroaggregative Escherichia coli from patients with and without diarrhoea in the United Kingdom. Eur J Clin Microbiol Infect Dis 26: 901–6
7. Jenkins C, Tembo M, Chart H, Cheasty T, Willshaw GA, et al. (2006a) Detection of enteroaggregative *Escherichia coli* in faecal samples from patients in the community with diarrhoea. J Med Microbiol 55: 1493–7
8. Boisen N, Scheutz F, Rasko DA, Redman JC, Persson S, et al. (2012) Genomic characterization of enteroaggregative *Escherichia coli* from children in Mali. J Infect Dis 205: 431–44.
9. Okeke IN, Wallace-Gadsden F, Simons HR, Matthews N, Labar AS, et al. (2010) Multi-locus sequence typing of enteroaggregative *Escherichia coli* isolates from Nigerian children uncovers multiple lineages. PLoS One 5:e14093.
10. Okeke IN, Nataro JP (2001) Enteroaggregative *Escherichia coli*. Lancet Infect Dis 1(5):304–13. Review
11. Nataro JP, Mai V, Johnson J, Blackwelder WC, Heimer R, et al. (2006) Diarrheagenic *Escherichia coli* infection in Baltimore, Maryland, and New Haven, Connecticut. Clin Infect Dis 43: 402–7.
12. Wilson A, Evans J, Chart H, Cheasty T, Wheeler JG, et al. (2001) Characterisation of strains of enteroaggregative *Escherichia coli* isolated during the infectious intestinal disease study in England. Eur J Epidemiol 17: 1125–30.
13. Itoh Y, Nagano I, Kunishima M, Ezaki T (1997) Laboratory investigation of enteroaggregative *Escherichia coli* O untypeable:H10 associated with a massive outbreak of gastrointestinal illness. J Clin Microbiol 35: 2546–50
14. Smith HR, Cheasty T, Rowe B (1997) Enteroaggregative *Escherichia coli* and outbreaks of gastroenteritis in UK. Lancet 350: 814–5.
15. Scavia G, Staffolani M, Fisichella S, Striano G, Colletta S, et al. (2008) Enteroaggregative *Escherichia coli* associated with a foodborne outbreak of gastroenteritis. J Med Microbiol 7: 1141–6.
16. Frank C, Werber D, Cramer JP, Askar M, Faber M, et al. (2011) Epidemic profile of Shiga-toxin-producing *Escherichia coli* O104:H4 outbreak in Germany. N Engl J Med 365: 1771–80.
17. Mellmann A, Harmsen D, Cummings CA, Zentz EB, Leopold SR, et al. (2011) Prospective genomic characterization of the German enterohemorrhagic *Escherichia coli* O104:H4 outbreak by rapid next generation sequencing technology. PLoS One. 6:e22751.
18. Bielaszewska M, Mellmann A, Zhang W, Köck R, Fruth A, et al. (2011) Characterisation of the *Escherichia coli* strain associated with an outbreak of haemolytic uraemic syndrome in Germany, 2011: a microbiological study. Lancet Infect Di 11: 671–6.
19. Rasko DA, Webster DR, Sahl JW, Bashir A, Boisen N, et al. (2011) Origins of the *E. coli* strain causing an outbreak of hemolytic-uremic syndrome in Germany. N Engl J Med. 365: 709–17.
20. King LA, Nogareda F, Weill FX, Mariani-Kurkdjian P, Loukiadis E, et al. (2012) Outbreak of Shiga toxin-producing Escherichia coli O104:H4 associated with organic fenugreek sprouts, France, June 2011. Clin Infect Dis. 54: 1588–94.
21. Buchholz U, Bernard H, Werber D, Böhmer MM, Remschmidt C, et al. (2011) German outbreak of *Escherichia coli* O104:H4 associated with sprouts. N Engl J Med. 365: 1763–70
22. Grad YH, Lipsitch M, Feldgarden M, Arachchi HM, Cerqueira GC, et al. (2012) Genomic epidemiology of the *Escherichia coli* O104:H4 outbreaks in Europe, 2011. Proc Natl Acad Sci U S A. 109: 3065–70.
23. Grad YH, Godfrey P, Cerquiera GC, Mariani-Kurkdjian P, Gouali M, et al. (2013) Comparative genomics of recent Shiga toxin-producing Escherichia coli O104:H4: short-term evolution of an emerging pathogen. MBio. 4:e00452–12.
24. Moran-Gilad J, Chand M, Brown C, Shetty N, Morris G, et al. (2012) Microbiological aspects of public health planning and preparedness for the 2012 Olympic Games. Epidemiol Infect 140: 2142–51.
25. Bankevich A, Nurk S, Antipov D, Gurevich AA, Dvorkin M, et al. (2012) SPAdes: a new genome assembly algorithm and its applications to single-cell sequencing. J Comput Biol 19: 455–77
26. Li H, Durbin R (2010) Fast and accurate long-read alignment with Burrows-Wheeler transform. Bioinformatics 26: 589–95.
27. Li H, Handsaker B, Wysoker A, Fennell T, Ruan J, et al. (2009) The Sequence Alignment/Map format and SAMtools. Bioinformatics 25: 2078–9.
28. McKenna A, Hanna M, Banks E, Sivachenko A, Cibulskis K, et al. (2010) The Genome Analysis Toolkit: a MapReduce framework for analyzing next-generation DNA sequencing data. Genome Res 20: 1297–303.
29. Price MN, Dehal PS, Arkin AP (2010) FastTree 2 - approximately maximum-likelihood trees for large alignments. PLoS One 5: e9490.
30. Inouye M, Conwa TC, Zobel J, Holt KE (2012) Short read sequence typing (SRST): multi-locus sequence types from short reads. BMC Genomics 13: 338
31. Carattoli A, Bertini A, Villa L, Falbo V, Hopkins KL, et al. (2005) Identification of plasmids by PCR-based replicon typing. J Microbiol Methods 63: 219–28.
32. Alikhan NF, Petty NK, Ben Zakour NL, Beatson SA (2011). BLAST Ring Image Generator (BRIG): Simple prokaryote genome comparisons. *BMC genomics* 12, 402.
33. Nataro JP, Deng Y, Maneval DR, German AL, Martin WC, et al. (1992) Infect Aggregative adherence fimbriae I of enteroaggregative *Escherichia coli* mediate adherence to HEp-2 cells and hemagglutination of human erythrocytes. Immun 60: 2297–304.
34. Czeczulin JR, Balepur S, Hicks S, Phillips A, Hall R, et al. (1997) Aggregative adherence fimbria II, a second fimbrial antigen mediating aggregative adherence in enteroaggregative *Escherichia coli*. Infect Immun 65: 4135–45
35. Bernier C, Gounon P, Le Bouguénec C (2002) Identification of an aggregative adhesion fimbria (AAF) type III-encoding operon in enteroaggregative *Escherichia coli* as a sensitive probe for detecting the AAF-encoding operon family. Infect Immun 70: 4302–11.
36. Boisen N, Struve C, Scheutz F, Krogfelt KA, Nataro JP (2008) New adhesin of enteroaggregative *Escherichia coli* related to the Afa/Dr/AAF family. Infect Immun 76: 3281–92.
37. Dallman T, Smith GP, O'Brien B, Chattaway MA, Finlay D, et al. (2012) Characterization of a verocytotoxin-producing enteroaggregative *Escherichia coli* serogroup O111:H21 strain associated with a household outbreak in Northern Ireland. J Clin Microbiol 50: 4116–9.
38. Boisen N, Ruiz-Perez F, Scheutz F, Krogfelt KA, Nataro JP (2009) Short report: high prevalence of serine protease autotransporter cytotoxins among strains of enteroaggregative *Escherichia coli*. Am J Trop Med Hyg 80: 294–301
39. Morin N, Santiago AE, Ernst RK, Guillot SJ, Nataro JP (2013) Characterization of the AggR regulon in enteroaggregative *Escherichia coli*. Infect Immun 81: 122–32.
40. Tam CC, Rodrigues LC, Viviani L, Dodds JP, Evans MR, et al. (2013) Burden and aetiology of diarrhoeal disease in infants and young children in developing countries (the Global Enteric Multicenter Study, GEMS): a prospective, case-control study. Gut. 61: 69–77.
41. Kotloff KL, Nataro JP, Blackwelder WC, Nasrin D, Farag TH, et al. (2013) Lancet 382: 209–22.
42. Ogura Y, Ooka T, Iguchi A, Toh H, Asadulghani M, et al. (2009) Comparative genomics reveal the mechanism of the parallel evolution of O157 and non-O157 enterohemorrhagic *Escherichia coli*. Proc Natl Acad Sci U S A. 106: 17939–44.
43. Wirth T, Falush D, Lan R, Colles F, Mensa P, et al. (2006) Sex and virulence in *Escherichia coli*: an evolutionary perspective. Mol Microbiol 60: 1136–51.
44. Spencer J, Smith HR, Chart H (1999) Characterization of enteroaggregative *Escherichia coli* isolated from outbreaks of diarrhoeal disease in England. Epidemiol Infect 123: 413–21.
45. Jenkins C, Chart H, Willshaw GA, Cheasty T, Smith HR (2006b) Genotyping of enteroaggregative *Escherichia coli* and identification of target genes for the detection of both typical and atypical strains. Diagn Microbiol Infect Dis 55: 13–9.
46. Jenkins C, van Ijperen C, Dudley EG, Chart H, Willshaw GA, et al. (2005) Use of a microarray to assess the distribution of plasmid and chromosomal virulence genes in strains of enteroaggregative *Escherichia coli*. FEMS Microbiol Lett 253: 119–24.
47. Hwang J, Mattei LM, VanArendonk LG, Meneely PM, Okeke IN (2010) A pathoadaptive deletion in an enteroaggregative *Escherichia coli* outbreak strain enhances virulence in a *Caenorhabditis elegans* model. Infect Immun 78: 4068–76.
48. Nüesch-Inderbinen MT, Hofer E, Hächler H, Beutin L, Stephan R (2013) Characteristics of enteroaggregative *Escherichia coli* isolated from healthy carriers and from patients with diarrhoea. Med Microbiol doi: 10.1099/jmm.0.065177-0. [Epub ahead of print]
49. Okeke IN, Lamikanra A, Czeczulin J, Dubovsky F, Kaper JB (2000) Heterogeneous virulence of enteroaggregative *Escherichia coli* strains isolated from children in Southwest Nigeria. J Infect Dis 181: 252–60.
50. Perry N, Jenkins C, Cheasty T, Wain J (2010) Diarrhoeagenic Escherichia coli from routine diagnostic faecal samples in England and Wales. J Med Microbiol. 59: 870–2.
51. Scheutz F, Nielsen EM, Frimodt-Møller J, Boisen N, Morabito S, et al. (2011) Characteristics of the enteroaggregative Shiga toxin/verotoxin-producing *Escherichia coli* O104:H4 strain causing the outbreak of haemolytic uraemic syndrome in Germany, May to June 2011. Euro Surveill 16(24).

Predominance of Norovirus and Sapovirus in Nicaragua after Implementation of Universal Rotavirus Vaccination

Filemón Bucardo[1], Yaoska Reyes[1], Lennart Svensson[2], Johan Nordgren[2]*

1 Department of Microbiology, University of León (UNAN-León), León, Nicaragua, **2** Division of Molecular Virology, Department of Clinical and Experimental Medicine, Linköping University, Linköping, Sweden

Abstract

Background: Despite significant reduction of rotavirus (RV) infections following implementation of RotaTeq vaccination in Nicaragua, a large burden of patients with diarrhea persists.

Methods: We conducted a community- and hospital-based study of the burden of RV, norovirus (NV) and sapovirus (SV) infections as cause of sporadic acute gastroenteritis (GE) among 330 children $\leq$ 5 years of age between September 2009 and October 2010 in two major cities of Nicaragua with a RotaTeq coverage rate of 95%.

Results: We found that NV, SV and RV infections altogether accounted for 45% of cases of GE. Notably, NV was found in 24% (79/330) of the children, followed by SV (17%, 57/330) and RV (8%, 25/330). The detection rate in the hospital setting was 27%, 15% and 14% for NV, SV and RV respectively, whereas in the community setting the detection rate of RV was $<$ 1%. Among each of the investigated viruses one particular genogroup or genotype was dominant; GII.4 (82%) for NV, GI (46%) for SV and G1P[8] (64%) in RV. These variants were also found in higher proportions in the hospital setting compared to the community setting. The GII.4.2006 Minerva strain circulating globally since 2006 was the most common among genotyped NV in this study, with the GII.4-2010 New Orleans emerging in 2010.

Conclusions: This study shows that NV has become the leading viral cause of gastroenteritis at hospital and community settings in Nicaragua after implementation of RV vaccination.

Editor: Li-Min Huang, National Taiwan University Hospital, Taiwan

Funding: This study was supported by grants from the Network for Research and Training in Tropical Diseases in Central America (NeTropica, Grant:05-N-2010) and Swedish Research Council (grants 10392 and 348-2011-7420). The funders had no role in study design, data collection and analysis, decision to publish, or preparation of the manuscript.

Competing Interests: The authors have declared that no competing interests exist.

* E-mail: johan.nordgren@liu.se

Introduction

Acute gastroenteritis (GE) is one of the leading causes of morbidity and mortality in children in the developing countries, with rotavirus (RV) and norovirus (NV) being the major causes of pediatric viral GE, altogether associated with approximately 800,000 deaths in young children every year [1–3]. In contrast, sapovirus (SV) infections are more rarely reported and generally considered to cause milder symptoms, with detection rates rarely reaching 10% [4–8].

A major reduction of severe RVGE has been observed in countries with high vaccine coverage but comprehensive analysis in several clinical trials indicates the vaccine efficacy to be lower in countries with high RV mortality [9,10]. In October 2006, the Nicaraguan Expanded Program of Immunization (EPI) initiated universal RV vaccination with the pentavalent RV vaccine from Merck (RotaTeq), which is orally administrated in a 3-dose regimen to children at 2, 4, and 6 months of age. Vaccine coverage rapidly reached over $>$ 90% in eligible Nicaraguan children [11]. A case control study evaluating RotaTeq in 2007–2008 in Nicaragua showed that vaccination was associated with a lower risk of RVGE in children younger than 2 years [12], but to a lesser extent than observed in clinical trials in Europe and USA [13]. The efficacy in Nicaragua against severe RV diarrhea was only 58%, which is similar to other studies from Asian and African countries [12,14,15]. In the post-vaccine period, a study found that 3.5% of outpatient children seeking care for diarrhea were positive for RV [16]. However, while RV incidence has decreased in Nicaragua, the overall number of GE cases of any etiology has remained at high levels after RV vaccine introduction [17]. A recent paper reports that a pre-vaccine community cohort experienced 36 episodes of watery diarrhea per 100 child-years, whereas a vaccine cohort experienced 25 episodes per 100 child-years, indicating a 60% persistence of watery diarrhea at community level during the vaccine era [18].

A non-specific effect of RV vaccine on GE of other etiologies has been suggested in a few studies [19–21]. However, this effect is still speculative and whether RV vaccination has any effect on NVGE or SVGE remains to be established.

In this study we investigated the virological causes behind the burden of diarrhea that persists after implementation of universal RV vaccination in Nicaragua. We thus explored the relative frequency of NV, SV and RV, both at hospital and community level in Nicaragua during 2009/2010 in the context of high RV vaccination rates. In addition we explored the association of these relative frequencies with RV vaccination status, dehydration status, and virus genotypes/genogroups.

Materials and Methods

Ethics statement

The study protocol and consent procedure was approved by the local ethical committee for biometrics research (Comite de Etica para Investigaciones Biomedicas [CEIB]; registration number: 61-2005, 73-2010). Informed written consent was given by parents or child guardians before samples were collected as described below. After the consent was given, personal details, as well as, epidemiological data were recorded in a paper file.

Study Design

Through a community- and hospital-based passive surveillance of sporadic acute diarrhea, a total of 330 children of ≤ 5 years of age with acute diarrhea were enrolled in a longitudinal, prospective manner from September 2009 to October 2010. In the hospital setting children (n = 175) were enrolled at the pediatric wards and emergency rooms from main hospitals of León and Jinotega, Nicaragua (Hospital Escuela "Oscar Danilo Rosales and Victoria Motta, respectively). Community children (n = 155) were outpatients consulting for diarrhea at two clinics of León.

Clinical assessment

All children involved in the study were clinically evaluated by pediatricians (hospital) or general practitioners (community) and classified by dehydration status, following the WHO protocol for integrated management of childhood illness (IMCI), into one of the following categories: "severe-dehydration", "some-dehydration", and "without-dehydration".

RotaTeq immunization assessment

The dates each child received vaccine doses in Nicaragua were registered by an EPI nurse on the child's vaccination-card. The RotaTeq immunization data used in this study were collected from the children's vaccination-cards. A child was considered "unvaccinated" if their vaccination card showed no recorded doses. If the child's vaccination card was not available, immunization status was considered unknown.

Collection of stool specimens

Fecal specimens were collected in sterile containers ≤ 24 h after admission, and transported either weekly (Jinotega) or daily (Leo at 4°C to the microbiology laboratory of UNAN-León. At the two outpatient clinics, fecal samples were collected by a nurse during the visit. Before transportation, samples were stored at 4°C at the collection site to ensure quality of virological testing. A 10% (wt/vol) suspension of stool material was prepared with phosphate-buffered saline (pH = 7.2), and two aliquots were frozen at 20°C for later examination of RV, NV and SV.

RV antigen detection

A direct enzyme immunoassay for detection of RV in fecal specimens, OXOID ProSpecT R240396 (Cambridge, UK), was used according to the manufacturer's instructions. The results were visually read and confirmed by absorbance measurements.

RNA extraction from stool specimens

Viral RNA was extracted from stool suspensions (200 µl) following the manufacturer's instructions using High Pure Viral RNA Kit (Roche Applied Science, Indianapolis, USA). A total of 50 µl of RNA was collected and stored at −20°C until reverse transcription (RT).

Reverse transcription

Reverse transcription (RT) was carried out as described previously [22]. Briefly, 28 µl of purified RNA was mixed with 50 pmol of random hexadeoxynucleotides [pd(N)6] (GE Healthcare Life Sciences), and the mixture was denatured at 97°C for 5 min and quickly chilled on ice for 2 min, followed by the addition of one RT bead (Amersham Biosciences, UK) and RNase-free water to a final volume of 50 µl. RT reaction mixtures were incubated for 30 min at 42°C to produce complementary DNA (cDNA).

RV G and P multiplex genotyping

The G and P genotypes of RVs recovered from stool samples were determined by PCR. The generic and genotype-specific primers used for detecting VP7 genotypes G1, G2, G3, G4, G8, G9, G10, and G12 were described previously [23,24]. Primers used for detecting VP4 genotypes P[4], P[6], P[8], and P[9] were also described previously [23,25]. Genotypes and full genomic analysis of RV found in RotaTeq vaccinated children from Jinotega has been described previously [26].

NV detection by real-time PCR

In brief, 2.5 µl of purified RNA was added to a reaction mixture consisting of 12.5 µl of FastStart Universal SYBR Green Master (ROX) (Roche Applied Science, IN, USA), 1 µl (10 pmol) of each non-labeled GI and GII primers (NVG1f1b and NVG1rlux, NVG2flux1 and COG2R), [27] and 8 µl of RNAse free water, to final volume of 25 µl. The real-time PCR reactions were performed in a 96-well reaction plate using the ABI 7500 Real Time PCR System (Applied Biosystems, Foster, CA). PCR was performed under the following conditions: 95°C for 5 min, followed by 40 cycles of 95°C for 15 s, 55°C for 30 s and 72°C for 1 min. Melting curve analysis, to confirm amplicon specificity, was performed immediately after PCR completion.

NV GI and GII genogrouping

All NV-positive samples were re-analyzed by genogroup specific SYBR Green real-time PCR, in separate tubes, following the procedure described for NV screening but using specific primers for either GI or GII [27]. A sample was considered of NV GI and/or GII if the Ct value was ≤ 40 and Tm of 76.1 ± 0.6°C for GI and 77.1 ± 0.6°C for GII.

NV genotyping

A subset of NV-positive samples with sufficient viral load were sequenced in the N-terminal region of the capsid gene as described [22]. The 380-bp and 378-bp amplicons obtained from GI and GII NVs, respectively were sequenced by Macrogen Inc. (Seoul, South Korea)., using NVG1f1b, G1SKR, NVG2flux1 and G2SKR primers as sequencing primers [27,28]. Sequence alignment was performed by using the ClustalW algorithm, version 1.83, with default parameters on the European Bioinformatics Institute server (EMBL-EBI). Phylogenetic analysis was performed using the MEGA 5.03 software package and the tree was constructed using the neighbor-joining method with the Kimura two-parameter model [29]. The significance of phylogenetic relationships was assessed by bootstrap resampling analysis (1,000 replications). The assignment of genotypes was done using pairwise nucleotide distance measurements [30].

SV detection by real-time PCR

SV screening was carried out following a modification of the method described by Chan et al 2006 [31]. In brief, 2.5 µl of purified RNA was added to a reaction mixture consisting of 12.5 µl of 2X RT-PCR Buffer and 1 µl 25X RT-PCR Enzyme Mix (AgPath-ID One-Step RT-PCR kit, Life Technologies, NY, USA), 1 µl (10 pmol) of each forward (CUSVF1 and CUSVF2) and reverse primer (CUSVR), 1 µl (10 pmol) of SV TaqMan Probe (TaqMan MGB was replaced with [6FAM] TGG TTY ATA GGY GGT AC [BHQ1]), 1.67 µl of detection enhancer and 4.33 µl of RNAse free water, to final volume of 25 µl. The real-time PCR reactions were performed on a 7500 Real-Time PCR System (Applied Biosystems, Foster City, CA). A sample with Ct value ≤ 40 was considered positive.

SV genogrouping

The cDNA of SV-positive specimens were amplified by an outer PCR using a primer pool that consisted of two forward (SV-F13 and SV-F14), and two reverse (SV-R13 and SV-R14) primers with PCR conditions as described elsewhere [32]. Genogroups, GI, GII, GIV and GV, were examined by nested PCR under identical conditions to the outer PCR using a primer pool that consisted of universal forward primers (SV-F13/-F14) and genogroup specific reverse primers (SV-G1-R, SV-G2-R, SV-G4-R and SV-G5-R). The 500-bp, 430-bp, 360-bp and 290-bp amplicons obtained from GI, GII, GIV and GV viruses, respectively, were visualized by 2% agarose gel electrophoresis followed by ethidium bromide staining. Co-infections with SV of different genogroups was confirmed by allele specific PCR.

SV genotyping 1 of

The N-terminal region of the capsid gene (~ 420 bp) was sequenced in a subset of 23 SV-positive samples. A total of 1 µ PCR product from the outer PCR reaction, described in SV genogrouping section, 10 pmol of each of forward (F22) and reverse (R2) primers [32] and RNase-free water were added to one Illustra PuReTaq Ready-To-Go PCR Bead (GE Healthcare, Uppsala, Sweden) to a final volume of 25 µl. The PCR reaction was performed following the conditions described previously [32]. The 420-bp amplicons obtained from SV-positive samples were sequenced by Macrogen Inc. (Seoul, South Korea) using F22 and R2 primers as sequencing primers. The assignment of genotypes was done using pairwise nucleotide distance measurements.

Statistical analysis

Relative frequencies between viral etiologies and genetic variants were analyzed for setting, clinical and epidemiological variables to investigate trends or statistical differences. Unadjusted Odds ratios (OR) were used to determine the degree of association and Fisher's exact test was used to compare frequencies of qualitative variables. Differences were considered to be statistically significant when the level of two-tailed significance was < 0.05.

The softwares SPSS (Statistical Program for Social Science version 14.0 for Windows; Chicago, IL) and GraphPad Prism (version 5.00 for Windows, GraphPad Software, San Diego California USA) were used for statistical analysis.

Nucleotide sequence accession numbers

The nucleotide sequences for NV, SV and RV determined in this work were submitted to GenBank and the following accession numbers were assigned for Norovirus: KF361389 to KF361442; Sapovirus: KF361366 to KF361388 and Rotavirus: JN129124, JN129096, JN129110, JN129054, JN129068, JN129082, JN128984, JN128998, JN129012, JN129026, JN129040.

Results

High detection rates of viruses among children with diarrhea vaccinated with RotaTeq

In total, viral GE was associated with 147 (45%) of the 330 diarrheal children investigated. The RV vaccine coverage observed in the current study was 95% (270/284; Table 1). Of these, 213 (79%), 43 (16%) and 14 (5%) had received 3, 2 and 1 vaccine dose(s) respectively. For 46 children, the vaccination status was not known.

Norovirus was the major cause of pediatric gastroenteritis

NV was observed in 79 (24%) of the 330 children with diarrhea investigated in this study. In the hospital setting, NV was observed in 27% (n = 47) of the children and in the community setting NV was observed in 21% (n = 32) (OR = 1.4, $p = 0.2$). NV was furthermore observed in 15 (26%) of 57 children with severe dehydration (Table 1). NVGE was not gender-dependent and most children with NVGE were less than 24 months of age with a mean age of 12.2 months (median = 10.1) (Table 1). The major peak for NVGE was observed in June 2010, corresponding to the early rainy season in Nicaragua (Fig. 1). Similar rates of NVGE (24% vs 21%) were observed in RV vaccinated compared to non-vaccinated children.

The majority of norovirus were of genotype GII.4

Genogroups analysis showed that a total of 71 (90%) NV-positive belonged to GII followed by GI with 7 (9%) and co-infection with both GI:GII in one case (Table 2). To investigate the relative predominance of NV genotypes in hospital and community settings a subset of 55 NV-positive were genotyped by nt sequencing analysis (Table 2). The globally dominant GII.4 genotype was observed in 82% (45/55) of all genotyped cases. The GII.4 genotype was observed in 30 (94%) of the 32 genotyped cases from the hospital and in 15 (65%) of the 23 genotyped cases from the community (Table 2) (OR = 8.0, $p = 0.012$). Other detected genotypes were; GII.6, GII.14, GII.9, GI.3 and GI.2 all found in lesser proportions and mainly in the community (Table 1). The pandemic variant GII.4-2006b also known as Minerva was dominant among GII.4 (35/45) and circulated in 2009 and 2010 with high detection rates during the rainy season of 2010. The other detected GII.4 variant, GII.4-2010 (10/45), also known as New Orleans emerged in 2010. The epidemiological peak of GII.4 Minerva and New Orleans variants corresponded with the peak of NVGE and peak of total GE cases (Fig. 1).

Sapovirus was the second major cause of pediatric gastroenteritis

SV was observed in 57 (17%) of the 330 children with diarrhea investigated in this study (Table 1). In the hospital setting, SV was observed in 15% (n = 27) of the children, and in the community setting SV was observed in 19% (n = 30) (OR = 0.76, $p = 0.38$). Most of the SV were observed in children with no or mild dehydration (48/57; 84%). Similar to NV, SVGE was not gender-

Table 1. Epidemiological profile and dehydration status of norovirus, sapovirus and rotavirus infections in a population with high RotaTeq coverage in Nicaragua, 2009–2010.

Parameter	Total	Norovirus n (%)	Sapovirus n (%)	Rotavirus n (%)
All children	330[a]	79 (24)	57 (17)	25 (8)
Site				
León	227	57 (25)	44 (19)	8 (4)
Jinotega	103	22 (21)	13 (13)	17 (16)
Setting				
Hospital	175	47 (27)	27 (15)	24 (14)
Community	155	32 (21)	30 (19)	1 (1)
Gender				
Male	190	45 (24)	34 (18)	13 (7)
Female	140	34 (24)	23 (17)	12 (9)
Age range (mo)				
≤ 6	64	16 (25)	8 (12)	4 (6)
7–12	108	31 (29)	21 (19)	9 (8)
13–24	107	25 (23)	24 (22)	7 (7)
25–60	51	7 (14)	4 (8)	5 (10)
RV vaccination status				
Vaccinated	270	64 (24)	51 (19)	16 (6)
Unvaccinated	14	3 (21)	0 (0)	2 (14)
Unknown	46	12 (26)	6 (13)	7 (15)
Dehydration status				
Severe dehydration[b]	57	15 (26)	9 (16)	16 (28)
Some dehydration	98	28 (29)	14 (14)	7 (7)
No dehydration	175	36 (21)	34 (19)	2 (1)

[a]Detection rates of norovirus, sapovirus and rotavirus is calculated per line in the table; thus for the total number of children per parameter
[b]All children with severe dehydration required intravenous rehydration.

dependent, with the majority of children with SVGE (45/57, 79%) being 7–24 months of age (Table 1) (OR = 2.3, p = 0.02), with the mean age of 12.7 months (median = 11.8). As for NVGE; the epidemiological peak of SVGE was in June 2010 corresponding to the early rainy season (Fig. 1). SV infections occurred in (51/270) children having received at least one RotaTeq dose and nil (0/14) in non-immunized children (OR = 6.8, p = 0.08) (Table 1).

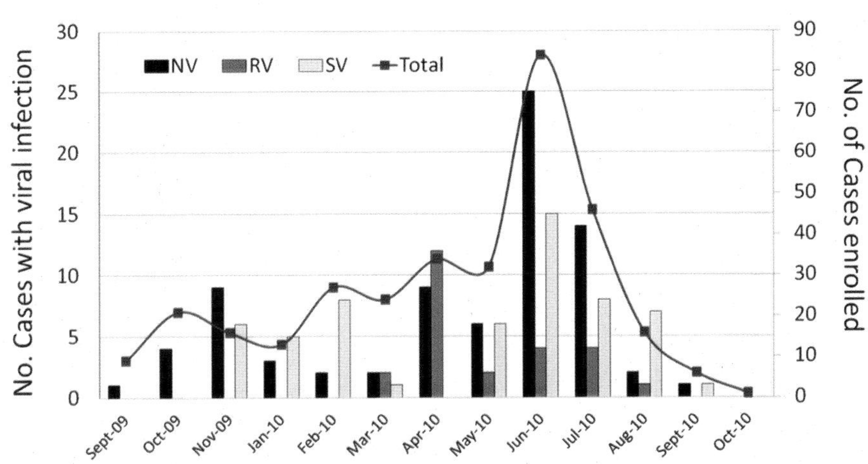

Figure 1. Temporal distribution of norovirus (NV), sapovirus (SV) and rotavirus (RV) infections in children with diarrhea ≤ 5 years of age, after national RotaTeq vaccination in Nicaragua, 2009–2010. Left Y axis; the black, grey and white bars represent monthly frequencies of NV, RV and SV, respectively. Right Y axis; the line represent monthly frequencies of gastroenteritis cases enrolled. The X axis represents seasonality, with the early rainy season typically starting in May and lasting until July.

Table. 2. Relative predominance between genetic variants of norovirus, sapovirus and rotavirus among children with gastroenteritis at hospital and community settings in Nicaragua, 2009–2010.

Genetic Variants	Both settings n (%)	Setting		OR[a] [95%, CI]; *p-value*[a]
		Hospital n (%)	Community n (%)	
Norovirus Genogroups				
GII	71 (90)	44 (94)	27 (84)	4.1 [0.74–22.5]; *0.12*
GI	7 (9)	2 (4)	5 (16)	0.25 [0.04–1.4]; *0.12*
GI:GII	1 (1)	1 (2)	0 (0)	NA[e]
Total	79 (100)	47 (100)	32 (100)	
Norovirus Genotypes				
GII.4[b]	45 (82)	30 (94)	15 (65)	8.0 [1.5–42]; *0.012*
GII Non-GII.4[c]	7 (13)	1 (3)	6 (26)	0.09 [0.01–0.82]; *0.017*
GI.3	2 (4)	1 (3)	1(4)	0.71 [0.04–12]; *1.0*
GI.2	1 (2)	0	1 (4)	NA
Total	55 (100)	32 (100)	23 (100)	
Sapovirus Genogroups				
GI	26 (46)	14 (52)	12 (40)	2.3[0.67–8.1]; *0.23*
GII	16 (28)	5 (19)	11 (37)	0.39 [0.11–1.4]; *0.21*
GIV	2 (3)	1 (4)	1 (3)	1.2 [0.07–21]; *1.0*
Mixed[d]	5 (9)	3 (11)	2 (7)	NA
Not genogrouped	8 (14)	4 (15)	4 (13)	NA
Total	57 (100)	27 (100)	30 (100)	
Sapovirus Genotypes				
GI/1	6 (27)	5 (36)	1 (12)	4.4 [0.42–47]; *0.34*
GI/2	8 (36)	7 (50)	1 (12)	8.0 [0.78–82]; *0.086*
GII/2	4 (14)	1 (7)	3 (25)	0.15 [0.01–1.8]; *0.26*
GII/3	5 (23)	1 (7)	4 (50)	0.1 [0.01–1.08]; *0.056*
Total	23 (100)	14 (100)	9 (100)	
Rotavirus Genotypes				
G1P[8]	16 (64)	16 (67)	0 (0)	NA
G3 P[8]	5 (20)	5 (21)	0 (0)	
G4 P[4]	1 (4)	1 (4)	0 (0)	
Not genotyped	3 (12)	2 (8)	1 (100)	
Total	25 (100)	24 (100)	1 (100)	

[a]Fisher's exact test with unadjusted odds ratio. Relative frequencies of genetic variants in hospital vs community setting. Mixed and non-typed infections were excluded from analysis.
[b]Only GII.4-2006 Minerva (n = 35) and GII.4-2009 New Orleans (n = 10) genetics variants were detected among GII.4.
[c]GII.6 (n = 3), GII.14 (n = 3) and GII.9 (n = 1).
[d]GI:GII (n = 3), GI:GIV (n = 1) and GI:GV(n = 1).
[e]Not applicable.

The most common SV genogroup was GI (46%), followed by GII (28%), GIV (3%) and mixed infections (9%). In 8 (14%) SV-positive samples, the genogroup could not be determined with the reagents used. To investigate if a particular genetic variant of SV contributed to the unusual high detection rate of SV in the current study, a subset of 23 SV-positives were genotyped by nt sequencing analysis (Table 2). In the hospital setting, GI/1 and GI/2 were the dominant genotypes (12/14), while SV of genotypes GII/2 and GII/3 were mainly found in community cases (7/9) (Table 2).

Rotavirus gastroenteritis was uncommon but severe in RotaTeq vaccinated children

RV was observed in 25 (8%) of the 330 children with diarrhea investigated. Interestingly, in the community setting, RV was observed in <1% (n = 1) of the cases whereas in the hospital setting RV was observed in 14% of the cases (n = 24) (OR = 24.5, $p < 0.001$), including 16 children with documented RV vaccination. Furthermore, the majority of RV infections were observed in children with severe dehydration (Table 1) (OR = 11.5, $p < 0.001$). In contrast to NV and SV infections however, there was an equal distribution of RV infections in all age groups (Table 1). Of note is also that the mean age for children with RVGE was high (14.6 months: median = 10.6). RVGE was observed in 16 (6%) of 270 children vaccinated with RotaTeq and in 2 (14%) of the 14 non-vaccinated children (OR = 0.38; p = 0.22). RV was also observed in 7 (15%) of 46 children with unknown vaccination status. In RV-positive children having received 3 and 2 RotaTeq doses, the RVGE episode occurred 193 and 65 days (median) post vaccination, respectively.

Rotavirus of genotypes G1P[8] and G3P[8] infected RotaTeq vaccinated children

Most RV genotypes (16/17), from hospitalized children of Jinotega were G1P[8], whereas the RV genotypes from León were G3P[8] (n = 4), G9P[4] (n = 1) and non-typeable (n = 3) with the reagents used. Full genome sequencing analysis of a G3P[8] RV strain (125L) from León, showed a Wa-like genome (G3-P[8]-I1-R1-C1-M1-A1-N1-T1-E1-H1). Similar genome constellations were previously observed after full genome sequencing of 12 RV-positive from Jinotega, of which 11 were G1P[8] and 1 was G3P[8]; as published elsewhere [26].

Co-infections with NV and SV

In total 14 (4%) children with GE shed more than one of the virus investigated. Of these, 11 shed SV-NV, 2 SV-RV, and 1 NV-RV, no triple virus infection was observed, but SVGI-SVGII-NVGI was observed. More than 50% (8/14) of the children with co-infections were observed in hospitalized children. Co-infections were confirmed by either secondary PCR or sequencing analysis.

Discussion

The burden of diarrhea after universal RV vaccination in Nicaragua remains high, despite reduction of RV infections and transmission in the community [12,16,18,33]. In the current study we investigated the role of NV, SV and RV in pediatric gastroenteritis in hospital and community settings in two cities with high RV vaccine coverage (>90%) in Nicaragua.

Our findings show that after RV vaccine implementation, NV has become the leading viral cause (24%) of medically attended acute GE among Nicaraguan children younger than 5 years of age. This is in agreement with recent studies carried out in Finland and USA [34–36]. SV was the second most common cause of acute GE (17%), followed by RV (8%). Altogether, these observations indicate that the etiology of viral gastroenteritis at hospital and community settings in Nicaragua has been altered by RV vaccine implementation and that NV and SV strongly contribute to the burden of diarrhea that still persists in the country [17,18]. Since a viral cause of GE was found in only approximately one half of the children investigated in this study, further surveillance studies of other etiologies are recommended to close this diagnostic gap in these settings [37,38].

NVGE has been generally described as a mild disease of short duration but new evidence suggests that the illness can be severe, especially among vulnerable populations [39,40]. The current study is in agreement with such new evidence as 27% of children in the hospital setting had NVGE and many of these required medical attention for mild and severe dehydration. The GII.4 genotypes comprised 94% of all genotyped NV in children in the hospital setting; compared to 65% in the community setting (p = 0.012). In a study carried out in Nicaragua in 2005, we observed that most NV cases requiring intravenous treatment were associated with GII.4 (Hunter), and that the same variant was less common in asymptomatic children [22,41]. Altogether, these observations suggest that besides vulnerable populations, not yet described virulence factors of GII.4 variants contribute to illness severity, a suggestion supported by a recent review of outbreaks associated with GII.4 viruses [39]. A potential bias of our comparison is that community samples were only collected from one city, León, and not Jinotega. However, due to the close geographical location of the cities which have good logistic connections and the long-term nature of the study, it is likely that GII.4 variants circulated in similar proportion in the communities of the two cities.

We further investigated the non-specific effect of RV vaccine against GE from other etiologies, previously suggested in one of the largest clinical trial of RotaTeq [13]. We found no significant differences between rates of NV infection and RV vaccination (24% vs 21%), and NV and SV together, were found in almost a half (24% and 19%, respectively) of the children with diarrhea having received one vaccination dose, with SV only observed in children vaccinated with RotaTeq. These observations strongly suggest that RV-vaccination do not reduce the incidence of NVGE and SVGE.

In previous surveillance studies of pediatric diarrhea in developed and developing countries, prevalence rates of SVGE barely reached 10% [4–8]. Despite significant progress on methods for SV detection, it remains poorly recognized as a cause of GE, probably because infection is generally believed mild and few cases need medical care [42]. In the current study, we report that SV infections were the second most common cause (17%) of pediatric GE in the vaccinated population investigated and that SV infections were detected less frequent in children with dehydration as compared to NV and RV. To demonstrate the clinical significance of SaV infections in RV5 vaccinated children; more studies (case – control) should be performed including more non-vaccinated children as well as asymptomatic children. A previous report from Nicaragua found asymptomatic shedding of SaV in ~9% of children < 5 years of age [8]. A possible explanation for the increased SV prevalence in this study (17%), as compared with a prevalence rate of 12% in 2005–2006 before RV-vaccination in Nicaragua [8] is that there is a higher relative likelihood of finding non-RV enteropathogens in this study where most children had been vaccinated for RV, compared to the time period before RV vaccination. Another reason could be the use of more sensitive methods enhancing detection of most genetic variants. The real-time PCR used in this study was proven to be 10-fold more sensitive than the conventional RT-PCR that uses first generation SV primers (JV33 and SR80) [31,43].

In line with previous studies we observed a decline of RVGE after introduction of universal RV vaccination [34–36], with RV observed in 14% of hospitalized children and less than 1% in community children with diarrhea. This data is also in line with the reduction of incidence of watery diarrhea in the community after RV vaccine introduction in Nicaragua [18]. These observations suggest that RotaTeq implementation has dramatically decreased the number of RVGE in primary care setting in Nicaragua, which is consistent with the low prevalence of RV at environmental level [33].

We investigated whether RV vaccinated children with severe RVGE in the current study were infected with RV strains different from those included in the vaccine. However, genomic analysis of a subset of the strains showed that all RV strains analyzed had genotype specificities typical for human G1P[8] and G3P[8] RVs, similar to genotypes present in the RotaTeq vaccine. This suggests that viral factors alone were not responsible for the vaccine failures in this study population. Another possible explanation could be a short duration of RotaTeq vaccine protection in some children. In this study we observed that RVGE occurred about 6 or 2 months post 3rd and 2nd vaccine dose respectively. A third possible explanation might be that host genetic factors in some children influence vaccine take. A particular attention has now been put on histo-blood group antigens, and remains to be elucidated [44].

To conclude, this study shows that NV has become the leading viral cause of pediatric viral gastroenteritis at hospital and community settings in Nicaragua after universal implementation of RotaTeq vaccine; and that NV together with SV infections strongly contribute to the high burden of diarrhea remaining after RV vaccination.

Acknowledgments

We would like to express our appreciation to Licdas. Angelica Castro and Cristel Escoto for help in collecting samples and epidemiological information in children from Jinotega, Dr. Gioconda Ramirez and Dra. Rafaela Briceno, for providing diarrhea surveillance data from Hospital Victoria Motta in Jinotega and HEODRA in León, respectively, Silvia Altamirano for valuable assistance on fieldwork activities, Eliana Espinoza, for collaboration on norovirus methods optimization and Patricia Blandon for her valuable assistance on laboratory activities.

Author Contributions

Conceived and designed the experiments: FB YR LS JN. Performed the experiments: FB YR. Analyzed the data: FB YR JN. Contributed reagents/materials/analysis tools: FB LS. Wrote the paper: FB YR LS JN.

References

1. Patel MM, Widdowson MA, Glass RI, Akazawa K, Vinje J, et al. (2008) Systematic literature review of role of noroviruses in sporadic gastroenteritis. Emerg Infect Dis 14: 1224–1231.
2. Parashar UD, Gibson CJ, Bresse JS, Glass RI (2006) Rotavirus and severe childhood diarrhea. Emerg Infect Dis 12: 304–306.
3. Tate JE, Burton AH, Boschi-Pinto C, Steele AD, Duque J, et al. (2012) 2008 estimate of worldwide rotavirus-associated mortality in children younger than 5 years before the introduction of universal rotavirus vaccination programmes: a systematic review and meta-analysis. Lancet Infect Dis 12: 136–141.
4. Johnsen CK, Midgley S, Bottiger B (2009) Genetic diversity of sapovirus infections in Danish children 2005-2007. J Clin Virol 46: 265–269.
5. Khamrin P, Maneekarn N, Peerakome S, Tonusin S, Malasao R, et al. (2007) Genetic diversity of noroviruses and sapoviruses in children hospitalized with acute gastroenteritis in Chiang Mai, Thailand. J Med Virol 79: 1921–1926.
6. Podkolzin AT, Fenske EB, Abramycheva NY, Shipulin GA, Sagalova OI, et al. (2009) Hospital-based surveillance of rotavirus and other viral agents of diarrhea in children and adults in Russia, 2005-2007. J Infect Dis 200 Suppl 1: S228–233.
7. Sakai Y, Nakata S, Honma S, Tatsumi M, Numata-Kinoshita K, et al. (2001) Clinical severity of Norwalk virus and Sapporo virus gastroenteritis in children in Hokkaido, Japan. Pediatr Infect Dis J 20: 849–853.
8. Bucardo F, Carlsson B, Nordgren J, Larson G, Blandon P, et al. (2012) Susceptibility of children to sapovirus infections, Nicaragua, 2005-2006. Emerg Infect Dis 18: 1875–1878.
9. Soares-Weiser K, Maclehose H, Bergman H, Ben-Aharon I, Nagpal S, et al. (2012) Vaccines for preventing rotavirus diarrhoea: vaccines in use. Cochrane Database Syst Rev 11: CD008521.
10. Vesikari T, Karvonen A, Ferrante SA, Ciarlet M (2010) Efficacy of the pentavalent rotavirus vaccine, RotaTeq(R), in Finnish infants up to 3 years of age: the Finnish Extension Study. Eur J Pediatr 169: 1379–1386.
11. Khawaja S, Cardellino A, Klotz D, Kuter BJ, Feinberg MB, et al. (2012) Evaluating the health impact of a public-private partnership: to reduce rotavirus disease in Nicaragua. Hum Vaccin Immunother 8: 777–782.
12. Patel M, Pedreira C, De Oliveira LH, Tate J, Orozco M, et al. (2009) Association between pentavalent rotavirus vaccine and severe rotavirus diarrhea among children in Nicaragua. JAMA 301: 2243–2251.
13. Vesikari T, Matson DO, Dennehy P, Van Damme P, Santosham M, et al. (2006) Safety and efficacy of a pentavalent human-bovine (WC3) reassortant rotavirus vaccine. N Engl J Med 354: 23–33.
14. Zaman K, Dang DA, Victor JC, Shin S, Yunus M, et al. (2010) Efficacy of pentavalent rotavirus vaccine against severe rotavirus gastroenteritis in infants in developing countries in Asia: a randomised, double-blind, placebo-controlled trial. Lancet 376: 615–623.
15. Madhi SA, Cunliffe NA, Steele D, Witte D, Kirsten M, et al. (2010) Effect of human rotavirus vaccine on severe diarrhea in African infants. N Engl J Med 362: 289–298.
16. Becker-Dreps S, Paniagua M, Zambrana LE, Bucardo F, Hudgens MG, et al. (2011) Rotavirus prevalence in the primary care setting in Nicaragua after universal infant rotavirus immunization. Am J Trop Med Hyg 85: 957–960.
17. Becker-Dreps S, Paniagua M, Dominik R, Cao H, Shah NK, et al. (2011) Changes in childhood diarrhea incidence in nicaragua following 3 years of universal infant rotavirus immunization. Pediatr Infect Dis J 30: 243–247.
18. Becker-Dreps S, Melendez M, Liu L, Zambrana LE, Paniagua M, et al. (2013) Community diarrhea incidence before and after rotavirus vaccine introduction in Nicaragua. Am J Trop Med Hyg 89: 246–250.
19. Pang XL, Koskenniemi E, Joensuu J, Vesikari T (1999) Effect of rhesus rotavirus vaccine on enteric adenovirus—associated diarrhea in children. J Pediatr Gastroenterol Nutr 29: 366–369.
20. Pang XL, Zeng SQ, Honma S, Nakata S, Vesikari T (2001) Effect of rotavirus vaccine on Sapporo virus gastroenteritis in Finnish infants. Pediatr Infect Dis J 20: 295–300.
21. Zeng SQ, Halkosalo A, Salminen M, Szakal ED, Karvonen A, et al. (2010) Norovirus gastroenteritis in young children receiving human rotavirus vaccine. Scand J Infect Dis 42: 540–544.
22. Bucardo F, Nordgren J, Carlsson B, Paniagua M, Lindgren PE, et al. (2008) Pediatric norovirus diarrhea in Nicaragua. J Clin Microbiol 46: 2573–2580.
23. Iturriza-Gomara M, Kang G, Gray J (2004) Rotavirus genotyping: keeping up with an evolving population of human rotaviruses. J Clin Virol 31: 259–265.
24. Samajdar S, Varghese V, Barman P, Ghosh S, Mitra U, et al. (2006) Changing pattern of human group A rotaviruses: emergence of G12 as an important pathogen among children in eastern India. J Clin Virol 36: 183–188.
25. Gentsch JR, Glass RI, Woods P, Gouvea V, Gorziglia M, et al. (1992) Identification of group A rotavirus gene 4 types by polymerase chain reaction. J Clin Microbiol 30: 1365–1373.
26. Bucardo F, Rippinger CM, Svensson L, Patton JT (2012) Vaccine-derived NSP2 segment in rotaviruses from vaccinated children with gastroenteritis in Nicaragua. Infect Genet Evol 12: 1282–1294.
27. Nordgren J, Bucardo F, Dienus O, Svensson L, Lindgren PE (2008) Novel light-upon-extension real-time PCR assays for detection and quantification of genogroup I and II noroviruses in clinical specimens. J Clin Microbiol 46: 164–170.
28. Kojima S, Kageyama T, Fukushi S, Hoshino FB, Shinohara M, et al. (2002) Genogroup-specific PCR primers for detection of Norwalk-like viruses. J Virol Methods 100: 107–114.
29. Kimura M (1980) A simple method for estimating evolutionary rates of base substitutions through comparative studies of nucleotide sequences. J Mol Evol 16: 111–120.
30. Zheng DP, Ando T, Fankhauser RL, Beard RS, Glass RI, et al. (2006) Norovirus classification and proposed strain nomenclature. Virology 346: 312–323.
31. Chan MC, Sung JJ, Lam RK, Chan PK, Lai RW, et al. (2006) Sapovirus detection by quantitative real-time RT-PCR in clinical stool specimens. J Virol Methods 134: 146–153.
32. Okada M, Yamashita Y, Oseto M, Shinozaki K (2006) The detection of human sapoviruses with universal and genogroup-specific primers. Arch Virol 151: 2503–2509.
33. Bucardo F, Lindgren PE, Svensson L, Nordgren J (2011) Low prevalence of rotavirus and high prevalence of norovirus in hospital and community wastewater after introduction of rotavirus vaccine in Nicaragua. PLoS One 6: e25962.
34. Payne DC, Vinje J, Szilagyi PG, Edwards KM, Staat MA, et al. (2013) Norovirus and medically attended gastroenteritis in U.S. children. N Engl J Med 368: 1121–1130.
35. Hemming M, Rasanen S, Huhti L, Paloniemi M, Salminen M, et al. (2013) Major reduction of rotavirus, but not norovirus, gastroenteritis in children seen in hospital after the introduction of RotaTeq vaccine into the National Immunization Programme in Finland. Eur J Pediatr 172: 739–746.
36. Koo HL, Neill FH, Estes MK, Munoz FM, Cameron A, et al. (2013) Noroviruses: The Most Common Pediatric Viral Enteric Pathogen at a Large University Hospital After Introduction of Rotavirus Vaccination. J Pediatric Infect Dis Soc 2: 57–60.
37. Tam CC, O'Brien SJ, Tompkins DS, Bolton FJ, Berry L, et al. (2012) Changes in causes of acute gastroenteritis in the United Kingdom over 15 years: microbiologic findings from 2 prospective, population-based studies of infectious intestinal disease. Clin Infect Dis 54: 1275–1286.
38. Simpson R, Aliyu S, Iturriza-Gomara M, Desselberger U, Gray J (2003) Infantile viral gastroenteritis: on the way to closing the diagnostic gap. J Med Virol 70: 258–262.
39. Desai R, Hembree CD, Handel A, Matthews JE, Dickey BW, et al. (2012) Severe outcomes are associated with genogroup 2 genotype 4 norovirus outbreaks: a systematic literature review. Clin Infect Dis 55: 189–193.
40. Glass RI, Parashar UD, Estes MK (2009) Norovirus gastroenteritis. N Engl J Med 361: 1776–1785.
41. Bucardo F, Nordgren J, Carlsson B, Kindberg E, Paniagua M, et al. (2010) Asymptomatic norovirus infections in Nicaraguan children and its association with viral properties and histo-blood group antigens. Pediatr Infect Dis J 29: 934–939.
42. Moreno-Espinosa S, Farkas T, Jiang X (2004) Human caliciviruses and pediatric gastroenteritis. Semin Pediatr Infect Dis 15: 237–245.

Genetic Diversity of Circulating Rotavirus Strains in Tanzania Prior to the Introduction of Vaccination

Sabrina J. Moyo[1,2*], Bjørn Blomberg[1,3], Kurt Hanevik[1,3], Oyvind Kommedal[4], Kirsti Vainio[5], Samuel Y. Maselle[2], Nina Langeland[1,6]

1 Department of Clinical Science, University of Bergen, Bergen, Norway, **2** Department of Microbiology and Immunology, Muhimbili University of Health and Allied Sciences, Dar es Salaam, Tanzania, **3** Centre for Tropical Infectious Diseases, Haukeland University Hospital, Bergen, Norway, **4** Department of Microbiology, Haukeland University Hospital, Bergen, Norway, **5** Division of Infectious Disease Control, Norwegian Institute of Public Health, Oslo, Norway, **6** Department of Medicine, Haukeland University Hospital, Bergen, Norway

Abstract

Background: Tanzania currently rolls out vaccination against rotavirus-diarrhea, a major cause of child illness and death. As the vaccine covers a limited number of rotavirus variants, this study describes the molecular epidemiology of rotavirus among children under two years in Dar es Salaam, Tanzania, prior to implementation of vaccination.

Methods: Stool specimens, demographic and clinical information, were collected from 690 children admitted to hospital due to diarrhea (cases) and 545 children without diarrhea (controls) during one year. Controls were inpatient or children attending child health clinics. Rotavirus antigen was detected using ELISA and positive samples were typed by multiplex semi-nested PCR and sequencing.

Results: The prevalence of rotavirus was higher in cases (32.5%) than in controls (7.7%, $P<0.001$). The most common G genotypes were G1 followed by G8, G12, and G4 in cases and G1, G12 and G8 in controls. The Tanzanian G1 variants displayed 94% similarity with the Rotarix vaccine G1 variant. The commonest P genotypes were P[8], P[4] and P[6], and the commonest G/P combination G1 P[8] (n = 123), G8 P[4] and G12 P[6]. Overall, rotavirus prevalence was higher in cool (23.9%) than hot months (17.1%) of the year ($P=0.012$). We also observed significant seasonal variation of G genotypes. Rotavirus was most frequently found in the age group of four to six months. The prevalence of rotavirus in cases was lower in stunted children (28.9%) than in non-stunted children (40.1%, $P=0.003$) and lower in HIV-infected (15.4%, 4/26) than in HIV-uninfected children (55.3%, 42/76, $P<0.001$).

Conclusion: This pre-vaccination study shows predominance of genotype G1 in Tanzania, which is phylogenetically distantly related to the vaccine strains. We confirm the emergence of genotype G8 and G12. Rotavirus infection and circulating genotypes showed seasonal variation. This study also suggests that rotavirus may not be an opportunistic pathogen in children infected with HIV.

Editor: Ana Paula Arez, Instituto de Higiene e Medicina Tropical, Portugal

Funding: This study was funded by the University of Bergen, Norway. The funders had no role in the study design, data collection and analysis, decision to publish, or preparation of the manuscript.

Competing Interests: The authors have declared that no competing interests exist.

* E-mail: Sabrina.moyo@med.uib.no

Introduction

Rotavirus is a major cause of severe dehydrating diarrhea both in developed and developing countries [1,2]. The WHO rotavirus surveillance networks estimates that more than a third of diarrhea hospitalizations among children under five years of age is attributed to rotavirus infection [3]. In 2008, rotavirus caused an estimated 453000 deaths in children younger than five years, more than half of which occurred in developing countries [4].

Due to the limited effect of sanitation-based strategies for preventing the spread of the virus, several rotavirus vaccines have been developed, out of which two oral vaccines (RotaTeq and Rotarix) have been licensed. The introduction of rotavirus vaccines in developed countries has significantly reduced diarrheal mortality and hospitalizations [5–10]. A live attenuated monovalent vaccine (Rotarix) was introduced in Tanzania early 2013 and is implemented in the national childhood vaccination schedule.

Rotaviruses are non-enveloped viruses of the genus Reoviridae [11]. The viral genome consists of double stranded segmented RNA enclosed in three protein layers. The middle-layer major capsid protein, VP6 determines the seven major groups (A through G) of rotavirus. Most human infections are caused by group A rotaviruses [12]. The outer capsid of rotavirus is composed of two structural proteins, VP4 (a protease cleaved protein, P protein) and VP7 (a glycoprotein, G protein), which independently elicit protective neutralizing antibodies and serve as the basis of a dual serotyping system [13–15]. At least 27 G genotypes and 35 P genotypes have been identified in human rotaviruses [16], whereof genotypes G1P[8], G2P[4], G3P[8], G4P[8], and G9P[8] are responsible for 80–90% of the childhood rotavirus disease burden globally [17]. Rotavirus G12 has recently been identified as an emerging genotype [9]. But from the African continent, G12 in combination with P[6] or P[8] has been reported from only South Africa, Malawi and Nigeria [18–20]. Rotavirus G8 genotype has been reported from humans worldwide with high prevalence in some African countries [17,21–28].

Rotavirus infection is common in both temperate and tropical climatic areas and shows distinct seasonality [29]. Before the discovery of the viral agent it was called 'winter diarrhea and winter gastroenteritis' in some parts of the world [29–31]. There is an increase in attention to the nature of rotavirus disease in relation to seasonality, and this has been well documented in temperate countries [32,33]. Recently two studies have also demonstrated the inverse relationship between temperature and rotavirus incidence in the tropics [29,34].

In Tanzania, it is estimated that rotavirus causes more than one third of diarrheal disease hospitalizations and each year it kills more than eight thousands children under five years of age [35]. In a previous study conducted in 2005–2006 [36], we reported high prevalence of rotavirus G9 among under-five children admitted with diarrhea in Dar es Salaam. The present study provides an update on the distribution of rotavirus G and P genotypes among children with diarrhea (cases) and compares it with that from children without diarrhea (controls) between August 2010 and July 2011. In addition we assessed the impact of HIV, clinical features and seasonal variation on rotavirus infection. The findings provide baseline information on rotavirus infection shortly before vaccine introduction in Tanzania.

Material and Methods

Ethics Statement

This study received ethical approval from the Senate Research and Publications Committee of Muhimbili University of Health and Allied Sciences in Dar es Salaam, Tanzania and from the Regional Committee for Medical and Health Research Ethics (REK) in Norway. Permission was also obtained from the respective hospital authorities where recruitment of study participants took place (i.e. MNH, Amana and Temeke Hospitals). Written informed consent was obtained from the parent, next of kin, caretaker, or guardian on behalf of all the minors/children enrolled in the study.

Study Population

This study was conducted between August 2010 and July 2011 in Dar es Salaam Tanzania, a city with a population of about five million. Sample collection was performed during two seasons, starting in August 2010 and in March 2011, aiming for minimum 300 cases and 300 controls in each period. The target for cases was reached in January 2011 and in June 2011, while enrollment of controls continued in February 2011 and July 2011. A total of 1266 stool specimens were collected from children below two years of age. Cases were children hospitalized due to diarrhea at three major hospitals of Dar es Salaam; Muhimbili National Hospital (MNH), Amana and Temeke Municipal Hospitals. MNH, with a bed capacity of 1200, is the largest hospital in the country and serves as a tertiary and national referral Hospital. Amana and Temeke are Municipal district Hospitals of Dar es Salaam. Controls included children below two years of age with no history of diarrhea for one month prior to the study enrollment. These were either children attending child health clinics for immunization and growth monitoring (CHC, n = 310) or children admitted to hospital due to diseases other than diarrhea (n = 235).

Inclusion Criteria Case Definition

Children admitted in the diarrhea wards with acute or persistent diarrhea were included in the study. Diarrhea was defined as three or more watery stools within 24 hours. An episode of diarrhea was considered over when two consecutive days pass without diarrhea. An episode of acute diarrhea was defined as diarrhea with duration between 24 hours and less than 14 days. Persistent diarrhea was defined as diarrhea for 14 days or more.

Controls included in the study were children without history of diarrhea for one month prior to enrollment. Controls were not matched by age and sex with cases.

Exclusion Criteria

Children above 24 months of age and cases that could not provide stool sample on the day of admission were not included in the study. Cases and controls whose parent or guardian did not consent to participate in the study were excluded.

Collection of Information from Children with Diarrhea (Cases) and from Children without Diarrhea (Controls)

Recruitment of cases was done during the admission of the child in the pediatric diarrhea wards of the study sites. A standardized questionnaire was used to collect demographic and clinical information, including age (date of birth), sex, place of residence, parent/guardian level of education and history of antibiotic use prior to admission. Consistency of stool (watery, bloody) and duration of diarrhea was also recorded. The child's length and weight measurements were recorded. Additional clinical information of patients, such as hydration status, as assessed on the day of admission by the attending clinician, was obtained from patient files together with HIV testing results. HIV testing was done by HIV-DNA PCR at the Hospital laboratory (MNH) or research laboratory at MUHAS, as previously described [37]. Potential controls were enrolled during the recruitment of cases. The questionnaire for controls did not have parameters for clinical characteristics such as type of diarrhea and presence of dehydration. In addition controls did not have diarrhea for one month prior to the study enrollment.

Weight and Length Measurements

All children were weighed using a 25 kg Salter hanging scales (CMS Weighing equipment, High Holborn, London, United Kingdom). Weight was recorded to the nearest 0.1 kilogram. Length was measured using standard length boards to the nearest millimeter. Weight for age (WAZ), length for age (LAZ) and weight for length (WLZ) Z-scores were calculated using EPI Info (USD, Inc., Stone Mountain, GA). Children were categorized to have normal nutritional status, mild or severe malnutrition using Z-scores according to WHO criteria [38].

Specimen Collection

A single stool specimen was collected on inclusion from each child using wide mouthed sterile plastic containers. One portion was frozen at −70°C the same day as it was collected.

Rotavirus Detection

Rotavirus antigens were detected using the commercially available ProSpecT Rotavirus ELISA kit (Oxoid, Hants, UK), with 10% fecal suspensions according to the manufacturer's instructions.

Extraction of RNA

Fifty μg of rotavirus antigen-positive stool specimen were mixed 1:10 with Bacterial Lysis buffer (Roche Applied Science, Mannheim, Germany), and centrifuged at 13.000 g for 3 minutes. RNA was extracted from 200 μL supernatant using the Magna Pure LC High Performance Total Nucleic Acid Isolation Kit (Roche Applied Science, Mannheim, Germany).

Reverse Transcription, G and P-typing of Rotaviruses

Reverse transcription, G and P typing was done as described in European Rotavirus Detection and Typing Methods version 4 [39]. Briefly a total of 40 μL of RNA extract was used as template for reverse transcription with random primers. Rotavirus G an P genotyping was performed using semi-nested type specific multiplex PCR's that could detect eight G genotypes (G1, G2, G3, G4, G8, G9, G10 and G12) and six P-types P[4], P[6], P[8], P[9], P[10] and P[11]. PCR products were subjected to electrophoresis on a 2% agarose gel, stained with Gel Red, and observed under ultraviolet light. The Rotavirus G and P genotypes were determined by their specific size on the agarose gel. The non-typeable rotavirus strains were further confirmed if they were rotavirus using a single round rotavirus VP6 specific PCR. Negative and positive controls were included in all PCR assays.

Sequencing of the VP7 and VP4 Gene of the Rotavirus Positive Strains

Partial sequencing of the first round PCR-amplicons for the VP7 gene was performed for all samples positive for rotavirus in order to confirm the PCR G- typing results as described in the European Rotavirus Detection and Typing Methods version 4 [39]. Randomly selected rotavirus positive isolates (33%) were subjected to partial sequencing of the VP4 gene to confirm PCR P-typing results. The sequencing of both VP4 and VP7 was done using purified first round PCR products, on an ABI3730 machine using BigDye (Applied Biosystems). The same primers as in the PCR were used, both forward and reverse primers for VP7 gene while only forward primers was used for VP4 gene.

Sequence and Phylogenetic Analysis of the VP7 Gene

Nucleotide sequences were analyzed using the RipSeq interpretation software (iSentio Ltd., Bergen, Norway) and by the nucleotide BLAST service (NCBI). The evolutionary distances between Tanzanian strains, vaccine strains and the reference strains from GenBank were investigated using pairwise comparison from multiple sequence alignments using the Genius software package (Biomatters) and the phylogenetic tree was constructed using the UPGMA and Kimura two-parameter methods [40]. A bootstrap resampling analysis was performed (1000 replicates) to test tree reliability.

Nucleotide Sequence Accession Numbers

The DNA sequences for the VP7 genes of the study strains were submitted directly to GenBank and were assigned accession numbers from KF976838 to KF976860.

The DNA sequences for the VP4 genes of the study strains were submitted directly to GenBank and were assigned accession numbers from KF976815 to KF976837.

Statistical Analysis

Weight for age, length for age and weight for length Z-scores were calculated using EPI Info (USD, Inc., Stone Mountain, GA, USA). Statistical analysis was performed using the Statistical Package for the Social Sciences (SPSS for IBM-PC, release 18.0; SPSS Inc., Chicago, IL, USA). Differences in proportions were tested using the chi-square (χ^2) test. A p-value of <0.05 was considered significant. The association between rotavirus positivity, genotypes, clinical and demographic characteristics was estimated as the odds ratio (OR) between rotavirus infected and rotavirus uninfected individuals in a logistic regression model. Factors from the univariate analysis were kept in the main logistic regression model. A separate regression model including HIV as a factor, employed manual, backwards, stepwise elimination of non-significant factors ($p \geq 0.05$).

Results

During the study period August 2010 to July 2011, a total of 1266 samples were collected. Among 1235 samples containing adequate material for rotavirus detection, 690 were from children with diarrhea and 545 were from controls (children without diarrhea). There were 717 (58.1%) males and 517(41.9%) females. Children were recruited from the districts Ilala (n = 634, 51.3%), Kinondoni (n = 360, 29.1%) and Temeke (n = 241, 19.5%).

Prevalence of Rotavirus Infection and Distribution of G and P Genotypes

Of the 1235 children with and without diarrhea included in the study, rotavirus was detected in 266 children (21.5%) using ELISA. The prevalence of rotavirus infection was significantly higher in cases (32.5%, 224/690) than in controls (7.7%, 42/545, $P<0.01$, OR = 5.8, 95%CI 4.045 to 8.192). The prevalence of rotavirus did not differ statistically between controls from Child Health Clinics (7.7%, 24/310) and hospital based controls (7.7%, 18/235, $P>0.05$).

Sequencing results detected rotavirus G8 in 33 cases, which were misallocated to G12 when G genotype was assessed by PCR alone. Therefore, all samples were G typed based on sequencing results. A total of 211 specimens, which were successfully sequenced were characterized to G genotypes, 190 cases and 21 controls. Out of eight rotavirus G genotypes searched for, only five G genotypes were found. The most commonly detected G genotype strains among cases were G1 (n = 131, 68.6%), followed by G8 (n = 33, 17.3%), G12 (n = 21, 11.05%), G4 (n = 4, 2.1%) and G9 (n = 1, 0.5%). Rotavirus genotype G1 was also common among children without diarrhea (controls) accounting for 66.7% followed by G12 (19.0%) and G8 (14.3%). Genotype G2, G3 and G10 were not detected.

A total of 236 samples were P genotyped using RT-PCR, 211 were cases and 25 were controls. One third of 236 samples underwent sequencing of the VP4 gene, which produced the same results as RT-PCR. Out of six P genotypes searched for, only three P genotypes were found. The commonest circulating P genotype in cases was P[8] (n = 141, 66.8%) followed by P[4] (n = 40, 19.0%) and P[6] (n = 30, 14.2%). Rotavirus P[9], P[10]and P[11] were not found. Table 1 shows G/P combinations for the 211 samples that were successfully typed for both G and P genotypes (among the 236 P-typed samples, 25 could not be G-typed). The commonest G/P combination in cases was G1P[8] accounting for 123 samples, followed by G8P[4] (n = 27) and G12P[6] (n = 21).

We found no rotavirus G or P genotype associated with diarrhea. The common G and P genotypes circulating in children with diarrhea were also common among children without diarrhea as shown in Table 1. We did not find samples with multiple strains of rotavirus.

Table 1. Sequencing results of rotavirus G and P genotypes circulating in children with diarrhea (cases) and children without diarrhea (controls) in Dar es Salaam, Tanzania (n = 211; 190 cases and 21 controls).

	G1	G4	G8	G9	G12	Total P types N (%)
Cases						
P4	7	2	27	0	0	36 (19.0%)
P6	1	2	6	0	21	30 (15.7%)
P8	123	0	0	1	0	124 (65.4%)
Total G types	131 (68.6%)	4 (2.1%)	33 (17.3%)	1 (0.5%)	22 (11.5%)	**190** (100%)
Controls						
P4	0	0	3	0	0	3 (14.3%)
P6	0	0	0	0	4	4 (19.0%)
P8	14	0	0	0	0	14 (66.7%)
Total G types	14 (66.7%)	0	3 (14.3%)	0	4 (19.0%)	**21** (100%)

Analysis of VP7 Nucleotide Sequences

Phylogenetic analysis based on VP7 nucleotide sequences showed that sequences varied by only 1–2% within the rotavirus G1 strains detected in Tanzania (Fig. 1A). These GI genotypes also showed 98–99% nucleotide similarity to G1 strains circulating worldwide such as in Malawi, Bangladesh, Belgium and USA with GenBank accession numbers JN591404, EF690754, EF690759, HQ392309 and HM773752. Notably, only 94% similarity was found between the Tanzanian G1genotype and the rotavirus vaccine-strains RotaTeq (GU565057) and Rotarix (JN849114).

The rotavirus G8 strains in this study had 98–99% nucleotide similarity with each other; they are also closely related (98%–99% nucleotide similarity) to circulating rotavirus G8 strains in Kenya, Malawi and USA with GenBank accession numbers EU488721, FJ386444, JN591405, GQ496281, JF693231, KC215513. The G12 genotypes in this study displayed nucleotide similarities above 99%. These rotavirus G12 strains were also closely related to circulating G12 strains in Malawi, India and Nepal with GenBank accession numbers EU573780, EF559260, AB263988 and AB275292.

Analysis of VP4 Nucleotide Sequences

Comparison of VP4 nucleotide sequences from Tanzanian strains and representatives of P-genotype strains from the GenBank database are shown in figure 1B. Tanzanian P[8] strains showed 98% nucleotide identity to each other and to circulating P[8] reference strains from Australia, Brazil, USA and Thailand with GenBank accession numbers JF490333, JX027920, DQ857918, HM773758 and DQ674980. Nucleotide identities between Tanzanian rotavirus P[4] strains and reference P[4] strains from Malawi and Kenya was 98%. GenBank accession numbers for P[4] reference strains are FJ386448 and HQ657141. Tanzanian rotavirus P[6] strains were closely related to each other with 99% nucleotide similarity and showed 98% nucleotide identity to reference P[6] strains from Malawi, South Africa and Bangladesh with GenBank accession numbers JN591402, HQ657163, EF033340, DQ490554, DQ146663.

Seasonality of Rotavirus Infection and Rotavirus G-types

The prevalence of rotavirus detected varied significantly by months in both cases and controls ($P<0.001$). When results were divided into cool and hot months of the year i.e. May through August vs. November through February, rotavirus prevalence (both in cases and controls) was significantly higher in cool than hot months (23.9% vs. 17.1%, $P = 0.012$, OR 1.52, 95% CI: 1.081 to 1.894: 1.09 to 2.11). As shown in Figure 1, there was also high number of rotavirus detected among cases in the beginning of the cool season i.e. April 2011 and between the cool and the hot season, which are periods that coincide with rain season.

We also observed significant variations of G genotypes detection in different months during the study period ($P<0.001$) as shown in Figure 2. The commonest genotype G1 was detected in most months of the study, with the highest peak in the month of April 2011, which is the beginning of the cool season and May 2011. Genotypes G8 and G12 were detected in most months of the study period, but genotype G9 was only detected in the month of October 2010.

We compared rotavirus prevalence in studies conducted in previous years in the same region but during different seasons of the year. We observed high prevalence in studies conducted during the cool months of the year [41,42] compared to studies conducted in hot months of the year, Table 2 [36,43].

Association between Rotavirus Infection and HIV Status

A total of 421 children were tested for HIV, of these 33 and 388 tested HIV positive and negative respectively. In univariate analysis, the prevalence of rotavirus infection was significantly lower in HIV-infected (15.4%, 4/26) than in HIV-uninfected children with diarrhea (cases) (55.3%, 42/76, $P = 0.001$, OR 0.152, 95% CI: 0.05–0.48). HIV status was not included in the final regression model; because it would introduce a high number of missing values as 54% rotavirus infected children were not tested for HIV. A separate regression model was performed including HIV status and other significant risk factors from the univariate analysis (length for age, place of residence and type of diarrhea). With stepwise, backwards removal of all non-significant factors ($P\geq0.05$), rotavirus infection remained significantly negatively associated with HIV infection ($P = 0.027$, OR 0.26, 95% CI: 0.08 to 0.85) and stunting ($P = 0.005$, OR 0.23, 95% CI: 0.08 to 0.63).

Among children without diarrhea (controls), the prevalence of rotavirus was significantly higher in HIV-infected (28.6%, 2/7) than in HIV-uninfected children (7.4%, 23/312, $P = 0.039$, OR 5.03, 95%CI: 0.92 to 27.35).

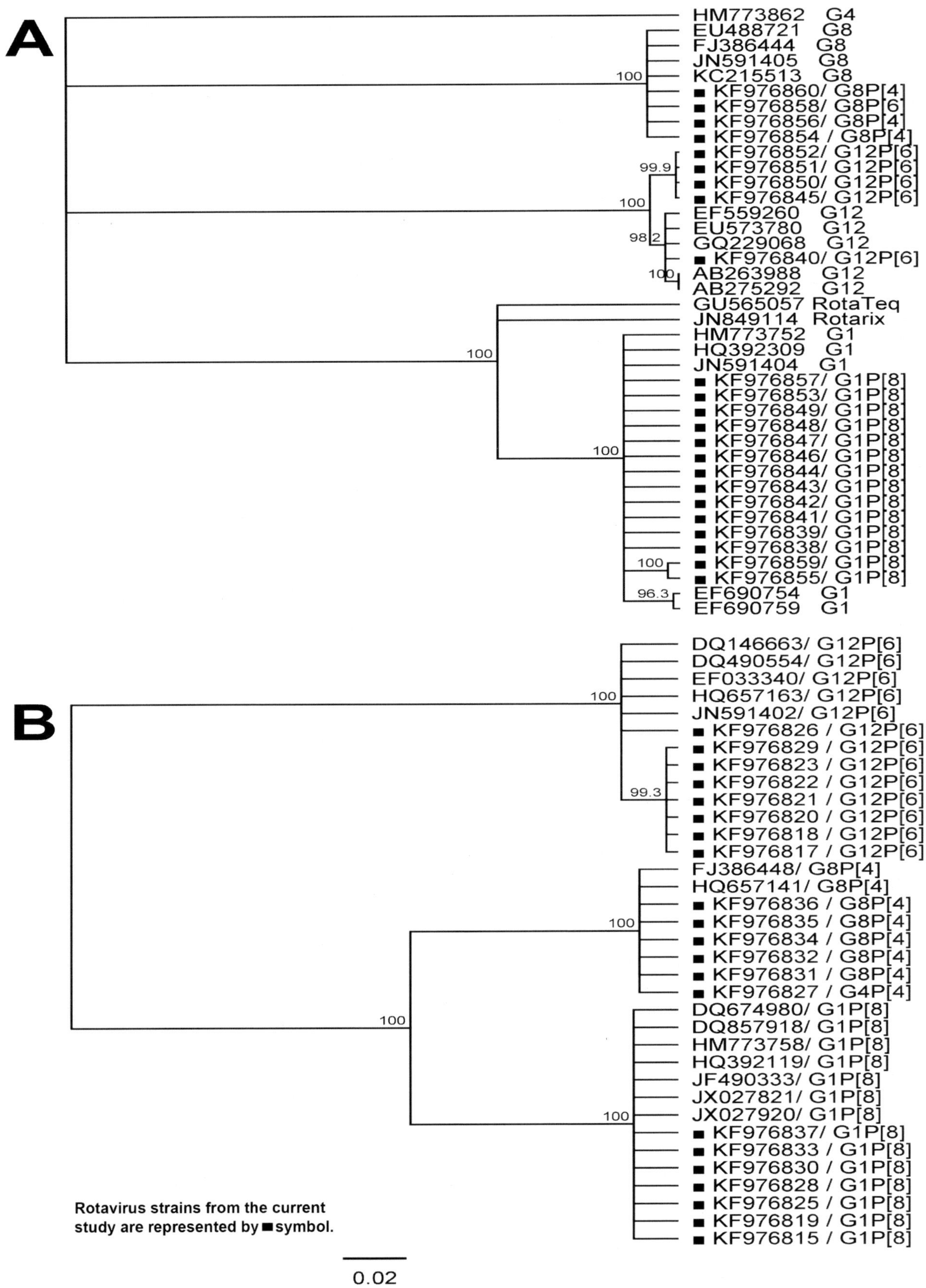

Figure 1. A and B. Phylogenetic trees of the rotavirus nucleotide sequence of the partial VP7 and VP4 genes. The phylogenetic tree: Phylogenetic trees based on the nucleotide sequence of the partial VP7 gene (figure 1A) and VP4 gene (figure 1B) of rotaviruses from Tanzania with known rotavirus reference strains from GenBank database and rotavirus vaccine strains i.e Rotateq and Rotarix. Reference strains, vaccine strains and

strains from this study are indicated by accession numbers. The Genius software package was used to build the tree with the UPGMA method and bootstrapped with 1,000 repetitions; The Kimura-2 substitution model was used. The bar indicates nucleotide substitutions per site.

Distribution of Rotavirus Infection and G/P Genotypes by Age and Sex

The median age of all rotavirus infected children (9.6 months) was significantly lower than that of rotavirus uninfected children (10.7 months, P = 0.003). There was no significant difference in the median age of rotavirus infected children with and without diarrhea (9.6 months vs. 9.7 months). Figure 3 shows that the prevalence of rotavirus infection in cases was significantly higher in the age group of 0–6 months compared to the age group ≥19 months (35.1% vs. 23.4%, P = 0.028, OR 2.14, 95% CI: 1.09 to 4.23). The prevalence of rotavirus infection did not differ significantly between age groups 7–12 and 13–18 months respectively, as compared to age group ≥19 months. The prevalence of rotavirus infection in controls did not differ significantly between age groups (P>0.05). Rotavirus genotypes G1 and G8 were detected in all age groups, whereas G4 was detected in the age of 0–12 months and one strain of G9 was detected from a child in the group of 0–6 months.

The proportion of rotavirus infection in all children with and without diarrhea did not differ significantly by sex as shown in Table 3.

The distribution of rotavirus G and P genotypes was not significantly associated with sex of the child, presence of dehydration, nutritional status or HIV status (P>0.05).

Discussion

Rotavirus is the leading cause of severe diarrhea both in developed and developing countries. This one-year surveillance study described the molecular epidemiology of rotavirus infection in children in Dar es Salaam, the major city of Tanzania with a population of about five million inhabitants. Children with diarrhea were six times more likely to be infected with rotavirus than those without diarrhea. The study confirms findings from other studies twenty years ago in the same location and elsewhere [42,44] indicating that rotavirus is still a major pathogen causing diarrhea in children in Tanzania. The presence of rotavirus among controls may represent reservoirs for transmission in the community.

In the current study, five G and three P genotypes were detected. Rotavirus G1[P8] was the most prevalent G/P combination and this genotype combination is reported to be responsible for 50–65% of rotavirus infections in children worldwide [45]. Since more than 60% of the study subjects were affected by this genotype combination, which is in the current vaccine introduced in Tanzania (Rotarix), we assume that the vaccine will be protective, given that the circulating genotype is stable. Rotavirus G8 was the second most common genotype in this study and this is the first time it is reported in Tanzania. Of note is the fact that all the G8 strains detected were initially genotyped as G12 by multiplex and semi-nested PCR using primers described in the European Rotavirus Detection and Typing Methods version 4 [39]. The G8 genotype-specific primers were compared to nucleotide sequences of the G8 viruses isolated in this study, and three to four primer mismatches were found predominantly in the 3′end. When G12 genotype-specific primers were compared to G8 sequences we found that the numbers of mismatches were fewer and in less critical positions than the unintended mismatches for the G8 specific primers. Consequently, in samples containing G8 genotype viruses, none of the primers had perfect match, and the G12 primers by chance obtained the strongest binding producing a false positive G12 result. Due to the higher mutation-rates in viral genomes, PCR based typing strategies will generally be more error-prone than typing based on sequencing. This can result in erroneous epidemiological data and a poor foundation for further vaccine research. Other studies have also documented mistyping of rotavirus strains by multiplex RT-PCR [20,46–48]. We suggest that caution should be taken when interpreting the results of rotavirus G genotypes based on multiplex PCR. Furthermore these findings emphasize the higher robustness obtained by sequencing for typing of rotaviruses.

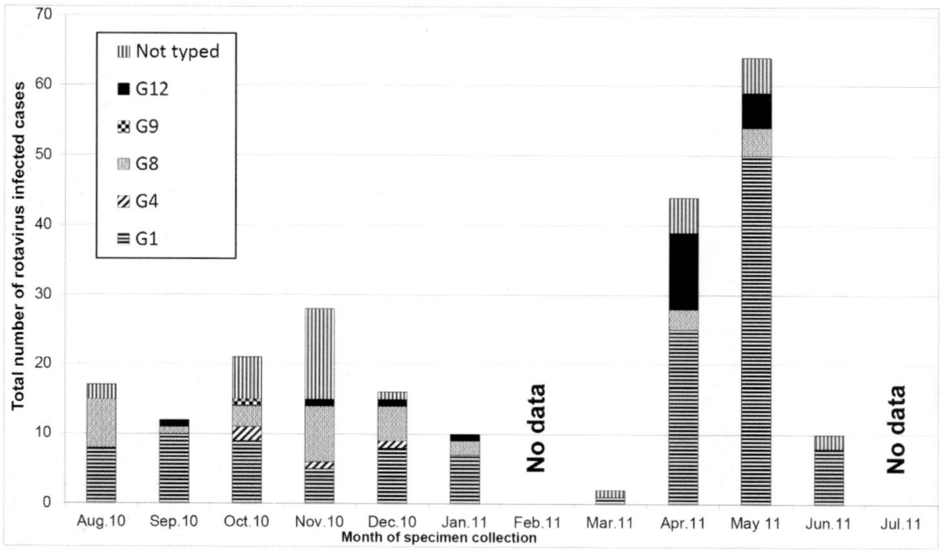

Figure 2. Seasonal variation of rotavirus infection and G genotypes among children admitted with diarrhea. The graph shows the total number of rotavirus infected children admitted due to diarrhea (cases) per month with G genotypes.

Table 2. Summary of studies on rotavirus in Dar es Salaam, Tanzania.

	Brookfield *et al* 1979[41]	Mhalu *et al* 1988[43]	Sam *et al* 1992[42]	Moyo *et al* 2007[36]	Current study 2014
Prevalence of rotavirus	31%	19.5%	43%	18.1%	32.5%
Type of subjects	Inpatients	Inpatients	Inpatients	Inpatients	Inpatients
Months of data collection	Mar1976–Sept 1976	Jan 1987–Feb 1987	May 1988–Aug 1988	Dec 2005–Feb 2006	Aug 2010–Jul 2011
Age group studied	<7 yrs	<3 yrs	<3 yrs	<5 yrs	<2 yrs
Method for detection	EM	Latex agglutination	EM+ latex agglutination	ELISA+PCR	ELISA+PCR

Genotype G12 was previously documented by sequencing only in three African countries, namely Malawi, South Africa and Nigeria [18–20]. The present study is the first documentation of genotype G12 in Tanzania.

Surprisingly we found only one strain of G9 in combination with P[8] in the current study, while this genotype predominated in the same study setting 8 years earlier [36]. This emphasizes the need for continuous rotavirus strain surveillance.

Apart from defining the serotype of rotavirus, G proteins are critical to vaccine development because they are targets for neutralizing antibodies that are believed to be important for protection. The two current rotavirus vaccines i.e RotaTeq (RV5) and Rotarix (RV1) can control infection against the five main rotavirus genotypes, which are G1, G2, G3, G4 and G9 [49]. Phylogenetic analysis was performed to show the relationship between the Tanzanian G1P[8] and vaccine strains in the Rotarix and RotaTeq vaccines. Our results revealed that the Tanzanian G1P[8] strains are distantly related to G1P[8] of the vaccine strains. This suggests that circulating G1P[8] strains may have changed over time through accumulated mutations making them different from original vaccine strains which were isolated over twenty six years ago [49,50]. In this study we report a significant increase in the prevalence of P[6] and P[4] rotavirus positive samples compared to the previous study in the same region [36]. Rotavirus samples with P[6] in this study were associated with a variety of G-genotypes (G4, G8, and G12). Phylogenetic analysis revealed that rotavirus P[6] in this study is closely related to P[6] from other African countries such as Malawi and South Africa. The high prevalence of rotavirus genotypes not included in the current rotavirus vaccines i.e. G8, G12, P[4] and P[6] in this study and other studies from developing countries may be one of the reasons for the reported lower vaccine efficacy in developing countries [51]. The Tanzanian G1P[8] variant may be able to escape from vaccine induced immunity [50]. However other possible contributing factors such as maternal antibodies and change in gut microbiota needs to be investigated [52,53]. No multiple rotavirus infection of G or P genotypes was detected in this study, which concurs with the previous findings in the same study setting [36]. In this study, rotavirus showed significant variation of prevalence in different months of the year with a peak

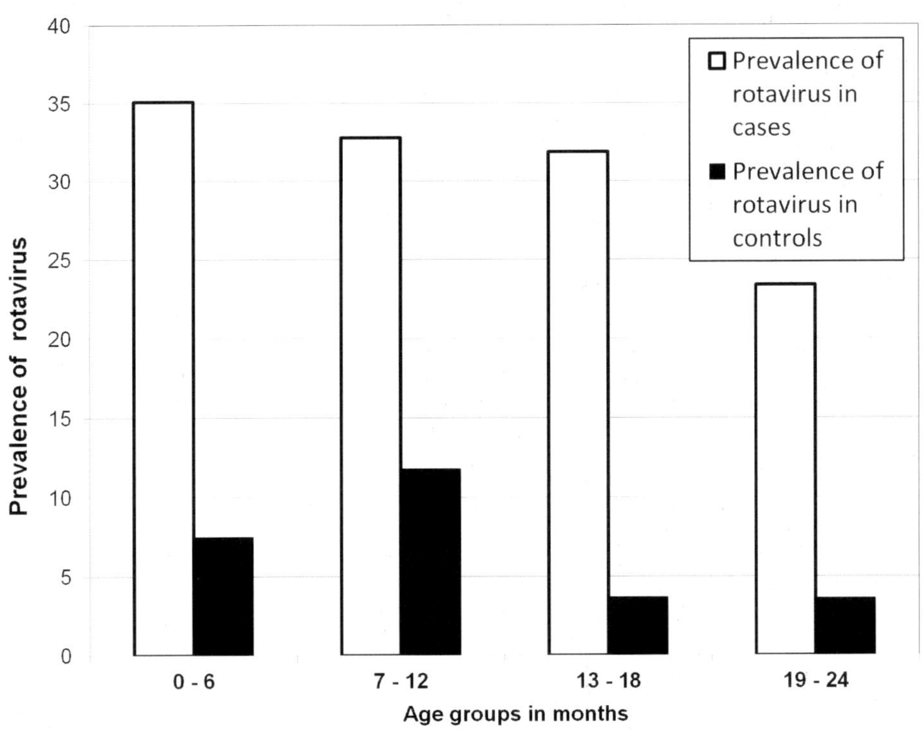

Figure 3. Prevalence of rotavirus infection in different age groups. The graph shows the prevalence of rotavirus from ELISA results per age group in cases and controls.

Table 3. Association between demographic/clinical characteristics and rotavirus infection among cases and controls in Dar es Salaam Tanzania.

				Rotavirus infection					
				Cases			Controls		
		N	N	*Univariate*		*Multivariate*[A]	*Univariate*		*Multivariate*[A]
Demographic/clinical characteristic		**Cases**	**Controls**	**n (%)**	**OR (95%CI)**	**OR (95%CI)**	**n (%)**	**OR (95%CI)**	**OR (95%CI)**
Sex	Male	422	296	140 (33.1)	1.09 (0.78–1.51)	1.06 (0.75–1.49)	26 (8.8)	1.40 (0.74–2.68)	1.58 (0.81–3.07)
	Female	268	249	84 (31.3)	1	1	16 (6.4)	1	
Parent/guardian level of education									
	Primary education	531	412	180 (34.0)	0.72 (0.47–1.10)	0.71 (0.46–1.11)	30 (7.2)	1.32 (0.66–2.67)	1.29 (0.62–2.66)
	Secondary education	137	128	37 (27.0)	0.91 (0.36–2.27)	1.05 (0.40–2.72)	12 (9.4)	0.0 (0.0)	0.0 (0.0)
	Higher education	22	5	7 (3.18)	1	1	0 (0.0)	1	1
Place of residence (district)									
	Temeke	150	91	65 (43.3)	0.61 (0.41–0.91)	0.49 (0.32–0.74)**	7 (7.7)	1.15 (0.48–2.75)	1.05 (0.43–2.56)
	Ilala	338	296	108 (32.0)	0.44 (0.28–0.70)	0.44 (0.28–0.71)**	26 (8.8)	0.72 (0.23–2.00)	0.82 (0.29–2.34)
	Kinondoni	201	158	51 (25.4)	1	1	9 (5.7)	1	1
Type of diarrhea									
	Acute diarrhea	613	na	212 (34.7)	2.87 (1.52–5.43)	2.81 (1.45–5.46)	na	na	na
	Persistent diarrhea	76	na	12 (15.8)	1	1	na	na	na
Hydration status on admission									
	Severe dehydration	157	na	46 (28.9)	1.42 (0.95–2.13)	1.23 (0.84–1.97)	na	na	na
	Some dehydration	362	na	132 (36.8)	0.91 (0.56–1.48)	0.92 (0.55–1.54)	na	na	na
	No dehydration	170	na	46 (27.1)	1	1	na	na	na
Nutrition status of the child									
	i)Underweight (WAZ)								
	Normal	300	326	107 (35.8)	1	1	30 (9.1)	1	1
	Malnourished	390	219	117 (30.0)	1.30(0.95–1.80)	1.01 (0.68–1.51)*	12 (5.5)	1.74 (0.87–3.47)	1.58 (0.65–3.87)
	ii)Stunting (LAZ)								
	Normal	223	242	89 (40.1)	1	1	21 (8.6)	1	1
	Malnourished	190	303	135 (28.9)	0.61(0.43–0.85)	0.61 (0.40–0.94)	21 (6.9)	1.40 (0.75–2.63)	1.07 (0.52–2.21)
	iii)Wasting(WLZ)								
	Normal	490	434	158 (32.2)	1	1	34 (7.8)	1	1
	Malnourished	200	111	66 (33.0)	0.96(0.68–1.36)	0.86 (0.55–1.35)	8 (7.2)	1.10 (0.50–2.45)	0.71 (0.27–1.88)

Note: na = not applicable for controls; N = total number of samples tested; n = number of positive rotavirus samples; A = multivariate logistic regression analysis included all variables in the table and age group in months;
* = P<0.05;
** = P<0.01.

of rotavirus infection during the cooler months of the year. The seasonal variation observed in the current study is further supported by findings from previous studies from the same region [36,41–43]. Studies conducted during cool months of the year [41,42] found high prevalence of rotavirus compared to studies conducted during hot months of the year [36,43]. Understanding seasonal patterns of rotavirus will be useful when considering the appropriate timing of immunization booster programs in settings, which have reported poor efficacy of rotavirus vaccine and have demonstrated strong seasonality. Rotavirus vaccine administration in the current Extended Program on Immunization schedule in developing countries is at 6, 10, and 14 weeks of age. However, if booster vaccination programs were to be considered for older children lacking immunity, vaccination during the pre-rotavirus season is recommended [34].

In this study we found significantly lower incidence of rotavirus in HIV-positive children compared to HIV-negative children with diarrhea. This supports findings of previous studies in Tanzania and other developing countries where rotavirus is detected less.

frequently or not detected at all among HIV-positive children with diarrhea [54–59]. On the other hand rotavirus was more prevalent among HIV-positive children than HIV-negative children without diarrhea. More studies are needed to clarify this issue.

Rotavirus diarrhea occurs at an earlier age among children in developing countries than children in industrialized countries. The mean age of rotavirus infection in this study compares with the mean age of rotavirus gastroenteritis in other developing countries which ranges from 6–9 months [60]. However the rotavirus prevalence of 27.8% in children less than three months is notably high with non-vaccine serotypes also found i.e. G8 and G12. This may have implications for the rotavirus vaccine introduced in the study setting; first, this age group may not fully benefit from the immunization programme, since the first dose is given at 6 weeks; secondly these infants may have acquired immunity from natural infection with rotavirus prior to immunization and therefore the ability to measure vaccine efficacy in the study setting may be impaired.

Conclusion

This study showed a switch from G9 genotype during the past 8 years to G1genotype dominance in this study, and a low similarity between the Tanzanian G1 genotype and the vaccine G1genotype. We have also observed unusual circulating genotypes G8 and G12 for the first time in Tanzania. Since early 2013, the rotavirus vaccine Rotarix has been introduced and included in the Extended Program of Immunization (EPI) in Tanzania. The present study represents pre-vaccination data and may be useful in the future when assessing the effectiveness of the vaccine. This study also showed seasonal variation in the prevalence of rotavirus. Rotavirus seasonality provides insights important for vaccination strategies, including potential shifts in seasonal peaks and duration of outbreaks. Our data also support the notion that rotavirus may not be an opportunistic pathogen in children infected with HIV.

Acknowledgments

We would like to thank Ms. Mary Nyange of MNH Central Pathology Laboratory for her technical support. We also thank Steinar Sornes from the Department of Clinical Science at the University of Bergen for his support in performing ELISA. We thank the parents/guardians who consented for their children to participate in the study.

Author Contributions

Conceived and designed the experiments: SJM NL BB SYM. Performed the experiments: SJM. Analyzed the data: SJM BB KH OK KV SYM NL. Contributed reagents/materials/analysis tools: SJM BB KH OK KV SYM NL. Wrote the paper: SJM BB KH OK KV SYM NL.

References

1. Parashar UD, Burton A, Lanata C, Boschi-Pinto C, Shibuya K, et al. (2009) Global mortality associated with rotavirus disease among children in 2004. J Infect Dis 200 Suppl 1: S9–S15.
2. Parashar UD, Gibson CJ, Bresee JS, Glass RI (2006) Rotavirus and severe childhood diarrhea. Emerg Infect Dis 12: 304–306.
3. Centers for Disease Control and Prevention (2011) Rotavirus surveillance–worldwide, 2009. MMWR Morb Mortal Wkly Rep 60: 514–516.
4. Tate JE, Burton AH, Boschi-Pinto C, Steele AD, Duque J, et al. (2012) 2008 estimate of worldwide rotavirus-associated mortality in children younger than 5 years before the introduction of universal rotavirus vaccination programmes: a systematic review and meta-analysis. Lancet Infect Dis 12: 136–141.
5. Wang FT, Mast TC, Glass RJ, Loughlin J, Seeger JD (2010) Effectiveness of the pentavalent rotavirus vaccine in preventing gastroenteritis in the United States. Pediatrics 125: e208–213.
6. de Palma O, Cruz L, Ramos H, de Baires A, Villatoro N, et al. (2010) Effectiveness of rotavirus vaccination against childhood diarrhoea in El Salvador: case-control study. BMJ 340: c2825.
7. Staat MA, Rice MA, Donauer S, Payne DC, Bresee JS, et al. (2010) Estimating the rotavirus hospitalization disease burden and trends, using capture-recapture methods. Pediatr Infect Dis J 29: 1083–1086.
8. Paulke-Korinek M, Rendi-Wagner P, Kundi M, Kronik R, Kollaritsch H (2010) Universal mass vaccination against rotavirus gastroenteritis: impact on hospitalization rates in austrian children. Pediatr Infect Dis J 29: 319–323.
9. Trimis G, Koutsoumbari I, Kottaridi C, Palaiologou N, Assimakopoulou E, et al. (2011) Hospital-based surveillance of rotavirus gastroenteritis in the era of limited vaccine uptake through the private sector. Vaccine 29: 7292–7295.
10. Becker-Dreps S, Paniagua M, Dominik R, Cao H, Shah NK, et al. (2011) Changes in childhood diarrhea incidence in nicaragua following 3 years of universal infant rotavirus immunization. Pediatr Infect Dis J 30: 243–247.
11. Martella V, Banyai K, Matthijnssens J, Buonavoglia C, Ciarlet M (2010) Zoonotic aspects of rotaviruses. Vet Microbiol 140: 246–255.
12. Kapikian AZ, Hoshino Y, Chanock RM (2001) Rotaviruses. In: Howley PM, editor. Fields virology 4th ed. Philadelphia, Pa.: Lippincott Williams & Wilkins. 1787–1833.
13. Hoshino Y, Sereno MM, Midthun K, Flores J, Kapikian AZ, et al. (1985) Independent segregation of two antigenic specificities (VP3 and VP7) involved in neutralization of rotavirus infectivity. Proc Natl Acad Sci U S A 82: 8701–8704.
14. Offit PA, Clark HF, Blavat G, Greenberg HB (1986) Reassortant rotaviruses containing structural proteins vp3 and vp7 from different parents induce antibodies protective against each parental serotype. J Virol 60: 491–496.
15. Laird AR, Gentsch JR, Nakagomi T, Nakagomi O, Glass RI (2003) Characterization of serotype G9 rotavirus strains isolated in the United States and India from 1993 to 2001. J Clin Microbiol 41: 3100–3111.
16. Matthijnssens J, Ciarlet M, McDonald SM, Attoui H, Banyai K, et al. (2011) Uniformity of rotavirus strain nomenclature proposed by the Rotavirus Classification Working Group (RCWG). Arch Virol 156: 1397–1413.
17. Santos N, Hoshino Y (2005) Global distribution of rotavirus serotypes/genotypes and its implication for the development and implementation of an effective rotavirus vaccine. Rev Med Virol 15: 29–56.
18. Cunliffe NA, Ngwira BM, Dove W, Nakagomi O, Nakagomi T, et al. (2009) Serotype g12 rotaviruses, Lilongwe, Malawi. Emerg Infect Dis 15: 87–90.
19. Page NA, de Beer MC, Seheri LM, Dewar JB, Steele AD (2009) The detection and molecular characterization of human G12 genotypes in South Africa. J Med Virol 81: 106–113.
20. Oluwatoyin Japhet M, Adeyemi Adesina O, Famurewa O, Svensson L, Nordgren J (2012) Molecular epidemiology of rotavirus and norovirus in Ile-Ife, Nigeria: high prevalence of G12P[8] rotavirus strains and detection of a rare norovirus genotype. J Med Virol 84: 1489–1496.
21. Chandrahasen C, Grimwood K, Redshaw N, Rich FJ, Wood C, et al. (2010) Geographical differences in the proportion of human group A rotavirus strains within New Zealand during one epidemic season. Journal of Medical Virology 82: 897–902.
22. Esona MD, Geyer A, Page N, Trabelsi A, Fodha I, et al. (2009) Genomic characterization of human rotavirus G8 strains from the African rotavirus network: relationship to animal rotaviruses. J Med Virol 81: 937–951.
23. Esona MD, Steele D, Kerin T, Armah G, Peenze I, et al. (2010) Determination of the G and P Types of Previously Nontypeable Rotavirus Strains from the African Rotavirus Network, 1996–2004: Identification of Unusual G Types. Journal of Infectious Diseases 202: S49–S54.

24. Gentsch JR, Laird AR, Bielfelt B, Griffin DD, Bányai K, et al. (2005) Serotype Diversity and Reassortment between Human and Animal Rotavirus Strains: Implications for Rotavirus Vaccine Programs. Journal of Infectious Diseases 192: S146–S159.
25. Kiulia NM, Kamenwa R, Irimu G, Nyangao JO, Gatheru Z, et al. (2008) The epidemiology of human rotavirus associated with diarrhoea in Kenyan children: a review. J Trop Pediatr 54: 401–405.
26. Matthijnssens J, Rahman M, Yang X, Delbeke T, Arijs I, et al. (2006) G8 Rotavirus Strains Isolated in the Democratic Republic of Congo Belong to the DS-1-Like Genogroup. Journal of Clinical Microbiology 44: 1801–1809.
27. Pietsch C, Petersen L, Patzer L, Liebert UG (2009) Molecular Characteristics of German G8P[4] Rotavirus Strain GER1H-09 Suggest that a Genotyping and Subclassification Update Is Required for G8. Journal of Clinical Microbiology 47: 3569–3576.
28. Steyer A, Poljšak-Prijatelj M, Bufon TL, Marčun-Varda N, Marin J (2007) Rotavirus genotypes in Slovenia: Unexpected detection of G8P[8] and G12P[8] genotypes. Journal of Medical Virology 79: 626–632.
29. Levy K, Hubbard AE, Eisenberg JN (2009) Seasonality of rotavirus disease in the tropics: a systematic review and meta-analysis. Int J Epidemiol 38: 1487–1496.
30. Cook SM, Glass RI, LeBaron CW, Ho MS (1990) Global seasonality of rotavirus infections. Bull World Health Organ 68: 171–177.
31. Pitzer VE, Viboud C, Simonsen L, Steiner C, Panozzo CA, et al. (2009) Demographic variability, vaccination, and the spatiotemporal dynamics of rotavirus epidemics. Science 325: 290–294.
32. D'Souza RM, Hall G, Becker NG (2008) Climatic factors associated with hospitalizations for rotavirus diarrhoea in children under 5 years of age. Epidemiol Infect 136: 56–64.
33. Atchison CJ, Tam CC, Hajat S, van Pelt W, Cowden JM, et al. (2010) Temperature-dependent transmission of rotavirus in Great Britain and The Netherlands. Proc Biol Sci 277: 933–942.
34. Jagai JS, Sarkar R, Castronovo D, Kattula D, McEntee J, et al. (2012) Seasonality of rotavirus in South Asia: a meta-analysis approach assessing associations with temperature, precipitation, and vegetation index. PLoS One 7: e38168.
35. PATH (2012) Vaccine Access and Delivery Global Program Rotavirus disease and vaccines in Tanzania. Seattle USA.
36. Moyo SJ, Gro N, Kirsti V, Matee MI, Kitundu J, et al. (2007) Prevalence of enteropathogenic viruses and molecular characterization of group A rotavirus among children with diarrhea in Dar es Salaam Tanzania. BMC Public Health 7: 359.
37. Ezeamama AE, Spiegelman D, Hertzmark E, Bosch RJ, Manji KP, et al. (2012) HIV infection and the incidence of malaria among HIV-exposed children from Tanzania. J Infect Dis 205: 1486–1494.
38. WHO (1977) The presentation and use of height and weight data for comparing the nutritional status of groups of children under the age of 10 years. Bull World Health Organ 55: 489–498.
39. EUROROTA (2009) European Rotavirus Detection and Typing Methods.
40. Kimura M (1980) A simple method for estimating evolutionary rates of base substitutions through comparative studies of nucleotide sequences. J Mol Evol 16: 111–120.
41. Brookfield DSK, Cosgrove BP, Bell EJ, Madeley CR (1979) Viruses demonstrated in children in Tanzania: studies in diarrhoea and measles. Journal of Infection 1: 249–255.
42. Sam NE, Haukenes G, Szilvay AM, Mhalu F (1992) Rotavirus infection in Tanzania: a virological, epidemiological and clinical study among young children. APMIS 100: 790–796.
43. Mhalu FS, Myrmel H, Msengi A, Haukenes G (1988) Prevalence of infection with rotavirus and enteric adenoviruses among children in Tanzania. NIPH Ann 11: 3–7.
44. Aminu M, Page NA, Ahmad AA, Umoh JU, Dewar J, et al. (2010) Diversity of rotavirus VP7 and VP4 genotypes in Northwestern Nigeria. J Infect Dis 202 Suppl: S198–204.
45. Arora R, Chitambar SD (2011) Full genomic analysis of Indian G1P[8] rotavirus strains. Infect Genet Evol 11: 504–511.
46. Aladin F, Nawaz S, Iturriza-Gomara M, Gray J (2010) Identification of G8 rotavirus strains determined as G12 by rotavirus genotyping PCR: updating the current genotyping methods. J Clin Virol 47: 340–344.
47. Iturriza-Gomara M, Kang G, Gray J (2004) Rotavirus genotyping: keeping up with an evolving population of human rotaviruses. J Clin Virol 31: 259–265.
48. Nordgren J, Nitiema LW, Sharma S, Ouermi D, Traore AS, et al. (2012) Emergence of unusual G6P[6] rotaviruses in children, Burkina Faso, 2009–2010. Emerg Infect Dis 18: 589–597.
49. Cortese MM, Parashar UD, Centers for Disease Control and Prevention (2009) Prevention of rotavirus gastroenteritis among infants and children: recommendations of the Advisory Committee on Immunization Practices (ACIP). MMWR Recomm Rep 58: 1–25.
50. Afrad MH, Hassan Z, Farjana S, Moni S, Barua S, et al. (2013) Changing profile of rotavirus genotypes in Bangladesh, 2006–2012. BMC Infect Dis 13: 320.
51. Madhi SA, Cunliffe NA, Steele D, Witte D, Kirsten M, et al. (2010) Effect of human rotavirus vaccine on severe diarrhea in African infants. N Engl J Med 362: 289–298.
52. Parashar UD, Glass RI (2009) Rotavirus vaccines–early success, remaining questions. N Engl J Med 360: 1063–1065.
53. Patel M, Shane AL, Parashar UD, Jiang B, Gentsch JR, et al. (2009) Oral rotavirus vaccines: how well will they work where they are needed most? J Infect Dis 200 Suppl 1: S39–48.
54. Cegielski JP, Msengi AE, Miller SE (1994) Enteric viruses associated with HIV infection in Tanzanian children with chronic diarrhea. Pediatr AIDS HIV Infect 5: 296–299.
55. Cunliffe NA, Gondwe JS, Kirkwood CD, Graham SM, Nhlane NM, et al. (2001) Effect of concomitant HIV infection on presentation and outcome of rotavirus gastroenteritis in Malawian children. Lancet 358: 550–555.
56. Liste MB, Natera I, Suarez JA, Pujol FH, Liprandi F, et al. (2000) Enteric virus infections and diarrhea in healthy and human immunodeficiency virus-infected children. J Clin Microbiol 38: 2873–2877.
57. Oshitani H, Kasolo FC, Mpabalwani M, Luo NP, Matsubayashi N, et al. (1994) Association of rotavirus and human immunodeficiency virus infection in children hospitalized with acute diarrhea, Lusaka, Zambia. J Infect Dis 169: 897–900.
58. Pavia AT, Long EG, Ryder RW, Nsa W, Puhr ND, et al. (1992) Diarrhea among African children born to human immunodeficiency virus 1-infected mothers: clinical, microbiologic and epidemiologic features. Pediatr Infect Dis J 11: 996–1003.
59. Rossit AR, de Almeida MT, Nogueira CA, da Costa Oliveira JG, Barbosa DM, et al. (2007) Bacterial, yeast, parasitic, and viral enteropathogens in HIV-infected children from Sao Paulo State, Southeastern Brazil. Diagn Microbiol Infect Dis 57: 59–66.
60. Bresee JS, Glass RI, Ivanoff B, Gentsch JR (1999) Current status and future priorities for rotavirus vaccine development, evaluation and implementation in developing countries. Vaccine 17: 2207–2222.

Mortality Trends Observed in Population-Based Surveillance of an Urban Slum Settlement, Kibera, Kenya, 2007–2010

Beatrice Olack[1]*, Daniel R. Feikin[2], Leonard O. Cosmas[2], Kennedy O. Odero[1], George O. Okoth[1], Joel M. Montgomery[2], Robert F. Breiman[2]

1 Kenya Medical Research Institute and Centers for Disease Control and Prevention Collaboration (KEMRI-CDC), Nairobi, Kenya, 2 Global Disease Detection Division, Kenya Office of the US Centers for Disease Control & Prevention, Nairobi, Kenya

Abstract

Background: We used population based infectious disease surveillance to characterize mortality rates in residents of an urban slum in Kenya.

Methods: We analyzed biweekly household visit data collected two weeks before death for 749 cases who died during January 1, 2007 to December 31, 2010. We also selected controls matched by age, gender and having a biweekly household visit within two weeks before death of the corresponding case and compared the symptoms reported.

Results: The overall mortality rate was 6.3 per 1,000 person years of observation (PYO) (females: 5.7; males: 6.8). Infant mortality rate was 50.2 per 1000 PYOs, and it was 15.1 per 1,000 PYOs for children <5 years old. Poisson regression indicates a significant decrease over time in overall mortality from (6.0 in 2007 to 4.0 in 2010 per 1000 PYOs; $p<0.05$) in persons ≥ 5 years old. This decrease was predominant in females (7.8 to 5.7 per 1000 PYOs; $p<0.05$). Two weeks before death, significantly higher prevalence for cough (OR = 4.7 [95% CI: 3.7–5.9]), fever (OR = 8.1 [95% CI: 6.1–10.7]), and diarrhea (OR = 9.1 [95% CI: 6.4–13.2]) were reported among participants who died (cases) when compared to participants who did not die (controls). Diarrhea followed by fever were independently associated with deaths (OR = 14.4 [95% CI: 7.1–29.2]), and (OR = 11.4 [95% CI: 6.7–19.4]) respectively.

Conclusions: Despite accessible health care, mortality rates are high among people living in this urban slum; infectious disease syndromes appear to be linked to a substantial proportion of deaths. Rapid urbanization poses an increasing challenge in national efforts to improve health outcomes, including reducing childhood mortality rates. Targeting impoverished people in urban slums with effective interventions such as water and sanitation interventions are needed to achieve national objectives for health.

Editor: Sten H. Vermund, Vanderbilt University, United States of America

Funding: This work was supported by the Centers for Disease Control and Prevention (CDC US). The funders had no role in study design, data collection and analysis, decision to publish, or preparation of the manuscript.

Competing Interests: The authors have declared that no competing interests exist.

* E-mail: bolack@kemricdc.org

Introduction

Africa is urbanizing at a faster rate than any other continent in the world [1]. By 2030, more than half of the population of sub-Saharan Africa is expected to live in urban areas [2]. More than 70% of urban residents in sub-Saharan Africa live in informal settlements or slums [3], where basic infrastructure cannot keep pace with urbanization rates [4]. These slums are characterized by dense population, poor sanitation, and contaminated water supplies, with potential adverse health impact for community residents [5], [6]. Consequently, such slums are often characterized by high incidence of a variety of communicable and non-communicable diseases [7] and injuries, leading to high rates of morbidity [8] and alarmingly high under-five mortality rates [9].

Mortality rate information is crucial for setting priorities for health interventions and research [10]. While recent studies have examined childhood mortality rates in rural or peri-urban areas [11], [12]. little is known about mortality in children and adults residing in informal urban settlements in Africa. Furthermore, data available on health status are often derived from hospital-based studies that neglect morbidity and mortality outside of health care systems accessed by a minority of people in African urban and rural settings [13], [14]. likely underestimating disease burden. In this paper, we describe the overall and age-specific mortality rates and trends over time in a well-defined population in Kibera, an urban slum in Nairobi, Kenya, by utilizing population-based surveillance data collected from January 2007 to December 2010.

Materials and Methods

The Kenya Medical Research Institute (KEMRI) and the US Centers for Disease Control and Prevention (CDC) have

Table 1. Characteristics of the study population.

Variable	PYO	Percentage
All	119119	
Sex		
Male	60647	50.9
Female	58472	49.1
Age in years		
<1	3210	2.7
1–4	17270	14.5
5–9	18035	15.1
10–17	18474	15.5
18–34	44784	37.6
35–49	14134	11.9
≥50	3211	2.7
Year of observation		
2007	28798	24.2
2008	29542	24.8
2009	30054	25.2
2010	30725	25.8

Table 2. Trend in mortality rates by gender, age and year in Kibera informal settlement, Kenya January 2009–December 2010.

	2007	2008	2009	2010	Overall	P-value
Sex						
Male	7.6	6.4	6.3	6.9	6.8	0.47
Female	7.8	5.5	4.8	5.0	5.7	<0.05*
Age in years						
<1	51.1	35.5	49.3	63.9	50.2	0.14
1–4	9.4	10.0	8.0	6.8	8.6	0.13
5–9	1.4	0.9	1.3	2.3	1.5	0.22
10–17	1.7	0.5	1.1	0.8	1.0	0.33
18–34	6.6	5.0	2.5	4.1	4.6	<0.05*
35–49	11.4	8.4	10.1	8.5	9.6	0.34
≥50	24.5	17.3	17.1	11.1	17.1	0.05
All Ages	7.7	6.0	5.6	6.0	6.3	<0.05*
<5	15.4	13.7	15.0	16.2	15.1	0.64
≥5	6.0	4.3	3.6	4.0	4.5	<0.05*

*Significant reductions in mortality rates over the years.

collaboratively conducted population-based infectious disease surveillance (PBIDS) since late 2005 in 2 villages (Gatwikera and Soweto West) in the Kibera slum, situated in Nairobi, Kenya. Population ranges between 25,000 and 29,000 people in the 0.37 km^2 surveillance area (mean population density = 77,000 persons/km^2). Consistent with conditions in most urban slums, the PBIDS site is characterized by sub-standard housing and poor security, insufficient garbage disposal, lack of formal sewers, overcrowding and inadequate water drainage.

PBIDS has been previously described [8]. Standardized home visit data were captured electronically with Personal Digital Assistants (PDA) by trained community interviewers who visited about 7000 enrolled households within the surveillance villages of Gatwikira and Soweto West every two weeks, asking standardized questions about illnesses and specific symptoms for each person in the household. Morbidity and vital events data were recorded for each person in the household. In the event of death, a household proxy was interviewed to collect relevant information about illnesses and health-seeking behaviour before death. Ill participants enrolled in the study could access free high quality care at a well staffed study clinic run in collaboration between Carolina for Kibera and KEMRI/CDC and located within 1 km of the surveillance area residence. Data used for the current analysis were abstracted from the PBIDS database for the years 2007–2010 (the study period). All participants registered into PBIDS were eligible for the study.

To be enrolled into PBIDS, participants must have resided in the area for at least 4 consecutive calendar months, and the household head consented to participation. Residency status in the surveillance area was used to determine start and stop dates for person-time (rate denominator) contribution. The difference between the start and stop dates were divided by 365.25 to generate person years contributed to the study [15].

Symptoms and care seeking behaviour occurring two weeks before death were determined from household interview data. Case definition for fever and diarrhoea symptoms are as earlier defined [13]. We used local language (Kiswahili or Dho-luo) terms when asking about presence of cough during the biweekly interviews.

Data analyses were performed using SAS (Statistical Analysis System, version 9.3, Cary, NC). A post hoc case control analysis was undertaken to determine the symptoms associated with death. Mortality rates were expressed as the number of deaths (overall or by age-group) of participants per 1,000 person years of observation (PYO) [15]. We defined infant mortality as deaths in children <12 months old, child mortality as deaths in children 12–59 months and under-five mortality rate as deaths in all children less than 60 months.

We compared age-group associated mortality rates using incidence rate ratios and used poisson regression to model for linear trend in the mortality rates. Pair-Matched Odds Ratio was used to evaluate whether an association exists between case status (for cases and controls) and death outcome. We used multivariate conditional logistic regression to evaluate whether illnesses reported by cases and controls differed and to determine which illness or group of illnesses are best predictors of the outcome variable (case status). Two and three way interactions were fitted and their significance tested using p-values. All insignificant interactions were dropped to obtain a well-fitting model.

Cases were all participants in PBIDS who died between January 2007 and December 2010 and had pre- mortem information from the biweekly household visit. Controls were participants who were alive at the time that their respective cases died. We selected age ranges which provided at least two controls per case with a target of three controls per case matched by gender, age and a biweekly household interview within 2-weeks before death of the corresponding case. To select controls, we used the following age ranges matched to each age category of cases: for each case <12 months old, matching controls were plus or minus 2 months of age around the age of the matching case; for each case 1-to-4 year of age, matching controls were within plus or minus 2 months of age; for each case aged 5 to 17 years old, matching controls were plus or minus 1 year of age, for each case aged 18 to 34 years old, matching controls were plus or minus 2 years of age. In selecting

Table 3. Distribution of reported symptoms by age among cases and controls two weeks before death in Kibera informal settlement, Kenya January 2007 to December 2010.

	Cough			Fever			Diarrhea		
Age in years	**Cases (%)**	**Controls (%)**	**OR (95% CI)**	**Cases (%)**	**Controls (%)**	**OR (95% CI)**	**Cases (%)**	**Controls (%)**	**OR (95% CI)**
<1	66 (47.1)	85 (20.2)	3.5 (2.3–5.3)	58 (41.4)	46 (11)	5.8 (3.6–9.1)	43 (30.7)	25 (6)	7.0 (4.1–12.0)
1–4	31 (24.6)	35 (9.3)	3.2 (1.9–5.5)	22 (17.5)	22 (5.8)	3.4 (1.8–6.4)	28 (22.2)	18 (4.8)	5.7 (3.0–10.8)
<5	**97 (36.5)**	**120 (15)**	**3.2 (2.4–4.4)**	**80 (30.1)**	**68 (8.5)**	**4.6 (3.2–6.6)**	**71 (26.7)**	**43 (5.4)**	**6.4 (4.2–9.6)**
5–9	4 (15.4)	4 (5.1)	3.4 (0.8–14.6)	8 (30.8)	3 (3.8)	11.1 (2.7–46.1)	2 (7.7)	1 (1.3)	6.4 (0.6–73.9)
10–17	3 (17.6)	1 (2)	10.7 (1.0–111.2)	6 (35.3)	0	NA	3 (17.6)	0	N/A
18–34	34 (18.7)	21 (3.8)	5.7 (3.2–10.2)	44 (24.2)	10 (1.8)	17.1 (8.4–34.8)	17 (9.3)	1 (0.2)	56.1 (7.4–424.9)
35–49	34 (27.9)	8 (2.2)	17.3 (7.7–38.7)	34 (27.9)	4 (1.1)	35.0 (12.1–101.1)	18 (14.8)	1 (0.3)	63.1 (8.3–478.5)
≥50	20 (37.7)	5 (3.2)	18.4 (6.4–52.6)	13 (24.5)	6 (3.8)	8.2 (2.9–22.9)	9 (17)	1 (0.6)	31.9 (3.9–258.7)
≥5	**95 (23.8)**	**39 (3.3)**	**9.2 (6.2–13.7)**	**105 (26.3)**	**23 (1.9)**	**18.2 (11.4–29.1)**	**49 (12.3)**	**4 (0.3)**	**41.7 (14.9–116.3)**
All Ages	**192 (28.8)**	**159 (8)**	**4.7 (3.7–5.9)**	**185 (27.8)**	**91 (4.6)**	**8.1 (6.1–10.7)**	**120 (18)**	**47 (2.4)**	**9.1 (6.4–13.2)**

the controls for each case >35 years old, matching controls were plus or minus 3 years of age.

Data collection was conducted as part of the KEMRI/CDC PBIDS protocol. The PBIDS protocol has been reviewed and approved by the Ethical Review Boards of the Kenya Medical Research Institute (KEMRI) (Protocol #932 and #1899) and the CDC's Institutional Review Board (#4566). Trained community interviewers obtained written informed consent for participants in the PBIDS study. For minors, consent was obtained from their parent or guardian.

Results

During the study period, PBIDS data comprised 46,022 individuals accumulating 119,119 person years. Children under five years contributed 17.2% of the total person time (Table 1). A total of 749 deaths were recorded during the study period, yielding an overall mortality rate of 6.3 (95% CI: 5.9, 6.8) per 1000 PYO. The mortality rate for children <5 years old, 15.1 (95% CI: 13.5, 16.9) per 1,000 PYO, was more than three-fold that for persons ≥ 5 years old (4.5 [95% CI: 4.1, 4.9] per 1,000 PYO). Half of the deaths (52%) in children under five were among infants. The infant mortality rate (50.2 [95% CI: 43.0, 58.6] per 1000 PYO) was >5-fold higher than the child mortality rate (8.6 [95% CI: 7.3, 10.1] per 1000 PYO).

There was a significant decline in overall annual mortality rates (7.7 in 2007 to 6.0 in 2010 per 1000 PYOs; $p<0.05$) over the four years. However, when stratified by age group, significant reductions over time were only shown for adults 18–34 year old (Table 2). The decline ($p<0.05$) in this age category was in both males and females. Over the course of the study period, a significant decline ($p<0.05$) in mortality rates was observed among all females regardless of age-but not among males (Table 2).

Males represented 55.1% of the total number of deaths. Overall mortality rates were significantly lower in females (5.7/1000 PYO) than in males (6.8/1000 PYO) (RR = 0.84 [95% CI: 0.73, 0.98], $P<0.05$). In persons ≥5 years old, females had significantly lower mortality rates (3.8 per 1000 PYO) than males (5.1 per 1000 PYO, RR = 0.75 [95% CI: 0.62, 0.91], $P<0.05$). Female infant mortality rates were 53.4 per 1000 PYO compared with 46.8 per 1000 PYO in male infants; however, this difference was not statistically significant, and there were no gender differences in child or overall under-five mortality rates.

Bi-weekly household visit data from the two weeks before death were available for 666 (89%) cases including 266 (40%) children under five years old and 400 (60%) persons ≥5 years old. There were 1996 controls for the 666 cases that had household morbidity data available. Among the cases 161 (61%) children under five years and 250 (63%) of persons aged >5 years reported at least one of the following cough, fever or diarrheal symptoms during the household visit, while among the controls 191 (24%) children under five years and 77 (6%) of persons aged >5 years reported at least one of the same symptoms. The percentages of cases and controls having fever were 27.8% and 4.6%. The corresponding percentages for cough were 28.8% and 8.0%, and 18.0% and 2.4% for diarrhea (Table 3). The percentage of cases and controls having both fever and cough were 16.7% and 3.3% respectively. The corresponding percentages for fever and diarrhea were 9.8% and 1.2%, and 9.9% and 1.6% for cough and diarrhea. We fitted a conditional logistic regression model for case/control status (death) including main effects for all three diseases and their three pair wise interaction terms. The 3-way interaction term was initially fit in the model and was non-significant, and thus subsequently dropped from the model. All three main effect variables for the diseases were significant (matched ORs = 11.4, 4.3, and 14.4 for fever, cough, and diarrhea, respectively) indicating that each disease is independently associated with death absent the other two (Table 4). The interaction terms for fever and cough ($p<0.001$) and for cough and diarrhea ($p = 0.001$) were both statistically significant and indicated that these two interactions were antagonistic (i.e. the risk factors reduce the effect of one another in each pair). The interaction term for fever and diarrhea was nonsignificant ($p = 0.38$). The matched ORs of death for fever and cough, fever and diarrhea, and cough and diarrhea versus no illness two weeks prior to death were 8.5, 105.4, and 11.9, respectively (Table 5). The matched OR of death with fever and cough versus cough alone was 2.0 ($p = 0.015$), but there was no evidence that deaths were more likely in persons with fever and cough versus fever alone. The matched OR of death was 9.3 for fever and diarrhea versus fever alone, and 7.3 for fever and diarrhea versus diarrhea alone. The matched OR of death for cough and diarrhea versus cough alone was 2.7 ($p = 0.014$) but

Table 4. Assesment of independent association of symptom(s) with death stratified by age group using conditional logistic regression.

Age in years	Symptom	Matched Odds Ratio (95% Wald Confidence Limits)	P-value
<1	Fever	8.2 (2.7–24.7)	0.0002
	Cough	2.6 (1.4–5)	0.0041
	Diarrhea	8.9 (2.4–32.5)	0.0010
	Fever and Cough	0.2 (0.1–0.9)	0.0336
1–4	Cough	3.5 (1.5–8.1)	0.0032
	Diarrhea	8.1 (2.4–27.6)	0.0008
	Cough and Diarrhea	0.2 (0–0.8)	0.0238
<5	Fever	4.6 (2.2–9.6)	<.0001
	Cough	2.8 (1.7–4.6)	<.0001
	Diarrhea	8.1 (3.4–19.6)	<.0001
	Fever and Cough	0.3 (0.1–0.9)	0.0276
	Cough and Diarrhea	0.3 (0.1–0.8)	0.0210
5–9	Fever	13 (1.4–119.3)	0.0236
10–17	None		
18–34	Fever	64.3 (8.6–481.1)	<.0001
	Cough	3.3 (1.2–9)	0.0171
	Fever and Cough	0 (0–0.4)	0.0076
35–49	Fever	Undefined	0.0024
	Cough	12.7 (3–52.7)	0.0005
	Diarrhea	Undefined	0.0006
≥50	Cough	Undefined	0.0008
	Diarrhea	40.2 (2.1–783.2)	0.0148
≥5	Fever	26.4 (10.8–64.6)	<.0001
	Cough	7.2 (3.8–13.6)	<.0001
	Diarrhea	34.8 (9.5–127.6)	<.0001
	Fever and Cough	0.1 (0–0.3)	0.0002
All Ages	Fever	11.4 (6.7–19.4)	<.0001
	Cough	4.3 (2.9–6.4)	<.0001
	Diarrhea	14.4 (7.1–29.2)	<.0001
	Fever and Cough	0.2 (0.1–0.4)	<.0001
	Cough and Diarrhea	0.2 (0.1–0.5)	0.0010

there was no evidence that deaths were more likely in persons with cough and diarrhea than in persons with diarrhea alone.

Among sick children and persons aged ≥5years, health care outside the home during the two weeks before death was sought for 121 (75%) children under-five and for 167 (67%) persons aged ≥5years. Male children <5 years old with cough or diarrhea or fever noted during the two weeks before death were slightly less likely (74%) to seek care at a health facility than females <5 years old with the same symptoms (77%) (OR = 0.86, [95% CI: 0.39–1.87]). Similarly, for persons ≥5 years of age, males with cough, diarrhea or fever were less likely (63%) to seek care than females (72%) (OR = 0.68, [95% CI: 0.39–1.20]). However, the differences were not statistically significant.

Discussion

The findings of our study indicate that essentially 5% (50 deaths per 1000 child-years) of infants die in the first year of life in this urban slum setting. In contrast with rural areas, where clinical services are often hard to access [14], six licensed health facilities within the surveillance villages are available in close proximity, and yet are often not timely utilized, even with illnesses serious enough to result in death [13]. This suggests that more work is needed to characterize health conditions in urban settings and understand health utilization determinants.

Comparison of illnesses among people living in this slum area and a sparsely populated rural in western Kenya suggest that rates of cough, febrile illness and diarrheal disease can be quite dissimilar [15]. Some etiologic agents for these syndromes appear to be disparate as well [16], [17]. Effective programs and interventions to improve health outcomes in urban slum settings may need to be configured quite differently than in rural areas. This is becoming an increasingly important issue as urbanization in Kenya continues to occur at approximately 7% annually [18] with people migrating from rural areas nearly universally into densely populated urban slums where sanitation, hygiene, and

Table 5. Conditional logistic regression model of death with reported symptom(s) as predictors.

Symptom(s)	Matched Odds Ratio (95% CI)	P-value
Fever, no cough, no diarrhea vs no illness	11.4 (6.7–19.4)	<.0001
Cough, no fever, no diarrhea vs no illness	4.3 (2.9–6.4)	<.0001
Diarrhea, no fever, no cough vs no illness	14.4 (7.1–29.2)	<.0001
Fever and cough, no diarrhea vs no illness	8.5 (5.5–13.1)	<.0001
Fever and diarrhea, no cough vs no illness	105.4 (32–346.8)	<.0001
Cough and diarrhea, no fever vs no illness	11.9 (5.6–25.3)	<.0001
Fever and cough, no diarrhea vs fever	0.7 (0.4–1.4)	0.3784
Fever and cough, no diarrhea vs cough	2 (1.1–3.4)	0.0151
Fever and diarrhea, no cough vs fever	9.3 (3–28.3)	<.0001
Fever and diarrhea, no cough vs diarrhea	7.3 (2.5–21.4)	0.0003
Cough and diarrhea, no fever vs cough	2.7 (1.2–6.1)	0.0140
Cough and diarrhea, no fever vs diarrhea	0.8 (0.3–2.1)	0.6890

water supplies are sub-optimal; in 2012, >60% of the Nairobi population resided in urban slums [19]. UNICEF's 2012 State of the World's Children Report emphasized that even where services are nearby, children growing up in poor urban settings face significant health risks [9].

The findings from this study suggest that mortality rates in the Nairobi urban slums were at par or higher than rates reported from an urban slum in India (6.2 per 1000 PYO) [10]. Data analyzed from 22 countries indicated that only five countries (Namibia, Eritrea, Madagascar, Uganda and Malawi) recorded declines in urban child mortality in line with the MDG target of about 4% per annum [20]. Although the Kenya Demographic and Health Survey from 2008 reported a decline in under-five mortality rates, continued urban migration without either infrastructural improvements or programs targeting unique urban health problems, may impede and potentially reverse progress in reducing childhood mortality. Consistent with that concern, the Nairobi Cross-sectional Slum Survey (NCSS), carried out by the African Population and Health Research Center (APHRC) in 2000 showed that urban under-five mortality has increased over time, and suggested that urban poor children have higher mortality than their rural counterparts [6]. The surveillance platform which provided data for this study includes free, high quality health care for acute illnesses for all surveillance participants. We believe that availability of high quality and free health services offered by the study clinic has impacted severe health outcomes; we are unable to confirm this because we do not have baseline disease incidence or mortality rates from the surveillance area before the program began. However, over the course of the study, there was a significant reduction in mortality rate among persons 18–34 years old. While free prevention services and treatment of children in urban areas are relatively ubiquitous, access for good quality and free care for adults is less common. We speculate that the introduction of free, high quality health care to residents within the surveillance community may have had differential benefits for adults, who otherwise had limited health utilization options. Further study will be needed to explore this potential benefit of health systems strengthening within impoverished informal settlements on severe illness and disease outcomes.

A limitation of this study is that the presence of the study clinic within the surveillance area may have led to underestimation of mortality rates for the majority of urban slum settings where a similar option does not exist. Also, it is difficult to compare our findings with most other studies providing mortality rates. Most childhood mortality calculations use the number of live births as the denominator. PBIDS did not collect data on births during the study period; however, since we conducted longitudinal surveillance within an area with known population size, we were able to use a rigorously defined denominator of people under surveillance to provide mortality rates per person years of observation. Nonetheless, it is likely that mortality rates were underestimated for very young children, early in infancy, since some (especially neonates) may die before they are officially enrolled into the system. While it was not possible to characterize mortality in the context of live-births, the description of the proportion of the population with death outcomes annually provides capacity to estimate overall raw numbers of deaths in similar settings where population size is known, and, therefore, to estimate the potential impact of interventions with known effectiveness on numbers of deaths averted.

We assumed that symptoms experienced two weeks prior death were associated with the death; however, the degree that this was indeed true was likely impacted by the timing of the household visit. Despite differences observed between cases and controls, it is likely that in many cases, symptoms reported during the biweekly visit were unrelated to the illness or event causing death. Formal verbal autopsies and pathologic studies are needed to shed more light on likely causes of death in this setting.

PBIDS provided an accurate denominator for calculating mortality rates across different age groups. The results of this analysis suggest that although health care for acute illnesses is accessible, high proportion of deaths may be associated with infectious disease symptoms, and these illnesses do not appear to have led to clinic visits.To derive well-targeted and effective interventions, further research among urban slum dwellers is needed to provide cause specific mortality rates and determinants, as well as data of impact of targeted public health interventions in similar settings.

Acknowledgments

We would like to acknowledge the following individuals and organisations for their contributions to this study. The IEIP Community Interviewers who worked tirelessly to collect this data, the IEIP data team for data management, Field Coordinators for continuous quality checks on data collected and participants in Soweto and Gatwikira who made this possible. This paper is published with the permission of the Director of the Kenya Medical Research Institute.

Author Contributions

Conceived and designed the experiments: BO DF RB . Analyzed the data: BO DF RB LC JM. Wrote the paper: BO RB. Actively supported the fieldwork phase of the study: KO GO. Read, edited, and approved the final manuscript: BO DF LC KO GO JM RB.

References

1. United Nations Human Settlements Programme (UN-HABITAT) (2008a) The state of the world's cities 2010/2011: Bridging the urban divide.
2. United Nations.Department of Economic and Social Affairs, Population Division (2002) World Urbanization Prospects: The 2001 Revision. New York. United Nations.
3. World Health Organization (WHO) (2005) Ecosystems and human well-being: health synthesis: a report of the Millennium Ecosystem Assessment. Geneva, Switzerland.
4. United Nations Human Settlements Programme (UN HABITAT) (2008b) The State of African *Cities* 2008: A framework for addressing urban challenges in Africa.
5. Zulu E, Dodoo FN, Ezeh CA (2002) Sexual risk-taking in the slums of Nairobi, Kenya, 1993–98. Population Studies 56:311–323.
6. African Population and Health Research Center (APHRC) (2002) Population and Health Dynamics in Nairobi's Informal Settlements. Nairobi (Kenya) African Population and Health Research Center.
7. Anand K, Shah B, Yadav K, Singh R, Mathur P, et al. (2007) Are the urban poor vulnerable to non-communicable diseases? A survey of risk factors for non-communicable diseases in urban slums of Faridabad. The National Medical Journal of India 20(3): 115–120.
8. Feikin DR, Audi A, Olack B, Bigogo GM, Polyak C, et al. (2010) Evaluation of the optimal recall period for disease symptoms in home-based morbidity surveillance in rural and urban Kenya. International Journal of Epidemiology 39(2): 450–458.
9. The United Nations Children's Fund (UNICEF) (2012) The state of the world's children 2012.Children in an urban world. New York.
10. Kanungo S, Tsuzuki A, Deen JL, Lopez AL, Rajendran K, et al. (2010) Use of verbal autopsy to determine mortality patterns in an urban slum in Kolkata, India. Bulletin of the World Health Organization 88: 667–674.
11. Fotso JC (2007) Urban-rural differentials in child malnutrition: trends and socioeconomic correlates in sub-Saharan Africa. Health Place.13 (1):205–23.
12. Anyamele OD (2009) Urban and rural differences across countries in child mortality in Sub-Saharan Africa. Journal of Health Care for the Poor and Underserved 20(4 Suppl): 90–98.
13. Breiman RF, Olack B, Shultz A, Roder S, Kimani K, et al. (2011) Healthcare-use for Major Infectious Disease Syndromes in an Informal Settlement in Nairobi, Kenya. Journal of Health Population and Nutrition 29:123–33.
14. Burton D, Flannery B, Onyango B, Larson C, Alaii J, et al. (2011) Health-seeking behavior for common infectious disease illnesses in rural Kenya. Journal of Health Population and Nutrition 29:61–70.
15. Feikin DR, Olack B, Bigogo GM, Audi A, Cosmas L, et al. (2011) The burden of common infectious disease syndromes at the clinic and household level from population-based surveillance in rural and urban Kenya. PLoS ONE 6(1): e16085.
16. Breiman RF, Cosmas L, Njuguna H, Audi A, Olack B, et al. (2012) Population-Based Incidence of Typhoid Fever in an Urban Informal Settlement and a Rural Area in Kenya: Implications for Typhoid Vaccine Use in Africa. PLoS ONE 7(1): e29119.
17. Tabu C, Breiman RF, Ochieng B, Aura B, Cosmas L, et al. (2012) Differing burden and epidemiology of Non-typhi Salmonella Bacteremia in Rural and Urban Kenya, 2006–2009. PLoS ONE 7(2): e31237.
18. United Nations Human Settlements Programme (UN-HABITAT) (2010) Strategic Urban Development Plan for Homa Bay Municipality (2008–2030) Strategic Planning for Environmental Governance and Poverty Alleviation.
19. United Nations Human Settlements Programme (UN-HABITAT) (2008c) UN HABITAT and the Kenya Slum Upgrading Programme Strategy Document.
20. Fotso JC, Ezeh AC, Madise NJ, Ciera J (2007) Progress towards the child mortality millennium development goal in urban Sub-Saharan Africa: the dynamics of population growth, immunization, and access to clean water. BMC Public Health 7:218.

Functional Analysis of a Missense Mutation in the Serine Protease Inhibitor *SPINT2* Associated with Congenital Sodium Diarrhea

Nicolas Faller, Ivan Gautschi, Laurent Schild*

Department of Pharmacology and Toxicology, University of Lausanne, Lausanne, Switzerland

Abstract

Membrane-bound serine proteases play important roles in different biological processes. Their regulation by endogenous inhibitors is poorly understood. A Y163C mutation in the *SPINT2* gene encoding the serine protease inhibitor Hepatocyte Growth Factor Inhibitor HAI-2 is associated with a congenital sodium diarrhea. The functional consequences of this mutation on HAI-2 activity and its physiological targets are unknown. We established a cellular assay in *Xenopus laevis* oocytes to study functional interactions between HAI-2 and candidate membrane-bound serine proteases expressed in the gastro-intestinal tract. We found that the wild-type form of HAI-2 is a potent inhibitor of nine gastro-intestinal serine proteases. The Y163C mutation in the second Kunitz domain of HAI-2 resulted in a complete loss of inhibitory activity on two intestinal proteases, prostasin and tmprss13. The effect of the mutation of the homologous Y68C in the first Kunitz domain of HAI-2 is consistent with a differential contribution of the two Kunitz domains of HAI-2 in the inhibition of serine proteases. By contrast to the Tyr to Cys, the Tyr to Ser substitution did not change the inhibitory potency of HAI-2, indicating that the thiol-group of the cysteine rather than the Tyr deletion is responsible for the HAI-2 loss of function. Our functional assay allowed us to identify membrane-bound serine proteases as cellular target for inhibition by HAI-2 wild type and mutants, and to better define the role of the Tyr in the second Kunitz domain in the inhibitory activity of HAI-2.

Editor: Andreas R. Janecke, Innsbruck Medical University, Austria

Funding: The work was supported by a grant from the Swiss National Science Foundation 323530-128871, MD-PhD Program of the Swiss Academy of Medical Sciences (to NF). The funders had no role in study design, data collection and analysis, decision to publish, or preparation of the manuscript.

Competing Interests: The authors have declared that no competing interests exist.

* E-mail: Laurent.Schild@unil.ch

Introduction

Membrane-bound or membrane-anchored serine proteases have lately emerged as a subfamily of 20 serine proteases that all share a conserved catalytic domain and a transmembrane domain [1]. They display diverse physiological and pathophysiological roles such as roles in skin and intestinal barrier integrity [2–5], processing of atrial natriuretic peptide [6], iron homeostasis [7–9], trophoblastic development [10], hearing [11,12] and ion homeostasis [13,14]. More elusive, however, are the identity and the roles of their physiological inhibitors.

The *SPINT1* and *SPINT2 genes* encode two Kunitz-type serine protease inhibitors called Hepatocyte Growth Factor Inhibitor HAI-1 and HAI-2. HAI-1, first purified from a stomach cancer cell line [15], is found as a complex with the membrane-bound serine protease matriptase in human milk [16]. Furthermore, genetic evidence supports an interaction between *SPINT1* and the *St14* gene encoding matriptase in mouse skin [17]. The membrane-bound HAI-2 and HAI-1, with their two inhibitory domains of Kunitz-type and their transmembrane domain, are highly homologous. However, HAI-2 lacks the LDL-receptor class A domain. HAI-2 was cloned from placental tissue, and from a gastric or pancreas cancer cell lines [18–20]. In cell-free *in vitro* systems, HAI-2 is a potent inhibitor of the membrane-bound serine proteases hepsin, prostasin, matriptase and tmprss13 [21–24].

The physiological role of *SPINT2* is incompletely characterized. In mice, *SPINT2* contributes to the appropriate development of the embryo as indicated by *SPINT2* knockout embryos showing clefting of the embryonic ectoderm, neural tube defects and defective placental branching morphogenesis; these defects can be rescued by the disruption of the *Prss8* and/or *St14* genes (encoding prostasin and matriptase respectively) [25–27]. In humans, various mutations in the *SPINT2* gene have been reported and shown to be linked to a syndromic form of congenital sodium diarrhea, indicating that *SPINT2* likely plays a role in intestinal ionic homeostasis [28,29]. Among these mutations, a missense mutation substitutes a conserved tyrosine in the second Kunitz domain for a cysteine (HAI-2 Y163C). It has been shown that this mutation decreases the ability of HAI-2 to inhibit the prototype gastro-intestinal serine protease trypsin [28,29]. The physiological partners of HAI-2 remain presently unknown.

Functional interactions between serine proteases and protease inhibitors are usually studied in cell-free *in vitro* systems. Here, we established a cellular assay using *Xenopus laevis* oocytes as a heterologous expression system to functionally assess the activity of candidate serine proteases and their inhibition by HAI-2 and its mutant Y163C. We found that HAI-2 was an efficient inhibitor of several membrane-bound serine proteases expressed in the GI tract. The *SPINT2* Y163C mutation associated with congenital

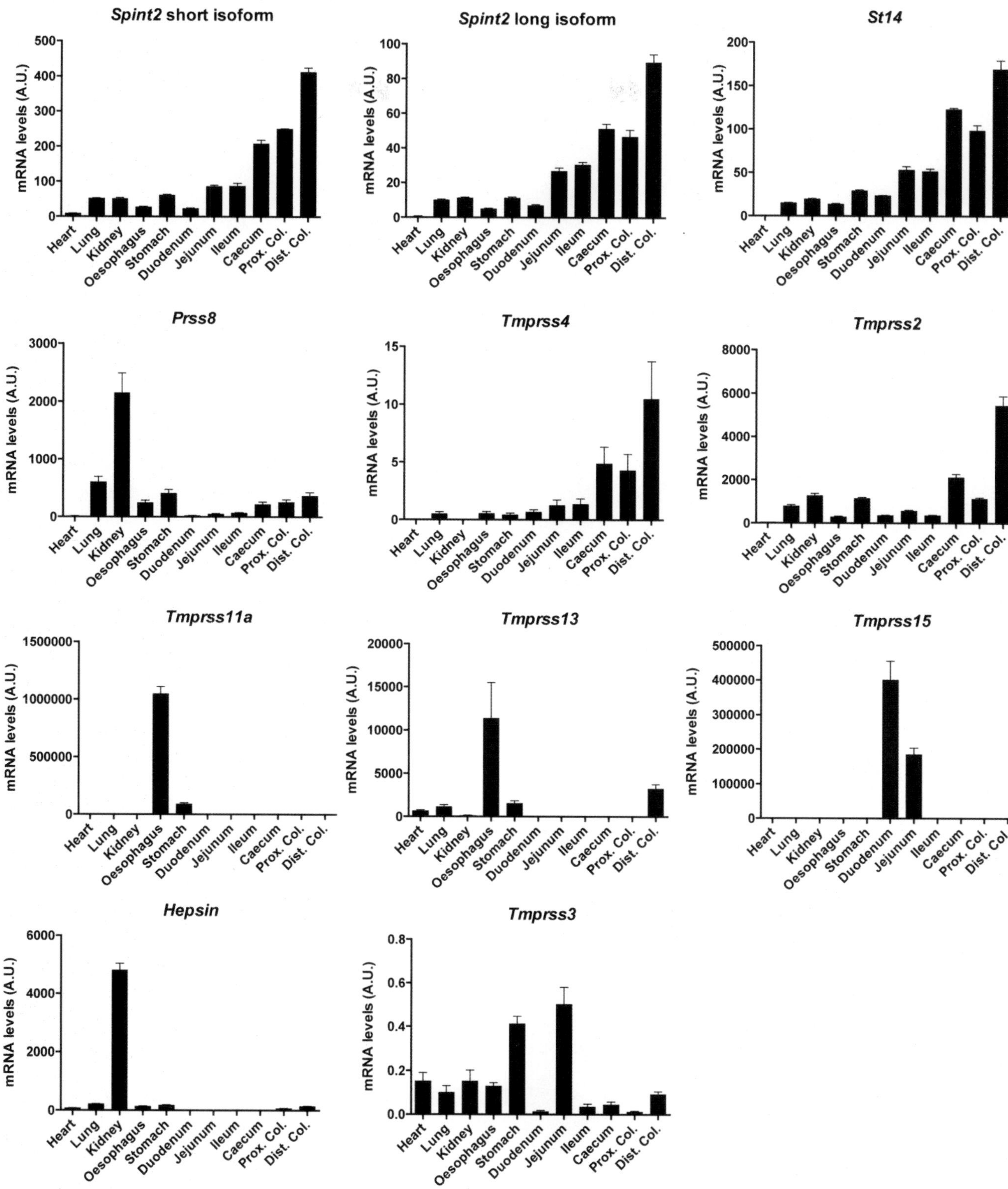

Figure 1. Tissue distribution of mRNA expression of *Spint2* and membrane-bound serine proteases. Quantitative RT-PCRs were performed on selected organs from three wild-type adult mice. From stomach to distal colon, tissues were scraped to get fractions enriched in mucosal cells. Each gene was assessed in duplicates in two independent experiments. Results are expressed as arbitrary units (A.U.) based on standard dilution curves (see Material and Methods).

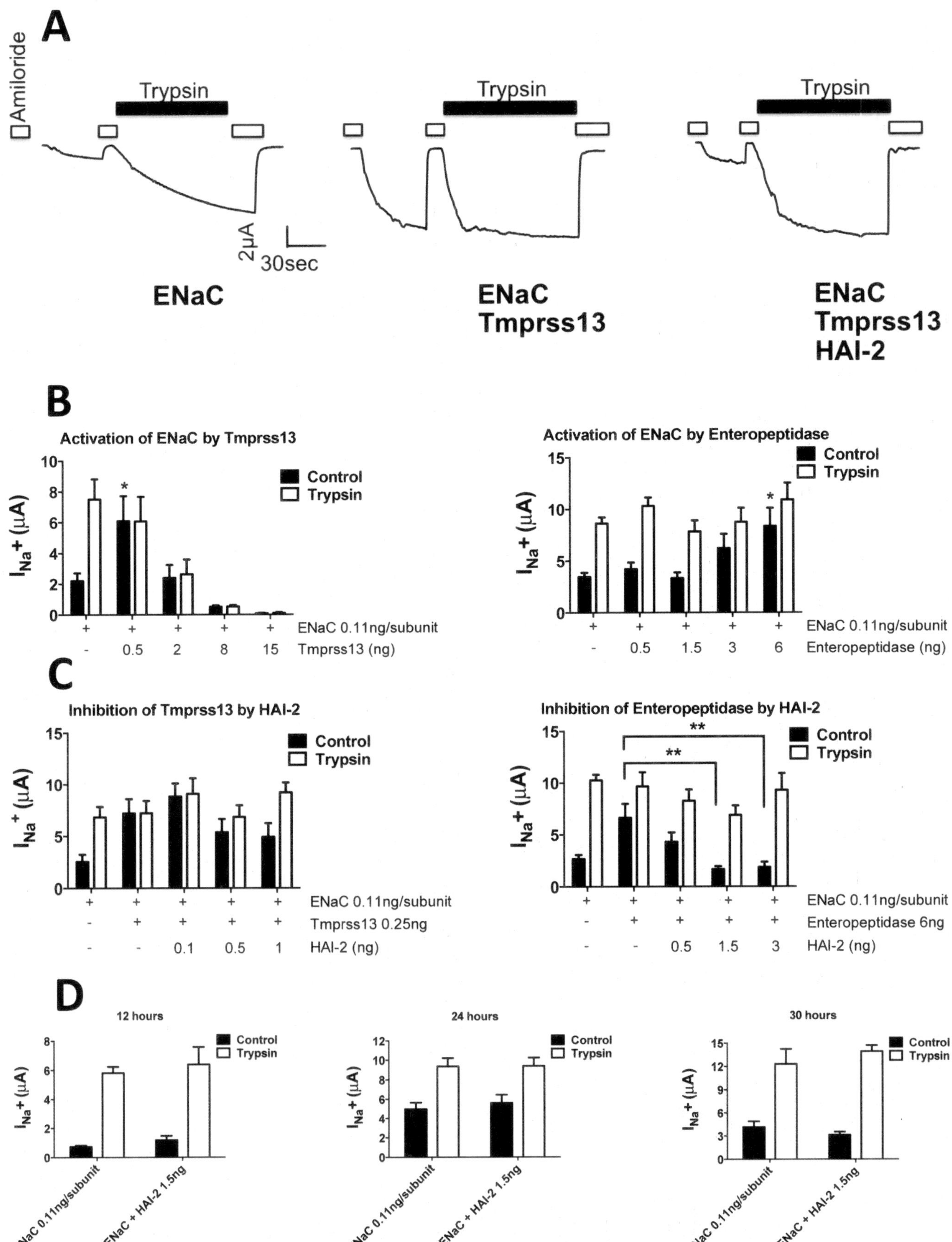
A
Amiloride
Trypsin
Trypsin
Trypsin
2µA
30sec
ENaC
ENaC
Tmprss13
ENaC
Tmprss13
HAI-2
B
Activation of ENaC by Tmprss13
Control
Trypsin
INa+ (µA)
ENaC 0.11ng/subunit
Tmprss13 (ng)
- 0.5 2 8 15
Activation of ENaC by Enteropeptidase
Control
Trypsin
ENaC 0.11ng/subunit
Enteropeptidase (ng)
- 0.5 1.5 3 6
C
Inhibition of Tmprss13 by HAI-2
Control
Trypsin
ENaC 0.11ng/subunit
Tmprss13 0.25ng
HAI-2 (ng)
- - 0.1 0.5 1
Inhibition of Enteropeptidase by HAI-2
Control
Trypsin
ENaC 0.11ng/subunit
Enteropeptidase 6ng
HAI-2 (ng)
- - 0.5 1.5 3
D
12 hours
24 hours
30 hours
Control
Trypsin
ENaC 0.11ng/subunit
ENaC + HAI-2 1.5ng

Figure 2. Validation of the functional assay using ENaC as a reporter gene. A, Representative recordings of amiloride-sensitive current (I_{Na}^+) in the presence (filled bars) or absence of trypsin (5 μg/ml), in *Xenopus* oocytes injected with 0.11 ng/subunit ENaC alone (left panel), with ENaC and 0.25 ng tmprss13 (middle panel) and with ENaC, tmprss13 and 1.5 ng spint2 cRNA (right panel). 10 μM amiloride was used to block the ENaC-mediated current. **B**, Effects of increasing the amounts of injected tmprss13 and enteropeptidase cRNAs on I_{Na}^+. I_{Na}^+ was measured in oocytes injected with ENaC with/without of tmprss13 or enteropeptidase as indicated. I_{Na}^+ was measured without (black bars) or with trypsin (5 μg/ml) perfused extracellularly (white bars) as a positive control for ENaC activation. **C**, Effects of increasing the amounts of injected spint2 cRNA to prevent the tmprss13- or enteropeptidase-mediated increase in I_{Na}^+ (left and right panels, respectively). **D**, Effect of spint2 on I_{Na}^+. I_{Na}^+ was measured 12, 24 and 30 hours after injection (left, middle and right panels, respectively) in three independent experiments. n = 6-9 measured oocytes per condition from 2 different batches for each experiment. Data are means ± SEM; *, $p<0.05$/**, $p<0.01$ compared to ENaC alone or ENaC + protease (as indicated) after two-way repeated measure ANOVA followed by Dunnett's multiple comparisons test.

sodium diarrhea induced a loss of inhibitory activity towards a limited number of serine proteases such as prostasin and tmprss13.

Material and Methods

Ethics Statement

Work done with animals was performed according to swiss national guidelines. Mice and *Xenopus laevis* were kept in an animal facility regulated by animal care rules of the University of Lausanne. All animals had access to food and water ad libitum. Protocols regarding sacrifice of the mice and surgical procedures on *Xenopus laevis* used in this study have been reviewed and approved by the Service de la Consommation et des Affaires Vétérinaires of the Canton of Vaud, Switzerland (authorization no. 2312 to LS).

Quantitative PCR analysis

Tissues were removed from three C57BL/6 8 week-old mice. Duodenal, jejunal, ileal, caecal and colonic (proximal and distal) tissues were longitudinally opened and mucosal side was scraped with a razorblade to obtain a fraction enriched in mucosal cells. To avoid contamination by squamous epithelium, colonic tissues was scraped a few millimeters above the anus. Total RNA was extracted from mouse tissues using the RNeasy kit from Qiagen according to the manufacturer's protocol. 500 ng RNA (RNA from the 3 mice was pooled together) was reverse transcribed into cDNA using the PrimeScript RTreagent kit (TaKaRa). RNA was treated with DNAse I (Promega) to remove any possible traces of genomic DNA before the cDNA synthesis. qRT-PCR experiments were carried out on an ABI PRISM 7500 equipment (Applied Biosystems). PCR was performed in 96-well plates (Applied Biosystems) in 20-μl reactions that contained 10 μl of FastSYBR Green Master Mix (Applied Biosystems), 125 nM of each primer and 4 μl of cDNA (diluted 30 times). For each gene, standard curves were obtained using tissues with the highest abundance and 1/1, 1/5, 1/25, 1/625 and 1/3125 dilutions. The analysis of the slope of the standard curves showed a PCR efficiency between 1.70 and 2. These values were used for absolute quantification. Relative quantification using reference genes such as *Actin* or *Gapdh* was not used because detection levels of those genes varied up to a difference of 4 cycles between different mouse tissues. Each gene was assessed in duplicates in two independent experiments.

Expression of human *Spint2* and human membrane-bound serine proteases in *Xenopus* oocytes

cDNA clones of human prostasin, tmprss4, matriptase, hepsin, tmprss2, tmprss11a, tmprss13, enteropeptidase and HAI-2 were obtained from the Mammalian Gene Collection (MGC). Human tmprss3 is a kind gift of Bernard Rossier (University of Lausanne). Membrane-bound serine proteases were selected based on their gastro-intestinal expression, as reported in the literature (see results). The other members of the membrane-bound serine proteases family were not tested because of a reported expression that appears to be restricted to specific tissues, even though we cannot rule out that they might display any gastro-intestinal expression. All cDNAs were subcloned into the pSD(BS)easy vector for expression in *Xenopus laevis* oocytes. A FLAG-tag sequence was added to HAI-2 using a single BstEII restriction site located in the sequence encoding the region between both Kunitz domains of HAI-2. PCR amplification was performed to add a tag of 8 histidines in the N-terminal part of tmprss13. Point mutations in HAI-2 cDNA were introduced by site–directed mutagenesis (Stratagene's QuickChange) to generate HAI-2 mutants Y68C, Y163C, Y68S, Y163S and double mutant Y68C/Y163C.

Stage V and VI healthy oocytes were isolated from ovarian tissue of *Xenopus laevis* and pressure–injected with 100 nl of cRNA solution. For the functional assay, oocytes were injected with α, β and γ subunits of rat ENaC cRNAs (0,11 ng of each subunit per oocyte) and with cRNAs of membrane-bound serine proteases and HAI-2 wild-type or mutants as indicated in the results section. In this heterologous expression system, we found that the effects of the serine proteases on ENaC as well as the effects of HAI-2 on the serine proteases were dose-dependent. To minimize artifacts due to overexpression, we determined for each serine protease the amount of cRNA to be injected for a robust proteolytic activation of ENaC similar to the activation by trypsin. We also determined the minimal amount of HAI-2 cRNA necessary to completely inhibit the effect of the protease. For the biochemical assay, oocytes were injected with cRNAs of His-tagged tmprss13 (1.7 ng) and FLAG-tagged HAI-2 (8.3 ng). This ratio tmprss13/HAI-2 is similar to the ratio used in the functional assay. Oocytes were kept at 19°C in a low Na^+ (for the functional experiments with ENaC) modified Barth solution (MBS) containing (in mM): 10 NaCl, 0.82 $MgSO_4$, 0.41 $CaCl_2$, 0.33 $Ca(NO_3)_2$, 80 *N*-methyl-D-glucamine (NMDG), 2 KCl and 5 HEPES or a normal Na^+ (for the biochemical experiments done without ENaC) modified Barth solution (MBS) containing (in mM): 85 NaCl, 1 KCl, 2.4 $NaHCO_3$, 0.82 $MgSO_4$, 0.41 $CaCl_2$, 0.33 $Ca(NO_3)_2$, and 10 HEPES, 4.08 NaOH.

Electrophysiology

Electrophysiological measurements were made 12 hours after injection except for experiments with tmprss3 and tmprss15, which were performed 30 hours after injection. ENaC-mediated Na^+ currents were measured in oocytes using the standard two-electrodes voltage clamp technique using a Dagan TEV voltage clamp amplifier (Dagan, Minneapolis, MN), the Digidata 1322 digitizer, and the PClamp 9 data-acquisition and analysis package (Axon Instruments, Molecular Devices, Sunnyvale, CA). The two electrodes contained 1 M KCl solution. All electrophysiological measurements were performed at room temperature (22°C) in a perfusion solution containing (in mM) 120 NaCl, 2.5 KCl, 1.8 $CaCl_2$-$2H_2O$, and 10 HEPES-H^+. The holding potential inside the oocytes was -100 mV.

Table 1. Increase in ENaC activity by membrane-bound serine proteases.

protease (ng of cRNA)	Fold increase in ENaC-mediated current
Tmprss2 (5 ng)	2.6±0.2 (trypsin: 3.5±0.3)
Tmprss11a (0.25 ng)	2.1±0.2 (trypsin: 3.7±0.3)
Enteropeptidase (6 ng)	2.6±0.3 (trypsin: 3.7±0.3)
Hepsin (0.05 ng)	2.5±0.3 (trypsin: 3.7±0.4)
Tmprss3 (2.5 ng)	2.6±0.3 (trypsin: 3.9±0.3)
Matriptase (1.5 ng)	2.6±0.3 (trypsin: 3.1±0.3)
Tmprss4 (2 ng)	2.4±0.4 (trypsin: 3±0.2)
Prostasin (1 ng)	3.6±0.4 (trypsin: 3.8±0.5)
Tmprss13 (0.25 ng)	5.2±0.8 (trypsin: 4.4±0.3)

Values were obtained from experiments in figure 3. Effect of trypsin is indicated in parentheses. Data are means ± SEM.

Data analysis

The epithelial sodium channel (ENaC) is highly sensitive to amiloride with an IC50 of 0.1 μM. ENaC activity was measured by the amiloride-sensitive Na^+ current (I_{Na}^+), defined as the difference between Na^+ current obtained in the presence (10 μM) and in the absence of amiloride. ENaC activity is increased by a variety of serine proteases including trypsin [13,30,31], making ENaC an ideal tool for monitoring serine protease activity. We used trypsin (Sigma-Aldrich Chemie) 5 μg/ml in the perfusion solution for 2–3 minutes to define a maximal proteolytic stimulation on ENaC activity as measured by the increase in I_{Na}^+. In each condition, sensitivity of ENaC to trypsin (defined as the relative trypsin-mediated increase in I_{Na}^+) can vary depending on whether proteases with or without HAI-2 wt/mutants are co-expressed with ENaC and was quantified by dividing, for each oocyte, I_{Na}^+ after trypsin treatment by I_{Na}^+ before trypsin treatment. A relative trypsin-mediated increase in I_{Na}^+ close to one reflects resistance of ENaC to trypsin because of the presence of an activating co-expressed protease. When HAI-2 fully inhibits the co-expressed protease, relative trypsin-mediated increase in I_{Na}^+ has a value (>1) similar to control oocytes injected with ENaC alone.

Statistical analysis

All data are represented as means ± SEM. Statistical significance was determined with one-way or two-way ANOVA followed by Dunnett or Tukey's multiple comparison tests and indicated in the legend of the figures.

Results

mRNA expression of *Spint2* and candidate membrane-bound serine protease along the mouse gastro-intestinal tract

We first identified potential targets for HAI-2 inhibition that are relevant for the pathogenesis of sodium diarrhea. We have limited our selection to members of the membrane-bound serine proteases family expressed in different gastro-intestinal (GI) tissues, because HAI-1, a highly conserved homolog of HAI-2 was reported as the physiological inhibitor of the membrane-bound serine protease matriptase. From the literature, nine membrane-bound serine proteases are expressed in GI tissues namely *Prss8* (encoding prostasin), *Tmprss4*, *St14* (encoding matriptase), *Hepsin*, *Tmprss2*, *Tmprss3*, *Tmprss11a*, *Tmprss13* and *Tmprss15* (encoding enteropeptidase) [11,21,32–44].

The mRNA expression levels of *Spint2* and of the candidate proteases were determined in mouse GI tissues, and compared to heart, lung and kidney. Since *Spint2* is mainly expressed in epithelial cells [21], we took intestinal tissue fractions enriched in mucosal cells. Fig.1 shows that *Spint2* mRNA is found along the entire GI tract, but its expression increases in the distal part. As already reported, the short isoform *of Spint2* lacking the first Kunitz domain appears more abundant than the long (full-length) isoform in mouse (opposite findings are known in human) [45]. *St14* mRNA has an expression pattern similar to *Spint2*. *Prss8*, *Tmprss4* and *Tmprss2* are easily detected in the small and large intestines with a higher abundance in the distal part. The other candidates show a more restricted expression distribution along the GI tract: *Tmprss11a* is essentially expressed in oesophagus, *Tmprss13* in oesophagus and colon, *Tmprss15* in duodenum and jejunum. Although *Hepsin* is very abundant in the kidney, low expression levels are observed in the colon. Finally, *Tmprss3* mRNA is detected at very low levels in all tissues, with a higher expression in stomach and jejunum.

Functional assay in *Xenopus laevis* oocytes

To test whether HAI-2 inhibits our selected intestinal serine proteases in a functional cellular assay, we used as a functional readout the epithelial sodium channel ENaC and its unique property to be stimulated by a wide variety of serine proteases [30]. This allowed us to quantitatively assess by an electrophysiological approach the proteolytic activity of a serine protease, as an increase in ENaC mediated Na current. *Xenopus laevis* oocytes were injected with cRNAs encoding ENaC and the above mentioned serine proteases with or without HAI-2. The activity of the serine protease monitored by the increase in epithelial sodium channel ENaC activity, was measured as an inward current sensitive to amiloride, a known blocker of ENaC [46,47]. The ENaC-mediated current was systematically compared with the maximal current obtained in the presence of trypsin, a well-established proteolytic agonist of ENaC. A typical electrophysiological recording is shown in figure 2A and illustrates the effect of the intestinal serine protease tmprss13 on ENaC-mediated currents (I_{Na}^+) and its inhibition by HAI-2. In an oocyte injected with ENaC alone, removing the ENaC blocker amiloride induces a discrete inward current which dramatically increases in the presence of trypsin (left tracing); co-injection of ENaC with tmprss13 increases the amiloride-sensitive current I_{Na}^+ to the level

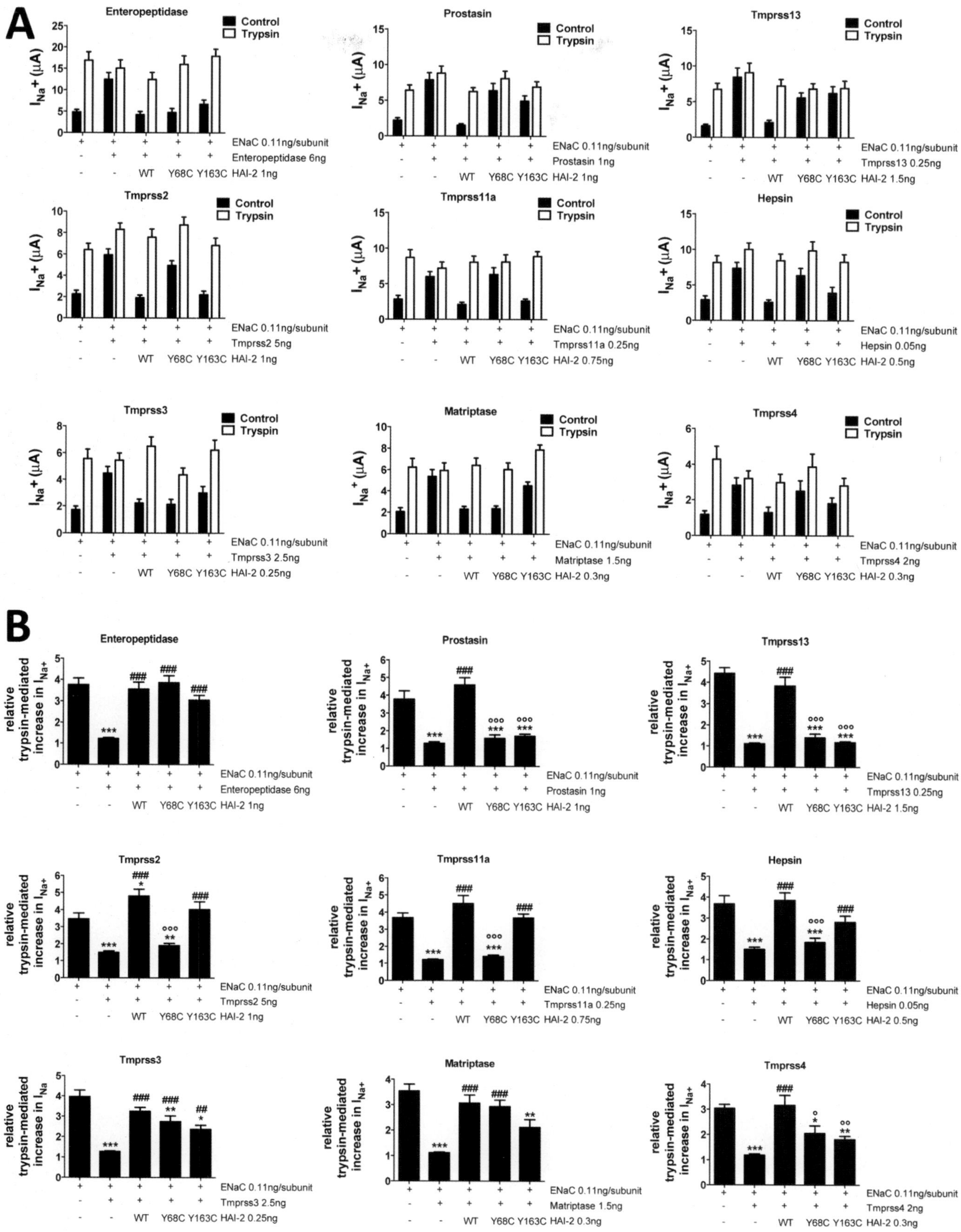

Figure 3. Functional analysis of interactions between HAI-2 (wt and mutants) and membrane-bound serine proteases. A, ENaC-mediated sodium currents (I_{Na}^{+}) were measured in *Xenopus* oocytes injected with ENaC with/without candidate serine protease and HAI-2 (wild-type or mutants Y68C and Y163C) as indicated. I_{Na}^{+} was measured without (black bars) or with trypsin (5 μg/ml) perfused extracellularly (white bars) as a

positive control for ENaC activation. n≥15 measured oocytes per condition from at least 2 different animals. Each protease was tested in at least two independent experiments. Data are means ± SEM. **B**, Relative trypsin-mediated increase in I_{Na}^+ was calculated by dividing, for each oocyte from experiments of panel A, I_{Na}^+ after treatment with trypsin by I_{Na}^+ before treatment with trypsin. Data are means ± SEM. */#/°, $p<0.05$, **/##/°°, $p<0.01$, ***/###/°°°, $p<0.001$, compared to ENaC alone, ENaC + protease or ENaC + protease + HAI-2 WT respectively after One-way ANOVA followed by Tukey's multiple comparisons test.

of I_{Na}^+ recorded in the presence of trypsin (middle tracing); finally, co-injection of ENaC tmprss13 and HAI-2 completely abolished the effect of tmprss13 on I_{Na}^+ (right tracing).

For some proteases such as tmprss13 we observed a dual effect on the activity of ENaC depending on the amounts of cRNA encoding the protease that were injected into the oocyte. Figure 2B compares the effects of increasing the amount of cRNA (i.e. the expression) of two proteases, tmprss13 (left panel) and enteropeptidase (right panel) on ENaC-mediated I_{Na}^+: co-injection of ENaC with 0.5 ng of tmprss13 cRNA increases I_{Na}^+ to the level obtained with trypsin but higher amounts of injected tmprss13 cRNA show a dose-dependent decrease in I_{Na}^+ in the presence and absence of trypsin. This observation is consistent with a progressive loss of ENaC activity at high levels of serine protease expression, likely due to an extensive proteolytic modification of the fully activated channel. For enteropeptidase a robust activation of ENaC activity to levels comparable with those obtained with trypsin could be obtained only with high doses of injected enteropeptidase cRNA up to 6 ng. We therefore systematically performed dose-response experiments for every serine protease tested to determine the minimal amount of the protease cRNA needed to stimulate ENaC-mediated I_{Na}^+ to levels comparable with those obtained for trypsin. All candidate serine proteases tested in our assay were functional as shown by the robust increase in ENaC-mediated I_{Na}^+ (see table 1 and figure 3). This effect varied from a 2 to 5 fold increase in ENaC activity depending on the protease and on the batch of oocytes used for the experiments.

Inhibition of serine proteases by HAI-2

We then evaluated the ability of HAI-2 to inhibit the different serine proteases shown in table 1. In preliminary experiments, as for the serine proteases, we determined the minimal amount of HAI-2 cRNA needed to completely reverse the effect of each protease tested. Typical experiments shown in figure 2C illustrate the inhibition of tmprss13 and enteropeptidase by HAI-2: 1 ng and 1.5 ng of HAI-2 cRNA are sufficient for a full inhibition of tmprss13 and enteropeptidase respectively as seen by a return of I_{Na}^+ to baseline and the recovery of the stimulatory effect of trypsin. We also verified that HAI-2 per se does not directly alter ENaC-mediated I_{Na}^+, neither the effect of trypsin on ENaC (fig.2D).

Effect of the congenital sodium diarrhea-associated mutation of HAI-2

We analyzed the Y163C mutation in the 2nd Kunitz domain of HAI-2 associated with congenital sodium diarrhea, and its effect on the inhibitory activity of the intestinal serine proteases. In addition, we have compared the Y163C mutation with its homologous Y68C mutation in the 1st Kunitz domain to assess the relative roles of the two Kunitz domains in the proteolytic activity of HAI-2. Figure 3A compares the effects of the HAI-2 wt, HAI-2/Y68C and HAI-2/Y163C mutants on the activity of the serine proteases listed in table 1. For these experiments we used similar amounts of injected cRNAs assuming that the three HAI-2 constructs have comparable levels of expression in the oocytes. These experiments show that the wild type form of HAI-2 reverses the increase in the I_{Na} mediated by the serine proteases, indicating that HAI-2 efficiently inhibits all membrane-bound serine proteases tested. This suggests that HAI-2 is a functional inhibitor of various intestinal membrane-bound serine proteases.

The Y68C and Y163C mutations in the 1st and 2nd Kunitz domains have differential effects depending on the serine protease: the Y68C or Y163C mutations have no effects on the ability of HAI-2 to inhibit enteropeptidase, whereas they result in a loss of the inhibitory function of HAI-2 on tmprss13. On other serine proteases such as tmprss11a, only the Y68C but not the Y163C abolished the activity on HAI-2. A partial loss of function was observed with the Y163C mutation on the inhibition of matriptase by HAI-2. The data on figure 3A are expressed as absolute values of ENaC-mediated I_{Na}^+ reflecting serine protease activities. In order to compensate for variations in ENaC expression and protease activation of I_{Na}^+ among the different batches of oocytes, we assessed in figure 3B the relative efficiency of HAI-2 wild type and mutants on the different serine protease by quantifying for each oocyte the trypsin response on I_{Na}^+ (ratio I_{Na}^+ after trypsin treatment/I_{Na}^+ before trypsin treatment). When the relative trypsin-mediated increase in I_{Na}^+ is equal to one, there is no trypsin response indicating full effect of the serine protease; whereas a trypsin response ≥3 (value similar to that obtained for oocytes injected with ENaC alone) indicates a full inhibitory effect of HAI-2 on the serine protease. As mentioned before, both Y68C and Y163C mutants of HAI-2 are fully functional on enteropeptidase. On prostasin and tmprss13 both mutations Y68C and Y163C result in a near complete loss of HAI-2 function. On tmprss2, tmprss11a and hepsin, only the Y68C mutation leads to a loss of HAI-2 inhibitory activity. A partial loss of function with the HAI-2 Y163C mutant, and full activity with the Y68C mutant are observed on tmprss3 and matriptase, A partial loss of function is seen with both mutants on tmprss4. These experiments indicate that either the Y68C in the 1st or the Y163C in the 2nd Kunitz domain are sufficient to induce a loss of function of HAI-2 on prostasin and tmprss13 proteases. These latter proteases appear thus as interesting potential partners of HAI-2 the regulation of Na^+ transport in the intestine. By contrast the Y68C mutation alone is sufficient to abolish the activity of tmprss11a, tmprss2 and hepsin, whereas the Y163C has no effect.

Effect of the double mutant HAI-2 Y68C/Y163C, and of serine substitutions

Four intestinal proteases, enteropeptidase, tmprss3, tmprss4 and matriptase are still partially, blocked by either HAI-2 Y68C or Y163C mutations. We assessed the effect of the double mutation HAI-2 Y68C/Y163C on these proteases. As shown in Fig.4, the Tyr to Cys mutations in both Kunitz domains nearly abolishes the inhibitory activity of HAI-2 on enteropeptidase, tmprss3, tmprss4 and matriptase, as shown on the measured ENaC-mediated I_{Na}^+ (fig.4A) or on the trypsin response (fig.4B).

To further understand the molecular basis of the Y68C and Y163C substitutions on the inhibitory capacity of HAI-2 towards a serine protease such as tmprss13, we asked whether this effect is due to the substitution of the tyrosine, which is highly conserved among HAI-2 orthologs from different species, or to the addition of a thiol group at position Y163. We mutated the Tyr68 and Tyr163 into a serine and assessed the effect of these mutations on

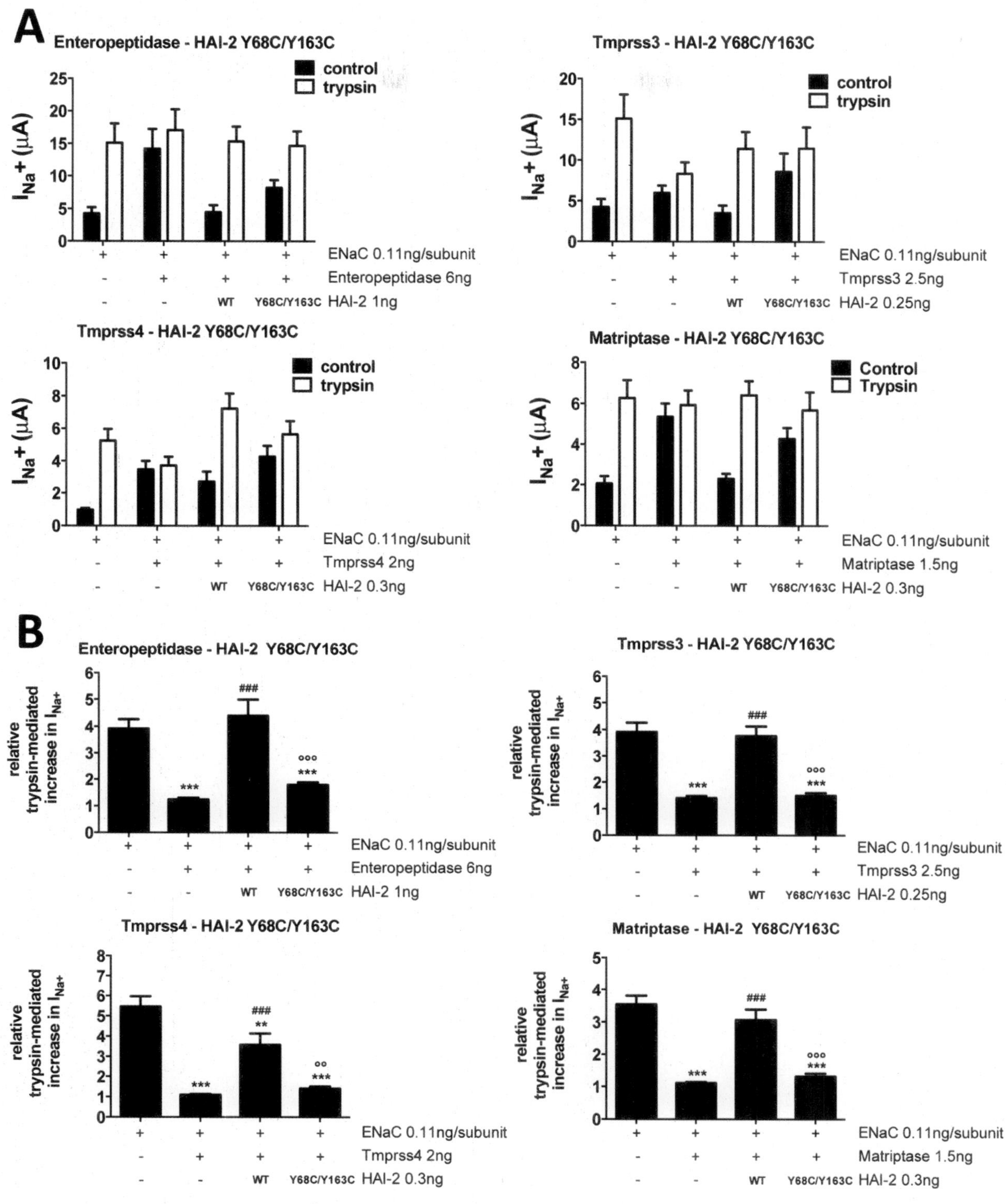

Figure 4. Effect of the double mutant HAI-2 Y68C/Y163C on enteropeptidase, Tmprss2, tmprss4 and matriptase. A, ENaC-mediated sodium currents (I_{Na}^{+}), were measured in *Xenopus* oocytes injected with ENaC with or without serine protease and HAI-2 (wild-type or double mutant Y68C/Y163C) as indicated. I_{Na}^{+} was measured without (black bars) and with trypsin (5 μg/ml) perfused extracellularly (white bars) as a positive control for ENaC activation. n≥11 measured oocytes from 4 different animals. Each protease was tested in two independent experiments. Data are means ± SEM. **B**, Relative trypsin-mediated increase in I_{Na}^{+} was calculated by dividing, for each oocyte from experiments of panel A, I_{Na}^{+} after treatment with trypsin by I_{Na}^{+} before treatment with trypsin. Data are means ± SEM. **/##/°°, p<0.01, ***/###/°°°, p<0.001, compared to ENaC alone, ENaC + protease or ENaC + protease + HAI-2 WT respectively after One-way ANOVA followed by Tukey's multiple comparisons test.

the ability of HAI-2 to inhibit tmprss13. In contrast to the cysteine mutants, the serine mutants HAI-2 Y68S and HAI-2 Y163S retain their activity and are able to fully inhibit the activity of tmprss13 on ENaC (Fig.5). This suggests that the presence of the additional cysteine with its thiol side chain in the 1st or 2nd Kunitz domains is

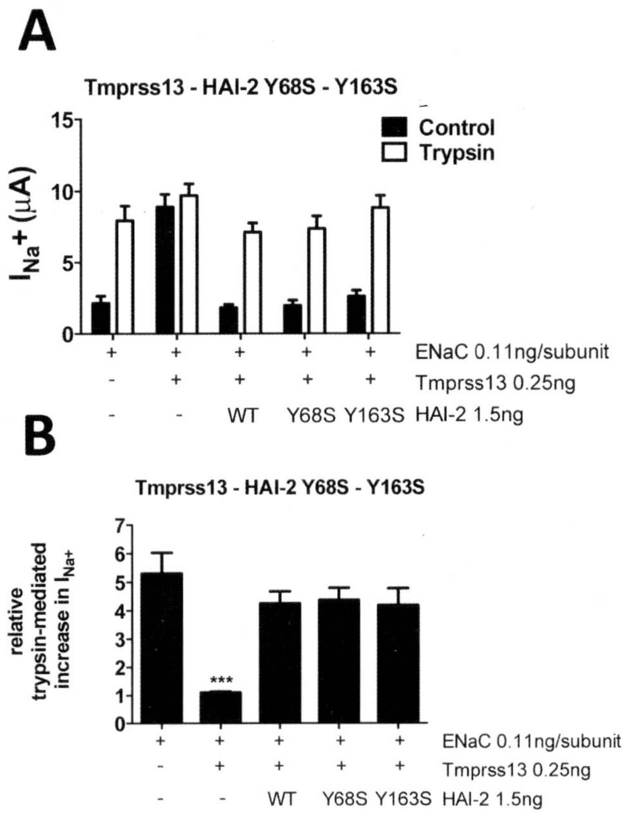

Figure 5. Effect of HAI-2 Y68S and Y163S mutations on tmprss13 activity. A, ENaC-mediated sodium currents (I_{Na}^+), were measured in *Xenopus* oocytes injected with ENaC, tmprss13 and HAI-2 (wild-type or mutant). I_{Na}^+ was measured without (black bars) and with trypsin (5 μg/ml) perfused extracellularly (white bars) as a positive control for ENaC activation. n≥14 measured oocytes from 4 different animals performed in two independent experiments. Data are means ± SEM. **B**, Relative trypsin-mediated increase in I_{Na}^+ was calculated by dividing, for each oocyte from experiments of panel A, I_{Na}^+ after treatment with trypsin by I_{Na}^+ before treatment with trpysin. Data are means ± SEM. ***, $p<0.001$, compared to ENaC alone, after One-way ANOVA followed by Tukey's multiple comparisons test.

responsible for the loss of the inhibitory activity of HAI-2 on tmprss13.

Discussion

In this study, we used a cellular assay to examine the functional interactions between HAI-2 wild type or mutants and different membrane-bound serine proteases expressed in the gastro-intestinal tract.

An *in vitro* cellular assay to assess the activity of membrane-bound serine proteases

This assay uses the ENaC channel as the readout protein for the proteolytic activity of intestinal membrane-bound serine proteases. ENaC is a target for stimulation by a large number of membrane-bound serine-proteases. Prostasin, tmprss4, matriptase and tmprss3 have already been shown to activate ENaC [13,34,40]. Here, we report the activation of ENaC by hepsin, tmprss11a, tmprss13, enteropeptidase and tmprss2 [48]. An important aspect to consider in this assay is the dual effect of serine proteases on ENaC activity. The expected stimulatory effect on ENaC was observed at low levels of serine protease expression, as for the proteolytic cleavage of α and γ ENaC subunits at the cell surface. However, increasing the level of expression of serine proteases like tmprss13 resulted in the inhibition of ENaC activity (see Fig.2), suggesting an extensive proteolytic cleavage of the fully active ENaC that becomes incompatible with a channel function. This stresses the necessity in this assay to perform dose-response curves for every serine protease in order to quantitatively assess their effects on ENaC by both an increase in ENaC activity and a resistance to trypsin. The physiological relevance of the dual effects of these intestinal serine-proteases on ENaC activity still needs to be addressed in *in vivo* models.

HAI-2 and membrane-bound serine proteases

We found that HAI-2 efficiently inhibits all intestinal proteases tested. The inhibition of hepsin, prostasin, matriptase and tmprss13 by HAI-2 has already been described [21–24] in cell-free assays. In addition, we also showed that HAI-2 inhibits tmprss4, tmprss2, tmprss3, tmprss11a and enteropeptidase.

The mutation of the conserved Tyr163 in the 2nd Kunitz domain (KD2) of HAI-2, as well as the corresponding Tyr mutation in the 1st Kunitz domain (KD1) alone or together resulted in a loss of function of HAI-2 against all the intestinal serine proteases tested in our assay. The crystal structure of the 1st Kunitz domain of the HAI-1 (HAI-1KD1) in complex with the catalytic domain of matriptase provides useful information at the atomic level on the possible mechanism underlying the loss of function of the HAI-2 Y163 or Y68C mutant [49]. The KD1 of HAI-1 structure adopts a pear-shape structure formed essentially by 2 loops that are stabilized by three disulfide bonds (figure 6). This binding mode of HAI-1 KD1 is common for the inhibition of other serine protease of Kunitz type [50]. The Tyr in KD1 conserved in HAI-1 and HAI-2 is in a close vicinity of cysteines (C259 and C283 in HAI-1) involved in a disulfide bond at the interface between the HAI-1 and matriptase (figure 6). By contrast to the Cys 259 and 283 of HAI-1 that interact with the catalytic triad of matriptase, the Tyr is surrounded by hydrophobic residues and does not participate directly to the interface between HAI-1 and matriptase. Simulation of the Tyr substitution by either Cys or Ser in the HAI1-KD1 that reproduces the Y68C or the Y68S in our experiments, resulted in a drop of the stability of the residues surrounding the Tyr by 2.8 kcal/mol and 3.3 kcal/mol (calculated with FoldX3.0) [51]. Such a decrease in the stability of the loop at the interface of the HAI-1 and matriptase does not seem to affect the binding of KDI with matriptase since in our experiments the Y68S HAI-2 mutant retains its inhibitory activity. Our experiments indicate that the Tyr to Cys substitution has a more profound effect on the conformation of the HAI-1 loops at the interface with matriptase. One interpretation is that the thiol group of the substituted Y68C or Y163C may bridge with either cysteines C47/C71 or C142/C166 of the HAI-2 loop normally involved in a disulfide bond that fits the protease binding site. Such aberrant disulfide bond is expected to disrupt the conformation of the Kunitz domain loops of HAI-2 and its interaction with the protease; this hypothesis is supported by our results showing that the Y68C and Y163C of the HAI-2 almost completely suppressed the inhibitory activity of HAI-2 on tmprss13 and prostasin. Interactions between HAI-2 and membrane-bound serine proteases are probably complex and not limited to the interaction between one Kunitz domain and the catalytic domain of the serine protease as shown by the crystal. In our experiments we expressed full-length HAI-2 (with 2 Kunitz domains) and serine proteases that may have several accessory domains potentially involved in protein-protein interaction.

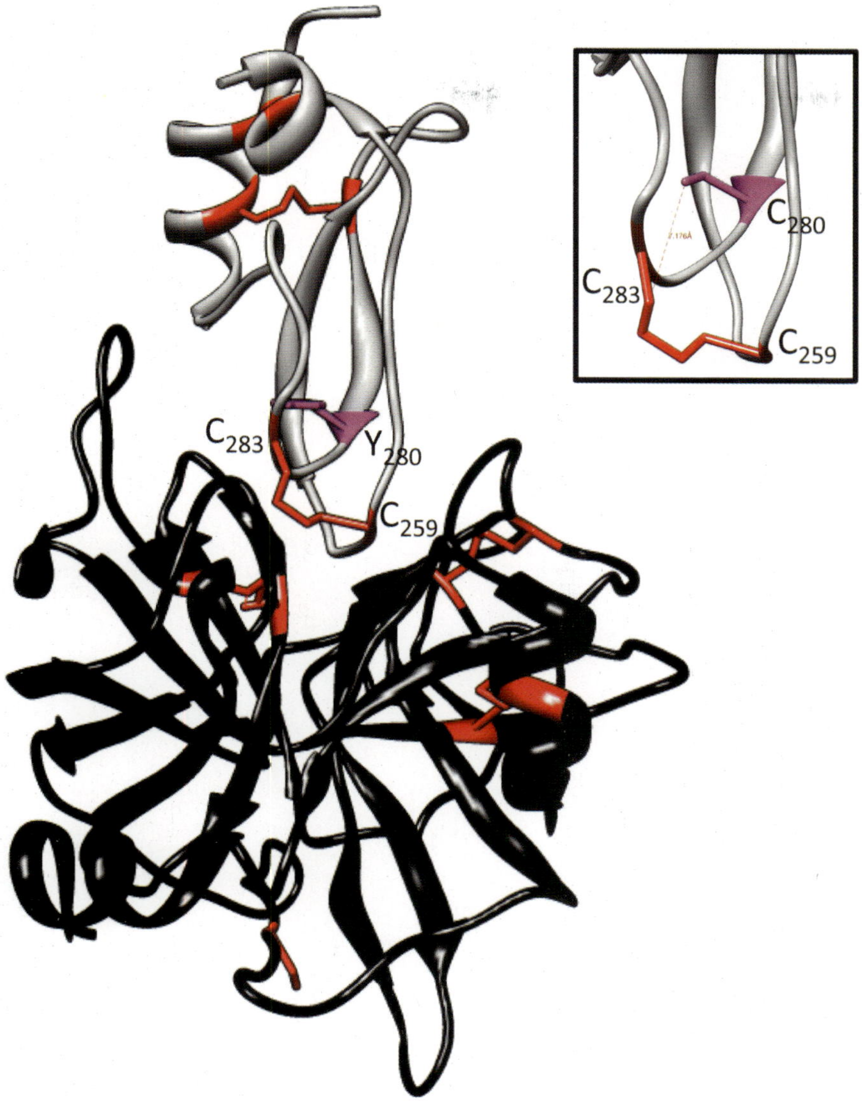

Figure 6. Structure of the catalytic domain of matriptase in complex with the 1st Kunitz domain of HAI-1. The crystal structure of the complex was solved by Zhao et al. [49] and the atomic coordinates used for the figure were obtained from the Protein Data Bank (code 4ISO). The 1st Kunitz domain of HAI-1 is shown in gray with the Tyr280 residue (magenta), and the cysteines (red) involved in disulfide bonds. The catalytic domain of the matriptase is represented in black with the cysteines (red) involved in disulfide bonds. *Insert*: substitution of the Tyr280 (magenta) in the KD1 of HAI-1with a cysteine pointing its side chain towards the Cys283.

The analysis of the cysteine mutations in either or both Kunitz domains of HAI-2, support a differential contribution of the KD1 and KD2 in the inhibition of target serine proteases. The KD2 of HAI-2 is clearly less efficient than the KD1 for inhibition of tmprss11, tmprss2 and hepsin. The KD1 and KD2 are equally efficient in inhibiting tmprss13 and prostasin. For matriptase or tmprss4, mutations of both Kunitz domains are required for a complete inhibition by HAI-2.

Among the intestinal serine proteases tested, we observed a loss of function of HAI-2 activity against prostasin and tmprss13 by the Y163C mutation associated with the congenital sodium diarrhea mutant. These two proteases represent potential targets of HAI-2 in regulating intestinal Na^+ transport. Prostasin shows significant mRNA levels in small intestine and colon like HAI-2, and recent genetic evidence shows that disruption of the *Prss8* (encoding prostasin) gene rescues the embryonic lethality of *Spint2* deficient mice [27]. Prostasin could also be a target of HAI-2 during embryonic development since children with the syndromic form of congenital sodium diarrhea also have dysmorphic features [28]. It should be mentioned that prostasin has been proposed to be an activator of ENaC in vivo [14] and notably in colon [52,53]. Tmprss13, whose physiological role is unknown, is also an interesting candidate target for inhibition by HAI-2. Tmprss13 is significantly expressed at the mRNA level in distal colon. The proteases matriptase, tmprss3 or tmprss4 were only partially inhibited by the HAI-2 Y163C. We cannot exclude that these serine proteases represent physiological targets for HAI-2 and play a role in the pathogenesis of congenital sodium diarrhea. The *Spint2* expression pattern is for instance particularly similar to the *St14* gene that encodes matriptase (as shown in this study and in

[21]). The functional targets of HAI-2 and the pathophysiological basis for the intestinal loss of Na^+ ions in congenital sodium diarrhea still remain to be identified.

In summary, we developed a cellular assay in *Xenopus* oocytes to study functional interactions between membrane-bound serine proteases and inhibitors using ENaC as a reporter gene. *SPINT2*, whose mutations have been linked to congenital sodium diarrhea, appears to be a potent inhibitor. Being no longer blocked by the Y68C and Y163C HAI-2 mutants, prostasin and tmprss13 are interesting candidate partners of HAI-2 for maintaining Na^+ homeostasis in the intestine. The functional effects of the cysteine or serine substitutions for the conserved Tyr in the KD1 and KD2 on the activity of HAI-2 are supported by the crystal structure of the complex formed by the HAI-1 homolog and matriptase.

Acknowledgments

We thank Stephan Kellenberger and Delphine Huser for critical reading of the manuscript, and Justyna Iwaszkiewicz for helpful comments and suggestions.

Author Contributions

Conceived and designed the experiments: NF LS. Performed the experiments: NF IG. Analyzed the data: NF IG LS. Contributed reagents/materials/analysis tools: NF IG LS. Wrote the paper: NF LS.

References

1. Szabo R, Bugge TH (2011) Membrane-anchored serine proteases in vertebrate cell and developmental biology. Annu Rev Cell Dev Biol 27: 213–235.
2. Leyvraz C, Charles RP, Rubera I, Guitard M, Rotman S, et al. (2005) The epidermal barrier function is dependent on the serine protease CAP1/Prss8. J Cell Biol 170: 487–496.
3. List K, Szabo R, Wertz PW, Segre J, Haudenschild CC, et al. (2003) Loss of proteolytically processed filaggrin caused by epidermal deletion of Matriptase/MT-SP1. J Cell Biol 163: 901–910.
4. Buzza MS, Netzel-Arnett S, Shea-Donohue T, Zhao A, Lin CY, et al. (2010) Membrane-anchored serine protease matriptase regulates epithelial barrier formation and permeability in the intestine. Proc Natl Acad Sci U S A 107: 4200–4205.
5. List K, Kosa P, Szabo R, Bey AL, Wang CB, et al. (2009) Epithelial integrity is maintained by a matriptase-dependent proteolytic pathway. Am J Pathol 175: 1453–1463.
6. Chan JC, Knudson O, Wu F, Morser J, Dole WP, et al. (2005) Hypertension in mice lacking the proatrial natriuretic peptide convertase corin. Proc Natl Acad Sci U S A 102: 785–790.
7. Finberg KE, Heeney MM, Campagna DR, Aydinok Y, Pearson HA, et al. (2008) Mutations in TMPRSS6 cause iron-refractory iron deficiency anemia (IRIDA). Nat Genet 40: 569–571.
8. Folgueras AR, de Lara FM, Pendas AM, Garabaya C, Rodriguez F, et al. (2008) Membrane-bound serine protease matriptase-2 (Tmprss6) is an essential regulator of iron homeostasis. Blood 112: 2539–2545.
9. Du X, She E, Gelbart T, Truksa J, Lee P, et al. (2008) The serine protease TMPRSS6 is required to sense iron deficiency. Science 320: 1088–1092.
10. Cui Y, Wang W, Dong N, Lou J, Srinivasan DK, et al. (2012) Role of corin in trophoblast invasion and uterine spiral artery remodelling in pregnancy. Nature 484: 246–250.
11. Scott HS, Kudoh J, Wattenhofer M, Shibuya K, Berry A, et al. (2001) Insertion of beta-satellite repeats identifies a transmembrane protease causing both congenital and childhood onset autosomal recessive deafness. Nat Genet 27: 59–63.
12. Guipponi M, Tan J, Cannon PZ, Donley L, Crewther P, et al. (2007) Mice deficient for the type II transmembrane serine protease, TMPRSS1/hepsin, exhibit profound hearing loss. Am J Pathol 171: 608–616.
13. Vallet V, Chraibi A, Gaeggeler HP, Horisberger JD, Rossier BC (1997) An epithelial serine protease activates the amiloride-sensitive sodium channel. Nature 389: 607–610.
14. Planes C, Randrianarison NH, Charles RP, Frateschi S, Cluzeaud F, et al. (2010) ENaC-mediated alveolar fluid clearance and lung fluid balance depend on the channel-activating protease 1. EMBO Mol Med 2: 26–37.
15. Shimomura T, Denda K, Kitamura A, Kawaguchi T, Kito M, et al. (1997) Hepatocyte growth factor activator inhibitor, a novel Kunitz-type serine protease inhibitor. J Biol Chem 272: 6370–6376.
16. Lin CY, Anders J, Johnson M, Dickson RB (1999) Purification and characterization of a complex containing matriptase and a Kunitz-type serine protease inhibitor from human milk. J Biol Chem 274: 18237–18242.
17. Szabo R, Kosa P, List K, Bugge TH (2009) Loss of matriptase suppression underlies spint1 _mutation-associated ichthyosis and postnatal lethality. Am J Pathol 174: 2015–2022.
18. Marlor CW, Delaria KA, Davis G, Muller DK, Greve JM, et al. (1997) Identification and cloning of human placental bikunin, a novel serine protease inhibitor containing two Kunitz domains. J Biol Chem 272: 12202–12208.
19. Kawaguchi T, Qin L, Shimomura T, Kondo J, Matsumoto K, et al. (1997) Purification and cloning of hepatocyte growth factor activator inhibitor type 2, a Kunitz-type serine protease inhibitor. J Biol Chem 272: 27558–27564.
20. Muller-Pillasch F, Wallrapp C, Bartels K, Varga G, Friess H, et al. (1998) Cloning of a new Kunitz-type protease inhibitor with a putative transmembrane domain overexpressed in pancreatic cancer. Biochim Biophys Acta 1395: 88–95.
21. Szabo R, Hobson JP, List K, Molinolo A, Lin CY, et al. (2008) Potent inhibition and global co-localization implicate the transmembrane Kunitz-type serine protease inhibitor hepatocyte growth factor activator inhibitor-2 in the regulation of epithelial matriptase activity. J Biol Chem 283: 29495–29504.
22. Shipway A, Danahay H, Williams JA, Tully DC, Backes BJ, et al. (2004) Biochemical characterization of prostasin, a channel activating protease. Biochem Biophys Res Commun 324: 953–963.
23. Herter S, Piper DE, Aaron W, Gabriele T, Cutler G, et al. (2005) Hepatocyte growth factor is a preferred in vitro substrate for human hepsin, a membrane-anchored serine protease implicated in prostate and ovarian cancers. Biochem J 390: 125–136.
24. Hashimoto T, Kato M, Shimomura T, Kitamura N (2010) TMPRSS13, a type II transmembrane serine protease, is inhibited by hepatocyte growth factor activator inhibitor type 1 and activates pro-hepatocyte growth factor. FEBS J 277: 4888–4900.
25. Mitchell KJ, Pinson KI, Kelly OG, Brennan J, Zupicich J, et al. (2001) Functional analysis of secreted and transmembrane proteins critical to mouse development. Nat Genet 28: 241–249.
26. Szabo R, Hobson JP, Christoph K, Kosa P, List K, et al. (2009) Regulation of cell surface protease matriptase by HAI2 is essential for placental development, neural tube closure and embryonic survival in mice. Development 136: 2653–2663.
27. Szabo R, Uzzun Sales K, Kosa P, Shylo NA, Godiksen S, et al. (2012) Reduced Prostasin (CAP1/PRSS8) Activity Eliminates HAI-1 and HAI-2 Deficiency-Associated Developmental Defects by Preventing Matriptase Activation. PLoS Genet 8: e1002937.
28. Heinz-Erian P, Muller T, Krabichler B, Schranz M, Becker C, et al. (2009) Mutations in SPINT2 cause a syndromic form of congenital sodium diarrhea. Am J Hum Genet 84: 188–196.
29. Salomon J, Goulet O, Canioni D, Brousse N, Lemale J, et al. (2014) Genetic characterization of congenital tufting enteropathy: epcam associated phenotype and involvement of SPINT2 in the syndromic form. Hum Genet 133: 299–310.
30. Rossier BC, Stutts MJ (2009) Activation of the epithelial sodium channel (ENaC) by serine proteases. Annu Rev Physiol 71: 361–379.
31. Chraibi A, Vallet V, Firsov D, Hess SK, Horisberger JD (1998) Protease modulation of the activity of the epithelial sodium channel expressed in Xenopus oocytes. J Gen Physiol 111: 127–138.
32. Vuagniaux G, Vallet V, Jaeger NF, Pfister C, Bens M, et al. (2000) Activation of the amiloride-sensitive epithelial sodium channel by the serine protease mCAP1 expressed in a mouse cortical collecting duct cell line. J Am Soc Nephrol 11: 828–834.
33. Adachi M, Kitamura K, Miyoshi T, Narikiyo T, Iwashita K, et al. (2001) Activation of epithelial sodium channels by prostasin in Xenopus oocytes. J Am Soc Nephrol 12: 1114–1121.
34. Vuagniaux G, Vallet V, Jaeger NF, Hummler E, Rossier BC (2002) Synergistic activation of ENaC by three membrane-bound channel-activating serine proteases (mCAP1, mCAP2, and mCAP3) and serum- and glucocorticoid-regulated kinase (Sgk1) in Xenopus Oocytes. J Gen Physiol 120: 191–201.
35. List K, Hobson JP, Molinolo A, Bugge TH (2007) Co-localization of the channel activating protease prostasin/(CAP1/PRSS8) with its candidate activator, matriptase. J Cell Physiol 213: 237–245.
36. Oberst MD, Singh B, Ozdemirli M, Dickson RB, Johnson MD, et al. (2003) Characterization of matriptase expression in normal human tissues. J Histochem Cytochem 51: 1017–1025.
37. Tsuji A, Torres-Rosado A, Arai T, Le Beau MM, Lemons RS, et al. (1991) Hepsin, a cell membrane-associated protease. Characterization, tissue distribution, and gene localization. J Biol Chem 266: 16948–16953.
38. Ganesan R, Kolumam GA, Lin SJ, Xie MH, Santell L, et al. (2011) Proteolytic activation of pro-macrophage-stimulating protein by hepsin. Mol Cancer Res 9: 1175–1186.
39. Vaarala MH, Porvari KS, Kellokumpu S, Kyllonen AP, Vihko PT (2001) Expression of transmembrane serine protease TMPRSS2 in mouse and human tissues. J Pathol 193: 134–140.

40. Guipponi M, Vuagniaux G, Wattenhofer M, Shibuya K, Vazquez M, et al. (2002) The transmembrane serine protease (TMPRSS3) mutated in deafness DFNB8/10 activates the epithelial sodium channel (ENaC) in vitro. Hum Mol Genet 11: 2829–2836.
41. Sales KU, Hobson JP, Wagenaar-Miller R, Szabo R, Rasmussen AL, et al. (2011) Expression and genetic loss of function analysis of the HAT/DESC cluster proteases TMPRSS11A and HAT. PLoS One 6: e23261.
42. Kim DR, Sharmin S, Inoue M, Kido H (2001) Cloning and expression of novel mosaic serine proteases with and without a transmembrane domain from human lung. Biochim Biophys Acta 1518: 204–209.
43. Kido H, Okumura Y, Takahashi E, Pan HY, Wang S, et al. (2008) Host envelope glycoprotein processing proteases are indispensable for entry into human cells by seasonal and highly pathogenic avian influenza viruses. J Mol Genet Med 3: 167–175.
44. Yuan X, Zheng X, Lu D, Rubin DC, Pung CY, et al. (1998) Structure of murine enterokinase (enteropeptidase) and expression in small intestine during development. Am J Physiol 274: G342–349.
45. Itoh H, Kataoka H, Hamasuna R, Kitamura N, Koono M (1999) Hepatocyte growth factor activator inhibitor type 2 lacking the first Kunitz-type serine proteinase inhibitor domain is a predominant product in mouse but not in human. Biochem Biophys Res Commun 255: 740–748.
46. Rossier BC, Pradervand S, Schild L, Hummler E (2002) Epithelial sodium channel and the control of sodium balance: interaction between genetic and environmental factors. Annu Rev Physiol 64: 877–897.
47. Schild L (2010) The epithelial sodium channel and the control of sodium balance. Biochim Biophys Acta 1802: 1159–1165.
48. Donaldson SH, Hirsh A, Li DC, Holloway G, Chao J, et al. (2002) Regulation of the epithelial sodium channel by serine proteases in human airways. J Biol Chem 277: 8338–8345.
49. Zhao B, Yuan C, Li R, Qu D, Huang M, et al. (2013) Crystal structures of matriptase in complex with its inhibitor hepatocyte growth factor activator inhibitor-1. J Biol Chem 288: 11155–11164.
50. Shia S, Stamos J, Kirchhofer D, Fan B, Wu J, et al. (2005) Conformational lability in serine protease active sites: structures of hepatocyte growth factor activator (HGFA) alone and with the inhibitory domain from HGFA inhibitor-1B. J Mol Biol 346: 1335–1349.
51. Guerois R, Nielsen JE, Serrano L (2002) Predicting changes in the stability of proteins and protein complexes: a study of more than 1000 mutations. J Mol Biol 320: 369–387.
52. Frateschi S, Keppner A, Malsure S, Iwaszkiewicz J, Sergi C, et al. (2012) Mutations of the serine protease CAP1/Prss8 lead to reduced embryonic viability, skin defects, and decreased ENaC activity. Am J Pathol 181: 605–615.
53. Malsure S, Wang Q, Charles RP, Sergi C, Perrier R, et al. (2014) Colon-Specific Deletion of Epithelial Sodium Channel Causes Sodium Loss and Aldosterone Resistance. J Am Soc Nephrol.

12

Probiotic *Lactobacillus rhamnosus* GG Enhanced Th1 Cellular Immunity but Did Not Affect Antibody Responses in a Human Gut Microbiota Transplanted Neonatal Gnotobiotic Pig Model

Ke Wen[1], Christine Tin[1], Haifeng Wang[1], Xingdong Yang[1], Guohua Li[1], Ernawati Giri-Rachman[1], Jacob Kocher[1], Tammy Bui[1], Sherrie Clark-Deener[2], Lijuan Yuan[1]*

1 Department of Biomedical Sciences and Pathobiology, Virginia-Maryland Regional College of Veterinary Medicine, Virginia Polytechnic Institute and State University, Blacksburg, Viginia, United States of America, **2** Department of Large Animal Clinical Sciences, Virginia-Maryland Regional College of Veterinary Medicine, Virginia Polytechnic Institute and State University, Blacksburg, Viginia, United States of America

Abstract

This study aims to establish a human gut microbiota (HGM) transplanted gnotobiotic (Gn) pig model of human rotavirus (HRV) infection and diarrhea, and to verify the dose-effects of probiotics on HRV vaccine-induced immune responses. Our previous studies using the Gn pig model found that probiotics dose-dependently regulated both T cell and B cell immune responses induced by rotavirus vaccines. We generated the HGM transplanted neonatal Gn pigs through daily feeding of neonatal human fecal suspension to germ-free pigs for 3 days starting at 12 hours after birth. We found that attenuated HRV (AttHRV) vaccination conferred similar overall protection against rotavirus diarrhea and virus shedding in Gn pigs and HGM transplanted Gn pigs. HGM promoted the development of the neonatal immune system, as evidenced by the significantly enhanced IFN-γ producing T cell responses and reduction of regulatory T cells and their cytokine production in the AttHRV-vaccinated pigs. The higher dose *Lactobacillus rhamnosus* GG (LGG) feeding (14 doses, up to 10^9 colony-forming-unit [CFU]/dose) effectively increased the LGG counts in the HGM Gn pig intestinal contents and significantly enhanced HRV-specific IFN-γ producing T cell responses to the AttHRV vaccine. Lower dose LGG (9 doses, up to 10^6 CFU/dose) was ineffective. Neither doses of LGG significantly improved the protection rate, HRV-specific IgA and IgG antibody titers in serum, or IgA antibody titers in intestinal contents compared to the AttHRV vaccine alone, suggesting that an even higher dose of LGG is needed to overcome the influence of the microbiota to achieve the immunostimulatory effect in the HGM pigs. This study demonstrated that HGM Gn pig is an applicable animal model for studying immune responses to rotavirus vaccines and can be used for studying interventions (i.e., probiotics and prebiotics) that may enhance the immunogenicity and protective efficacy of vaccines through improving the gut microbiota.

Editor: Shan Lu, University of Massachusetts Medical Center, United States of America

Funding: This work was supported by a grant (R01AT004789) to Lijuan Yuan from the National Center of Complementary and Alternative Medicine, National Institutes of Health, Bethesda, MD. The funders had no role in study design, data collection and analysis, decision to publish, or preparation of the manuscript.

Competing Interests: The authors have declared that no competing interests exist.

* E-mail: lyuan@vt.edu

Introduction

Gnotobiotic (Gn) pig models have been extensively used in studies of human rotavirus (HRV) because of the similar susceptibility to the Wa strain (G1P1A[8]) HRV infection and clinical manifestations in neonatal Gn pigs as in human infants [1-4]. Our previous studies demonstrated that probiotic *Lactobacillus acidophilus* NCFM (LA) at the appropriate dose was effective in reducing rotavirus diarrhea as well as enhancing immunogenicity of oral rotavirus vaccines in Gn pigs [5]. LA regulated rotavirus vaccine-induced immune responses in a dose-dependent manner in Gn pigs [5,6]. Low dose LA (5 doses; up to 10^6 colony-forming-unit (CFU)/dose) significantly enhanced effector T cell responses and down-regulated regulatory T (Treg) cell responses; high dose LA (14 doses; up to 10^9 CFU/dose) significantly down-regulated effector T cell responses and up-regulated Treg cell responses [6]. Intermediate dose LA (9 doses, up to 10^6 CFU/dose) significantly enhanced rotavirus-specific antibody secreting cell (ASC) and memory B cell responses induced by rotavirus vaccines in Gn pigs [5]. LA also dose-dependently regulated innate immune responses of cytokine producing dendritic cells and Toll-like receptor expressing antigen presenting cells [7]. The probiotic *Lactobacillus rhamnosus* (LGG) strain also enhanced the immunogenicity of rotavirus vaccines in Gn pigs at the appropriate dose in our previous study (Manuscript in preparation). LGG, but not LA has been evaluated in several human clinical trials as a vaccine adjuvant [8], including rotavirus vaccine [9] and influenza vaccine [10], therefore we chose LGG for the present study.

Interactions between probiotics and host immune responses can be influenced by gut microbiota, which is lacking in Gn pigs. A previous study of pigs showed that the gut microbiota composition in human gut microbiota (HGM) transplanted pigs resembles that from the human donor [11]. *Bifidobacteria* from human stool could not colonize the gut of HGM transplanted ex-germfree mice [12] but succeeded in colonization of HGM transplanted pigs [11]. Furthermore, the colonization and evolutional development of microbiota in the gut of HGM transplanted pigs was similar to that observed in humans [11]. Of most importance to human health, HGM transplanted pigs had a healthy gut immune system and similar immunity to pathogens as those in humans [13], which supports the applicability of HGM transplanted pigs in studying immune responses to human pathogens and vaccines. Therefore, to verify the functions of probiotic adjuvants demonstrated in the previous studies, the current study establishes a HGM transplanted neonatal Gn pig model of HRV infection and diarrhea to closely mimic the real context of rotavirus vaccination in infants and to test LGG's dose effects on the immune response profiles induced by the AttHRV vaccine.

Materials and Methods

Ethics statement

All animal experiments were performed in strict accordance with federal and university guidelines. Specifically, we adhered to the recommendations in the Guide for the Care and Use of Laboratory Animals of the National Institutes of Health and the American Veterinary Medical Association Guidelines on Euthanasia. The animal protocol was approved by the Institutional Animal Care and Use Committee at Virginia Tech (Protocol# 10-168-CVM and 13-187-CVM). Ethical Committee approval was received from Virginia Tech Institutional Review Board for the newborn human stool sample collection (IRB number 11-1049).

Probiotic Bacteria and rotavirus

Lactobacillus rhamnosus GG strain (ATCC 53103) was used in the current study and propagated in lactobacilli MRS broth (Weber, Hamilton, NJ). LGG inoculums were prepared and titrated as we previously described [14].

The cell culture-adapted human rotavirus Wa strain (G1P1A[8]), derived from the 35th passage in African green monkey kidney cells (MA104, ATCC# CRL-2378.1), was used as the AttHRV vaccine for inoculation of Gn pigs at a dose of 5×10^7 fluorescent focus-forming units (FFU) [15]. AttHRV was also used as the detector antigen in the enzyme-linked immunosorbent assay (ELISA) [5] and as the stimulating antigen in the intracellular IFN-γ staining assay as described previously [16].

The virulent HRV (VirHRV) Wa strain was passaged through Gn pigs and the pooled intestinal contents from the 27th passage were used to challenge Gn pigs at a dose of 10^5 FFU. The median infectious dose (ID_{50}) and median diarrhea dose (DD_{50}) of the VirHRV in Gn pigs were determined as approximately 1 FFU [17].

Human gut microbiota inoculum

Human gut microbiota was obtained from stool samples of a healthy male infant born in the United States who was delivered by C-section, solely breast-fed, and did not exhibit any signs of digestive disorders or receive any medication prior to stool sample collection. A freshly passed stool was diluted 20-fold and homogenized in sterile and pre-reduced 0.1 M potassium phosphate buffer (PBS, pH 7.2) containing 15% glycerol (v/v) to produce a 5% human fecal suspension, which was then aliquoted into 15 ml sterile tubes and injected with nitrogen for 1 min and stored at −80°C. After completing sample collection daily between 17 to 23 days of age, the fecal samples were then thawed, mixed and homogenized to make a large stock for the entire experiment. The stock was divided into 15 ml aliquots, injected with nitrogen, and stored at −80°C. In order to remove glycerol prior to feeding to piglets, the fecal samples were thawed and washed with at least ten-fold volumes of PBS, centrifuged at 2000 rpm/min for 10 min at 4°C, and then diluted to the original volume with PBS.

Death of neonatal pigs caused by opportunistic bacteria infection after transplanting HGM from an apparently healthy 11 years old human donor has been reported previously [18]. Therefore, before the study, the stool samples collected from the solely breast fed, healthy infant at 17–23 days of age were subjected to multi-step safety testing. First, the stool suspension was plated on blood agar plates to observe any sign of hemolytic activity which can be an indication of the presence of pathogenic bacteria. No hemolytic activity was observed. The stool sample was then screened by Viral Chips and the genomes were sequenced on an Illumina MiSeq^{TM} at the Viral Diagnostics and Discovery Center, University of California, San Francisco. The sequencing results confirmed that no known viruses are present in this sample. Lastly, a bioassay was conducted. High doses of the stool inoculum (2.5-, 5-, and 10-times of the normal dosage of the stool inoculum) were tested in newborn Gn pigs and no adverse effect, except for mild diarrhea, was observed.

Treatment groups and inoculation of Gn pigs

Gn pigs were derived and maintained as we previously described [6]. The pigs in the HGM groups were orally fed with 1 ml/dose of the 5% fecal suspension starting at 12 hrs after birth daily for 3 days to establish HGM transplanted Gn pigs. HGM transplanted Gn pigs were randomly assigned to five treatment groups: (1) Mock control with no treatment, (2) 14 doses of LGG (LGG14X) alone, (3) AttHRV alone, (4) AttHRV plus 9 doses of LGG (AttHRV+LGG9X), and (5) AttHRV plus 14 doses of LGG (AttHRV+LGG14X) (see Table 1 for the number of pigs for non-HGM group and HGM groups). Detailed probiotic dosing schedules for the intermediate dose (LGG9X) and high (LGG14X) dose were described in our previous publication [5]. Pigs from both non-HGM and HGM transplanted groups were vaccinated with the AttHRV vaccine following the same protocol as we previously described [6]. At post-inoculation day (PID) 28, subsets of HGM pigs from the three AttHRV groups and the non-HGM AttHRV group, all HGM pigs from the mock control and LGG14X groups were orally challenged with 10^5 FFU VirHRV. After HGM inoculation from 0 to 12 of days of age and from postchallenge days (PCD) 0 to 7, pigs were examined daily for clinical signs (diarrhea) and fecal swabs were collected daily as we previously described [15]. Mononuclear cells (MNCs) were isolated from ileum, spleen, and peripheral blood of pigs euthanized on PID 28 or PCD 7 as we previously described [6,15].

Detection of rotavirus and LGG shedding and assessment of rotavirus diarrhea

Rectal swabs were collected for 7 days after VirHRV challenge to assess rotavirus diarrhea and shedding. Pigs with daily fecal scores of ≥2 were considered diarrheic. Fecal consistency was scored as follows: 0, normal; 1, pasty; 2, semiliquid; and 3, liquid. Daily scores were added up for each challenged pig from PCD 0 to 7 to get the cumulative fecal score and then the average cumulative fecal score for all the pigs in each group was calculated. Virus shedding was detected by ELISA and cell culture immunofluorescence (CCIF) assay in processed rectal swab fluids as described previously [19,20].

Feces and LIC were collected and processed as described previously [19,20]. Bacterial DNA was extracted using the Wizard

Table 1. Number of pigs in non-HGM group and HGM groups at beginning of study and at euthanasia on PID 28 and PCD 7.

Treatment groups	Total at PID 0	Excluded	PID 28	PCD 7
Non-HGM group				
AttHRV	18	0	6	12
HGM groups				
HGM only	4	1	0	3
HGM+LGG14x	4	0	0	4
HGM+AttHRV	12	4	4	4
HGM+AttHRV+LGG9x	13	3	6	4
HGM+AttHRV+LGG14x	10	1	4	5

Genomic DNA Purification Kit (Promega, Madision, WI) according to the manufacturer's instruction. The extracted DNA was then used for enumerating LGG numbers by real-time PCR. Pure LGG with known numbers quantified as described in the previous study [14] was used as the standard to calculate relative numbers of LGG in the samples. Real-time quantitative PCR was carried out with RT^2 SYBR® Green qPCR Mastermix (QIAGEN Inc., Valencia, CA). PCR cycling conditions were 5 min at 94°C, and then 40 cycles of 15 s at 94°C, 15 s at 60°C, and 30 s at 72°C. The reaction mixtures each contained 2 µl of the sample DNA and 18 µl of the master mix, which included the appropriate sense and antisense primers. The sense primer for LGG is 5′-CGCCCTTAACAGCAGTCTTCAAAT-3′ and the antisense primer is 5′-ACGCGCCCTCCGTATGCTTAAACC-3′ [21].

Flow cytometry

The frequencies of specific subsets of effector and regulatory T cells were determined by using intracellular cytokine staining and flow cytometry as we previously described [6,16]. Their absolute numbers were calculated based on their frequencies among MNCs and the total number of MNCs isolated from each tissue in ileum, IEL, spleen and blood of Gn pigs.

Assessment of rotavirus-specific IgA responses in serum and small intestinal contents and IgG responses in serum

Sera were collected at PID0, PID13, PID22, PID28 and PCD7, and the small intestinal contents (SIC) were collected at PID28 and PCD7 to measure rotavirus-specific IgA and IgG responses using indirect isotype-specific antibody ELISA as previously described [22,23].

Statistical analysis

Kruskal-Wallis rank sum test was performed to compare all data, except for proportions of virus shedding and diarrhea among treatment groups, which were compared using Fisher's exact test. Statistical significance was assessed at $p<0.05$. All statistical analysis was performed using SAS program 9.2 (SAS Institute, INC, USA).

Results

Similar clinical signs in AttHRV-vaccinated pigs with or without HGM transplantation after VirHRV challenge

Comparisons of clinical signs and fecal virus shedding of AttHRV-vaccinated pigs with or without HGM transplantation after VirHRV challenge are summarized in Fig. 1A. Compared to the Gn pigs, except for the significantly higher cumulative fecal scores and virus shedding titers in the HGM transplanted Gn pigs, both pig groups had similar incidence of diarrhea (67% and 75% for Gn and HGM pig groups, respectively) and fecal virus shedding (50% for both pig groups), similar mean duration of diarrhea and fecal virus shedding, as well as similar onset of fecal virus shedding. Both pig groups shed low titers of virus (< 200 FFU/ml); however, the HGM pigs shed significantly higher virus titers (6-fold) compared to the Gn pigs (Fig. 1A).

High dose LGG feeding significantly enhanced the fecal and intestinal LGG counts in HGM transplanted Gn pigs

Two LGG dosing regimens were included to investigate the effectiveness of different LGG feeding regimens in modulating the LGG counts in the feces and intestine of the HGM transplanted pigs (Fig. 1B). AttHRV+LGG14X pigs had significantly higher LGG titers in feces at PID 23 than AttHRV+LGG9X and AttHRV pigs; this high dose LGG feeding also resulted in higher (not significantly) LGG counts in feces at PID 5 and PID 10 and in large intestine contents (LIC) at PID 28 and PCD 7 compared to the other two groups. AttHRV+LGG9X and AttHRV only pigs had similar LGG counts from PID 5 to PCD 7. Since AttHRV only pigs were not fed LGG, the data indicate that the LGG detected in those pigs was a component of the donor HGM with successful colonization of the Gn pig intestine. Notably, the magnitude of increases of LGG counts in the AttHRV+LGG14X group (22-fold) was greater than the AttHRV+LGG9X group (14 fold) from PID 5 to PID 10, reflecting the difference in the LGG dosing regimens.

HGM colonization significantly promoted the development of Th1 type immune responses and down-regulated Treg cell responses

To study interactions among HGM, neonatal immune system and rotavirus vaccine, and to evaluate the effect of HGM on the development of neonatal immune system in the context of rotavirus vaccination, we compared the total numbers and frequencies of effector (Fig. 2) and Treg cell (Fig. 3) subsets in the intestinal [ileum and intraepithelial lymphocytes (IEL)] and systemic (spleen and blood) lymphoid tissues of the AttHRV-vaccinated pigs with and without HGM. HGM did not significantly alter the total numbers of CD3+CD4+ and CD3+CD8+ T cells in any tissues tested at PID 28, suggesting that AttHRV provided sufficient antigen stimulation for the expansion of the T cell compartment of the neonatal immune system in Gn pigs without HGM. However, AttHRV-vaccinated pigs with HGM had significantly higher frequencies of IFN−γ+CD4+ T

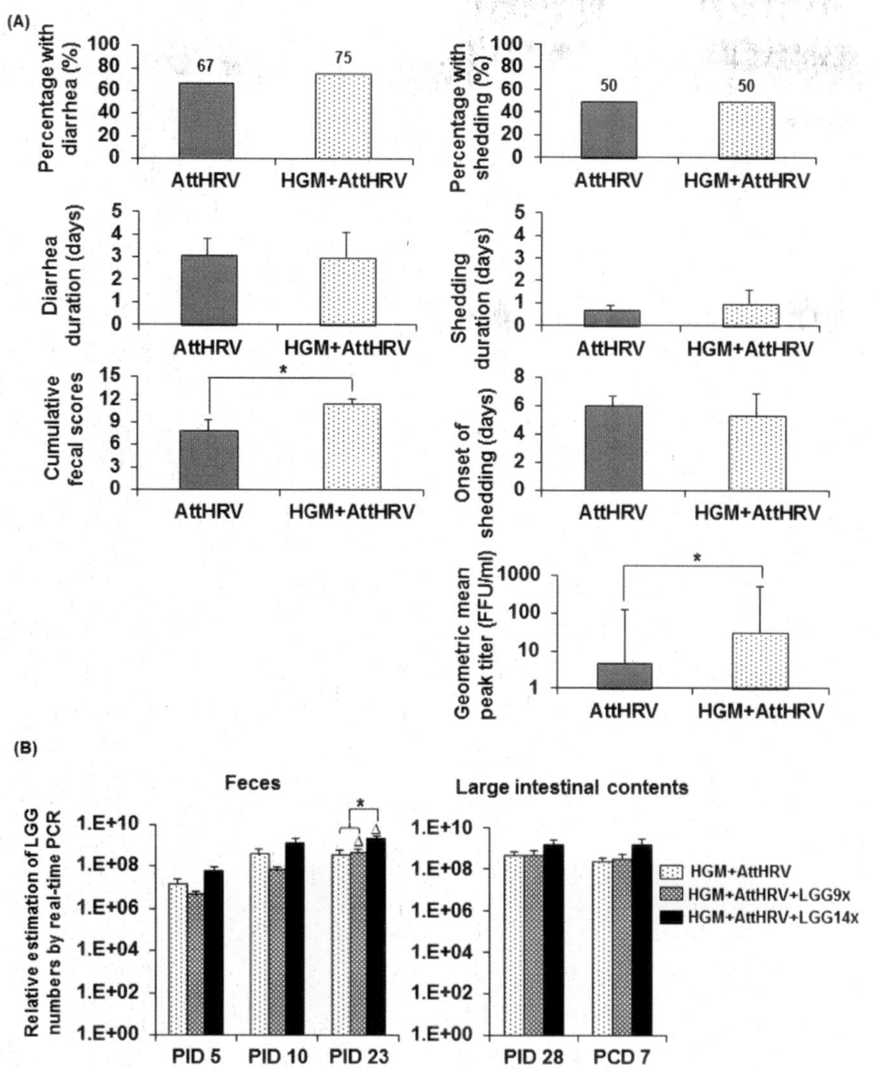

Figure 1. Clinical sign and virus shedding in AttHRV vaccinated pigs with or without HGM transplantation (A) and LGG shedding in fecal samples and large intestinal contents of HGM transplanted Gn pigs fed with or without LGG (B). After VirHRV challenge, pigs were monitored for 7 days for incidence of diarrhea, fecal score and virus shedding. Data are presented as mean ± standard error of the mean (n = 12 for AttHRV group; n = 4 for HGM+AttHRV group). The sign "*" in (A) indicates significant difference between groups (Kruskal-Wallis test, $p<0.05$). LGG amounts at different time points were determined by strain-specific real-time PCR and are presented as mean counts/ml ± standard error of the mean (n = 7–10 for fecal samples and n = 3–6 for large intestinal content samples). The sign "*" in (B) indicates significant differences between groups at the same time points and the symbol "Δ" indicates significant increases in LGG numbers compared to PID 5 for the same group (Kruskal-Wallis test, $p<0.05$).

cells among CD3+ cells in blood and IFN−γ+CD8+ T cells among CD3+ cells in all tissues at PID 28 compared to AttHRV-vaccinated pigs without HGM. HGM+AttHRV pigs also had significantly higher numbers of IFN−γ+CD3+CD8+ T cells in spleen at PID 28 than AttHRV only pigs. Postchallenge, HGM significantly increased total numbers of CD3+CD8+ cells in spleen and significantly enhanced IFN−γ producing CD8+ T cell responses measured in both frequencies and numbers in spleen and blood of AttHRV-vaccinated pigs.

Consistent with the enhanced Th1 type immune responses, HGM down-regulated or significantly down-regulated the frequencies of CD4+CD25−FoxP3+ Treg cells in all tissues of AttHRV-vaccinated pigs. HGM+AttHRV pigs had significantly lower numbers of Treg cells in spleen and blood at PID 28 and in ileum, IEL and blood at PCD 7 compared to AttHRV only pigs. Furthermore, HGM decreased or significantly decreased the frequencies of IL-10 or TGF-β producing Treg cells in all tissues (with one exception in IL-10 producing Treg cells in blood at PCD7) of AttHRV-vaccinated pigs.

High dose LGG significantly enhanced rotavirus-specific IFN-γ producing T cell responses but did not affect Treg cells in AttHRV-vaccinated pigs with HGM

To investigate the dose effect of LGG as an adjuvant in enhancing the immunogenicity of the rotavirus vaccine, we measured the virus-specific effector T cell responses in AttHRV-vaccinated HGM pigs fed with or without the 9 and 14 doses of LGG at challenge (PID 28) and postchallenge (PCD 7) (Fig. 4). The AttHRV+LGG14X pigs had significantly higher frequencies of rotavirus-specific IFN-γ producing CD4+ T cells in IEL and spleen and IFN-γ producing CD8+ T cells in ileum, IEL and blood compared to both the AttHRV and AttHRV+LGG9X pig

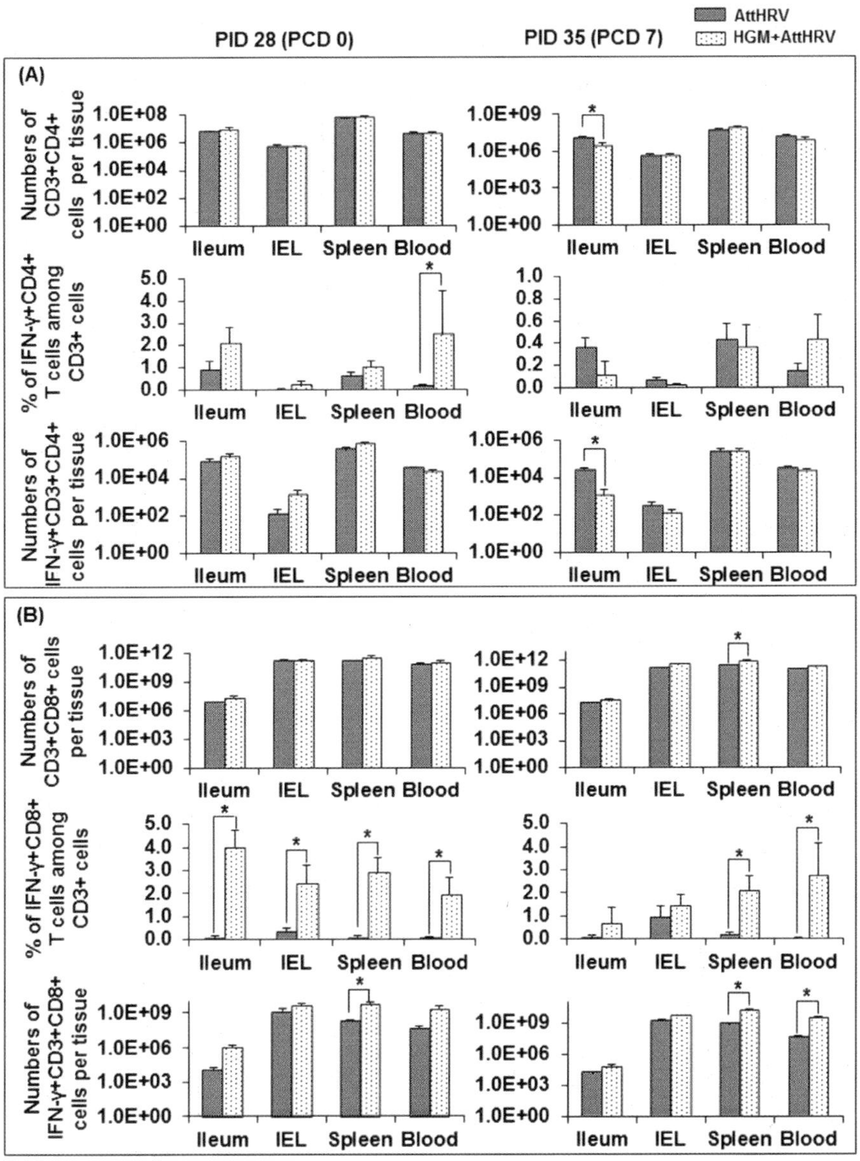

Figure 2. T cell responses in AttHRV vaccinated pigs with or without HGM transplantation. MNCs were stimulated with semi-purified AttHRV antigen *in vitro* for 17 hrs. Brefeldin A was added for the last 5 hrs to block secretion of cytokines produced by the T cells. HRV-specific IFN-γ producing CD4+ and CD8+ T cells was detected by intracellular staining and flow cytometry as we previously described [16]. The frequencies of IFN−γ+CD4+/CD8+ T cells were expressed as percentages among total CD3+ T cells (A and B, middle panel). All mean frequencies are reported after subtraction of the background frequencies. The absolute numbers of CD3+CD4+/CD8+ cells and IFN−γ+CD3+CD4+/CD8+ cells per tissue (A and B, top and bottom panels) were calculated based on the frequencies of CD3+CD4+/CD8+ cells and IFN−γ+CD3+CD4+/CD8+ cells, respectively, and the total number of MNCs isolated from each tissue. Data are presented as mean number or frequency ± standard error of the mean (n = 4–12). The sign "*" indicates the significant difference between groups (Kruskal–Wallis test, $p<0.05$).

groups at PID 28. The AttHRV+LGG14X pigs also had significantly increased frequencies of rotavirus-specific IFN-γ producing CD4+ T cells in ileum and blood compared to the AttHRV+LGG9X pigs at PID 28. Postchallenge, AttHRV+LGG14X pigs had significantly higher frequencies of IFN-γ producing CD4+ T cells in ileum than the AttHRV and AttHRV+LGG9X pigs. The AttHRV+LGG14X pigs also had significantly increased frequencies of rotavirus-specific IFN-γ producing CD8+ T cells in ileum and IEL compared to the AttHRV only pigs at PCD 7. The AttHRV+LGG9X pigs had slightly (not significantly) increased IFN-γ producing CD4+ and CD8+ T cell responses in all tissues at PCD 7.

No significant differences were observed in the frequencies of CD4+CD25−FoxP3+ Treg cells and the frequencies of their cytokine production in any tissues among the three AttHRV-vaccinated HGM pig groups with or without LGG feeding at PID 28 or PCD 7 (data not shown).

Similar rotavirus-specific antibody responses associated with similar protection rate against rotavirus infection among all three groups of AttHRV-vaccinated HGM pigs with or without LGG feeding

In the HGM pigs, AttHRV vaccination with and without LGG induced significantly higher rotavirus-specific serum IgA responses

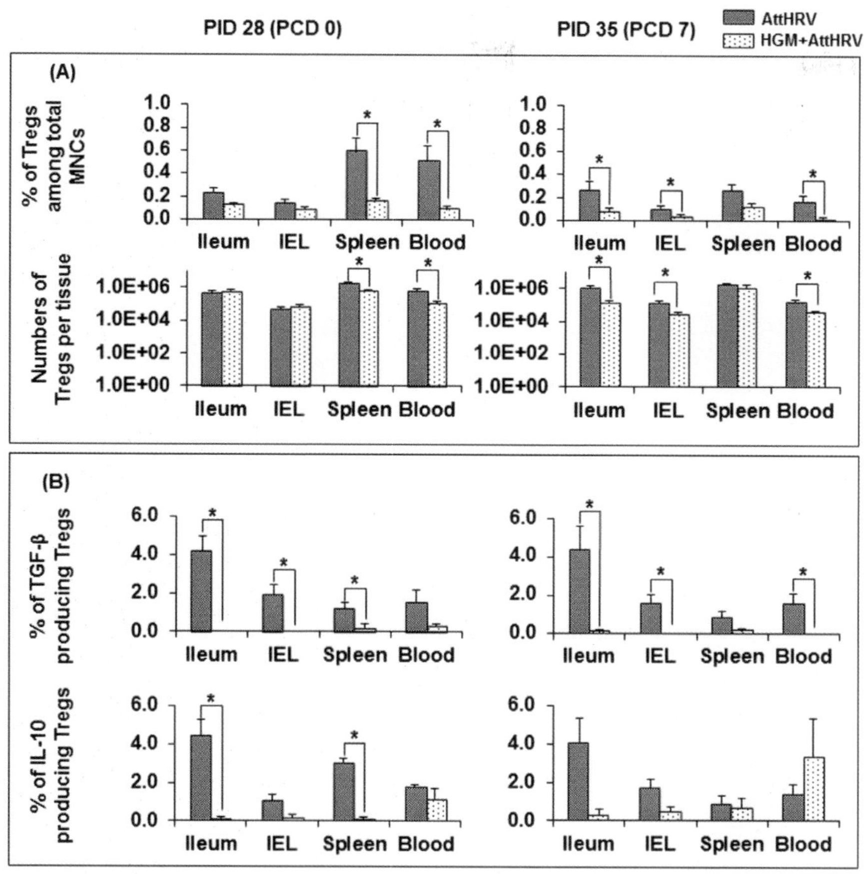

Figure 3. Treg responses in AttHRV vaccinated pigs with or without HGM transplantation. MNCs were stained freshly without *in vitro* stimulation. The frequencies of Tregs were expressed as the percentages among gated MNCs (A, top panel). The absolute numbers of Tregs per tissue were calculated based on the frequencies of Tregs and the total number of MNCs isolated from each tissue (A, bottom panel). The frequencies of IL−10+ or TGF−β+ Tregs were expressed as the percentages of IL−10+ or TGF−β+ cells among the Tregs (B). Data are presented as mean number or frequency ± standard error of the mean (n = 4–9). See Fig. 2 legend for statistical analysis.

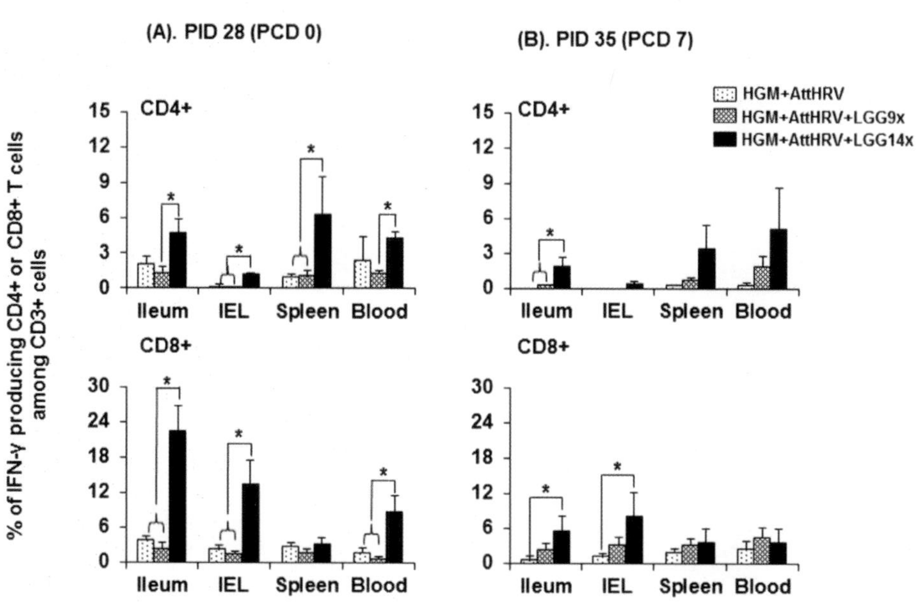

Figure 4. Rotavirus-specific IFN-γ producing T cell responses in HGM transplanted Gn pigs fed with different doses of LGG. Data are presented as mean frequency ± standard error of the mean (n = 4–6). See Fig. 2 legend for detection of rotavirus-specific IFN-γ producing T cell and statistical analysis.

at PID22, PID28 and PCD7 and serum IgG responses from PID12 to PCD7 compared to the unvaccinated pig groups (Fig. 5). Of interest, pigs from all three AttHRV groups with and without LGG feeding had similar rotavirus-specific serum IgA and IgG titers at each examined time point from PID0 to PID28 (Fig. 5). Consistent with this data, LGG feeding also did not significantly alter rotavirus-specific IgA responses in small intestinal contents at PID28, although AttHRV+LGG14X pigs had a trend for higher IgA titers than the AttHRV+LGG9X and AttHRV-only pigs at PID28 (Fig. 5). Postchallenge, however, the AttHRV+LGG9X and AttHRV+LGG14X pigs had significantly higher rotavirus-specific IgA titers in serum; AttHRV+LGG9X pigs also had significantly higher rotavirus-specific IgA titers in small intestinal contents compared to the AttHRV only pigs at PCD7 (Fig. 5). Serum IgG titers did not differ significantly among the three AttHRV groups at PCD7 (Fig. 5).

When analyzing the dynamics of antibody responses, pigs from all three AttHRV vaccinated groups had the highest rotavirus-specific serum IgA and IgG titers at PCD7, which were significantly higher than those examined at all previous time points (Fig. 5). All AttHRV pigs from the three groups also had significantly higher rotavirus-specific serum IgA and IgG responses at PID22 and PID28 compared to PID0 or PID12, and had significantly higher rotavirus-specific serum IgG titers at PID12 compared to those at PID0 (Fig. 5). Thus, LGG feedings did not significantly influence the magnitude and dynamics of rotavirus-specific antibody responses induced by the AttHRV vaccine in HGM pigs at PID28, but LGG enhanced the anamnestic antibody responses upon VirHRV challenge. The similar antibody responses were associated with similar corresponding protection against rotavirus fecal shedding observed in the three AttHRV pig groups upon VirHRV challenge (Table 2). There were no statistically significant differences in the percent of diarrhea and fecal virus shedding, mean days to onset and mean duration of diarrhea and virus shedding among the three AttHRV pig groups, likely due to the small number of pigs in each group. However, there was a trend for shorter mean duration of diarrhea and lower cumulative fecal scores in the LGG fed pigs, which is consistent with the moderate effect of LGG in reducing rotavirus diarrhea observed in Gn pigs [24] and in human infants [25].

Safety of the HGM in newborn Gn pigs

Although the multi-step safety testing was done to confirm the safety of the collected stool samples, 2–3 pigs in each litter became ill (poor appetite, lethargic, fever, vomiting, and/or diarrhea) during the experiments and had to be euthanized prior to the scheduled time point, despite treatment with 50% dextrose (8ml/dose) by mouth every 8 hrs. The mean mortality rate in the HGM pigs was 20.9% (Table 1). The necropsy reports from the Anatomic Pathology Laboratory, Virginia Tech Animal Laboratory Services, gave the final diagnoses as mild enteritis and mild hepatitis. The bacterial culture identified *Klebsiella oxytoca*, *Enterococcus faecalis*, and *Staphyloccus epidermdis* in the pigs. *Klebsiella oxytoca* was considered the likely primary pathogen. These early euthanized pigs were excluded from this study.

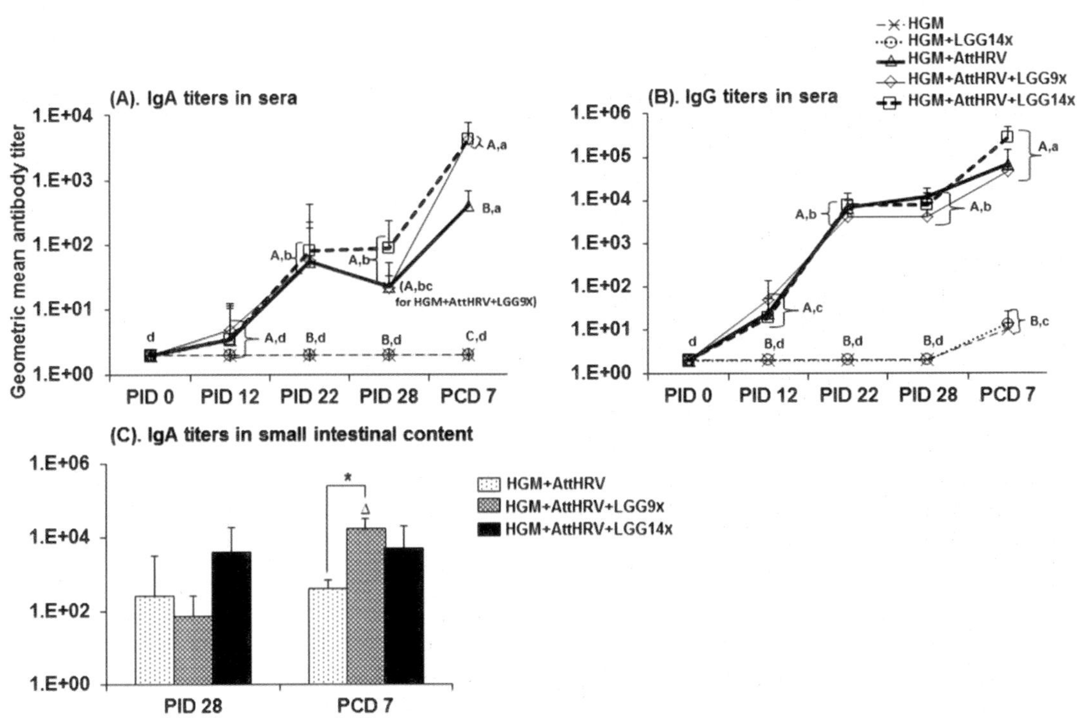

Figure 5. Rotavirus-specific serum IgA and IgG antibody responses (A and B) and rotavirus-specific IgA antibody responses in small intestine contents (C) of Gn pigs transplanted with HGM and fed different doses of LGG. Rotavirus-specific antibody titers were measured by an indirect isotype-specific antibody ELISA and presented as geometric mean titers for each treatment group + standard error of the mean (n = 3–10 for serum samples and n = 3–6 for small intestine content samples). Different capital letters (A, B, or C) indicate significant differences in antibody titers compared among different groups at the same time points; different lower case letters (a, b, c, d) indicate significant difference between different time points in the same group (Kruskal–Wallis test, $p<0.05$), whereas shared letters indicate no significant difference. The sign "*" indicates significant differences in IgA titers in small intestine contents between groups at the same time points and the symbol "Δ" indicates significant increases in IgA titers at PCD7 compared to PID28 for the same group (Kruskal–Wallis test, $p<0.05$).

Table 2. Clinical signs and rotavirus fecal shedding in AttHRV-vaccinated HGM pigs after VirHRV challenge.

Treatment groups	n	Clinical signs				Fecal virus shedding (by CCIF and/or ELISA)			
		% with diarrhea*, a	Mean days to onset**	Mean duration (days) **, b	Mean cumulative scores**, c	% virus shedding*	Mean days to onset**	Mean duration (days)**, b	Geometric mean peak titer (FFU/ml) **,e
AttHRV+LGG9x	4	100^A	2.3 (1.3^d)^A	1.0 (0.0)^A	9.6 (0.2)^B	50^A	5.5 (1.4)^A	0.5 (0.3)^A	7.5^A
AttHRV+LGG14x	5	60^A	4.0 (1.6)^A	2.2 (1.1)^A	10.3 (1.3)^{AB}	60^A	5.0 (1.3)^A	1.2 (0.6)^A	4.4^A
AttHRV	4	75^A	2.8 (1.8)^A	3.0 (1.1)^A	11.5 (0.6)^A	50^A	5.3 (1.6)^A	1.0 (0.6)^A	29.9^A

[a]Pigs with daily fecal scores of ≥2 were considered diarrheic. Fecal consistency was scored as follows: 0, normal; 1, pasty; 2, semiliquid; and 3, liquid.
[b]For durations of diarrhea and virus shedding, if no diarrhea or virus shedding until the euthanasia day (PCD7), the duration (days) were recorded as 0 and the onset (days) were as 8 for statistical analysis.
[c]Mean cumulative score calculation included all the pigs in each group.
[d]Standard error of the mean.
[e]FFU, fluorescent focus forming units. Geometric mean peak titers were calculated among pigs that shed virus.
*Fisher's exact test or ** Kruskal-Wallis rank sum test was used for comparisons. Different letters indicate significant differences among treatment groups ($p<0.05$), while shared letters indicate no significant difference.

Discussion

Gnotobiotic pigs offer distinct advantages for investigating enteric virus infections and vaccines and for dissecting immunomodulatory functions of probiotics. Gnotobiotic status prevents confounding factors from preexisting gut microflora and maternal antibodies that are present in conventionally reared animals or in humans. However, gnotobiotic animals also have some disadvantages. The major drawback is that the germ-free status causes underdeveloped intestinal lymphatic constituents and leads to the decreasing number of gut-associated lymphoid tissues [26–28]. Intestinal colonization of germfree animals with commensal microbes significantly promoted the development of mucosal and systemic immune systems [29–31]. Our current study demonstrated that HGM transplantation significantly promoted the activation of Th1 effector cells in both intestinal and systemic lymphoid tissues as evidenced by the increased numbers and significantly increased frequencies of IFN-γ producing CD8+ T cells in ileum, IEL, spleen and blood of the AttHRV vaccinated pigs at PID28. However, HGM did not significantly alter the total numbers of CD3+CD4+ and CD3+CD8+ T cells in any tissues of the AttHRV-vaccinated pigs at PID28, suggesting that exposure to the live AttHRV vaccine alone provided sufficient antigen stimulation for the expansion of the T cell compartment of the neonatal immune system in Gn pigs without HGM.

Our previous studies [5,6] using Gn pigs demonstrated that probiotic *L. acidophilus* regulated T cell and B cell immune responses in a dose-dependent manner. We also found that the probiotic LGG dose-dependently regulated T cell and B cell immune responses in Gn pigs (manuscript in preparation). Due to competition between LGG and other bacterial species for colonizing the gut in HGM transplanted pigs, LGG doses higher than that used for Gn pigs were needed to effectively regulate immune responses in HGM pigs. We found that 14 LGG feedings (up to 10^9 CFU/dose), but not 9 feedings (up to 10^6 CFU/dose), enhanced virus-specific IFN-γ producing T cell responses in AttHRV vaccinated pigs transplanted with HGM; AttHRV+LGG14X pigs also had a trend for higher IgA titers than the AttHRV+LGG9X and AttHRV-only pigs at PID28, which suggests that an even higher dose of LGG may be needed to achieve the desired adjuvant effect in the HGM pigs [5]. In a recent study [32], Zhu et al. fed piglets with the total LGG (ATCC 7469) dose of 7×10^{10} CFU, which was called "low dose" but higher than the highest dose (total 2.2×10^9 CFU) of LGG used in our studies. They found that 7×10^{10} CFU of LGG down regulated ileal IL-17A, enhanced ileal TGF-β1 and IL-10 mRNA but had no effect on IFN-γ, IL-12, and IL-4 mRNA expression in the small intestine [32], an immunoregulatory profile suggesting that the LGG dose was too high for an immunostimulatory profile desired by our purpose of using LGG as an adjuvant [5,6]. Collectively, these studies suggest that all probiotic strains differentially regulate immune responses in each specific narrow dose range. Further studies are needed to identify the appropriate LGG dose and dosing regimen as a vaccine adjuvant to effectively enhance virus-specific antibody responses in the HGM pigs. The interplay between HGM, probiotics and host immune system is complex, yet it reflects the real-world situation of human infants vaccinated with rotavirus vaccines and treated with probiotics. The results from the HGM pigs provide more relevant reference for human clinical practice. However, using the HGM pig model, like human clinical trials, is more difficult than the Gn pig model to reach clear conclusions, and future experiments will be required to include a larger number of subjects in each treatment group to establish the correlations between T cell and B cell responses and protection.

Because Gn pigs derived by hysterectomy (unsuckled) are devoid of maternal antibodies due to the impervious nature of the sow placenta to immunoglobulin, it is expected that Gn pigs are highly prone to opportunistic pathogen infections from transplanted HGM. One early study reported that in two litters of HGM pigs, 17 of 24 died due to the opportunistic pathogen *Klebsiella pneumoniae* present in the HGM from an apparently healthy human donor of 11 years of age [18]. With these safety concerns in mind, the HGM inoculum we used in this study was screened carefully; however, 20.9% of the pigs still became ill within several days after the oral administration of the HGM from the infant donor. Bacterial cultures from the euthanized pigs identified *Klebsiella oxytoca* as the likely cause of the illness. To build safe inoculum pools of HGM from donor stools, a more comprehensive screening procedure is needed. In addition to the screening steps we performed in this study, high-depth and high-throughput sequencing analysis and species-specific PCR for detection of potential pathogenic bacterial species for pigs such as *Klebsiella* spp. should be performed.

AttHRV vaccination with or without HGM transplantation conferred similar levels of protection in Gn pigs against diarrhea, virus shedding, and overall clinical signs upon VirHRV challenge, even though HGM pigs had significantly higher Th1 type effector T cell responses and lower Treg cell responses compared to Gn pigs. Furthermore, high dose LGG feeding increased the fecal and intestinal LGG counts, suggesting that sufficient doses of LGG fed to pigs with preexisting HGM and prior colonization by LGG were able to further enhance the fecal and intestinal counts of LGG. High dose LGG feeding also significantly enhanced the intestinal and circulating virus-specific effector T cell responses, but did not significantly enhance intestinal or serum virus-specific antibody responses in HGM pigs at the time of challenge (PID28) and did not significantly enhance the protective efficacy of the AttHRV vaccine. The magnitude of virus-specific serum and intestinal IgA antibody responses induced by rotavirus vaccines is an important indicator of protective efficacy of the vaccines [5,22]. The results from this study highlighted again the importance of antibody responses. It is worth noting that only the AttHRV+ LGG9X pigs had significant increases in the intestinal IgA antibody response from PID 28 to PCD 7. The AttHRV+ LGG14X pigs had significantly higher intestinal virus-specific IFN-γ producing CD4+ T cell responses than the AttHRV+ LGG9X pigs at PID 28 and PCD 7, indicating that AttHRV+ LGG14X pigs had a skewed Th1 type response in the intestine that suppressed the virus-specific intestinal IgA antibody responses. Nonetheless, there is a disagreement between the increased immunogenicity (as indicated by the increased level of intestinal IFN-γ producing T cells) of the AttHRV vaccine in the HGM over the Gn pigs and the similar levels of protection upon VirHRV challenge. A plausible explanation is that certain strains of bacteria in the HGM facilitated the replication of VirHRV in the gut leading to increased challenge virus load. We noticed that the mean peak virus shed in feces postchallenge in the HGM pigs were 6-fold higher than the Gn pigs. Our study of a porcine epithelial cell line (IPEC-J2 cells) showed that treatment of the cells with *L. acidophilus* prior to rotavirus infection significantly increased the amount of rotavirus antigens and the virus titers [20]. In two other previous studies, Gn pigs inoculated with the VirHRV and fed with *L. acidophilus* plus *L. reuteri* or inoculated with the AttHRV and fed with *L. acidophilus*, shed higher titers of the viruses in feces than the pigs not receiving lactobacilli feeding [33,34]. Several other studies have also shown that gut microbiota enhanced the replication or virus entry of enteric viruses and their pathogenesis [35–37] and that elimination of microbiota delayed rotavirus infection and significantly reduced rotavirus infectivity in mice [37].

In previously reported studies using HGM pigs, HGM from a healthy 3-month old baby [38] or older human donors at 10, 14, 27–28, or 50–70 years of age [11,13,18,38,39] were used to transplant gut microbiota to newborn pigs. Considering the dramatic shifts in composition and diversity of the fecal microbiota that occur with age from infancy to adulthood [40], our HGM transplanted pig model more closely mimics the colonization and evolution of HGM in infants from a very early age and is a more applicable model for studying HRV, which causes gastroenteritis in infants.

In conclusion, both Gn pig and HGM Gn pig models are applicable models for the evaluation of rotavirus vaccines and therapeutics, but each model has its advantages and drawbacks. The Gn pigs have the advantage of being devoid of confounding factors from the gut microbiota, whereas HGM Gn pigs have the advantage of more closely mimicking real-world situations. This current study demonstrated that HGM Gn pig model is an appropriate model for studying HRV infection and vaccines and for evaluation of the immunomodulatory effects of probiotics. To the best of our knowledge, this is the first study to establish the neonatal HGM transplanted Gn pig model of HRV infection and immunity. The findings also have implications in using Gn animal models with HGM for studies of other pathogens and diseases.

Acknowledgments

We thank Pete Jobst, Andrea Pulliam, Mariah Weiss, Kimberly Allen, and Shannon Viers for animal care, Dr. Marlice Vonck and Betsy Midkiff for veterinary service. The AttHRV and VirHRV strains were from Dr. Linda J. Saif, The Ohio State University.

Author Contributions

Conceived and designed the experiments: LY KW. Performed the experiments: KW CT HW XY GL EGR JK TB SCD. Analyzed the data: KW CT HW LY. Wrote the paper: KW CT LY.

References

1. Saif LJ, Ward LA, Yuan L, Rosen BI, To TL (1996) The gnotobiotic piglet as a model for studies of disease pathogenesis and immunity to human rotaviruses. Arch Virol Suppl 12: 153–161.
2. Yuan L, Saif LJ (2002) Induction of mucosal immune responses and protection against enteric viruses: rotavirus infection of gnotobiotic pigs as a model. Vet Immunol Immunopathol 87: 147–160.
3. Yuan L, Saif LJ (2003) Rotavirus-like particle vaccines evaluated in a pig model of human rotavirus diarrhea and in cattle. In: Desselberger U, Gray J, editors. Viral Gastroenteritis. Netherlands: Elsevier Sciences. pp. 357–368.
4. Levast B, Schulz S, Hurk S, Gerdts V (2013) Animal models for neonatal diseases in humans. Vaccine 31: 2489–2499.
5. Liu F, Wen K, Li G, Yang X, Kocher J, et al. (2013) Dual Functions of Lactobacillus acidophilus NCFM at The Intermediate Dose In Protection Against Rotavirus Diarrhea In Gnotobiotic Pigs Vaccinated With A Human Rotavirus Vaccine. J Pediatr Gastroenterol Nutr.
6. Wen K, Li G, Bui T, Liu F, Li Y, et al. (2012) High dose and low dose Lactobacillus acidophilus exerted differential immune modulating effects on T cell immune responses induced by an oral human rotavirus vaccine in gnotobiotic pigs. Vaccine 30: 1198–1207.
7. Yuan L, Wen K, Liu F, G L (2013) Dose Effects of LAB on Modulation of Rotavirus Vaccine Induced Immune Responses. Availabe: http://www.intechopen.com/books/lactic-acid-bacteria-r-d-for-food-health-and-livestock-

purposes/dose-effects-of-lab-on-modulation-of-rotavirus-vaccine-induced-immune-responses. Accessed 2013 January 30.
8. Licciardi PV, Tang ML (2011) Vaccine adjuvant properties of probiotic bacteria. Discov Med 12: 525–533.
9. Isolauri E, Joensuu J, Suomalainen H, Luomala M, Vesikari T (1995) Improved immunogenicity of oral D x RRV reassortant rotavirus vaccine by Lactobacillus casei GG. Vaccine 13: 310–312.
10. Davidson LE, Fiorino AM, Snydman DR, Hibberd PL (2011) Lactobacillus GG as an immune adjuvant for live-attenuated influenza vaccine in healthy adults: a randomized double-blind placebo-controlled trial. Eur J Clin Nutr 65: 501–507.
11. Pang X, Hua X, Yang Q, Ding D, Che C, et al. (2007) Inter-species transplantation of gut microbiota from human to pigs. ISME J 1: 156–162.
12. Hirayama K (1999) Ex-germfree mice harboring intestinal microbiota derived from other animal species as an experimental model for ecology and metabolism of intestinal bacteria. Exp Anim 48: 219–227.
13. Che C, Pang X, Hua X, Zhang B, Shen J, et al. (2009) Effects of human fecal flora on intestinal morphology and mucosal immunity in human flora-associated piglet. Scand J Immunol 69: 223–233.
14. Zhang W, Wen K, Azevedo MS, Gonzalez A, Saif LJ, et al. (2008) Lactic acid bacterial colonization and human rotavirus infection influence distribution and frequencies of monocytes/macrophages and dendritic cells in neonatal gnotobiotic pigs. Vet Immunol Immunopathol 121: 222–231.
15. Yuan L, Ward LA, Rosen BI, To TL, Saif LJ (1996) Systematic and intestinal antibody-secreting cell responses and correlates of protective immunity to human rotavirus in a gnotobiotic pig model of disease. J Virol 70: 3075–3083.
16. Yuan L, Wen K, Azevedo MS, Gonzalez AM, Zhang W, et al. (2008) Virus-specific intestinal IFN-gamma producing T cell responses induced by human rotavirus infection and vaccines are correlated with protection against rotavirus diarrhea in gnotobiotic pigs. Vaccine 26: 3322–3331.
17. Ward LA, Rosen BI, Yuan L, Saif LJ (1996) Pathogenesis of an attenuated and a virulent strain of group A human rotavirus in neonatal gnotobiotic pigs. J Gen Virol 77 (Pt 7): 1431–1441.
18. Wei H, Shen J, Pang X, Ding D, Zhang Y, et al. (2008) Fatal infection in human flora-associated piglets caused by the opportunistic pathogen Klebsiella pneumoniae from an apparently healthy human donor. J Vet Med Sci 70: 715–717.
19. Azevedo MS, Yuan L, Jeong KI, Gonzalez A, Nguyen TV, et al. (2005) Viremia and nasal and rectal shedding of rotavirus in gnotobiotic pigs inoculated with Wa human rotavirus. J Virol 79: 5428–5436.
20. Liu F, Li G, Wen K, Bui T, Cao D, et al. (2010) Porcine small intestinal epithelial cell line (IPEC-J2) of rotavirus infection as a new model for the study of innate immune responses to rotaviruses and probiotics. Viral Immunol 23: 135–149.
21. Ahlroos T, Tynkkynen S (2009) Quantitative strain-specific detection of Lactobacillus rhamnosus GG in human faecal samples by real-time PCR. J Appl Microbiol 106: 506–514.
22. To TL, Ward LA, Yuan L, Saif LJ (1998) Serum and intestinal isotype antibody responses and correlates of protective immunity to human rotavirus in a gnotobiotic pig model of disease. J Gen Virol 79 (Pt 11): 2661–2672.
23. Parreno V, Hodgins DC, de Arriba L, Kang SY, Yuan L, et al. (1999) Serum and intestinal isotype antibody responses to Wa human rotavirus in gnotobiotic pigs are modulated by maternal antibodies. J Gen Virol 80 (Pt 6): 1417–1428.
24. Liu F, Li G, Wen K, Wu S, Zhang Y, et al. (2013) Lactobacillus rhamnosus GG on Rotavirus-Induced Injury of Ileal Epithelium in Gnotobiotic Pigs. J Pediatr Gastroenterol Nutr 57: 750–758.
25. Szajewska H, Wanke M, Patro B (2011) Meta-analysis: the effects of Lactobacillus rhamnosus GG supplementation for the prevention of healthcare-associated diarrhoea in children. Aliment Pharmacol Ther 34: 1079–1087.
26. Pleasants JR, Johnson MH, Wostmann BS (1986) Adequacy of chemically defined, water-soluble diet for germfree BALB/c mice through successive generations and litters. J Nutr 116: 1949–1964.
27. Tlaskalova-Hogenova H, Sterzl J, Stepankova R, Dlabac V, Veticka V, et al. (1983) Development of immunological capacity under germfree and conventional conditions. Ann N Y Acad Sci 409: 96–113.
28. Stepankova R, Sinkora J, Hudcovic T, Kozakova H, Tlaskalova-Hogenova H (1998) Differences in development of lymphocyte subpopulations from gut-associated lymphatic tissue (GALT) of germfree and conventional rats: effect of aging. Folia Microbiol (Praha) 43: 531–534.
29. Atarashi K, Tanoue T, Shima T, Imaoka A, Kuwahara T, et al. (2011) Induction of colonic regulatory T cells by indigenous Clostridium species. Science 331: 337–341.
30. Kunisawa J, Kiyono H (2011) Peaceful mutualism in the gut: revealing key commensal bacteria for the creation and maintenance of immunological homeostasis. Cell Host Microbe 9: 83–84.
31. Gaboriau-Routhiau V, Rakotobe S, Lecuyer E, Mulder I, Lan A, et al. (2009) The key role of segmented filamentous bacteria in the coordinated maturation of gut helper T cell responses. Immunity 31: 677–689.
32. Zhu YH, Li XQ, Zhang W, Zhou D, Liu HY, et al. (2014) Dose-dependent Effects of Lactobacillus rhamnosus on Serum IL-17 Production and Intestinal T Cell Responses in Pigs Challenged with Escherichia coli. Appl Environ Microbiol.
33. Zhang W, Azevedo MS, Wen K, Gonzalez A, Saif LJ, et al. (2008) Probiotic Lactobacillus acidophilus enhances the immunogenicity of an oral rotavirus vaccine in gnotobiotic pigs. Vaccine 26: 3655–3661.
34. Zhang W, Azevedo MS, Gonzalez AM, Saif LJ, Van Nguyen T, et al. (2008) Influence of probiotic Lactobacilli colonization on neonatal B cell responses in a gnotobiotic pig model of human rotavirus infection and disease. Vet Immunol Immunopathol 122: 175–181.
35. Kuss SK, Best GT, Etheredge CA, Pruijssers AJ, Frierson JM, et al. (2011) Intestinal microbiota promote enteric virus replication and systemic pathogenesis. Science 334: 249–252.
36. Kane M, Case LK, Kopaskie K, Kozlova A, MacDearmid C, et al. (2011) Successful transmission of a retrovirus depends on the commensal microbiota. Science 334: 245–249.
37. Uchiyama R, Chassaing B, Zhang B, Gewirtz AT (2014) Antibiotic treatment suppresses rotavirus infection and enhances specific humoral immunity. J Infect Dis (epub ahead of print doi:10.1093/infdis/jiu037)
38. Zhang Q, Widmer G, Tzipori S (2013) A pig model of the human gastrointestinal tract. Gut Microbes 4: 193–200.
39. Shen J, Zhang B, Wei H, Che C, Ding D, et al. (2010) Assessment of the modulating effects of fructo-oligosaccharides on fecal microbiota using human flora-associated piglets. Arch Microbiol 192: 959–968.
40. Avershina E, Storro O, Oien T, Johnsen R, Pope P, et al. (2013) Major faecal microbiota shifts in composition and diversity with age in a geographically restricted cohort of mothers and their children. FEMS Microbiol Ecol.

13

Two Novel EHEC/EAEC Hybrid Strains Isolated from Human Infections

Rita Prager[9], **Christina Lang**[9], **Philipp Aurass, Angelika Fruth, Erhard Tietze, Antje Flieger***

Divison of Enteropathogenic Bacteria and *Legionella*, National Reference Centre for *Salmonella* and other Bacterial Enteric Pathogens, Robert Koch-Institut, Wernigerode, Germany

Abstract

The so far highest number of life-threatening hemolytic uremic syndrome was associated with a food-borne outbreak in 2011 in Germany which was caused by an enterohemorrhagic *Escherichia coli* (EHEC) of the rare serotype O104:H4. Most importantly, the outbreak strain harbored genes characteristic of both EHEC and enteroaggregative *E. coli* (EAEC). Such strains have been described seldom but due to the combination of virulence genes show a high pathogenicity potential. To evaluate the importance of EHEC/EAEC hybrid strains in human disease, we analyzed the EHEC strain collection of the German National Reference Centre for *Salmonella* and other Bacterial Enteric Pathogens (NRC). After exclusion of O104:H4 EHEC/EAEC strains, out of about 2400 EHEC strains sent to NRC between 2008 and 2012, two strains exhibited both EHEC and EAEC marker genes, specifically were *stx2* and *aatA* positive. Like the 2011 outbreak strain, one of the novel EHEC/EAEC harbored the Shiga toxin gene type *stx2a.* The strain was isolated from a patient with bloody diarrhea in 2010, was serotyped as O59:H$^-$, belonged to MLST ST1136, and exhibited genes for type IV aggregative adherence fimbriae (AAF). The second strain was isolated from a patient with diarrhea in 2012, harbored *stx2b*, was typed as Orough:H$^-$, and belonged to MLST ST26. Although the strain conferred the aggregative adherence phenotype, no known AAF genes corresponding to fimbrial types I to V were detected. In summary, EHEC/EAEC hybrid strains are currently rarely isolated from human disease cases in Germany and two novel EHEC/EAEC of rare serovars/MLST sequence types were characterized.

Editor: Michael Hensel, University of Osnabrueck, Germany

Funding: This work was supported by the Robert Koch Institute. The funders had no role in study design, data collection and analysis, decision to publish, or preparation of the manuscript.

Competing Interests: The authors have declared that no competing interests exist.

* E-mail: fliegera@rki.de

[9] These authors contributed equally to this work.

Introduction

Escherichia coli bacteria on the one hand belong to the normal flora of the human intestine but on the other hand may cause disease. Pathogenic *E. coli* variants harbor specific genes encoding virulence determinants [1]. For example, enterohemorrhagic *E. coli* (EHEC) are an intestinal pathovar that cause about 1,000 to 1,500 cases of diarrhea or bloody diarrhea in Germany per year and about 70 cases of the severe pathology hemolytic uremic syndrome (HUS) [2]. For the large outbreak of bloody diarrhea/HUS in Germany in 2011, 53 deaths, 833 HUS cases, and about 3,000 cases of gastroenteritis were recorded [3]. Although Shiga toxin-positive strains inducing HUS in many cases belong to the serovar O157:H7/H$^-$ and others such as O26:H11/H$^-$, O103:H2/H$^-$, O111:H8/H$^-$, O145:H28/H$^-$, the outbreak was caused by an *E. coli* strain of the rare serotype O104:H4 characterized by the presence of EHEC pathovar markers as well as genes of another pathovar, enteroaggreagative *E. coli* (EAEC). So called mixed *E. coli* pathovars or hybrid strains have been seldom described and show a high virulence potential [4–16].

Important virulence determinants of classical EHEC are the Shiga toxin Stx, a type III-protein secretion system coded on a pathogenicity island, the locus of enterocyte effacement (LEE), and the EHEC toxin Ehx encoded by the gene *ehxA*. Stx is responsible for severe pathologies as observed for HUS, LEE induces intimate attachment of the bacteria to the intestinal epithelia, and Ehx is a pore-forming toxin [1,17]. An Stx gene, especially for the more toxic type Stx2, but not LEE- or Ehx-related genes were found in the 2011 EHEC/EAEC outbreak strain [4,5,7,9,12,13].

Classical EAEC do not possess *stx* genes but encode aggregative adherence fimbriae (AAF) on the virulence plasmid pAA which cause the characteristic stacked brick-like adherence of the bacteria to host cells [18,19]. So far, five different types of such fimbriae are known and the 2011 outbreak strain coded type I aggregative fimbriae [4,6,7,20–23]. The virulence plasmid of EAEC not only encodes the aggregative adherence fimbrial subunit genes but in many cases also an ABC transporter complex Aat involved in the export of the antiaggregation protein dispersin (Aap), and the AraC-like regulator AggR which drives their expression but also expression of chromosomally localized genes [24–27]. EAEC have first been found associated with persistent diarrhea mainly in children in developing countries but are increasingly recognized as a cause of diarrhea in industrial countries [25,28].

Analysis of the 2011 outbreak strain uncovered that its core genome is related to an earlier described classical EAEC of serovar O104:H4 designated 55989 and suggested additional acquisition of some EHEC features [5,9,12,13,16,29,30]. Further, genome sequencing determined the relation of the outbreak strain to another O104:H4 EHEC/EAEC isolated from HUS cases in 2001. It was hypothesized that the two EHEC/EAEC strains and the EAEC strain of the same serovar share a common ancestor [9]. Differences between the three strains which all belong to the MLST sequence type ST678 were further noted in the antibiotic resistance profile, the plasmid profile, and the macrorestriction/pulsed-field electrophoresis (PFGE) pattern [4,5,7,9].

To evaluate the significance of EHEC/EAEC hybrid strains in human disease, we here analyzed strains from the EHEC strain collection of the German National Reference Centre for *Salmonella* and other Bacterial Enteric Pathogens (NRC). In the repository of EHEC strains collected between 2008 and 2012, two strains exhibiting both EHEC and EAEC marker genes were found. These were further analyzed in our study and compared to the 2011 outbreak strain, classical EAEC and EHEC.

Materials and Methods

Strains

The strains used in the study are listed in Table 1. Strains were grown on nutrient agar (Oxoid GmbH, Germany) or in tryptic soy broth (TSB) (BD-BBL, Germany), if not stated otherwise. Testing of hemolytic activity was performed on enterohemolysin agar (Sifin GmbH, Germany).

Triplex PCR for Detection of *stx1*, *stx2*, and *aatA*

For simultaneous detection of *stx1/2* (EHEC marker) and *aatA* (EAEC marker), colony PCR was performed. *stx1/2* primer sequences have been used from Cebula et al. (LP30: CAG TTA ATG TGG TGG CGA AGG, LP31: CAC CAG ACA ATG TAA CCG CTG and LP43 ATC CTA TTC CCG GGA GTT TAC G, LP44: GCG TCA TCG TAT ACA CAG GAG C) [31]. *aatA* primers designed in this study are directed to conserved regions within the gene (aatA_fw: TCG GCT TAT GAA GCA AAA ATG; aatA_rv: GAT AAC GTC GTC TTG TCC ATT C). Each reaction contained 2.5 µl of 10×PCR buffer (NEB), 1 unit of Taq DNA polymerase (NEB), 5 pmol of each forward and reverse primers, 200 µM of each deoxynucleoside triphosphate (Bioline) and distilled water up to a total reaction volume of 15 µl. A small amount of a single bacterial colony resuspended in 10 µl distilled water and heated for 10 min at 95°C was used as DNA template. DNA amplification was carried out in a PCR thermal cycler. The following PCR conditions were used: 94°C for 5 min, followed by 30 cycles of 30 seconds at 94°C, 1 min at 55°C, and 1 min at 72°C with a final extension of 5 min at 72°C. Separate PCR analysis for *stx1/2* or *aatA* was performed at comparable conditions but as a duplex or single assay, respectively.

PCR Analysis for Differentiation of AAF Fimbriae

The AAF variants AAF/I, AAF/II, AAF/III and AAF/IV (or Hda) were determined by PCR amplification of the corresponding subunits and usher genes (*aggA, aggC, aafA, aafC, agg3A, agg3C, hdaA, hdaC*) as described previously [20,21,23,32–34]. A PCR assay was developed for detection of the AAF/VA subunit gene. The primers (aaf5_fw: TAT CAT TGC GAG TCT GGT ATT CA and aaf5_rv: TAA TTT AAG CTG AAG AAT CCA GTC AA) were designed from homologous regions of the annotated AAF/VA gene region from GenBank-deposited pAA plasmid or aaf5A sequences from *E. coli* O111:H21 (accession AB513347, [6]), *E. coli* O127:H21 (accession AB571097), and *E. coli* O6:H$^-$ (accession AB571098). PCR reaction conditions were as described above for the *aatA* PCR assay, except that an annealing temperature of 54°C was used.

E. coli Serotyping

Serotyping was performed using antisera against *E. coli* O-antigens 1–181 and *E. coli* H-antigens 1–56 by use of a microtitre agglutination method as described elsewhere [35].

Determination of *fliC* Genotype

Non-motile (NM or H$^-$) strains were analyzed for their flagellar (*fliC*) genotypes by restriction fragment length polymorphism (RFLP) of PCR-products (RFLP-PCR) as described by Prager et al. [35].

Determination of *stx2* Subtype and Occupation Analysis of Typical Stx-associated Bacteriophage Insertion Sites

The *stx2* subtypes were determined according to Scheutz et al. [36] and occupation of the *wrbA* and *argW* sites for the Stx-associated bacteriophage were tested as described in Shaikh and Tarr [37] and Shringi et al. [38].

Analysis of Large Plasmids

The determination of plasmid profiles was carried out according to Prager et al. [39].

Southern Blotting for Identification of pAA Plasmid

Experiments were performed as outlined in Prager et al. using an *aatA* probe [40].

Analysis of Phylogenetic Type

Phylo-groups A, B1, B2 and D were determined by the multiplex PCR based on the amplification of the genes *chuA*, *yjaA* and the DNA fragment TspE4.C2 according to Clermont et al. [41].

Analysis of Antibiotic Resistance Profile

Antimicrobial susceptibility of strains was tested against 16 substances by a broth micro dilution method determining the minimum inhibitory concentration according to the guidelines of the European Committee on Antimicrobial Susceptibility Testing (EUCAST) and breakpoints were applied as recommended (www.eucast.com). Antibiotics tested were ampicillin, chloramphenicol, cefoxitin, cefotiam, gentamicin, kanamycin, mezlocillin, mezlocillin/sulbactam, oxytetracyclin, sulfamethoxazol, streptomycin, trimethoprim/sulfamethoxazol, ceftazidim, cefotaxim, ciprofloxacin, and nalidixic acid. *Escherichia coli* ATCC 25922 served as quality control strain.

Adherence to Hep-2 Cells

A Hep-2 cell adherence assay was performed as previously described [42,43] with modifications. Briefly, bacteria were grown to exponential growth phase in TSB (Difco), then inoculated 1:100 in 5 ml TSB containing 1% D-mannose and incubated for 20 h statically at 37°C. Equal growth of the cultures was confirmed by reading OD600. Hep-2 cells, grown to 70 to 90% optical confluence in 24 well plates (in DMEM/10% FCS, GE Healthcare), were washed with PBS and the medium was replaced with DMEM containing 1% D-mannose. Subsequently, 40 ul of the bacterial cultures were added per well. After 3 h of incubation, cells were washed three times with PBS, followed by fixation in ice-cold 70% ethanol on ice for 15 min. Next, samples were stained with Giemsa staining solution (1/20 diluted 0.4% stock solution, diluted in PBS) for 20 min at room temperature. Samples were then rinsed with water, air dried, and mounted for microscopy at 600-fold magnification on a Nikon Eclipse inverted microscope.

Table 1. Characteristics of EHEC/EAEC, EAEC, and EHEC strains analyzed in the study.

Pathovar/notes	Isolate number	Date/year of isolation	Symptoms	Serovar	Phylo group	MLST ST	*aatA*	AAF type	*stx1*	*stx2*	*eaeA*	*ehxA*	Plasmids [MDa]	Antibiotic resistance
Novel EHEC/EAEC, this study	**10-06235**	**12.11.2010**	**Bd**	**O59:H$^-$ (*fliC*$_{H19}$)**	**B1**	**1136**	**+**	***hdaA/C* (type IV)**	**–**	**+**	**–**	**–**	**50, 60*, 70**	**SMZ, STR, SXT**
Novel EHEC/EAEC, this study	**12-05829**	**5.12.2012**	**diarrhea**	**Orough:H$^-$ (*fliC*$_{H8}$)**	**B1**	**26**	**+**	**unknown**	**–**	**+**	**–**	**–**	**40, 75*, 80**	**susceptible**
EHEC/EAEC HUSEC 041 Germany [48]	01-09591	2001	Bd, HUS	O104:H4	B1	678	+	*agg3A/C* (type III)	–	+	–	–	3,4; 5,5; 46*; 60;	AMP, MEZ, NAL, SMZ, STR
EHEC/EAEC outbreak 2011 Germany [7]	11-02027	19.5.2011	Bd, Hc, HUS	O104:H4	B1	678	+	*aggA/C* (type I)	–	+	–	–	55*, 60	AMP, CAZ, CTM, CTX, MEZ, MSU, NAL, OTE, SMZ, STR, SXT
EAEC, this study	05-08045	3.11.2005	diarrhea	O106:H$^-$ (*fliC*$_{H18}$)	D1	414	+	*aafA/C* (type I)	–	–	–	–	80	NAL
EAEC, this study	06-06057	31.8.2006	unknown	O92:H33	A1	34	+	*aggA/C* (type I)	–	–	–	–	60	AMP, MEZ, NAL, OTE, SMZ, SXT
EAEC, this study	10-03550	21.7.2010	unknown	O111:H21	B1	40	+	*aaf5A/agg3C* (type V)	–	–	–	–	60	AMP, CTM
EAEC, this study	10-06623	28.10.2010	unknown	O173:H6	B1	278	+	*hdaA/C* (type IV)	–	–	–	–	98	susceptible
EAEC, this study	11-08343	28.10.2011	Bd	O59:H$^-$ (*fliC*$_{H19}$)	B1	1136	+	*hdaA/C* (type IV)	–	–	–	–	55, 60*	susceptible
EHEC Reference strain EDL933 [62,63]	CDC EDL933	1982	Raw Hamburger meat	O157: H7	B1	11	–	n.a.	+	+	+	+	61	n.d.

MLST sequence types were assigned or cited according to the MLST database at the University College Cork, Ireland [46]. Abbreviations: Bd = bloody diarrhea, Hc = hemorrhagic colitis, n.d. = not determined, n.a. = not applicable, AMP = ampicillin, CTM = Cefotiam, MEZ = mezlocillin, MSU = mezlocillin/sulbactam, OTE = oxytetracyclin, SMZ = sulfamethoxazol, STR = streptomycin, SXT = trimethoprim/sulfamethoxazol, CAZ = ceftazidim, CTX = cefotaxim, and NAL = nalidixic acid.
*-pAA plasmid.

Cytotoxicity Assay

Toxicity towards Vero cells was determined as described previously [44] with modifications. Briefly, strains were grown to exponential phase in TSB (Difco), then diluted 1:100 in 5 ml TSB, and incubated for 20 h at 37°C with agitation (180 rpm). Next, 100 ul of 8-fold to 512-fold DMEM (GE Healthcare) diluted cell free culture supernatants of the TSB-grown strains were added to washed confluent Vero cell monolayers in 100 ul DMEM/10% FCS in 96 well plates in triplicates. For each experiment fresh culture supernatants were produced and equal growth of the bacterial cultures was confirmed by OD600 readings. After 48 h of incubation at 37°C, supernatants were analyzed for LDH release by means of the CytoTox96 Non-Radioactive Cytotoxicity Assay (Promega) according to the manufacturer's protocol. All values shown are corrected by the background reading of the diluted culture supernatants. In all assays, 256-fold diluted *E. coli* culture supernatants were determined as best discriminative and are therefore shown.

Macrorestriction Analysis/Pulsed-field Gel Electrophoresis

The macrorestriction analysis by pulsed-field gel electrophoresis (PFGE) using the restriction enzyme XbaI was carried out as specified by Prager et al [45].

Multi Locus Sequence Typing

The multiple locus sequence typing (MLST) was performed as described in Prager et al [45]. The MLST alleles and sequence types (ST) were assigned in concordance with the *E. coli* MLST database at http://mlst.ucc.ie/mlst/mlst/dbs/Ecoli/ [46].

Results

Identification of Two EHEC Strains with Additional EAEC Marker Genes from Human Infections

After the large outbreak caused by EHEC/EAEC O104:H4 in 2011, we analyzed whether additional EHEC/EAEC were among the strains deposited in the EHEC collection of the German National Reference Centre for *Salmonella* and other Bacterial Enteric Pathogens (NRC). Between 2008 and 2012 4059 EHEC samples from mainly human origin were analyzed at NRC. After exclusion of O104:H4 EHEC/EAEC, 2435 strains were investigated for the presence of *stx1, stx2, eaeA*, and *ehxA* genes. 268 *eaeA*- and *ehxA*-negative EHEC strains of O-serotypes commonly associated with EAEC, rare EHEC O-serotypes, and untypable EHEC strains were chosen for further analysis of EAEC marker genes. As a first step in our study, analysis of the diagnostic EAEC marker gene *aatA* was employed [47]. We detected two strains, one from 2010 (strain 10-06235) and another from 2012 (strain 12-05829), showing a positive PCR amplification for *stx2* and *aatA* and therefore represent novel EHEC/EAEC hybrids (Fig. 1A). To facilitate future analysis of EHEC/EAEC hybrid strains, we designed a primer pair for detection of *aatA* which can be combined with the earlier published primers for the *stx1/2* duplex PCR in a novel triplex PCR approach [31]. We tested known EHEC/EAEC and a variety of classical EAEC for correct determination of *aatA* presence (Tab. 1). As shown in Fig. 1B, all of the tested EAEC or EHEC/EAEC strains yielded an *aatA* amplificate (Fig. 1B). Further presence of *stx1* and/or *stx2* was correctly detected in the here investigated EHEC or EHEC/EAEC strains (Fig. 1B). In summary, our data show that EHEC/EAEC strains are infrequently associated with human disease in Germany. Further, we found two novel potential EHEC/EAEC strains and we developed a triplex PCR to facilitate future detection of EHEC/EAEC.

Strain 10-06235 Belongs to the Rare Serovar O59:H$^-$ and to Rare ST1136, and Represents a Novel EHEC/EAEC with Type IV Aggregative Fimbriae

To characterize the novel EHEC/EAEC candidates, we first analyzed the strain from 2010 (strain 10-06235) which was isolated from a patient with bloody diarrhea. It belonged to the serovar O59:H$^-$ and to ST1136 [46]. In the *E. coli* MLST database at http://mlst.ucc.ie/mlst/mlst/dbs/Ecoli/only one strain of unknown serotype isolated from a patient with urinary tract infection in Rio de Janeiro/Brasil in 2006 (strain HMMC322, source_lab Beatriz M. Moreiro) has been assigned to this sequence type. Among the intestinal pathogenic *E. coli* strains within the strain collection of NRC, only one other strain of serovar O59:H$^-$ (strain 11-08343) was found between 1993 and 2012 demonstrating the rare occurrence of this serovar in human infections in Germany. This strain, isolated from a patient with bloody diarrhea in 2011, was a classical EAEC strain and did not possess an *stx* gene (Fig. 1B). Both O59:H$^-$ strains showed a flagellar *fliC* genotype $fliC_{H19}$ (data not shown) and the presence of type IV aggregative AAF fimbriae as determined by amplification of the *hdaA* and *hdaC* genes (Fig. 2A and data not shown). In contrast, the *aggA*, *aggC* or *agg3A* and *agg3C* genes, representing the genes for type I or type III AAF found in the 2011 O104:H4 outbreak strain or in HUSEC041, another EHEC/EAEC of serovar O104:H4 isolated from a HUS patient in 2001, respectively, were not detected (Fig. 2A) [48]. The genes corresponding to type II or type V AAF were not amplified in the O59:H$^-$ strains (data not shown and Fig. 2B). As expected from the detection of AAF genes, the O59:H$^-$ as well as the O104:H4 strains showed the characteristic aggregative adherence to Hep-2 cells (Fig. 2C). We therefore conclude that the O59:H$^-$ strain from 2010 indeed represents a novel EHEC/EAEC belonging to a rare serovar and ST.

The Novel O59:H$^-$ EHEC/EAEC Strain Possesses a Shiga Toxin Gene of the Subtype *stx2a* and Further Genes Characteristic for EHEC and EAEC

Next, we analyzed the Shiga toxin gene type associated with the novel EHEC/EAEC and found that the O59:H$^-$ strain exhibited the subtype *stx2a* [36]. PCR analysis revealed occupation of the *argW* but not the *wrbA* site suggesting integration of the Stx-associated bacteriophage into the *argW* site (data not shown) [38]. The *stx2AB* gene sequence of the O59:H$^-$ strain (GenBank accession: KJ158456) differed only by two nucleotides at position 129 (A/G) and 867 (T/C) in *stx2A* from the sequence of the 2011 O104:H4 outbreak strain (GenBank accession: CP003289). The StxA and StxB protein sequences of both strains were identical. We compared the toxicity of Stx released by the novel EHEC/EAEC to that of the 2011 O104:H4 outbreak strain and the classical EHEC EDL933. Although the toxicity of the new EHEC/EAEC strains towards Vero cells was lower than that of the prototypic EHEC O157:H7 strain EDL933, it was in each of the novel EHEC/EAEC strains significantly higher than the toxicity of Stx-negative control strains; indicating that the hybrid EHEC/EAEC strains produced biologically active Stx2 (Fig. 3). We further analyzed additional marker genes of classical EHEC and EAEC by means of PCR [4]. The following genes frequently associated with EHEC were detected for both of the O59:H$^-$ strains: *iha* (gene for IrgA adhesion homolog), $lpfA_{O26}$ (gene for structural subunit of long polar fimbriae (LPF) of EHEC O26), $lpfA_{O113}$ (gene for structural subunit of LPF of EHEC O113), and *irp2* (gene for a component of iron uptake system on high pathogenicity island) (Tab. 2). In addition to the already mentioned AAF genes *hdaA* and *hdaC* (Fig. 2A), the presence of

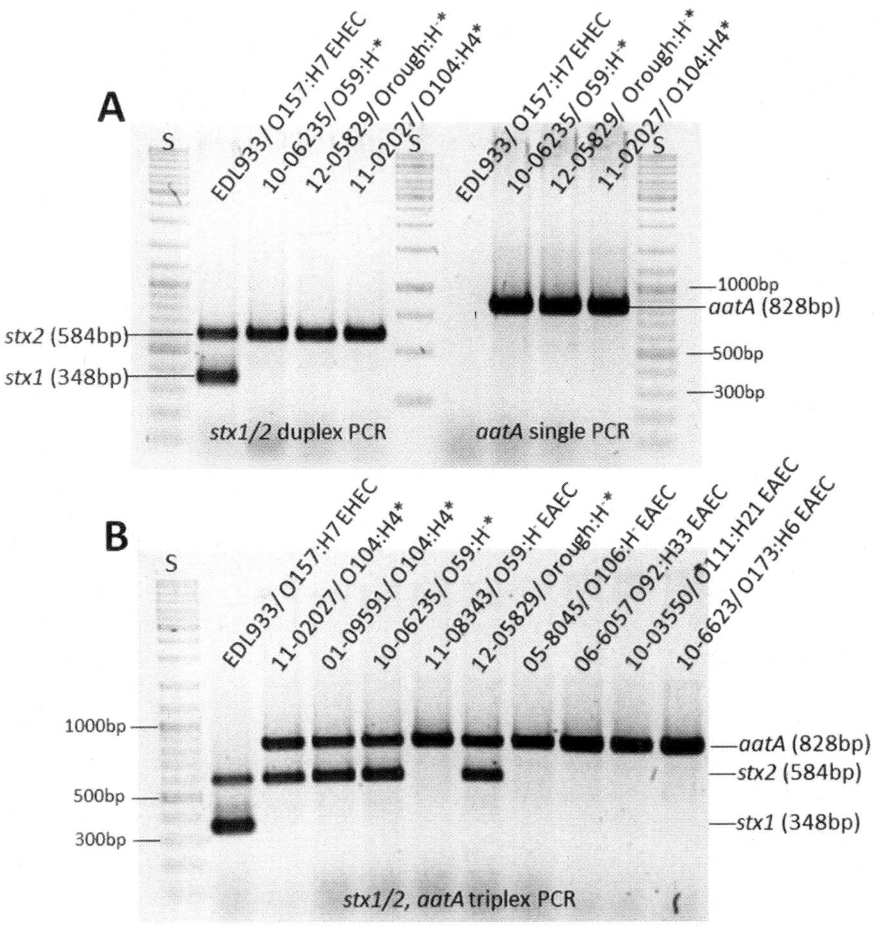

Figure 1. Identification of two novel EHEC/EAEC strains. (**A**) Duplex *stx1/2* PCR analysis (left side of panel) and single *aatA* PCR analysis (right side of panel) of EHEC EDL933, known EHEC/EAEC 11-02027 (O104:H4 outbreak 2011), and the two novel EHEC/EAEC: 10-06235 (O59:H$^-$) and 12-05829 (Orough:H$^-$). (**B**) Novel Triplex PCR analysis for simultaneous detection of *stx1/2* and *aatA* in different EHEC, EHEC/EAEC, and EAEC strains. S = bp standard; *EHEC/EAEC.

the following EAEC markers was determined in both O59:H$^-$ strains: *aggR* (transcriptional regulator gene), *aap* (dispersin gene), *set1a* (*Shigella* enterotoxin subunit A gene), *set1b* (*Shigella* enterotoxin subunit B gene), *pic* (coding for Pic, a protein involved in intestinal colonization), *sigA* (gene for the SPATE protein, i.e. the cytotoxic serin protease autotransporter of Enterobacteriaceae, [49]) and *iucA* (gene for the siderophore aerobactin). *astA*, the gene for EAEC heat stable enterotoxin 1, EAEST1, was not detected in these strains (Tab. 2).

The Novel O59:H$^-$ EHEC/EAEC Strain Possesses Three Large Plasmids and Resistance towards Three Antibiotic Classes

The novel O59:H$^-$ EHEC/EAEC strain was analyzed for the presence of plasmids and three large plasmids of ~50, ~60, ~70 MDa were detected (Fig. 4A). The classical O59:H$^-$ EAEC strain possessed two large plasmids of ~50 and ~60 MDa (Fig. 4A) and the 2011 O104:H4 outbreak strain two large plasmids of ~55 and ~60 MDa. Southern blot analysis using an *aatA* probe identified in both O59:H$^-$ strains the ~60 MDa plasmid (i.e. the second largest plasmid in the EHEC/EAEC strains and the larger plasmid in the EAEC strain) as the pAA plasmid (Fig. 4B). Having in mind the unusual multidrug resistance of the O104:H4 outbreak strain from 2011 towards a variety of antibiotics, including sulfonamides, streptomycin, trimethoprim/sulfonamide, ampicillin, 3rd generation cephalosporines, and others [4,5,7], we also analyzed the O59:H$^-$ strains for their resistance phenotype. In the case of the novel O59:H$^-$ EHEC/EAEC, we found resistance towards sulfonamides, streptomycin, and trimethoprim/sulfonamide. The O59:H$^-$ EAEC was susceptible to all antibiotics investigated. Clearly, the 2011 outbreak strain showed resistance towards more (at least seven) substance classes than the O59:H$^-$ strains which were resistant towards three substance classes or completely susceptible (Tab. 1).

PFGE Analysis Shows that the O59:H$^-$ EHEC/EAEC Isolate is not Closely Related to the O59:H$^-$ EAEC Isolate

PFGE analysis was used to determine the degree of genetic relatedness between the two O59:H$^-$ strains. As already suggested by the presence or absence of *stx2*, the different plasmid profiles, and antibiotic resistance phenotypes, the EHEC/EAEC and the EAEC were not closely related. PFGE analysis showed differing restriction patterns for both strains with about 71% similarity and therefore corroborated our earlier findings (Fig. 5).

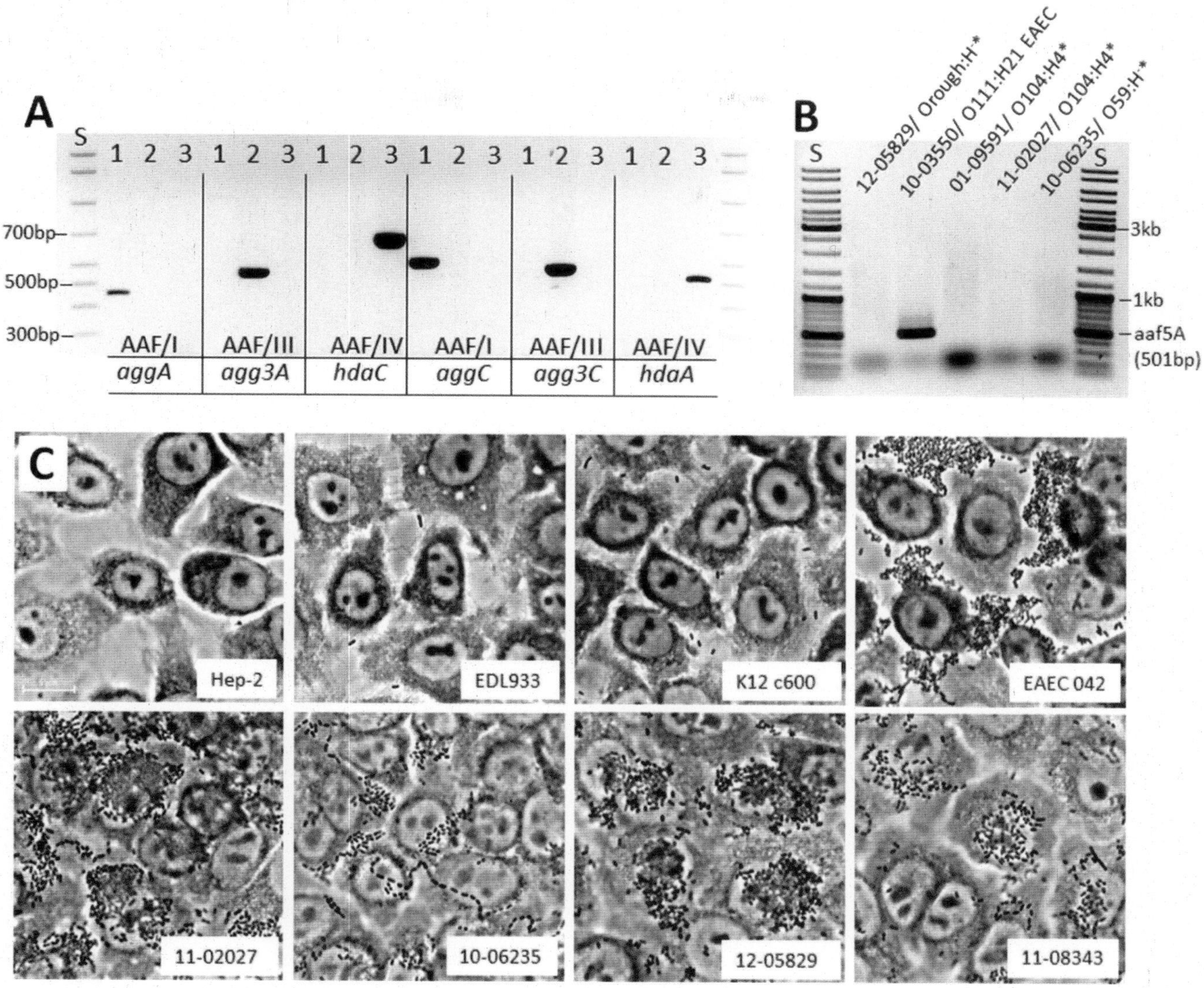

Figure 2. The novel O59:H$^-$ EHEC/EAEC codes for AAF/IV fimbriae and both novel EHEC/EAEC show aggregative adherence. (A) PCR-based determination of AAF type I, III, and IV genes of the EHEC/EAEC O59:H$^-$ strain (3) compared to two known EHEC/EAEC O104:H4 (1 - outbreak 2011 and 2 - HUSEC 041) strains. **(B)** PCR-based determination of AAF/V-coding gene *aaf5A* of different EHEC/EAEC strains and an O111:H21 EAEC strain as positive control. **(C)** Aggregative adherence of the two novel EHEC/EAEC strains to Hep-2 cells. The controls EHEC EDL933 (O157:H7) and *E. coli* K12c600 without aggregative adherence and the aggregative adherence reference strains EAEC 042 (O44:H18), EHEC/EAEC 11-02027 (O104:H4 outbreak 2011) were analyzed in addition to the EHEC/EAEC 10-06235 (O59:H$^-$), EHEC/EAEC 12-05829 (Orough:H$^-$), and the EAEC 11-08343 (O59:H$^-$) strains. Images were taken at 600-fold magnification. S = bp standard; *EHEC/EAEC.

Strain 12-05829 was Typed as Orough:H$^-$, Belongs to ST26, and Shows an Aggregative Phenotype

We next analyzed the strain from 2012 (strain 12-05829) which comprised the *stx2* and *aatA* genes (Fig. 1A). The strain was isolated from a patient with diarrhea. It could not be attributed to any known serovar due to its rough character and lacking motility. The strain showed a flagellar *fliC* genotype $fliC_{H8}$ (data not shown). ST26 was assigned [46] and according to the MLST database, only two *E. coli* strains of the serovar O40:H8, one from a human without disease symptoms (Wunsiedel/Germany, strain 6840/96, source_lab H. Karch) and another from a patient with diarrhea (Wuerzburg/Germany, strain 3199/98, source_lab H. Karch), have been found associated with this sequence type and no clonal complex has been defined yet. Within the strain collection of NRC, 11 other EHEC strains of the serovar O40:H8 have been found. All were negative for *aatA* as analyzed by PCR (data not shown). For the novel *aatA*-positive Orough:H$^-$ strain from 2012 not any of the known type I–V AAF-encoding genes was detected but aggregative adherence to Hep-2 cells was found (data not shown and Fig. 2B and C). Therefore, we conclude that this novel EHEC/EAEC isolate likely possesses so far unclassified AAF [25], [34]. The strain harbored an *stx2* gene of type *stx2b*, showed toxicity towards Vero cells (Fig. 3), and three large plasmids of ~40, ~75 and ~80 MDa (Fig. 4A and data not shown). Southern Blot analysis of its plasmid profile indicated that the ~75 MDa DNA represents the pAA plasmid (Fig. 4B). Strain 12-05829 was susceptible to all of the antibiotics used in the study (Tab. 1).

We analyzed strain 12-05829 for additional marker genes of classical EHEC and EAEC [4]. The following genes associated with EHEC were detected: $lpfA_{O26}$ (gene for structural subunit of long polar fimbriae (LPF) of EHEC O26), $lpfA_{O113}$ (gene for structural subunit of LPF of EHEC O113), *terA* (gene of tellurite

Table 2. Characteristics of the novel EHEC/EAEC strains analyzed in the study compared to the O59:H$^-$ EAEC and the O104:H4 2011 outbreak strain.

				genes frequently associated with EHEC						genes frequently associated with EAEC								
Pathovar/notes	**Isolate number**	**Serovar**	**AAF type**	***stx***	***iha***	***lpfA$_{O26}$***	***lpfA$_{O113}$***	***irp2***	***terA***	***aatA***	***aap***	***set1a***	***set1b***	***pic***	***sigA***	***iucA***	***astA***	***aggR***
Novel EHEC/EAEC, this study	**10-06235**	**O59:H$^-$ (*fliC$_{H19}$*)**	*hdaA/C* (type IV)	2a	+	+	+	+	−	+	+	+	+	+	+	+	−	+
EAEC, this study	11-08343	O59:H$^-$ (*fliC$_{H19}$*)	*hdaA/C* (type IV)	−	+	+	+	+	−	+	+	+	+	+	+	+	−	+
Novel EHEC/EAEC, this study	**12-05829**	**Orough:H$^-$ (*fliC$_{H8}$*)**	unknown	2b	−	+	+	+	+	+	−	−	−	−	−	−	+	−
EHEC/EAEC outbreak 2011 Germany [7]	11-02027	O104:H4	*aggA/C* (type I)	2a	+	+	+	+	+	+	+	+	+	+	+	+	−	+

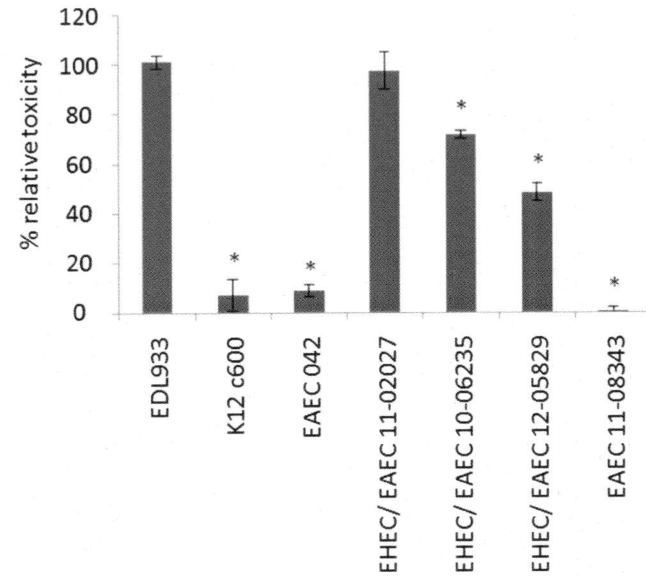

Figure 3. Toxicity of the two novel EHEC/EAEC strains towards Vero cells. As a positive control EHEC EDL933 and as negative controls *E. coli* K12c600 and EAEC 042 were incubated with Vero cells. Further EHEC/EAEC 11-02027 (O104:H4 outbreak 2011), EHEC/EAEC 10-06235 (O59:H$^-$), EHEC/EAEC 12-05829 (Orough:H$^-$), and EAEC 11-08343 (O59:H$^-$) were analyzed. Toxicity of EHEC EDL933 served as a quantitative reference and was set to 100%. Bars represent means and standard deviations of triplicate samples and 256-fold diluted culture preparations. Asterisks indicate significantly lower cytotoxicity compared to the EDL933 reference strain, however all EHEC/EAEC strains were significantly more cytotoxic then the *E. coli* K12 control, the EAEC 042, as well as EAEC 11-08343 (O59:H$^-$) strains (two tailed student's t-test type 1, $p<0.01$; $p<0.03$ for EHEC/EAEC 12-05829 compared to *E. coli* K12).

resistance gene cluster), and *irp2* (gene of component of iron uptake system on high pathogenicity island) (Tab. 2). Further, the presence of *astA* (gene for EAEC heat stable enterotoxin 1 EAEST1), an EAEC marker, was determined. The EAEC markers *aggR* (transcriptional regulator gene) and *aap* (dispersin gene) as well as some others were not detected (Tab. 2).

Discussion and Conclusion

We here identified and characterized two novel EHEC/EAEC hybrid strains which were isolated from humans in Germany in

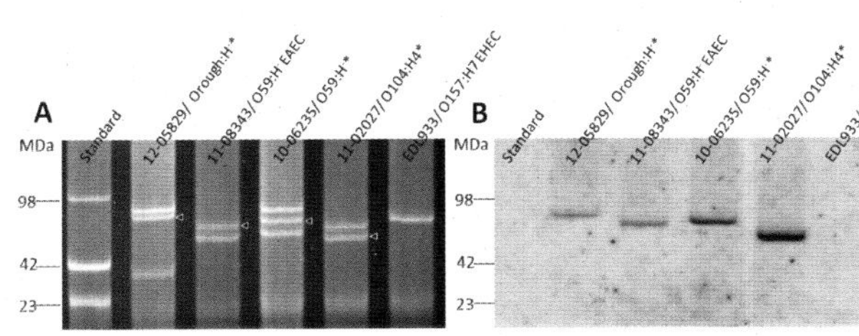

Figure 4. Plasmid profile of the two novel EHEC/EAEC strains and identification of the pAA plasmid. (**A**) EHEC/EAEC 12-05829 (Orough:H$^-$), EAEC 11-08343 (O59:H$^-$), EHEC/EAEC 10-06235 (O59:H$^-$), EHEC/EAEC 11-02027 (O104:H4 outbreak 2011), and EHEC EDL933 (O157:H7) were analyzed for their plasmid profile. *E. coli* reference strain 39R861 plasmids served as molecular mass standard. (**B**) Southern hybridization with plasmid DNA of the same strains as mentioned in (A) was performed using a digoxigenin-labelled *aatA* gene probe. *EHEC/ EAEC; ?pAA plasmid.

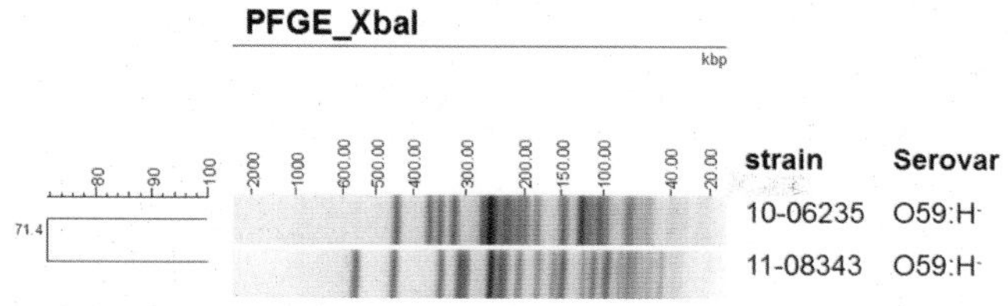

Figure 5. Pulsed-field gel analysis after XbaI macrorestriction shows that the EHEC/EAEC O59:H$^-$ (upper lane) and EAEC O59:H$^-$ (lower lane) are not closely related.

2010 and in 2012. Since the large outbreak due to EHEC/EAEC O104:H4 2011 in Germany, attention was drawn on these mixed *E. coli* pathovars and so far such strains have been seldom described. Nevertheless, at least eight other O104:H4 EHEC/EAEC strains have been documented, for example a strain designated HUSEC041 causing HUS in Germany in 2001, two French strains from 2004 and 2009, and five additional strains causing HUS in France in 2011. Those strains clearly differ from the 2011 outbreak strain, for example in their PFGE macrorestriction profile, AAF type, antibiotic resistance, plasmid profile, virulence gene sets, or SNPs on the genomic level [9,16,50–52]. The relatively frequent occurrence of EHEC/EAEC among the serovar O104:H4 strains suggests that either certain EAEC serovars/strains might be more susceptible to acquire EHEC determinants, such as an *stx*-harboring phage, or that there are certain EHEC/EAEC ancestors which successfully adapted to survive specific selection conditions.

Although it has been shown that the *stx1* phage is easily transferred to *E. coli* K-12 in the intestinal tract of mice [53], just a few other *E. coli* serovars are reported to reveal strains with EHEC/EAEC features. An O111:H2 strain causing HUS in France in 1996 exhibits *stx2*, AAF and was *eaeA* and *ehxA* negative and the first described EHEC/EAEC [10,11,54]. Further, an O86:H$^-$ strain with *stx2* and AAF marker genes but no *eaeA* was isolated from a pediatric patient with HUS and bloody diarrhea in Japan in 1999 [55]. An O111:H21 strain associated with a household outbreak in Northern Ireland in 2011 including a HUS case in a child was characterized on the genomic level. It was *eaeA* negative and it belongs to ST40, a sequence type comprising a diversity of *E. coli* pathovars, such as STEC, EAEC, EPEC, and non-pathogenic *E. coli* [6]. The strain possesses *stx2c* and a recently described type of AAF, designated type V AAF [6] (see also below). Of note, hybrid *E. coli* pathovars showing EHEC properties combined with features of yet other pathotypes were recently reported [56,57].

In our study, we found two novel EHEC/EAEC strains associated with human disease; one of those belonged to the rare serovar O59:H$^-$ (flagellar genotype *fliCH19*) and the rare MLST ST1136. The other strain was a non-motile strain with rough LPS belonging to the rare MLST ST26. Since two other strains of ST26 were found in the MLST database which were serotyped as O40:H8, we tested the Orough:H$^-$ strain for genetic elements coding for the surface antigens related to those in the O40:H8 strains. Accordingly, the *fliC* genotype was *fliCH8*. Screening the literature on *E. coli* of O-serotype O59 or O40 revealed only a few publications addressing the characterization of the antigenic polysaccharides or using the strain as a reference strain to evaluate survival of *E. coli* [58–61]. Our finding therefore confirms that EHEC/EAEC in the so far known cases belong to *E. coli* serovars rarely described to cause humans disease.

EHEC/EAEC strains show a high virulence potential. This is illustrated by the O104:H4 outbreak in 2011 where an extraordinarily high number, more than 20%, of the registered patients, developed the severe pathology HUS [7,3]. In the case of classical EHEC, the proteins coded by the LEE locus and most importantly the adhesin EaeA promote intimate attachment to the host cells and therefore facilitate Stx application and action [1]. The so far described EHEC/EAEC strains do not possess *eaeA* and it is argued that attachment driven by AAF may be at least as effective as that mediated by EaeA. The ability of EHEC/EAEC strains to form adhesive aggregates may even increase Stx quantities at a specific site and therefore the toxic capacity of the bacteria [8,10,14,15]. This notion is underlined by an observation involving the 2011 O104:H4 strain. Studies determined that the pAA plasmid can be lost in the human gut and the authors hypothesized that loss of the adhesive aggregative properties attenuates virulence, a point which might have contributed to the limited number of secondary infections [14].

So far five different types of AAF have been assigned to specific gene components coded on the pAA plasmid [6,20–23]. In a study which analyzed 17 EAEC isolates from Danish diarrhea patients, type I AAF turned out to be the most common AAF type found in 9 of the isolates, an AAF type also present in the 2011 outbreak strain [4,7,20]. Further, Boisen et al. described that 8 strains could not be assigned to other known AAF types II and III although showing aggregative adherence, suggesting that so far unknown types of AAF do exist. Indeed, for five strains, it was found that the pilin gene cluster showed several important differences from the other AAF types which was the reason to classify them into AAF/IV [20]. The recently described O111:H21 EHEC/EAEC strain was classified as an AAF/V-harboring strain [6]. However, it was not described how the novel AAF type discriminates from the ones previously assigned and how this type may be detected by means of PCR. AAF/V so far represented by the major pilin subunit gene *aaf5a* of EHEC/EAEC O111:H21 [6], *E. coli* O127:H21 (GenBank accession AB571097), and *E. coli* O6:H$^-$ (GenBank accession AB571098) showed no homology to the major pilin subunit gene of AAF/I to AAF/IV on the DNA level. About 30% homology to related proteins of AAF/III was found on the protein level and similarities were especially present in the N-terminal regions of the proteins. Therefore, we have designed a PCR assay amplifying the *aaf5A* gene (Fig. 2B). No type I–V AAF fimbriae could be assigned to the novel Orough:H$^-$ EHEC/EAEC strain by the here used PCR-based AAF gene detection. Therefore, other AA fimbrial subunits such as those not yet known or completely distinct aggregation factors may be present in this strain, as suggested by Harrington et al. [25]. Future experiments involving genome or pAA sequence analysis may give an insight into the nature of the aggregation determinants.

Due to the high virulence potential of EHEC/EAEC as outlined above, it is necessary to keep track of EHEC/EAEC causing human disease and to characterize their virulence determinants. To facilitate recognition of EHEC/EAEC strains in the future, we developed a triplex PCR assay for concomitant detection of *stx1*, *stx2*, and *aatA*. This assay extends on the duplex *stx* PCR assay previously described to amplify both *stx1* and *stx2* [31] by adding a primer pair for *aatA* detection (Fig. 1B).

In conclusion, we described two novel EHEC/EAEC strains isolated from human disease cases in Germany in 2010 and 2012; one of those originating from a bloody diarrhea. Those strains belong to MLST sequence types and/or serotypes seldom associated with human disease and in addition to *stx2* harbor EAEC characteristics which qualify them to cause severe disease.

Acknowledgments

We thank Gerlinde Bartel, Simone Dumschat, Susanne Karste, Bettina Leiste, Sieglinde Schidlo, Ute Siewert, Ute Strutz for excellent technical assistance. We are indebted to students of the master module molecular infection epidemiology of the Technical University Braunschweig (Germany) for support in EHEC/EAEC analysis.

Author Contributions

Conceived and designed the experiments: RP CL PA A. Flieger. Performed the experiments: RP CL PA A. Fruth ET. Analyzed the data: RP CL PA A. Fruth ET A. Flieger. Contributed reagents/materials/analysis tools: RP A. Fruth ET A. Flieger. Wrote the paper: A. Flieger. Editing of the manuscript: RP CL PA A. Fruth ET A. Flieger.

References

1. Kaper JB, Nataro JP, Mobley HL (2004) Pathogenic Escherichia coli. Nat Rev Microbiol 2: 123–140.
2. Robert-Koch-Institut (2013) Infektionsepidemiologisches Jahrbuch meldepflichtiger Krankheiten für 2012. Berlin, Germany.
3. Robert-Koch-Institut (2011) Final presentation and evaluation of the epidemiological findings in the EHEC O104:H4 outbreak, Germany 2011. Berlin, Germany: Robert-Koch-Institut.
4. Bielaszewska M, Mellmann A, Zhang W, Kock R, Fruth A, et al. (2011) Characterisation of the Escherichia coli strain associated with an outbreak of haemolytic uraemic syndrome in Germany, 2011: a microbiological study. Lancet Infect Dis 11: 671–676.
5. Brzuszkiewicz E, Thurmer A, Schuldes J, Leimbach A, Liesegang H, et al. (2011) Genome sequence analyses of two isolates from the recent Escherichia coli outbreak in Germany reveal the emergence of a new pathotype: Entero-Aggregative-Haemorrhagic Escherichia coli (EAHEC). Arch Microbiol 193: 883–891.
6. Dallman T, Smith GP, O'Brien B, Chattaway MA, Finlay D, et al. (2012) Characterization of a verocytotoxin-producing enteroaggregative Escherichia coli serogroup O111:H21 strain associated with a household outbreak in Northern Ireland. J Clin Microbiol 50: 4116–4119.
7. Frank C, Werber D, Cramer JP, Askar M, Faber M, et al. (2011) Epidemic profile of Shiga-toxin-producing Escherichia coli O104:H4 outbreak in Germany. N Engl J Med 365: 1771–1780.
8. Karch H, Denamur E, Dobrindt U, Finlay BB, Hengge R, et al. (2012) The enemy within us: lessons from the 2011 European Escherichia coli O104:H4 outbreak. EMBO Mol Med 4: 841–848.
9. Mellmann A, Harmsen D, Cummings CA, Zentz EB, Leopold SR, et al. (2011) Prospective genomic characterization of the German enterohemorrhagic Escherichia coli O104:H4 outbreak by rapid next generation sequencing technology. PLoS One 6: e22751.
10. Morabito S, Karch H, Mariani-Kurkdjian P, Schmidt H, Minelli F, et al. (1998) Enteroaggregative, Shiga toxin-producing Escherichia coli O111:H2 associated with an outbreak of hemolytic-uremic syndrome. J Clin Microbiol 36: 840–842.
11. Morabito S, Karch H, Schmidt H, Minelli F, Mariani-Kurkdjian P, et al. (1999) Molecular characterisation of verocytotoxin-producing Escherichia coli of serogroup O111 from different countries. J Med Microbiol 48: 891–896.
12. Rasko DA, Webster DR, Sahl JW, Bashir A, Boisen N, et al. (2011) Origins of the E. coli strain causing an outbreak of hemolytic-uremic syndrome in Germany. N Engl J Med 365: 709–717.
13. Rohde H, Qin J, Cui Y, Li D, Loman NJ, et al. (2011) Open-source genomic analysis of Shiga-toxin-producing E. coli O104:H4. N Engl J Med 365: 718–724.
14. Zhang W, Bielaszewska M, Kunsmann L, Mellmann A, Bauwens A, et al. (2013) Lability of the pAA Virulence Plasmid in O104:H4: Implications for Virulence in Humans. PLoS One 8: e66717.
15. Jandhyala DM, Vanguri V, Boll EJ, Lai Y, McCormick BA, et al. (2013) Shiga toxin-producing Escherichia coli O104:H4: an emerging pathogen with enhanced virulence. Infect Dis Clin North Am 27: 631–649.
16. Grad YH, Lipsitch M, Feldgarden M, Arachchi HM, Cerqueira GC, et al. (2012) Genomic epidemiology of the Escherichia coli O104:H4 outbreaks in Europe, 2011. Proc Natl Acad Sci U S A 109: 3065–3070.
17. Thomas S, Holland IB, Schmitt L (2013) The Type 1 secretion pathway - The hemolysin system and beyond. Biochim Biophys Acta.
18. Nataro JP, Kaper JB, Robins-Browne R, Prado V, Vial P, et al. (1987) Patterns of adherence of diarrheagenic Escherichia coli to HEp-2 cells. Pediatr Infect Dis J 6: 829–831.
19. Vial PA, Robins-Browne R, Lior H, Prado V, Kaper JB, et al. (1988) Characterization of enteroadherent-aggregative Escherichia coli, a putative agent of diarrheal disease. J Infect Dis 158: 70–79.
20. Boisen N, Struve C, Scheutz F, Krogfelt KA, Nataro JP (2008) New adhesin of enteroaggregative Escherichia coli related to the Afa/Dr/AAF family. Infect Immun 76: 3281–3292.
21. Czeczulin JR, Balepur S, Hicks S, Phillips A, Hall R, et al. (1997) Aggregative adherence fimbria II, a second fimbrial antigen mediating aggregative adherence in enteroaggregative Escherichia coli. Infect Immun 65: 4135–4145.
22. Nataro JP, Deng Y, Maneval DR, German AL, Martin WC, et al. (1992) Aggregative adherence fimbriae I of enteroaggregative Escherichia coli mediate adherence to HEp-2 cells and hemagglutination of human erythrocytes. Infect Immun 60: 2297–2304.
23. Bernier C, Gounon P, Le Bouguenec C (2002) Identification of an aggregative adhesion fimbria (AAF) type III-encoding operon in enteroaggregative Escherichia coli as a sensitive probe for detecting the AAF-encoding operon family. Infect Immun 70: 4302–4311.
24. Dudley EG, Thomson NR, Parkhill J, Morin NP, Nataro JP (2006) Proteomic and microarray characterization of the AggR regulon identifies a pheU pathogenicity island in enteroaggregative Escherichia coli. Mol Microbiol 61: 1267–1282.
25. Harrington SM, Dudley EG, Nataro JP (2006) Pathogenesis of enteroaggregative Escherichia coli infection. FEMS Microbiol Lett 254: 12–18.
26. Morin N, Santiago AE, Ernst RK, Guillot SJ, Nataro JP (2013) Characterization of the AggR regulon in enteroaggregative Escherichia coli. Infect Immun 81: 122–132.
27. Nataro JP, Yikang D, Yingkang D, Walker K (1994) AggR, a transcriptional activator of aggregative adherence fimbria I expression in enteroaggregative Escherichia coli. J Bacteriol 176: 4691–4699.
28. Wilson A, Evans J, Chart H, Cheasty T, Wheeler JG, et al. (2001) Characterisation of strains of enteroaggregative Escherichia coli isolated during the infectious intestinal disease study in England. Eur J Epidemiol 17: 1125–1130.
29. Chaudhuri RR, Sebaihia M, Hobman JL, Webber MA, Leyton DL, et al. (2010) Complete genome sequence and comparative metabolic profiling of the prototypical enteroaggregative Escherichia coli strain 042. PLoS One 5: e8801.
30. Touchon M, Hoede C, Tenaillon O, Barbe V, Baeriswyl S, et al. (2009) Organised genome dynamics in the Escherichia coli species results in highly diverse adaptive paths. PLoS Genet 5: e1000344.
31. Cebula TA, Payne WL, Feng P (1995) Simultaneous identification of strains of Escherichia coli serotype O157:H7 and their Shiga-like toxin type by mismatch amplification mutation assay-multiplex PCR. J Clin Microbiol 33: 248–250.
32. Elias WP, Uber AP, Tomita SK, Trabulsi LR, Gomes TA (2002) Combinations of putative virulence markers in typical and variant enteroaggregative Escherichia coli strains from children with and without diarrhoea. Epidemiol Infect 129: 49–55.
33. Vila J, Vargas M, Henderson IR, Gascon J, Nataro JP (2000) Enteroaggregative escherichia coli virulence factors in traveler's diarrhea strains. J Infect Dis 182: 1780–1783.
34. Elias WP, Suzart S, Trabulsi LR, Nataro JP, Gomes TA (1999) Distribution of aggA and aafA gene sequences among Escherichia coli isolates with genotypic or phenotypic characteristics, or both, of enteroaggregative E. coli. J Med Microbiol 48: 597–599.
35. Prager R, Strutz U, Fruth A, Tschape H (2003) Subtyping of pathogenic Escherichia coli strains using flagellar (H)-antigens: serotyping versus fliC polymorphisms. Int J Med Microbiol 292: 477–486.
36. Scheutz F, Teel LD, Beutin L, Pierard D, Buvens G, et al. (2012) Multicenter evaluation of a sequence-based protocol for subtyping Shiga toxins and standardizing Stx nomenclature. J Clin Microbiol 50: 2951–2963.
37. Shaikh N, Tarr PI (2003) Escherichia coli O157:H7 Shiga toxin-encoding bacteriophages: integrations, excisions, truncations, and evolutionary implications. J Bacteriol 185: 3596–3605.
38. Shringi S, Schmidt C, Katherine K, Brayton KA, Hancock DD, et al. (2012) Carriage of stx2a differentiates clinical and bovine-biased strains of Escherichia coli O157. PLoS One 7: e51572.
39. Prager R, Annemuller S, Tschape H (2005) Diversity of virulence patterns among shiga toxin-producing Escherichia coli from human clinical cases-need for more detailed diagnostics. Int J Med Microbiol 295: 29–38.
40. Prager R, Fruth A, Busch U, Tietze E (2011) Comparative analysis of virulence genes, genetic diversity, and phylogeny of Shiga toxin 2 g and heat-stable enterotoxin STIa encoding Escherichia coli isolates from humans, animals, and environmental sources. Int J Med Microbiol 301: 181–191.
41. Clermont O, Bonacorsi S, Bingen E (2000) Rapid and simple determination of the Escherichia coli phylogenetic group. Appl Environ Microbiol 66: 4555–4558.
42. Scaletsky IC, Michalski J, Torres AG, Dulguer MV, Kaper JB (2005) Identification and characterization of the locus for diffuse adherence, which encodes a novel afimbrial adhesin found in atypical enteropathogenic Escherichia coli. Infect Immun 73: 4753–4765.
43. Scaletsky IC, Silva ML, Trabulsi LR (1984) Distinctive patterns of adherence of enteropathogenic Escherichia coli to HeLa cells. Infect Immun 45: 534–536.
44. Roberts PH, Davis KC, Garstka WR, Bhunia AK (2001) Lactate dehydrogenase release assay from Vero cells to distinguish verotoxin producing Escherichia coli from non-verotoxin producing strains. J Microbiol Methods 43: 171–181.
45. Prager R, Fruth A, Siewert U, Strutz U, Tschape H (2009) Escherichia coli encoding Shiga toxin 2f as an emerging human pathogen. Int J Med Microbiol 299: 343–353.
46. Wirth T, Falush D, Lan R, Colles F, Mensa P, et al. (2006) Sex and virulence in Escherichia coli: an evolutionary perspective. Mol Microbiol 60: 1136–1151.

47. Schmidt H, Knop C, Franke S, Aleksic S, Heesemann J, et al. (1995) Development of PCR for screening of enteroaggregative Escherichia coli. J Clin Microbiol 33: 701–705.
48. Mellmann A, Bielaszewska M, Kock R, Friedrich AW, Fruth A, et al. (2008) Analysis of collection of hemolytic uremic syndrome-associated enterohemorrhagic Escherichia coli. Emerg Infect Dis 14: 1287–1290.
49. Boisen N, Ruiz-Perez F, Scheutz F, Krogfelt KA, Nataro JP (2009) Short report: high prevalence of serine protease autotransporter cytotoxins among strains of enteroaggregative Escherichia coli. Am J Trop Med Hyg 80: 294–301.
50. Grad YH, Godfrey P, Cerquiera GC, Mariani-Kurkdjian P, Gouali M, et al. (2013) Comparative genomics of recent Shiga toxin-producing Escherichia coli O104:H4: short-term evolution of an emerging pathogen. MBio 4: e00452-00412.
51. Jourdan-da Silva N, Watrin M, Weill FX, King LA, Gouali M, et al. (2012) Outbreak of haemolytic uraemic syndrome due to Shiga toxin-producing Escherichia coli O104:H4 among French tourists returning from Turkey, September 2011. Euro Surveill 17.
52. Monecke S, Mariani-Kurkdjian P, Bingen E, Weill FX, Baliere C, et al. (2011) Presence of enterohemorrhagic Escherichia coli ST678/O104:H4 in France prior to 2011. Appl Environ Microbiol 77: 8784–8786.
53. Acheson DW, Reidl J, Zhang X, Keusch GT, Mekalanos JJ, et al. (1998) In vivo transduction with shiga toxin 1-encoding phage. Infect Immun 66: 4496–4498.
54. Boudailliez B, Berquin P, Mariani-Kurkdjian P, Ilef D, Cuvelier B, et al. (1997) Possible person-to-person transmission of Escherichia coli O111–associated hemolytic uremic syndrome. Pediatr Nephrol 11: 36–39.
55. Iyoda S, Tamura K, Itoh K, Izumiya H, Ueno N, et al. (2000) Inducible stx2 phages are lysogenized in the enteroaggregative and other phenotypic Escherichia coli O86:HNM isolated from patients. FEMS Microbiol Lett 191: 7–10.
56. Bielaszewska M, Schiller R, Lammers L, Bauwens A, Fruth A, et al. (2014) Heteropathogenic virulence and phylogeny reveal phased pathogenic metamorphosis in Escherichia coli O2:H6. EMBO Mol Med 6: 347–357.
57. Toval F, Kohler CD, Vogel U, Wagenlehner F, Mellmann A, et al. (2014) Characterization of Escherichia coli isolates from hospital inpatients or outpatients with urinary tract infection. J Clin Microbiol 52: 407–418.
58. Gervilla R, Felipe X, Ferragut V, Guamis B (1997) Effect of high hydrostatic pressure on Escherichia coli and Pseudomonas fluorescens strains in ovine milk. J Dairy Sci 80: 2297–2303.
59. Guo H, Kong Q, Cheng J, Wang L, Feng L (2005) Characterization of the Escherichia coli O59 and O155 O-antigen gene clusters: the atypical wzx genes are evolutionary related. FEMS Microbiol Lett 248: 153–161.
60. Sau A, Misra AK (2012) Convergent synthesis of the tetrasaccharide repeating unit of the cell wall lipopolysaccharide of Escherichia coli O40. Beilstein J Org Chem 8: 2053–2059.
61. Zhao G, Perepelov AV, Senchenkova SN, Shashkov AS, Feng L, et al. (2007) Structural relation of the antigenic polysaccharides of Escherichia coli O40, Shigella dysenteriae type 9, and E. coli K47. Carbohydr Res 342: 1275–1279.
62. O'Brien AD, Lively TA, Chang TW, Gorbach SL (1983) Purification of Shigella dysenteriae 1 (Shiga)-like toxin from Escherichia coli O157:H7 strain associated with haemorrhagic colitis. Lancet 2: 573.
63. Wells JG, Davis BR, Wachsmuth IK, Riley LW, Remis RS, et al. (1983) Laboratory investigation of hemorrhagic colitis outbreaks associated with a rare Escherichia coli serotype. J Clin Microbiol 18: 512–520.

14

Coliform Bacteria as Indicators of Diarrheal Risk in Household Drinking Water: Systematic Review and Meta-Analysis

Joshua S. Gruber*, Ayse Ercumen, John M. Colford, Jr.

Division of Epidemiology, University of California, Berkeley, California, United States of America

Abstract

Background: Current guidelines recommend the use of *Escherichia coli* (EC) or thermotolerant ("fecal") coliforms (FC) as indicators of fecal contamination in drinking water. Despite their broad use as measures of water quality, there remains limited evidence for an association between EC or FC and diarrheal illness: a previous review found no evidence for a link between diarrhea and these indicators in household drinking water.

Objectives: We conducted a systematic review and meta-analysis to update the results of the previous review with newly available evidence, to explore differences between EC and FC indicators, and to assess the quality of available evidence.

Methods: We searched major databases using broad terms for household water quality and diarrhea. We extracted study characteristics and relative risks (RR) from relevant studies. We pooled RRs using random effects models with inverse variance weighting, and used standard methods to evaluate heterogeneity and publication bias.

Results: We identified 20 relevant studies; 14 studies provided extractable results for meta-analysis. When combining all studies, we found no association between EC or FC and diarrhea (RR 1.26 [95% CI: 0.98, 1.63]). When analyzing EC and FC separately, we found evidence for an association between diarrhea and EC (RR: 1.54 [95% CI: 1.37, 1.74]) but not FC (RR: 1.07 [95% CI: 0.79, 1.45]). Across all studies, we identified several elements of study design and reporting (e.g., timing of outcome and exposure measurement, accounting for correlated outcomes) that could be improved upon in future studies that evaluate the association between drinking water contamination and health.

Conclusions: Our findings, based on a review of the published literature, suggest that these two coliform groups have different associations with diarrhea in household drinking water. Our results support the use of EC as a fecal indicator in household drinking water.

Editor: Sudha Chaturvedi, Wadsworth Center, United States of America

Funding: The authors have no funding or support to report.

Competing Interests: The authors have declared that no competing interests exist.

* Email: jsgruber@gmail.com

Introduction

Globally, drinking water has been established as a primary transmission pathway for diarrhea pathogens. [1,2] In industrialized countries, centrally treated drinking water distribution systems have largely eliminated outbreaks of waterborne diseases, such as typhoid fever and cholera. [3] In developing countries, there is a large body of evidence that improving the microbial quality of drinking water by household treatment and safe storage reduces diarrhea. [4–6] Yet, evidence directly linking diarrheal illness to measured fecal contamination in drinking water remains inconclusive. [3,7,8]

In general, it is not feasible to test water for all known waterborne pathogens to assess whether it is safe for drinking. [2,9–11] Instead, since the early 1900s there has been heavy reliance on fecal indicator organisms as measures of drinking water quality. [1,12] Current World Health Organization (WHO) guidelines recommend *Escherichia coli* (EC) and/or thermotolerant ("fecal") coliforms (FC) as indicators of the effectiveness of disinfection processes, and as index organisms for the potential presence of fecal contamination and waterborne pathogens; [2,10,12,13] previous WHO guidelines use categories of EC and FC concentrations to define levels of disease risk from drinking water. [14] While EC are considered the most suitable indicator organism due to their specificity to fecal sources of contamination, FC are also recommended as an acceptable surrogate; this recommendation exists despite the recognition that the FC group includes coliform species of environmental origin, and is therefore not likely specific to fecal contamination. [2,12,13] Despite heavy reliance on EC and FC to assess the microbiological safety of drinking water, it has yet to be shown that either of these specific indicators is associated with waterborne illness. [8]

A previous systematic review and meta-analysis evaluated the evidence for the link between household drinking water quality, measured by fecal indicator organisms, and health; [8] the authors found no evidence of an association between diarrhea and indicators of drinking water contamination (EC, FC and *fecal streptococci*). This review, however, was limited by the availability, size and quality of articles published at the time the search was conducted (2001). [8] Specifically, the previous review included only three relatively small studies that reported using EC, and therefore focused mostly on FC as a measure of water quality. Given the limited number of studies available to the authors, they were also unable to evaluate the performances of EC and FC separately. Since the previous review, several studies have been published using EC as a measure of water quality (n = 6) [15–21], motivating our updated review with this newly available evidence. In addition, this larger body of evidence allows us to evaluate the performance of EC and FC separately; we hypothesized that the two coliform groups would have different associations with diarrhea given their different specificities for fecal contamination. Given the widespread use of EC and FC as measures of water quality by researchers and policy makers, and the limited evidence regarding the association of these proxy measures with actual disease outcomes, we believe that our systematic review and meta-analysis will make a significant contribution to the body of knowledge on the performance of indicator organisms in household drinking water, and have implications for their recommended use for future guidelines and research. In addition, based on the findings of our systematic review, we are able to make several recommendations for the design and reporting of future studies that assess the relationship between drinking water contamination and health.

Methods

Search Strategy

We searched MEDLINE, EMBASE, and Web of Knowledge databases for relevant articles. We used broad search terms for water, water quality and indicator organisms, diarrhea and household (point-of-use) sampling (Table 1). Titles and abstracts from the search were examined, and the full texts of relevant articles were reviewed. The bibliographies of relevant articles identified from full-text reviews were scanned to identify additional relevant studies. Searches were limited to articles published in peer-reviewed journals, in English, Spanish, German or Turkish (languages spoken by the authors). No restrictions were placed on date of publication. The final search was conducted on February 27, 2013. A protocol was not registered for this systematic review.

Inclusion and Exclusion Criteria

We reviewed articles that reported data on the association between exposure to *Escherichia coli* (EC) or thermotolerant ("fecal") coliforms (FC) in household drinking water, and the occurrence of diarrhea under non-outbreak conditions; we excluded other, less commonly used indicator organisms (e.g., total coliforms, *fecal streptococci*). Our inclusion criterion was that the study collected exposure and outcome data at the household level or at the point of use; studies were excluded if they only reported measures of source water quality (e.g., shared wells, distribution system "nodes"), or used ecologic outcome data (e.g., health ministry reports). No further restrictions were placed on: definitions of diarrhea, recall period, study design, age groups, study location (developed/developing country), study setting (urban/rural), or drinking water source (as long as exposure to indicator bacteria was measured at the point of use).

Study Reporting and Data Extraction

For each relevant study two authors (JG and AE) independently extracted basic study characteristics, including year of publication, sample size, age groups, study location, setting and design, indicator organism and enumeration methods, and diarrhea definition and enumeration methods into standardized forms, and resolved any discrepancies. Where possible, a relative risk (RR) such as odds ratio, cumulative incidence ratio, incidence density ratio or prevalence ratio was extracted from relevant studies. When no effect measure was reported by the authors, raw data were extracted to calculate an appropriate RR and confidence interval using standard methods. [22] If authors reported both raw data and unadjusted RRs we confirmed the reported estimates using the raw data; we used the RRs reported by the authors, unless otherwise noted. If authors reported results for both indicators (EC and FC) the results were treated as two separate studies in the meta-analysis. All RRs were extracted such that a value greater than unity indicated increased risk of illness among the group exposed to contaminated water. We also noted whether authors controlled for additional variables (by study design, stratified analysis or regression methods) and whether they accounted for correlation (clustering) of outcomes in their analysis.

Exposure Thresholds

There are multiple ways to define comparison groups in water quality studies. For example, authors often use a threshold to define exposed and non-exposed groups based on indicator organism counts measured in 100 ml samples of water (i.e., exposed: ≥10 EC/100 ml; non-exposed: <10 EC/100 ml; with RRs calculated to compare these two groups); however, threshold levels can vary between studies. Current WHO guidelines recommend that drinking water that is safe for human consumption should have no detectable EC or FC in any 100 ml sample (i.e., a 1 EC/FC threshold); however, there is also evidence from the literature that much higher indicator organism concentrations are required to cause disease. For example, a study conducted in the Philippines on source water quality [23] previously reported a "threshold effect", where no association with diarrhea was found at the 1 EC, 10 EC or 100 EC cutoffs, but an association was found at the 1000 EC cutoff; it is plausible that a similar threshold effect could be present for point-of-use drinking water. Given the limited number of studies included in the previously published systematic review and meta-analysis, the authors made no attempt to differentiate indicator organism-diarrhea associations at different threshold levels. [8] In our review, we attempted to extract RRs for different thresholds at the 1 EC or FC, 10 EC or FC, 100 EC or FC and 1000 EC or FC levels, when the authors reported these data.

Categorical Exposures

As an alternative approach to exposure categorization, previous WHO guidelines defined disease risk from drinking water based on categories of indicator organism counts measured in 100 ml samples of water: 0 EC or FC, safe; 1–10 EC or FC, low risk; 11–100 EC or FC, intermediate risk; 101–1000 EC or FC, high risk;> 1000 EC or FC, very high risk. [14] Investigators commonly use these guidelines to define exposure categories in studies of drinking water quality; each category is treated as an independent exposure group, and RRs are calculated for each elevated category relative to the 0 EC or FC exposure group. In our review, we extracted RRs for these categorical exposures to explore the presence of a dose-response (increased disease risk associated with increasing exposure levels) and to evaluate previous WHO guidelines that defined health risk based on these exposure categories. Within

Table 1. Systematic Review Search Terms. [a]

Water Exposure	Household Sampling	Disease Outcome
water quality	household	Diarrhea
water microbiology	point of use	Diarrheoa
water pollution	Pou	gastrointestinal illness
water contamination	point-of-use	gastrointestinal disease
water supply	drinking water	gastrointestinal infection
drinking water	consumption	Dysentery
"indicator bacteria"	tap water	"HCGI"
"indicator organism"	well water	"highly credible gastrointestinal illness"
"thermotolerant coliforms"	domestic	"AGI"
"thermo-tolerant coliforms"		"AGII"
"fecal coliforms"		"acute gastrointestinal illness"
escherichia coli		
"e. coli"		
"fecal bacteria"		
"fecal contamination"		
"microbiological indicators"		

[a]Search terms combined using Boolean logic: within column terms combined using "or" statements; "and" statements were used to combine terms between columns.

studies that evaluated dose-responses, we extracted p-values for tests of trend. In studies that did not report p-values for tests of trend but reported results for different categorical exposure levels, we extracted the appropriate data, where possible, and conducted our own tests of trend using previously published methods that estimate a log-linear dose-response while accounting for correlations between RRs from a single study (*glst* command: STATA 12, STATA Corp, College Station Texas). [24]

Meta-analysis

For consistency with the previously published review, we conducted meta-analyses to calculate a summary measure pooled across all studies which provided an extractable RR, combining all EC and FC studies. [8] The previous review was not explicit about which results were used for meta-analyses if data could be extracted at multiple thresholds. In our review, we estimated a summary measure across all studies using the lowest extractable threshold from each study (e.g., if a study reported raw data that could be combined at the 1 EC, 10 EC and 100 EC thresholds, we included the RR calculated for the 1 EC threshold in the main meta-analysis). In addition, we conducted a sub-group analysis to explore the type of indicator organism used in each study as a source of heterogeneity in the main analysis; for this sub-group analysis we stratified studies by indicator used (EC and FC) and re-pooled summary measures separately for each indicator. In a secondary meta-analysis, we explored evidence for a threshold effect in household drinking water (see "Exposure Thresholds" above). For this analysis, we restricted meta-analyses to studies that reported extractable RRs at the 1 EC, 10 EC and 100 EC thresholds, respectively – this analysis was only feasible for studies that reported extractable data for all three threshold levels.

Summary measures were calculated by meta-analysis using random effects models with inverse variance weighting (STATA 12). [25] Heterogeneity across studies was evaluated using the Mantel-Haentzel χ^2 test; we considered a p-value on the χ^2 statistic <0.2 as evidence of heterogeneity. We used funnel plots to evaluate publication bias; plot asymmetry was interpreted as evidence of "small study bias", for which publication bias is a likely contributor. [26,27]

Results

Systematic Review

Database searches were completed on February 27, 2013, from which we identified 5,801 titles and abstracts; 20 relevant articles were identified for review (Figure 1). Of the 20 relevant articles, 14 presented data in an extractable format (see Methods) and were included in meta-analyses. One article [28] presented results for both EC and FC; these results were treated as separate studies in the meta-analyses (resulting in 15 total studies).

Study Characteristics: All Studies

The 20 relevant studies were published between 1977 and 2012 (Table 2). Two studies were conducted in a developed country (Canada), the rest in low-resource settings; no studies were conducted among populations with access to centralized water-treatment and distribution systems. The study settings included a mix of urban/peri-urban (n = 7) and rural (n = 13), and the study populations included a range of age groups (Table 2). The included articles used cohort (n = 14) and case-control (n = 6) study designs (Tables 3 and 4). We identified one randomized control trial [16] that reported data on the direct association between water quality and diarrhea; we considered this study a cohort design for the purposes of the review since water quality was not randomized. We note that, while cohort designs traditionally measure an exposure and then follow a population over time to measure outcomes, the cohort designs we identified in this review measured exposure (EC or FC): (i) simultaneously with outcomes through cross-sectional sampling; (ii) at intervals during ongoing diarrhea surveillance, or; (iii) the timing and analysis of water samples relative to diarrhea measurement was mixed or not clearly reported (Tables 3 and 4). The included case-control studies measured exposure after disease occurrence by design; however one study [19] utilized a nested case control design with

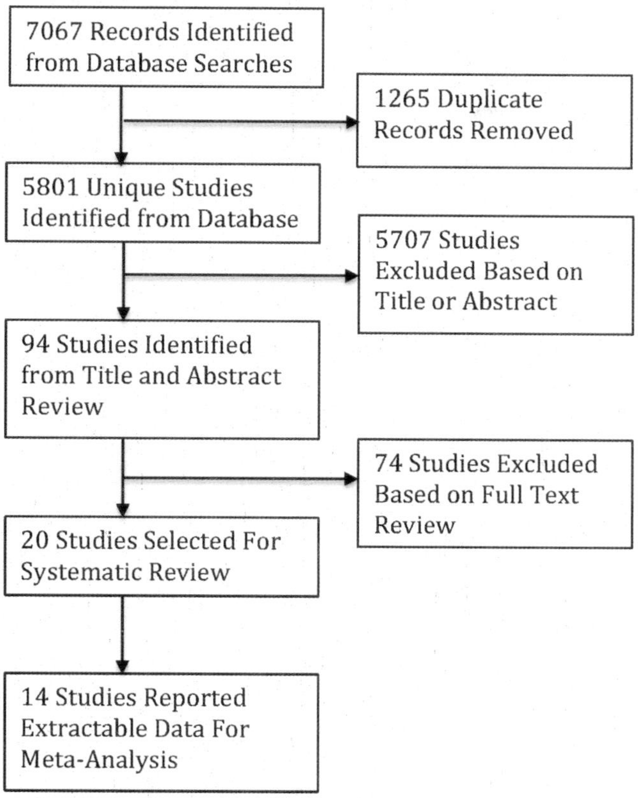

Figure 1. Systematic review flow chart.

risk set sampling in which disease and EC exposure were measured on the same day.

Included studies measured EC (n = 9), FC (n = 10), or both (n = 1) in drinking water samples collected at the point of use. Overall, studies varied in their reporting of enumeration and incubation methods, and we could not always confirm the indicator organism enumerated based on the reported information (Tables 3 and 4). In at least one study, authors reported using EC, but a description of their methods suggested they measured FC. [29] With this exception, we relied on the authors' reporting or deferred to the categorization used by the previous review. [8]

Most studies used a definition of diarrhea that is consistent with current recommendations: three or more loose or watery stools in a 24-hour period (Tables 3 and 4). [30,31] Four studies included the presence of blood or mucus in stool as part of their definition of diarrhea, [15,17,18,32] and two studies [15,17] reported dysentery as an outcome separate from "general" diarrhea; we did not include dysentery as a separate outcome in our review. Cohort studies in low-resource settings relied primarily on household surveillance and self-reported symptoms (e.g., maternal recall) for outcome assessment, using a range of recall periods (daily, up to one month; Tables 3 and 4); the two Canadian studies relied on monthly calendars maintained in the household and reported by telephone. Case-control studies mostly identified cases through hospitals and clinics, and selected controls from community samples; however, two studies identified cases and controls based on concurrent [19] or prior [33] household diarrhea surveillance conducted by the investigators.

Among the studies identified in our review, eight studies reported results that controlled for potential confounders; the other 12 studies found no evidence for confounding, or did not report attempting to control for confounding (Tables 5 and 6) – we did not differentiate between these studies in meta-analyses. In general, reporting on the independence of observations or methods to account for clustered outcomes was poor (Tables 5 and 6). Only five of the 20 studies reported using methods to account for correlated outcomes (e.g., generalized estimating equations; GEE). In general, the RRs and confidence intervals we calculated from available raw data were consistent with those reported by the authors, whether or not they reported accounting for correlated outcomes. However, in one of these studies, that reported using GEE, we calculated confidence intervals from extracted raw data that were substantially more conservative than those reported by the authors; [15] we included the more conservative confidence intervals for this study in our meta-analyses (Table 5).

Disease-Indicator Associations

Tables 5 and 6 summarize results from EC and FC studies, respectively. Among the ten EC studies, eight reported data that quantified the relationship between indicator exposure and diarrhea (Table 5). Of the eight studies with quantitative results, six reported threshold results at the 1 EC/100 ml cutoff [15,18,20,21,28,33] and all six reported RRs greater than unity; however, only one study was able to rule random error out as an explanation for their results (Table 5). [15] The remaining two studies, among the eight that quantified a relationship between EC and diarrhea, reported significant relationships between diarrhea and linear increases in exposure to mean log10 EC concentrations; the results were very consistent across these two studies (Table 5). [16,19] The two studies that did not have extractable, quantifiable results reported that no "association" or "correlation" was found between EC and diarrhea. [17,34] However, we could not confirm whether the authors' conclusions were based on the size of the effect estimate (i.e., similar to unity), precision (i.e., "non-significant" confidence intervals or *p*-values), or both.

Among the 11 FC studies (including FC results from Genthe et al. 1997 as separate from their EC results), nine studies reported data that quantified the relationship between indicator exposure and diarrhea (Table 6). Results from these nine FC studies were less consistent than results from EC studies. Using the lowest extractable threshold, five studies reported estimates that suggest increases in the risk of diarrhea with exposure to FC [32,35–38], and four reported effects equivalent to unity or reduced diarrhea risk with exposure to FC. [28,39–41] Henry and Rahim (1990) reported FC effects for two distinct study areas differentiated by "adequate" versus "poor" sanitation infrastructure; while a single summary measure for this study suggested an increased risk of diarrhea with exposure to FC, the results from the two separate study populations were very different (Table 6; FC counts were associated with an increase in illness in the area with improved sanitation and a reduction in illness in the area with unimproved sanitation). Of the two FC studies that did not report extractable data, results were also mixed: one reported no difference in FC isolation from water in case and control households, [29] the other reported that households with diarrhea had higher overall geometric mean FC levels compared to control households. [42]

Summary Measures

For consistency with the previous review, we conducted meta-analyses across all studies (combining both EC and FC studies), using the lowest extractable threshold for each study (Tables 5 and 6). Across all studies, our summary estimate suggests a non-significant increase in diarrhea risk from exposure to drinking water contaminated with EC or FC (RR 1.26 [95% CI: 0.98,

Table 2. Selected Characteristics of Included Studies.

First Author	Year	Location	Setting	Study Size[a]	Ages	Indicator
deAceituno	2012	Honduras	Rural	1020	All	EC
Levy	2012	Ecuador	Rural	115	NR	EC
Gundry	2009	S. Africa/Zimbabwe	Rural	254	1–2 y	EC
Brown	2008	Cambodia	Rural	1196	All	EC
Jensen	2004	Pakistan	Rural	209	<5 y	EC
Bhargava	2003	Bangladesh	Rural	99	1–10 y	FC
Strauss	2001	Canada	Rural	647	All	EC
Raina	1999	Canada	Rural	531	All	EC
Genthe	1997	S. Africa	Urban	316	"Pre-school"	Both
Jagals	1997	S. Africa	Urban	100	NR	FC
Vanderslice	1993	Philippines	Urban	254	<2 y	FC
Knight	1992	Malaysia	Rural	196	4–59 m	FC
Han	1991	Myanmar	Urban	208	6–29 m	FC
Henry	1990	Bangladesh	Rural	92	6–18 m	FC
Henry and Rahim	1990	Bangladesh	Urban	137	1–6 y	FC
Echeverria	1987	Thailand	Urban	NR	<5 y	FC[b]
Esrey	1986	Lesotho	Rural	545	1–60 m	FC
Lloyd-Evans	1984	Gambia	Urban	20	6–36 m	EC
Black	1982	Bangladesh	Rural	40	5–18 m	EC
Rajasekaran	1977	India	Rural	1091	<5 y	FC

EC: Escherichia Coli; FC: Fecal Coliform.
[a]May not reflect the analytic sample used by the authors;
[b]Authors report EC but methods suggest FC.

1.63]; Figure 2). However, we also found evidence of significant heterogeneity ($X^2 = 36.13$, degrees of freedom (d.f.) $= 12$, $p < 0.001$), and evidence of publication bias (Figure 3).

In order to explore a potential source of heterogeneity across all studies, we stratified results by indicator organism (EC vs. FC) and re-estimated summary measures in these sub-groups. Across all EC studies, the summary measure suggests a significant association between exposure to EC in household drinking water and diarrhea (RR: 1.54 [95% CI: 1.37, 1.74]); Figure 4). While we found no evidence of heterogeneity across EC studies ($X^2 = 1.65$, d.f. $= 5$, $p = 0.90$), and minimal evidence of publication bias (Figure 5), we note that the EC summary measure was disproportionately influenced by one study [15] ("% weight", Figure 4). We therefore conducted a sensitivity analysis by repeating the EC analysis without the study by Brown et al. Removing this study did not impact the magnitude of the summary measure, but did reduce the precision of the estimate (RR 1.48 [95% CI: 1.02, 2.15]); Figure S1); there was no evidence of heterogeneity after removing Brown et al. from the analysis ($X^2 = 1.59$, d.f. $= 4$, $p = 0.81$). Across all FC studies, our summary effect measure suggests no association between FC exposure in drinking water and diarrhea (RR: 1.07 [95% CI: 0.79, 1.45]); Figure 4); we also found evidence of significant heterogeneity ($X^2 = 2.30$, d.f. $= 6$, $p = 0.06$), and publication bias (Figure 6).

Threshold Effects

Two EC studies provided extractable data that allowed us to explore threshold effects at three different levels (1 EC, 10 EC, and 100 EC per 100 ml; Table 5) [15,18]. RRs were calculated by comparing outcomes in the exposed group (≥EC threshold) to outcomes in the control group (<EC threshold). In one study, [15] increasing the threshold from 1EC to 10EC suggested a slight increase in diarrhea risk; there was no further increase in risk when the threshold was increased to 100EC (Table 5). In the other study, increasing the threshold beyond 1EC did not increase the magnitude of the effect estimates (Table 5). [18] We pooled estimates across these two studies, and found no evidence that increasing thresholds beyond WHO drinking water guidelines (1 EC/100 mL) was associated with an increased risk of diarrhea (Figure 7). [2] A third EC study reported finding no threshold effect at 1000 EC/100 ml, but did not report a RR. [19]

Categorical Exposure and Dose-Response

Four EC studies reported investigating a dose-response relationship. [15,18,19,21] Only three of these studies evaluated the presence of a dose-response using similar exposure categories (<1 EC (referent), 1–10 EC, 11–100 EC, 100+, or 101–1000 EC and 1000+; Table 5). Of these three studies, one did not report extractable data, but reported finding no evidence of a dose-response effect. [19] Results from the other two studies [15,18] suggest a qualitative dose response (increased risk of diarrhea with increasing exposure categories; Table 5); formal tests of trend, however, had mixed results (Brown et al: $p<0.001$ provides evidence of a dose response; Jensen et al: $p = 0.26$ does not provide evidence of a dose response). A fourth study [21] used different EC exposure categorizations. The results from this study qualitatively suggested increasing risk across 0.1–1.5 EC and 1.6–700 EC exposure categories; however, the authors found no evidence of a linear trend ($p = 0.45$; Table 5).

Table 3. Summary of EC Study Exposure and Outcome Measurements.

First Author	Year	Study Design	Outcome [a]	Recall	Measured EC Relative to Outcome	Enumeration Method	Medium	Temp (°C)[f]
deAceituno	2012	RCT	Diarrhea	7-day	After (<1 week)	MPN	IDEXX Colilert	NR
Levy	2012	CC	Diarrhea	Daily	Same Day	MF	BD Difco ml agar[e] (EPA 1604)	30
Gundry	2009	Cohort	Diarrhea	Daily	Before (<2 weeks)	MPN	IDEXX Colilert	NR
Brown	2008	Cohort	Diarrhea	7-day	After (<1 week)	MF	"selective medium"[d]	NR
Jensen	2004	Cohort	Diarrhea	7-day	Before/After (<3 days)	MF	Hach m-ColiBlue 24 Broth PourRite	35
Strauss	2001	Cohort	AGII[b]	Monthly Diary	Twice over 28-d surveillance	MF	m-FC-BCIG agar	44.5
Raina	1999	Cohort	GI Illness[c]	Monthly Diary	5 times over 1-y surveillance	NR	"standard methods" (MOE 1992)	NR
Genthe	1997	CC	Diarrhea	Hospital	After	NR	"standard methods" (APHA 1989)	NR
Lloyd-Evans	1984	CC	Diarrhea	7-day	After (1–2 months)	MF	Millipore (DHSS 1969)	NR
Black	1982	Cohort	Diarrhea	NR	After (<1 month)	Plating	MacConkey's Agar	37

EC: *Escherichia Coli*; CC: Case Control; MF: Membrane Filtration; MPN: Most Probable Number; NR: Not Reported; C: Celsius; DHSS: Department of Health & Social Security: *The bacteriological examination of water* supplies; APHA: American Public Health Association: *Standard Methods for the Examination of Water and Wastewater*; MOE: *Ministry of Environment: Ontario's Drinking Water Objectives.*
[a]Unless noted, used a definition consistent with World Health Organization recommendation of 3 or more loose/watery stools in 24 hour period;
[b]Acute Gastrointestinal Illness: 1) vomiting or liquid diarrhea or 2) nausea or soft, loose diarrhea combined with abdominal cramps;
[c]Diarrhea with or with out vomiting;
[d]selective medium: "containing chromogenic and fluorogenic b-glucuronide and b-galactoside substrates";
[e]Multiple EC enumeration methods used – we report the method with the largest sample size and for which the authors report an extractable RR;
[f]Incubation temperature.

Table 4. Summary of FC Study Exposure and Outcome Measurements.

First Author	Year	Study Design	Outcome [a]	Recall	Measured FC Relative to Outcome	Enumeration Method	Medium	Temp (°C)[e]
Bhargava	2003	Cohort	GI Morbidity [b]	1-month	After (<1 month)	MF	*DIFCO* m-FC media	45
Genthe	1997	CC	Diarrhea	Hospital	After	NR	"standard methods" (APHA 1989)	NR
Jagals	1997	CC	Diarrhea [c]	Clinic	After	MF	"standard methods" (APHA 1992)	44.5
Vanderslice	1993	Cohort	Diarrhea [c]	7-day	2–5 times over 1 year	MF	m-FC agar (APHA 1985)	44.5
Knight	1992	CC	Diarrhea	Clinic	After (4–14 days)	MF	*Paqualab* (ELE International 1986)	NR
Han	1991	Cohort	Diarrhea	7-day	Averaged over surveillance	MF	m-FC agar (WHO 1983)	NR
Henry	1990	Cohort	Diarrhea	7-day	Averaged over surveillance	NR	"standard methods" (APHA 1981)	NR
Henry and Rahim	1990	Cohort	Diarrhea	14-day	Unclear (<6 months)	dip-slides	*ORION Hygicult* Agar Slides [d]	37
Echeverria	1987	CC	Diarrhea	Hospital	After	MF	m-FC agar (APHA 1975)	44
Esrey	1986	Cohort	Diarrhea [c]	24-hour	Unclear	MF	Faecal Coliform Broth (AJPH 1975)	NR
Rajasekaran	1977	Cohort	Diarrhea	NR	Unclear (<15 days)	MPN	IMViC (APHA 1965)	44

FC: Fecal Coliform; CC: Case Control; GI: Gastrointestinal; MF: Membrane Filtration; MPN: Most Probable Number; NR: Not Reported; C: Celsius; APHA: American Public Health Association: *Standard Methods for the Examination of Water and Wastewater*; WHO: World Health Organization: *Guidelines for Drinking Water Quality*; IMViC: Indole, methyl red, Voges–Proskauer and citrate [a] [a] Unless otherwise noted, study used a definition consistent with current World Health Organization recommendation of 3 or more loose/watery stools in a 24 hour period; [b] Morbidity included: diarrhea, dysentery, vomiting, stomachache, acidity, typhoid, cholera; [c] Did not report a definition; [d] Report enumerating *Enterobacteriaceae* – included as FC for consistency with previous review. [e] Incubation temperature

Table 5. EC Study Results.

First Author	Year	Adjusted Analysis	RR	Threshold Results [a] RR (95% CI)	Categorical/Dose Response: [b]RR (95% CI)	Alternate Results: RR (95% CI)
deAceituno	2012	Yes	OR [c]	-	-	Log10 increase: 1.26 (1.08,1.46)
Levy	2012	NR	OR [c]	1000 EC: "no effect"	no "dose-response" (1–10 EC, 11–100 EC, 101–1,000 EC, 1,000+ EC)	Log10 increase: 1.29 (1.02,1.65)
Gundry	2009	Yes	NR	-	-	"no association"
Brown [d]	2008	No	PR [c]	1 EC: 1.55 (1.36,1.76) 10 EC: 1.70 (1.52,1.90) 100 EC: 1.67 (1.51,1.84) 1000 EC: 1.37 (1.21,1.54)	1–10 EC: 0.98 (0.81–1.20) 11–100 EC: 1.35 (1.13–1.61) 101–1000 EC: 1.83 (1.58–2.11) 1001+EC: 1.81 (1.54–2.11) [e]	-
Jensen	2004	No	IDR	1 EC: 1.32 (0.77,2.27) 10 EC: 1.25 (0.83,1.88) 100 EC: 1.23 (0.85,1.80)	1–10 EC: 1.17 (0.55–2.47) 11–100 EC: 1.26 (0.70–2.28) 100+EC: 1.45 (0.81–2.59) [f]	-
Strauss	2001	Yes	OR [c]	1 EC: 1.52 (0.33,6.92)	0.1–1.5 EC: 0.85 (0.10,7.19) 1.6–700 EC: 2.69 (0.34,21.56) [g]	-
Raina	1999	Yes	OR [c]	1 EC: 2.11 (0.90,4.94)	-	-
Genthe	1997	Yes	OR	1 EC: 1.26 (0.59,2.72)	-	-
Lloyd-Evans	1984	No	OR	1 EC: 3.86 0.33,45.57)	-	-
Black	1982	NR	NR	-	-	"no correlation found"

EC: *Escherichia Coli*; RR: Relative Risk; OR: Odds Ratio; PR: Prevalence Ratio; IDR: Incidence Density Ratio; NR: Not Reported; CI: Confidence Interval;
[a]Compares risk in groups exposed to ≥EC value, to <EC value;
[b]Reference group is <1 EC for all categories;
[c]Authors report using methods to account for correlated (clustered) outcomes;
[d]RRs and 95% CIs calculated from raw data;
[e]*p*-value for linear trend <0.01;
[f]p-value for linear trend =0.26;
[g]p-value for linear trend =0.45.

Table 6. FC Study Results.

First Author	Year	Adjusted Analysis	RR	Threshold Results [a] RR (95% CI)	Alternate Results RR (95% CI)
Bhargava	2003	Yes	NA	-	ML Coefficient: 0.204 (SE: 0.08) *p-value* <0.05
Genthe	1997	Yes	OR	1 FC: 0.84 (0.46,1.52)	
Jagals	1997	NR	NA	-	Geometric mean FC higher in homes with diarrhea (compared to control homes)
Vanderslice	1993	Yes	NA	-	Probit coefficient: −0.002 *p-value* >0.10
Knight	1992	Yes	OR	1 FC: 1.45 (0.57,4.76)	-
Han	1991	No	PR	Medium: 0.72 (0.56,0.94) [b]	Medium-High: 0.73 (0.52,1.02) [c] High: 0.72 (0.52,1.00) [c]
Henry	1990	No	IDR	Low: 1.03 (0.75,1.42) [b]	-
Henry and Rahim	1990	No	CIR	10^4 FC: 1.26 (0.59,2.72) [d]	Improved Area: 2.58 (0.70,9.54) [d] Unimproved Area: 0.86 (0.34–2.18) [d]
Echeverria	1987	NR	NR	-	FC isolated from water as often in homes with diarrhea as in control homes
Esrey	1986	No	PR	10 FC: 1.53 (0.69,3.40) 100 FC: 1.46 (0.62,3.45)	10–100 FC: 1.41 (0.53,3.76) [e]>100 FC: 1.64 (0.64,4.18) [e]
Rajasekaran	1977	No	PR	10 FC: 2.93 (1.10,7.81)	-

FC: Fecal Coliform; RR: Relative Risk; OR: Odds Ratio; PR: Prevalence Ratio; IDR: Incidence Density Ratio; NR: Not Reported; CI: Confidence Interval; ML: maximum likelihood
[a]Compares risk in groups exposed to ≥FC value, to <FC value;
[b]Based on median of samples or arbitrary cutoffs;
[c]Compared to "Low" group – Authors do not report specific FC concentrations used to determined categories;
[d]Reference group is <1000 colony forming units FC per gram;
[e]Reference group <10 FC.

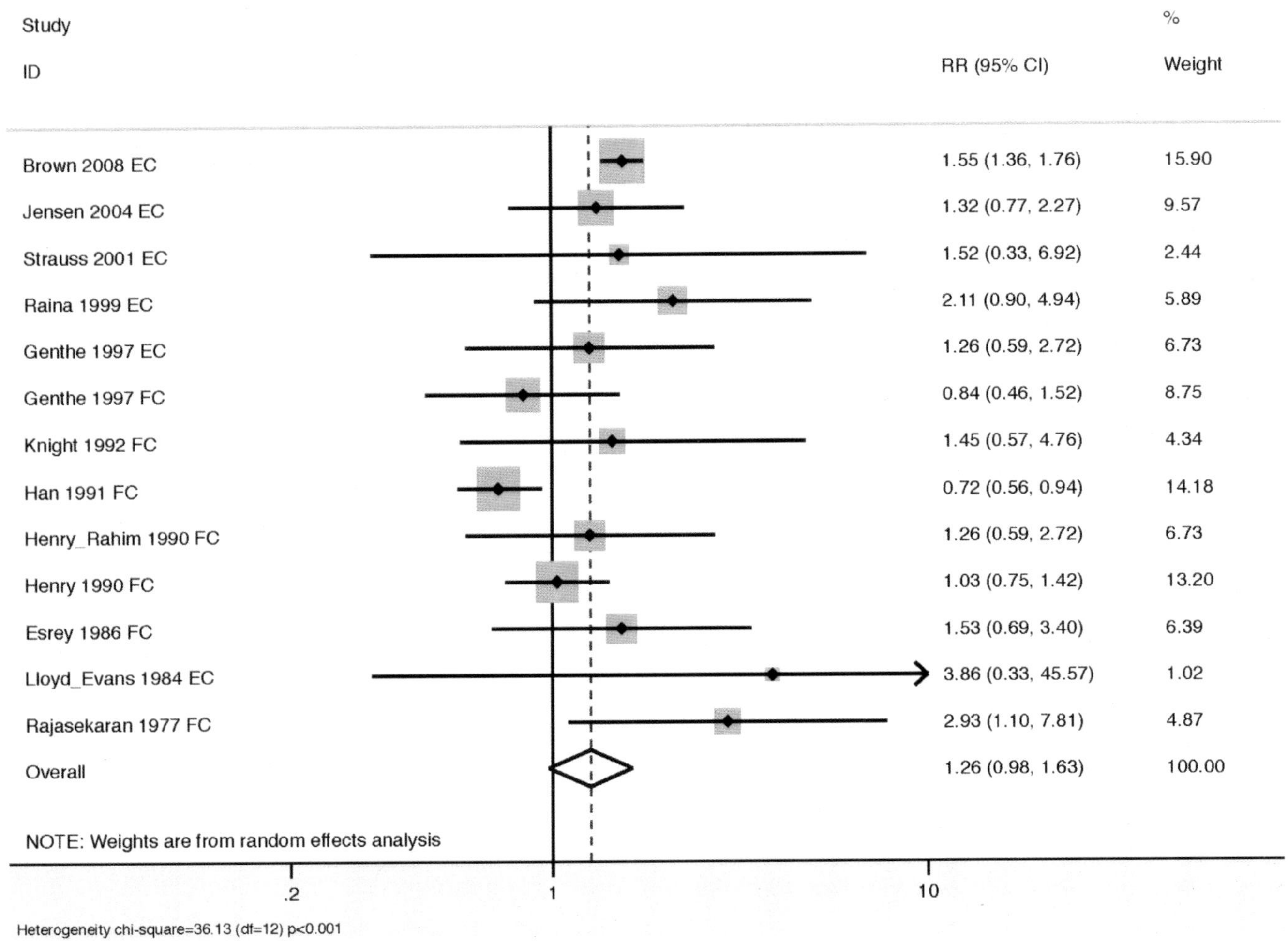

Figure 2. Forest plot for all included studies.

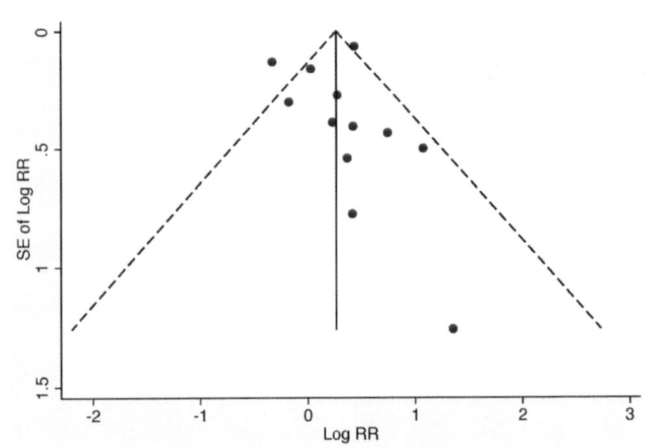

Figure 3. Funnel plot for all included studies (EC and FC studies). Studies are plotted relative to size (SE of Log RR), and reported log relative risk (Log RR); studies higher on the vertical axis are larger, and studies further to the right have larger RRs. The solid vertical line is the log of the summary RR for all studies, and the dotted lines are "pseudo 95% confidence intervals" for the summary measure. The absence of smaller studies with small or null RRs (lower left region of the plot) creates plot asymmetry, and provides evidence of possible publication bias.

Discussion

Summary of Findings

We conducted a systematic review and meta-analysis to evaluate the relationship between diarrheal illness and the presence of EC or FC indicators in household drinking water. Consistent with a prior review, [8] we did not find conclusive evidence for an association between contaminated drinking water and diarrhea when EC and FC results were combined (previous review: RR 1.12 [95% CI: 0.85, 1.48]; our review: RR 1.26, [95% CI: 0.98, 1.63]; Figure 2). We also found evidence of significant heterogeneity and publication bias across all studies (Figure 2, Figure 3). After stratifying studies by EC and FC to explore the choice of indicator organism as a source of heterogeneity, we found that EC studies reported consistent effect estimates that suggest an increased risk of diarrhea with exposure to contaminated drinking water with no evidence of heterogeneity (pooled RR 1.54 [95% CI: 1.37, 1.74]; Table 5, Figure 4). In contrast, FC studies reported mixed results with significant heterogeneity and provided minimal evidence of an association with diarrhea (pooled RR 1.07 [95% CI: 0.79, 1.45]; Table 6, Figure 4). We found no evidence that exposure thresholds greater than 1 EC/100 mL (e.g., 10 EC/100 mL, 100 EC/100 mL) were associated with increased diarrheal disease, but this evidence is based on a limited number of studies. Results regarding a dose-response relationship between EC in household drinking water and diarrhea were limited and

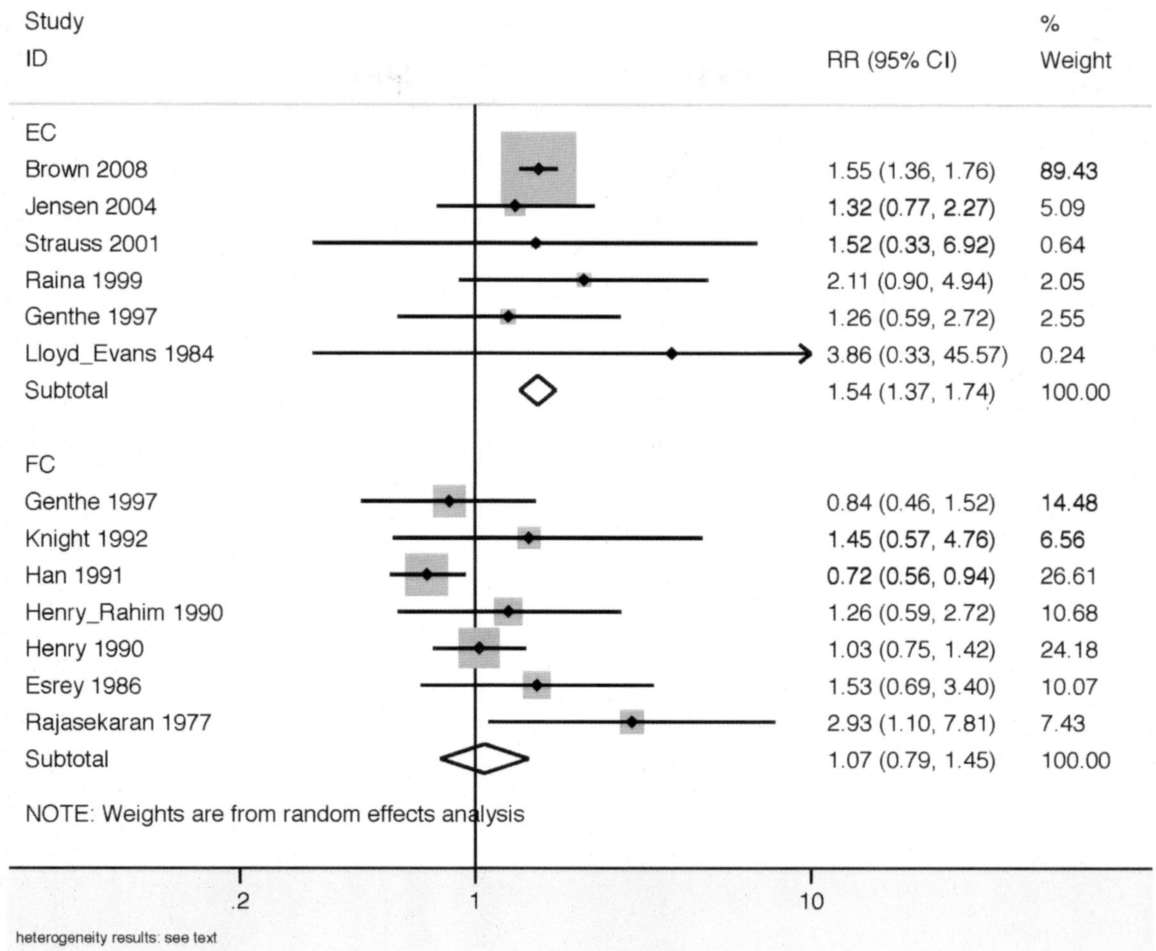

Figure 4. Forest plot for all studies stratified by indicator organism. Top panel, EC: *Escherichia coli*; Bottom panel, FC: thermotolerant ("fecal") coliforms.

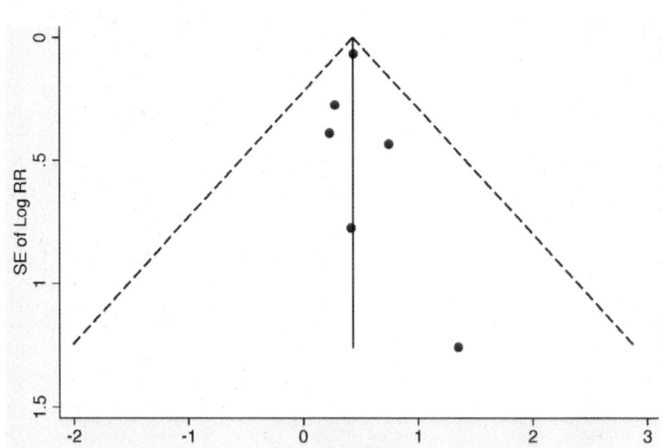

Figure 5. Funnel plot for EC studies. Studies are plotted relative to size (SE of Log RR), and reported log relative risk (Log RR); studies higher on the vertical axis are larger, and studies further to the right have larger RRs. The solid vertical line is the log of the summary RR for all studies, and the dotted lines are "pseudo 95% confidence intervals" for the summary measure. Studies on this plot are generally symmetrical, with the exception of one small study with a large RR, providing minimal evidence of publication bias.

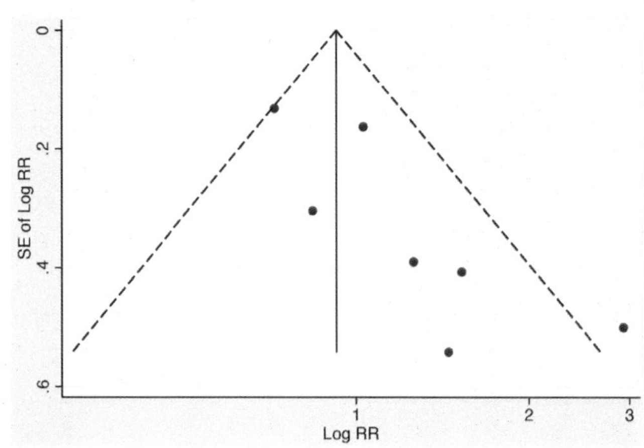

Figure 6. Funnel plot for all FC studies. Studies are plotted relative to size (SE of Log RR), and reported log relative risk (Log RR); studies higher on the vertical axis are larger, and studies further to the right have larger RRs. The solid vertical line is the log of the summary RR for all studies, and the dotted lines are "pseudo 95% confidence intervals" for the summary measure. The absence of smaller studies with small or null RRs (lower left region of the plot) creates plot asymmetry, and provides evidence of possible publication bias.

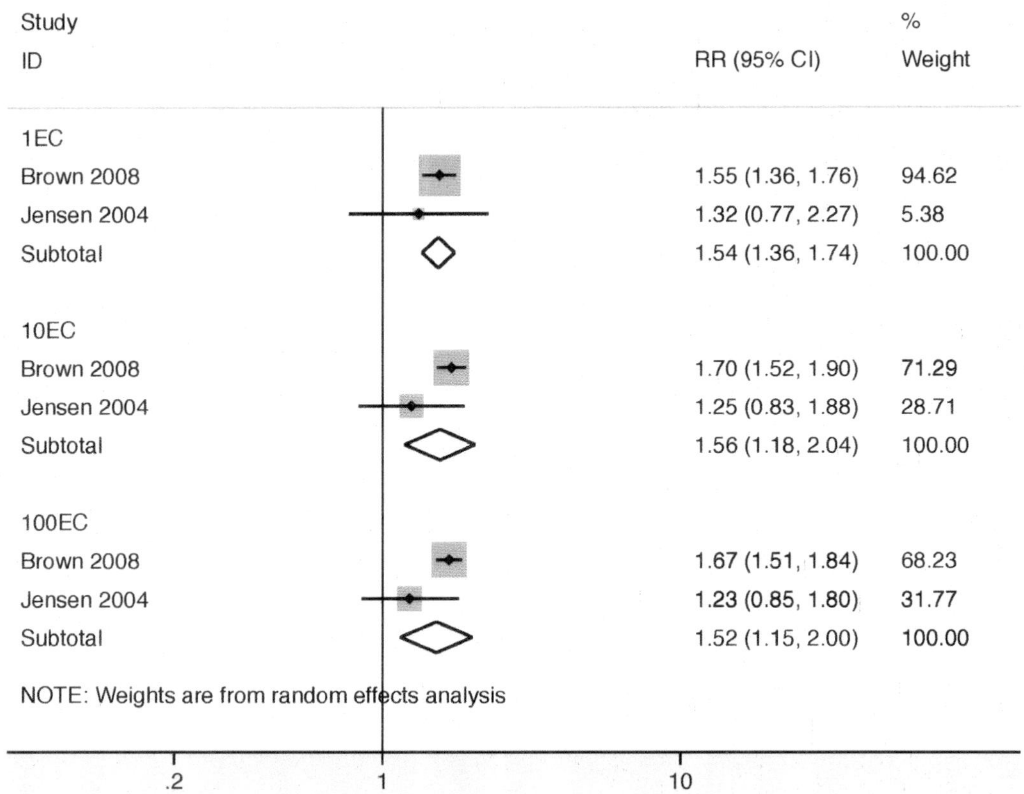

Figure 7. Forest plot for two studies with extractable data at multiple thresholds. Data were pooled across the two studies at the 1 EC/ 100 ml threshold (top panel), 10 EC/100 ml threshold (middle panel), and 100 EC/100 ml threshold (bottom panel). EC: *Escherichia coli.*

inconclusive. In addition to the results of the meta-analysis, we identified several elements of study design and reporting that could improve future studies evaluating the relationship between water quality and health.

Implications for Choice of Indicator Organism to Assess Microbiological Safety of Drinking Water

Current guidelines recommend two specific uses for indicator organisms: (i) fecal indicators (index organisms), used to indicate the presence of fecal contamination, potential pathogens, and possible health risk, and; (ii) process indicators used to evaluate the effectiveness of a water treatment process. [1,2,13]. While the performance of coliform bacteria as process indicators has been described previously, [2,43] and is outside the scope of this review, the results from our review have implications for the use of EC and FC as index organisms in household drinking water. Currently, EC is considered the "most suitable" fecal indicator; however, FC is generally recognized as a suitable surrogate. [1,2,12,13] Our findings support the continued use of EC as a fecal indicator (index organism) to assess water quality at the point of use, but do not support the use of FC as a surrogate as it does not demonstrate a clear association with diarrheal disease outcomes.

Our findings that EC and FC perform differently as indicators of diarrhea risk from contaminated drinking water are not surprising. While EC is generally of fecal origin, [10] and likely to be present simultaneously with diarrheagenic pathogens in recently contaminated drinking water, FC are known to include coliforms of environmental origin (e.g., *Klebsiella*), in addition to EC. [1,2,13] The consistency with which FC methods will be specific to human pathogens will therefore vary with the environments in which water samples are being collected. Indeed, our results show that the magnitude and direction of the effect estimates for FC were highly inconsistent (Figure 4, Table 6); even within a single study [37] the authors found highly divergent results using FC in two separate study areas (Table 6). In contrast, the magnitude and direction of effect estimates across the EC studies included in our review were consistent across diverse study regions, and when pooled provided evidence of a significant association with diarrhea; these results are consistent with the higher specificity of EC for fecal contamination, compared to FC (Table 5, Figure 4). The presence of a dose-response between EC and diarrhea could have provided further evidence to support our findings that drinking water contaminated with EC is associated with diarrhea. However, dose-response results from our review were inconclusive, and represent an avenue for future research.

While our summary measures suggest that the presence of EC in household drinking water is significantly associated with diarrhea, it is important to note that only one individual EC study in our review was able to rule out chance as a possible explanation of their findings [15]. It has been demonstrated that indicator levels can vary considerably even over short periods of time in both household and source water, [44,45] and that pathogens and indicator organisms have inconsistent correlations. [46] The studies in this review relied on intermittent grab samples to classify household water quality. Even daily grab samples likely provided only a crude assessment of a household's exposure to fecal contamination and diarrheagenic pathogens, which likely contributed to the lack of precision in the individual studies included in our review. While the imprecision of results from individual studies supports a previous assertion that fecal indicator organisms are "blunt" tools to characterize water quality, [19] our findings suggest that they have continued utility in health and water research. Indeed, while recent WHO drinking water guidelines have shifted focus from recommendations using specific indicator levels to define water safety to a more integrated approach centered on water safety plans, these recommendations are largely directed towards the management of water distribution systems. [2,13] In practice, regional organizations and researchers working in areas without access to drinking water distribution systems rely heavily on indicator organisms to assess the risk of disease from drinking water, and to measure the effectiveness of household water treatment and safe storage interventions; this is particularly true in resource poor settings with limited access to advanced laboratory facilities. Our results suggest that EC have continued value in both of these applications.

Threshold Effects for Diarrhea Risk

The findings from our review do not support the existence of a "threshold effect" in contaminated household drinking water. A previous study evaluating the effect of contaminated *source* water on diarrhea [23] found no evidence of an association between EC and diarrhea at the 1 EC threshold level; however, significant associations with diarrhea were observed at the 1000 EC threshold level. The authors concluded that their findings of a "threshold effect" supported earlier assertions that relaxing drinking water guidelines (beyond the 1 EC threshold) might be acceptable in developing countries. [47] Contrary to these findings, in our review of household drinking water we found consistently elevated risks of diarrhea at the 1 EC threshold, with a significant summary measure when pooled across all studies. These results support current WHO guidelines recommending that all drinking water intended for human consumption contain zero EC/100 ml, regardless of location. [2] Beyond the 1 EC threshold, our results did not suggest increased risk of diarrhea at elevated cutoffs, but this evidence was based on a limited number of studies.

Recommendations for Future Water Quality Studies

The studies included in our review covered several decades, and varied considerably with respect to methodological quality and completeness of reporting. In this section, we highlight several findings from our systematic review that could improve the design and reporting of future studies that seek to evaluate the relationship between water quality and health.

The studies in our systematic review used very consistent definitions of diarrhea, relying primarily on self- or caregiver reporting of diarrhea symptoms (Tables 3 and 4). However, we note that diarrhea recall periods and identification strategies varied greatly (e.g., daily recall, one-month recall, cases presenting to clinics; Tables 3 and 4). Reliance on self-reported diarrhea symptoms as a health measure could have introduced bias into individual studies through two primary mechanisms, which have implications for the use of self-reported diarrhea as an outcome in future studies. First, as with any self-reported, subjective outcome, there is a potential for differential reporting relative to exposure status [48]. If study-specific reporting biases were differential with respect to drinking water contamination, it is possible that the results of individual studies (and therefore our review) could be biased. However, there is no reason to suspect that individuals would be aware of the indicator status of their drinking water when reporting diarrhea symptoms, which would decrease the potential for this bias. Second, longer follow-up periods can bias diarrhea reporting due to poor outcome recall, which could have biased findings towards the null if non-differential with respect to exposure, and/or compounded biases associated with differential reporting in individual studies. [49] The inclusion of objective health outcome measures (e.g., pathogen-specific antibody responses) could improve future studies by reducing reliance on self-reported diarrhea symptoms and their associated biases. [50,51] In addition, while our review focused exclusively on diarrhea, expanding the range of water-related health outcomes studied and reviewed (e.g., indicators of growth and malnutrition) could also improve our understanding of the health impacts of drinking water contamination beyond gastrointestinal illnesses.

Very few studies in our review were able to establish temporality between exposures (indicator organism) and outcomes (diarrhea), and therefore mostly relied on the assumption that drinking water samples were representative of an exposure period that was relevant to measured disease outcomes. While this assumption might be reasonable, or the only option given the practicalities of field conditions, it does leave open the possibility of reverse causality (i.e., diarrhea caused by other environmental pathways led to increased fecal contamination of drinking water). The design of future water quality studies should attempt to measure exposure in advance of disease outcomes, and all studies should be explicit about the timing of exposure and disease measurements in their reporting. These recommendations would all but preclude the use of "traditional" case-control studies, where cases and controls (i.e., disease status) are identified first, followed by visits to households to collect water samples to ascertain exposure status. Instead, a cohort design that measures exposure to contaminated drinking water first, followed by surveillance visits after an appropriate incubation period to measure health outcomes, is a more suitable study design. Decisions regarding follow-up frequency, recall period, and measures of disease occurrence (i.e., incidence, prevalence) will vary depending on study context and logistics, but should be carefully considered and explicitly reported. [49,52]

In studies evaluating the relationship between drinking water quality and health, confounding bias is a concern: there are numerous factors that could cause both drinking water contamination and diarrhea in a given study setting. Overall, the studies in our review were not consistent in reporting adjusted results (Tables 5 and 6), and there was no consistent set of factors used across studies when authors did report attempting to control for confounding. Incomplete control of confounding in the included studies could have biased individual study results, and therefore the findings of our review. Future studies should be explicit about their attempts to measure and control for confounding factors. Additionally, several studies did not account for correlated outcomes in their analyses, which could have influenced the precision of summary estimates. However, for EC studies we note the consistency of the direction and magnitude of the associations reported across diverse study locations, and across studies that did and did not adjust for confounding and/or account for clustering. Regardless, reporting on these issues could be improved upon in future studies.

Our systematic review included published, peer-reviewed studies. As with any systematic review, publication bias, where smaller studies with small or null ("non-positive") results are systematically excluded from the published literature, could have impacted our findings. In our review, we found evidence of publication bias among FC studies (smaller studies with smaller effect sizes appear to be absent from the funnel plot; lower left region, Figure 6); however, inclusion of smaller FC studies with RRs at or less than unity would have strengthened our findings of no association between FC and diarrhea. We found minimal evidence to suggest publication bias among EC studies (Figure 5);

however, we cannot rule out publication bias as a possible explanation of our findings – the funnel plot suggests that most studies were balanced around the summary measure with the exception of one small study with a large positive finding. Taken together, there is evidence that smaller studies with small ("non-positive") effects sizes are systematically missing from the literature on the relationship between water quality and diarrheal illness.

In our review, we pooled RRs across relevant studies using meta-analysis to investigate the association of fecal indicator measures in drinking water with diarrhea. The limitations of meta-analysis have been discussed [53]; we caution against interpreting the summary measures from our review as "true" underlying causal effects, but rather consider them additional pieces of evidence regarding the relationship between fecal indicators in drinking water and diarrhea. The evidence from our pooled summary measures, taken together with biologic plausibility and the consistency of results across studies, provides evidence to support a relationship between diarrhea and the presence of EC in point-of-use drinking water; we do not, however, find evidence to support an equivalent relationship between diarrhea and FC.

Conclusions

We reviewed the available literature to identify studies that evaluated the relationship between microbial indicators of drinking water quality and diarrhea. We found that studies using *Escherichia coli* (EC) as an indicator of household drinking water quality reported consistent effect estimates, that when pooled suggested a significant association with increased diarrheal illness. Results from studies using thermotolerant ("fecal") coliforms (FC), on the other hand, were inconsistent, and suggested no association with diarrhea when pooled. In this review, we also note several areas where the design and reporting of the included studies could have been improved, and make recommendations for future studies. The results from our review suggest that EC has value as a fecal indicator organism, but that use of FC should be considered carefully in contexts where an association with diarrheal disease outcomes is important.

Acknowledgments

The authors would like to acknowledge Professor Kara Nelson for generously reviewing this manuscript, and providing key feedback.

Author Contributions

Conceived and designed the experiments: JG JC. Performed the experiments: JG AE. Analyzed the data: JG. Contributed reagents/materials/analysis tools: JG AE. Wrote the paper: JG AE JC.

References

1. Dufour AP (2003) Assessing microbial safety of drinking water: Improving approaches and methods: International Water Assn.
2. WHO (2011) Guidelines for drinking-water quality, fourth edition. Geneva: World Health Organization.
3. Cutler D, Miller G (2005) The role of public health improvements in health advances: The twentieth-century United States. Demography 42: 1–22.
4. Arnold BF, Colford JM Jr (2007) Treating water with chlorine at point-of-use to improve water quality and reduce child diarrhea in developing countries: a systematic review and meta-analysis. The American journal of tropical medicine and hygiene 76: 354.
5. Clasen T, Schmidt WP, Rabie T, Roberts I, Cairncross S (2007) Interventions to improve water quality for preventing diarrhoea: systematic review and meta-analysis. bmj 334: 782.
6. Fewtrell L, Kaufmann RB, Kay D, Enanoria W, Haller L, et al. (2005) Water, sanitation, and hygiene interventions to reduce diarrhoea in less developed countries: a systematic review and meta-analysis. The Lancet infectious diseases 5: 42–52.
7. National Research Council (2004) Indicators for Waterborne Pathogens. Washington, DC: The National Academies Press.
8. Gundry S, Wright J, Conroy R (2004) A systematic review of the health outcomes related to household water quality in developing countries. J Water Health 2: 1–13.
9. Gerba C (2000) Indicator Microogranisms. Environmental Microbiology. San Diego, CA: Academic Press.
10. Leclerc H, Mossel D, Edberg S, Struijk C (2001) Advances in the bacteriology of the coliform group: their suitability as markers of microbial water safety. Annual Reviews in Microbiology 55: 201–234.
11. Reynolds KA, K.D Mena, Gerba CP (2008) Risk of waterborne illness via drinking water in the United States. Reviews of Environmental Contamination and Toxicology 192: 117–158.
12. Tallon P, Magajna B, Lofranco C, Leung KT (2005) Microbial indicators of faecal contamination in water: a current perspective. Water, Air, and Soil Pollution 166: 139–166.
13. Ashbolt NJ, Grabow WOK, Snozzi M (2001) Indicators of microbial water quality. In: Fewtrell L, Bartram J, editors.Water Quality: Guidelines, Standards and Health. London, UK: IWA Publishing,.
14. WHO (1997) Guidelines for drinking-water quality, 2nd edition. Geneva: World Health Organization.
15. Brown JM, Proum S, Sobsey MD (2008) Escherichia coli in household drinking water and diarrheal disease risk: evidence from Cambodia. Water Science and Technology 58: 757–763.
16. de Aceituno AMF, Stauber CE, Walters AR, Sanchez REM, Sobsey MD (2012) A Randomized Controlled Trial of the Plastic-Housing BioSand Filter and Its Impact on Diarrheal Disease in Copan, Honduras. American Journal of Tropical Medicine and Hygiene 86: 913–921.
17. Gundry SW, Wright JA, Conroy RM, Du Preez M, Genthe B, et al. (2009) Child dysentery in the Limpopo Valley: A cohort study of water, sanitation and hygiene risk factors. Journal of Water and Health 7: 259–266.
18. Jensen PK, Jayasinghe G, van der Hoek W, Cairncross S, Dalsgaard A (2004) Is there an association between bacteriological drinking water quality and childhood diarrhoea in developing countries? Trop Med Int Health 9: 1210–1215.
19. Levy K, Nelson KL, Hubbard A, Eisenberg JN (2012) Rethinking indicators of microbial drinking water quality for health studies in tropical developing countries: case study in northern coastal Ecuador. Am J Trop Med Hyg 86: 499–507.
20. Raina PS, Pollari FL, Teare GF, Goss MJ, Barry DA, et al. (1999) The relationship between E. coli indicator bacteria in well-water and gastrointestinal illnesses in rural families. Can J Public Health 90: 172–175.
21. Strauss B, King W, Ley A, Hoey JR (2001) A prospective study of rural drinking water quality and acute gastrointestinal illness. BMC Public Health 1: 8.
22. Rothman K, Greenland S, (1998) Modern Epidemiology. Philadelphia: Lippincott-Raven Publishers.
23. Moe C, Sobsey M, Samsa G, Mesolo V (1991) Bacterial indicators of risk of diarrhoeal disease from drinking-water in the Philippines. Bulletin of the World Health Organization 69: 305.
24. Greenland S, Longnecker MP (1992) Methods for trend estimation from summarized dose-response data, with applications to meta-analysis. American Journal of Epidemiology 135: 1301–1309.
25. Egger M, Smith G Davey, Altman D (2001) Systematic Reviews in Healthcare. Meta-analysis in Context. London: BMJ Books.
26. Egger M, Smith GD, Schneider M, Minder C (1997) Bias in meta-analysis detected by a simple, graphical test. bmj 315: 629–634.
27. Sterne JAC, Egger M (2001) Funnel plots for detecting bias in meta-analysis: Guidelines on choice of axis. Journal of Clinical Epidemiology 54: 1046–1055.
28. Genthe B, Strauss N, Seager J, Vundule C, Maforah F, et al. (1997) The effect of type of water supply on water quality in a developing community in South Africa. Water Science and Technology 35: 35–40.
29. Echeverria P, Taylor DN, Seriwatana J (1987) Potential sources of enterotoxigenic Escherichia coli in homes of children with diarrhoea in Thailand. Bulletin of the World Health Organization 65: 207–215.
30. Baqui AH, Black RE, Yunus M, Hoque ARA, Chowdhury H, et al. (1991) Methodological issues in diarrhoeal diseases epidemiology: definition of diarrhoeal episodes. International journal of epidemiology 20: 1057.
31. WHO (2013) Diarrhoeal disease; fact sheet.

32. Rajasekaran P, Dutt PR, Pisharoti KA (1977) Impact of Water Supply on the Incidence of Diarrhoea and Shigellosis Among Children in Rural Communities in Madurai. Indian J Med Res 66: 189–199.
33. Lloyd-Evans N, Pickering HA, Goh SGJ, Rowland MGM (1984) Food and Water Hygiene and Diarrhoea in Young Gambian Children: a Limited Case Control Study. Transactions of the Royal Society of Tropical Medicine and Hygiene 78: 209–211.
34. Black RE, Brown KH, Becker S, Alim AR, Merson MH (1982) Contamination of weaning foods and transmission of enterotoxigenic Escherichia coli diarrhoea in children in rural Bangladesh. Trans R Soc Trop Med Hyg 76: 259–264.
35. Bhargava A, Bouis HE, Hallman K, Hoque BA (2003) Coliforms in the water and hemoglobin concentration are predictors of gastrointestinal morbidity of Bangladeshi children ages 1–10 years. American journal of human biology 15: 209–219.
36. Esrey SA, Habicht J, Casella G, Miliotis MD, Kidd AH, et al. (1986) Infection, Diarrha, and Growth Rates of Young Children Following the Installation of Village Water Supplies in Lesotho. Interanation Symptosium on Water-Related Health Issues November: 11–16.
37. Henry FJ, Rahim Z (1990) Transmission of diarrhoea in two crowded areas with different sanitary facilities in Dhaka, Bangladesh. J Trop Med Hyg 93: 121–126.
38. Knight SM, Toodayan W, Caique WC, Kyi W, Barnes A, et al. (1992) Risk factors for the transmission of diarrhoea in children: a case-control study in rural Malaysia. Int J Epidemiol 21: 812–818.
39. Han AM, Oo KN, Aye T, Hlaing T (1991) Bacteriologic studies of food and water consumed by children in Myanmar: 2 Lack of association between diarrhoea and contamination of food and water. J Diarrhoeal Dis Res 9: 91–93.
40. Henry F, Huttly S, Patwary Y, Aziz K (1990) Environmental sanitation, food and water contamination and diarrhoea in rural Bangladesh. Epidemiology and infection London, New York NY 104: 253–259.
41. Vanderslice J, Briscoe J (1993) All Coliforms Are Not Created Equal - a Comparison of the Effects of Water Source and in-House Water Contamination on Infantile Diarrheal Disease. Water Resources Research 29: 1983–1995.
42. Jagals P, Grabow WOK, Williams E (1997) The effects of supplied water quality on human health in an urban development with limited basic subsistence facilities. Water Sa 23: 373–378.
43. Sobsey MD (1989) Inactivation of health-related microorganisms in water by disinfection processes. Water Science & Technology 21: 179–195.
44. Levy K, Hubbard AE, Nelson KL, Eisenberg JN (2009) Drivers of water quality variability in northern coastal Ecuador. Environmental science & technology 43: 1788–1797.
45. Levy K, Nelson KL, Hubbard A, Eisenberg JN (2008) Following the water: a controlled study of drinking water storage in northern coastal Ecuador. Environmental health perspectives 116: 1533.
46. Wu J, Long S, Das D, Dorner S (2011) Are microbial indicators and pathogens correlated? A statistical analysis of 40 years of research. J Water Health 9: 265–278.
47. Feachem RG, McGarry MG, Mara DD (1977) Water, wastes and health in hot climates: John Wiley and Sons Ltd.
48. Wood L, Egger M, Gluud LL, Schulz KF, Jüni P, et al. (2008) Empirical evidence of bias in treatment effect estimates in controlled trials with different interventions and outcomes: meta-epidemiological study. bmj 336: 601–605.
49. Arnold BF, Galiani S, Ram PK, Hubbard AE, Briceño B, et al. (2013) Optimal recall period for caregiver-reported illness in risk factor and intervention studies: A multicountry study. American journal of epidemiology 177: 361–370.
50. Crump JA, Mendoza CE, Priest JW, Glass RI, Monroe SS, et al. (2007) Comparing serologic response against enteric pathogens with reported diarrhea to assess the impact of improved household drinking water quality. American Journal of Tropical Medicine and Hygiene 77: 136.
51. Schmidt W-P, Cairncross S (2009) Household Water Treatment in Poor Populations: Is There Enough Evidence for Scaling up Now? Environmental science & technology 43: 986–992.
52. Schmidt W-P, Arnold BF, Boisson S, Genser B, Luby SP, et al. (2011) Epidemiological methods in diarrhoea studies—an update. Int J Epidemiol 40: 1678–1692.
53. Berk RA, Freedman DA (2003) Statistical assumptions as empirical commitments: Law, Punishment, and Social Control: Essays in Honor of Sheldon Messinger, 2nd edn. Aldine de Gruyter.

The Analysis of Factors Associated with Progression of Isolated Terminal Ileal Lesions

Zhang Fangbin[1]*, Hao Weiwei[1], Zhao Wugan[2], Zheng Cong[1], Chu Yanjun[1], Xu Feng[1]

1 Department of Gastroenterology, The First Affiliated Hospital of Zhengzhou University, Zhengzhou, People's Republic of China, **2** Department of Pathology, The First Affiliated Hospital of Zhengzhou University, Zhengzhou, People's Republic of China

Abstract

Objective: To assess the factors associated with the progression of isolated terminal ileal lesions (ITILs) at colonoscopy in Chinese patients.

Methods: Patients diagnosed with ITILs were enrolled. The ileoscopy was performed by two experienced gastroenterologists every 52 weeks. A logistic regression analysis was used to elucidate the factors associated with Crohn's disease (CD) and mucosal healing. A log rank test was used to assess the differences of the cumulative proportion of CD and mucosal healing in different groups at different times.

Results: (1) A total of 34 patients were included and no patient had taken nonsteroidal anti-inflammatory drug in the last 6 months; eight (23.5%) patients had a clinical diagnosis of CD, 14 (41.2%) patients achieved mucosal healing, and 12 (35.3%) patients showed no significant changes in the lesions at last follow-up. (2) The logistic regression analysis showed that only abdominal pain was a factor in the ITIL disease outcomes. (3) The cumulative proportion of CD in the abdominal pain group after 3 years was statistically higher than that in the non-abdominal pain group (42.7% *vs.* 6.2%, $\chi^2 = 10.129$, $P = 0.001$). However, the cumulative proportion of mucosal healing in the non-abdominal pain group was statistically higher than that in the abdominal pain group (73.3% *vs.* 5.6%, $\chi^2 = 5.225$, $P = 0.022$). (4) The numbers of lesions observed on the initial colonoscopy exams and the initial histologic findings were not related to the ITIL disease outcomes.

Conclusions: Clinical symptoms may be related to ITIL disease outcomes. Patients with abdominal pain had a high likelihood of CD, whereas those without abdominal pain had a high likelihood of mucosal healing.

Editor: John Green, University Hospital Llandough, United Kingdom

Funding: This study was sponsored by research funding for the doctoral program of higher education of China and the Youth Innovation Fund of the First Affiliated Hospital of Zhengzhou University. The funders had no role in study design, data collection and analysis, decision to publish, or preparation of the manuscript.

Competing Interests: The authors have declared that no competing interests exist.

* E-mail: dr_mingren@163.com

Introduction

Ileal intubation is increasingly recognized as being valuable in patients with abdominal pain, diarrhea or bloody stools—particularly where inflammatory bowel disease is a consideration. [1–3] This has led to an increased identification of patients (about 0.1–0.3%) who are not easily classified—those with Isolated ileal abnormalities, which we have coined isolated terminal ileal lesions (ITILs). [4,5] It is likely that a proportion of these patients are suffering from a restricted form or so-called forme fruste of Crohn's disease (CD). Currently, the clinical significance of this entity is unclear. [2,6,7].

The present study evaluated the clinical course of patients with ITILs to determine the clinical significance of these lesions.

Materials and Methods

Subjects

Patients diagnosed with ITILs at the Gastroenterology clinic of the First Affiliated Hospital of Zhengzhou University Hospital from 2005 to 2010 were actively recruited to this study with the goal of evaluating the natural history of terminal ileal lesions. All patients underwent gastroscopy and double contrast small bowel radiography to evaluate their upper gastrointestinal and small intestinal mucosa.

Subjects were excluded if they fulfilled any of the following criteria: (1) a follow-up of less than 2 years; (2) a history of nonsteroidal anti-inflammatory drug or glucocorticoid use within the 6 months before the study; (3) erosions in other parts of the colon in addition to the terminal ileum; (4) oral or genital ulcerations suggestive of Behçet disease; (5) infectious colitis (except tuberculosis); (6) a prior history of CD or ulcerative colitis; (7) a history of colorectal cancer or surgery; (8) a history of systemic lupus erythematosus or vasculitis; or (9) poor adherence to the study: rejection of colonoscopies during the follow-up.

Study Design

Clinical data, including sex, age, clinical symptoms and medical records were recorded. The patient information was collected by a clinician. All patients were asked to ingest 2 L of polyethylene glycol solution in the evening before the ileoscopy. The ileoscopy was performed by two experienced gastroenterologists at weeks 0, 52, 104, 156, 208, 260, 312, 364, 416, 468, and 520. Two biopsy specimens were obtained from the most severe area of the lesion in each subject. All of the biopsy specimens were evaluated separately by two experienced pathologists. In cases in which they did not agree on an evaluation, a discussion with a senior gastrointestinal pathologist was employed.

Drug therapy was directed toward the dominant symptoms: a selective smooth-muscle relaxant for abdominal pain, loperamide for diarrhea, and lactulose syrup or polyethylene glycol for constipation. (Table 1) The treatments were withdrawn when the clinical symptoms resolved and reintroduced when the clinical symptoms recurred. Patients with positive occult blood test, mild abdominal discomfort, or surveillance after colorectal polypectomy underwent no any treatment during the total duration of follow-up.

The symptoms were assessed daily by asking the patient to complete a diary regarding the following: abdominal pain, discomfort, stool frequency, and stool consistency.

Assessment of overall symptom relief was measured weekly. (Table 2) Patients were assessed for symptom recurrence weekly by telephone interview and monthly at a clinic visit.

The patients recorded the overall clinical symptom relief in a diary by answering 'yes' or 'no' to the following question: 'Do you consider that over the past week you have had satisfactory relief from your symptoms?' 'Satisfactory' meant that compared with their typical experience of the disorder in the past, the patient felt that during the past week their clinical symptoms had been alleviated to the extent that they would take medication to maintain that state.

At scheduled doctor visits, response to initial treatment was designated when patients' overall satisfactory relief from symptoms for at least 2 of the 4 previous weeks; those whose overall satisfactory relief from symptoms for less than 2 weeks in the 4 previous weeks were considered nonresponders.

Patients requesting urgent restoration of medication treatment because of recurring/worsening symptoms before or at a scheduled telephone contact during the withdrawal period were considered to have relapsed.

Statistical Analyses

Statistical analysis was performed using SPSS software, version 16.0 (SPSS Inc., Chicago, Ill, USA). To elucidate the factors associated with developing CD and mucosal healing, a logistic regression analysis was used and results were expressed as odds ratios (OR) with 95% confidence intervals (CI). A Kaplan–Meier plot and a log-rank test were used to visualize and to test differences between CD and mucosal healing in probability of remaining in the study. A χ^2 test was used to compare the endoscopic findings, pathologic findings on the initial colonoscopy exams and disease outcomes of ITILs. A *P*-value less than 0.05 was considered to be significant.

Ethical Considerations

The ethics committee of the participating center approved the study (reference numbers: 20050401GS-7 (University of Zhengzhou)). The study was conducted according to the principles expressed in the Declaration of Helsinki. Written informed consent was obtained from all participants at recruitment.

Results

Subject Characteristics

During the study period, 32,197 patients underwent colonoscopic examinations at the Gastrointestinal Endoscopy Center. Of these, 43 were assigned an endoscopic diagnostic code for ITILs. Of these 43 patients, seven patients (16.3%) with a follow-up of less than 2 years and two patients (4.7%) with poor compliance were excluded, the data of these 9 patients wasn't analyzed in this study; the remaining 34 patients (79.1%) met the study criteria. These 34 patients including in this study have no a history of nonsteroidal anti-inflammatory drug (such as aspirin) or glucocorticoid use within the 6 months before the study. These 34 patients including in this study have no family history of IBD.

The patient sample consisted of 19 men and 15 women with a mean age of 33.3±11.1 years (range 22–62 years), and the mean follow-up was 3 years (range 2–5 years). The indications for colonoscopy included abdominal pain in 10 (29.4%) patients, stools >3 times daily in nine patients (26.5%), abdominal pain and diarrhea in four patients (11.8%), abdominal pain and constipation in two patients (5.9%), positive occult blood test in two patients (5.9%), mild abdominal discomfort in two patients (5.9%), constipation in one patient (2.9%), diarrhea in one patient (2.9%), and surveillance after colorectal polypectomy in three patients (8.8%). Table 3 shows the demographic characteristics of the 34 patients.

According to the Rome III criteria, [9] two of the 34 patients (5.9%) with abdominal pain and diarrhea and two of the 34 patients (5.9%) with abdominal pain and constipation met criteria for irritable bowel syndrome (IBS), two of the 34 patients (5.9%) with abdominal discomfort were considered functional bloating,

Table 1. Possible Drugs for a Dominant Symptom in Patients.

Symptom	Drug	Dose
Abdominal Pain	Pinaverium bromide	50 mg qd to qid ac
	Amitriptyline	Start 25–50 mg hs, then adjust
	Paroxetine hydrochloride	Start 20 mg hs, then adjust
Diarrhea	Loperamide	2–4 mg when necessary/maximum 12 mg/d
	Pinaverium bromide	50 mg qd to qid ac
Constipation	Lactulose syrup	10–20 g bid
	Polyethylene glycol	17 g in 8 oz water qd
	Mosapride	5 mg tid ac

qd, quaque die; bid, bis in die; qid, quater in die; hs, hora somni; ac, ante cibum; oz, ounce.

Table 2. Overall Relief Assessment.

Abdominal pain	
	0 = none (no symptoms)
	1 = mild (presence of symptoms but well-tolerated)
	2 = moderate (symptoms interfere with but do not prevent normal daily activities such as work and/or sleep)
	3 = severe (symptoms prevent normal daily activities such as work and/or sleep)
Stool frequency	
	the daily number of bowel movements was recorded
Stool consistency [8]	
	1 = separate hard lumps, like nuts
	2 = sausage-like, but lumpy
	3 = like a sausage but with cracks in the surface
	4 = like a sausage, smooth and soft
	5 = soft blobs with clear-cut edges
	6 = fluffy pieces with ragged edges, a mushy stool
	7 = watery, no solid pieces

one of the 34 patients (2.9%) with constipation was considered functional constipation, one of the 34 patients (2.9%) with diarrhea was considered functional diarrhea, two of the 34 patients (5.9%) with abdominal pain and diarrhea were considered unspecified functional bowel disorder.

Clinical Findings

Of the 34 patients, eight (23.5%) were eventually diagnosed with CD on follow-up, 14 (41.2%) achieved mucosal healing, and 12 (35.3%) showed no significant changes in the lesions. Of the 31 patients categorized as symptomatic (symptom onset at least 3 days per month in the last 3 months), eight (26%) had a clinical diagnosis of CD during the follow-up; the mean interval between the first visit and the appearance of typical CD symptoms was 2.0 years (range 1.0–4.0 years). Of the three patients categorized as asymptomatic (without symptom or symptom onset less than 3 days per month in the last 3 months), 2 (66.7%) achieved mucosal healing, and one (33.3%) showed no significant changes in the lesions.

Table 3. The Demographic Characteristics of the 34 Patients.

Sex (male:female)	19:15
Mean age at diagnosis (y)	33±11 (22–62)
Duration of follow-up (y)	3 (2–5)
Symptoms	
Abdominal pain	10 (29%)
Stools >3 times daily	9 (26%)
Abdominal pain and diarrhea	4 (12%)
Abdominal pain and constipation	2 (6%)
Positive occult blood test	2 (6%)
Mild abdominal discomfort	2 (6%)
Constipation	1 (3%)
Diarrhea	1 (3%)
Surveillance after colorectal polypectomy	3 (9%)
Colonoscopy	3±1 (2–5)

Of the 31 symptomatic patients, 29 (93.5%, 29/31) underwent drug therapy based on their dominant symptoms, 26 (89.7%, 26/29) attained recovery during the initial treatment period, 23 (88.5%, 23/26) experienced symptoms relapse during the withdrawal period, and 20 (87.0%, 20/23) attained recovery during the retreatment period.

Of the 12 patients who showed no significant changes in the lesions, all attained recovery during the initial treatment period, 10 (83.3%, 10/12) experienced symptom relapse during the withdrawal period, and nine (90.0%, 9/10) attained recovery during the retreatment period.

Endoscopic and Pathologic Findings

Normal mucosa was observed on the gastroscopies and radiological exams in the 34 patients.

All of the 34 patients underwent ileoscopy. On the initial colonoscopy exams, each case demonstrated one to several discrete, focal erosions within an otherwise normal small bowel mucosa. The erosions were located less than 5 cm proximal to the ileocecal valve. Most of the erosions were surrounded by normal or edematous mucosa and were covered by thin or faint exudates. (Fig. 1a, 1b, and 1c) The size of the erosions was estimated to be 2 to 3 mm. Of the 34 patients, 10 patients (29.4%) had a single erosion, and 24 patients (70.6%) had several erosions.

Of the eight patients with a clinical diagnosis of CD, typical longitudinal ulcerations existed in seven patients, irregular ulcerations existed in one patient (Fig. 2a and 2b), narrowing or stricture on imaging in four patients, perianal disease in one patient, and multiple episodes of small bowel obstruction in one patient.

The initial histologic findings in the patients included mucosal edema (7), erosions (8), acute or chronic inflammatory cells (11) and architectural alterations (3). The 8 patients with a final diagnosis of CD had non-caseating granulomas (3), architectural alterations (9) cryptitis (3), or focal chronic (lymphocytes and plasma cells) inflammation (7).

All of the patients responded to inflammatory bowel disease (IBD) treatments (1 patient was treated with infliximab and

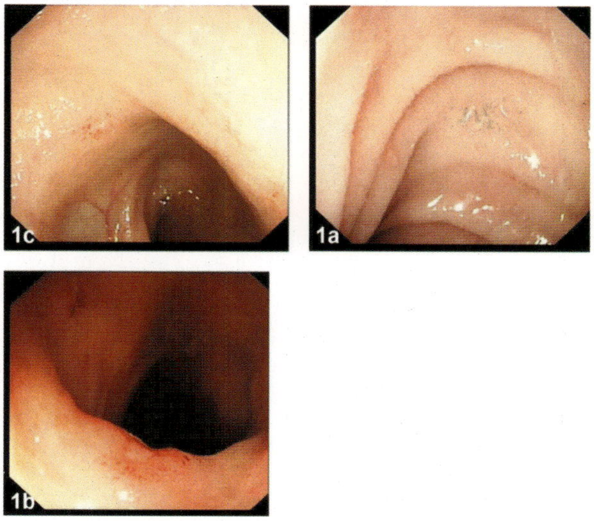

Figure 1. Initial colonoscopic images in the 34 patients. Erosions surrounded by normal mucosa (1a), edematous mucosa (1b), and covered by thin or faint exudates (1a, 1b, and 1c).

azathioprine, two patients were treated with azathioprine, and five patients were treated with 5-amino salicylic acid) and were still on maintenance therapy for CD at the most recent follow-up.

Clinical Symptoms and Outcomes

We conducted a logistic regression analysis to assess the factors associated with progression of isolated terminal ileal lesions in the 34 patients. The independent variables were age, sex, clinical symptoms, and duration of follow-up; the dependent variables were developing CD and mucosal healing. In this regression model, only abdominal pain was significantly associated with developing CD and mucosal healing (developing CD: OR 13.1 95% CI, 1.4–124.5, $P=0.025$; mucosal healing OR = 38.1 95% CI, 3.5–414.0, $P=0.003$).

The 34 patients were divided into an abdominal pain group and an non-abdominal pain group based on their clinical symptoms; the abdominal pain group contained 16 patients (10 patients with abdominal pain, four patients with abdominal pain and diarrhea, and two patients with abdominal pain and constipation), and the non-abdominal pain group contained 18 patients (nine patients with stools >3 times daily, two patients with positive occult blood tests, two patients with mild abdominal discomfort, three patients with surveillance after colorectal polypectomy, one patient with constipation, and one patient with diarrhea). In the abdominal pain group, seven patients were eventually diagnosed with CD on follow-up, Including two patients with IBS. The median interval between the first visit and the presentation of typical CD symptoms was 2 years (range 1–4 years). In the remaining nine patients with abdominal pain, eight showed no significant changes compared with their initial colonoscopic findings, and one patient achieved mucosal healing after anti-tuberculosis therapy for 9 months. In the non-abdominal pain group, 13 patients achieved mucosal healing. The median interval between the first visit and mucosal healing was 3 years (range 1–5 years). In the remaining five patients without abdominal pain, four showed no significant changes, and one patient with a positive occult blood test developed CD in the 3rd year of follow-up.

Of the 34 patients, sex and age were not significantly different between the abdominal pain and non-abdominal pain groups. The

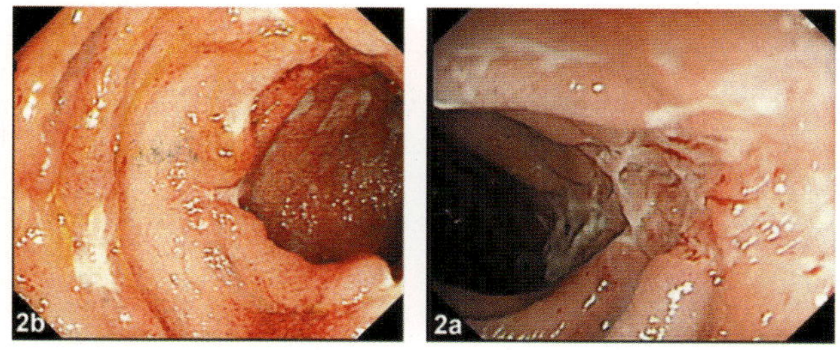

Figure 2. Colonoscopic images in the patients who developed CD. Typical longitudinal ulcerations of CD covered with mucous exudates (2a), and irregular ulcerations existed of CD covered with mucous exudates (2b). CD, Crohn's disease.

Kaplan–Meier method showed that the cumulative proportions of CD in the abdominal pain group in the 1st, 2nd, and 3rd years of follow-up were 6.2%, 31.2% and 42.7%, respectively, whereas in the non-abdominal pain group, the proportions were 0, 0, and 6.2%, respectively. The log-rank test showed that the cumulative proportion of CD in the abdominal pain group after 3 years was statistically higher than that in the non-abdominal pain group (42.7% *vs.* 6.2%, $\chi^2=10.129$, $P=0.001$). (Fig. 3) The cumulative proportions of mucosal healing in the non-abdominal pain group in the 1st, 2nd, 3rd, and 4th years of follow-up were 6.2%, 27.8%, 55.6% and 73.3%, respectively, whereas the proportions in the abdominal pain group were 5.6%, 5.6%, 5.6% and 5.6%, respectively. The cumulative proportion of mucosal healing in the non-abdominal pain group after 4 years was statistically higher

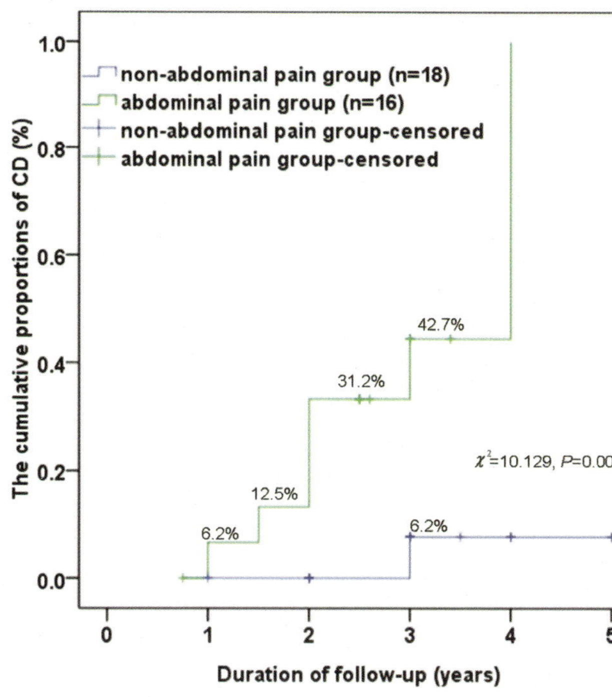

Figure 3. The cumulative proportions of CD in the 34 patients. The cumulative proportions of CD in the abdominal pain group in the 1st, 2nd, and 3rd years of follow-up were 6%, 31% and 43%, respectively, and the proportions in the non-abdominal pain group were 0, 0, and 6%, respectively. Moreover, the cumulative proportion of CD in the abdominal pain group after 3 years was statistically higher than that in the non-abdominal pain group (43% *vs.* 6%, $\chi^2=10.129$, $P=0.001$). CD, Crohn's disease.

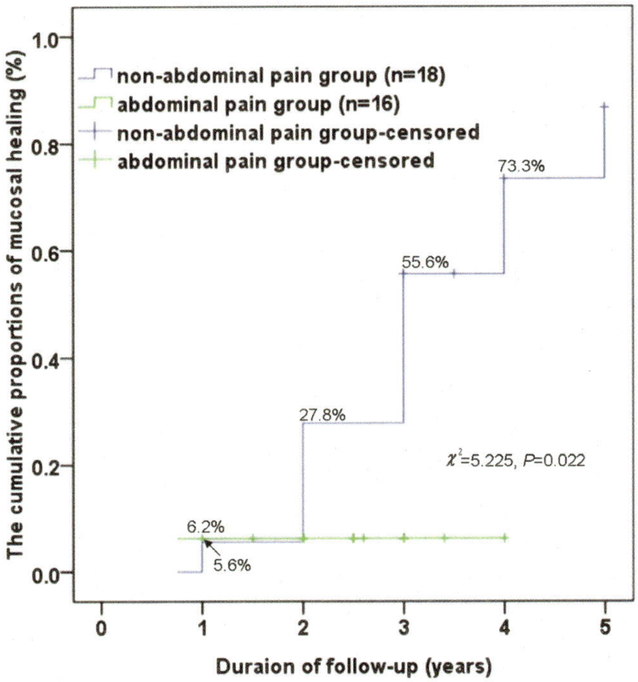

Figure 4. The cumulative proportions of mucosal healing in the 34 patients. The cumulative proportions of mucosal healing in the non-abdominal pain group in the 1st, 2nd, 3rd, and 4th years of follow-up were 6%, 28%, 56% and 73%, respectively, and the proportions in the abdominal pain group were 6%, 6%, 6% and 6%, respectively. Moreover, the cumulative proportion of mucosal healing in the non-abdominal pain group after 4 years was statistically higher than that in the abdominal pain group (73% *vs.* 6%, $\chi^2 = 5.225$, $P = 0.022$).

than that in the abdominal pain group (73% *vs.* 6%, $\chi^2 = 5.225$, $P = 0.022$). (Fig. 4)

Endoscopic Findings, Pathologic Findings and Outcomes

Next, we analyzed the association between the initial endoscopic findings and ITIL disease outcomes. We found that the numbers of lesions on the initial colonoscopy exams did not differ in the patients who were eventually diagnosed with CD on follow-up, achieved mucosal healing, and showed no significant changes in the lesions (2 (1–3) *vs.* 2.5 (1–3) *vs.* 2.5 (1–3), $\chi^2 = 1.252$, $P = 0.535$). Similarly, the initial histologic findings did not differ in these three groups (the proportion of patients with mucosal edema 25.0% (2/8) *vs.* 21.4% (3/14) *vs.*16.7% (2/12), $\chi^2 = 0.427$, $P = 1.000$; the proportion of patients with erosions 12.5% (1/8) *vs.* 21.4% (3/14) *vs.* 33.3% (4/12), $\chi^2 = 1.144$, $P = 0.678$; the proportion of patients with acute or chronic inflammatory cells 25.0% (2/8) *vs.* 50.0% (7/14) *vs.*16.7% (2/12), $\chi^2 = 3.304$, $P = 0.207$; and the proportion of patients with architectural alterations 12.5% (1/8) *vs.* 0 (0/14) *vs.* 16.7% (2/12), $\chi^2 = 2.543$, $P = 0.317$).

Discussion

Through a prospective study, we aimed to assess the factors associated with progression of ITILs in 34 Chinese patients.

ITILs are not uncommonly seen during routine screening colonoscopy, the frequency was about 0.1–0.3% and 0.1% (34/32,197) in this study. [4,5] The clinical significance of the ITILs is unclear. Goldstein et al. reported that eight of 28 patients (28.6%) developed typical CD at an average interval of 3.6 years. [7] Then, Courville et al. reported that 10 of 29 patients (34.5%) developed typical CD at an average interval of 2.2 to 12.6 years. [10] A recent study by Chang et al. reported that 1 of 93 patients (1.1%) developed typical CD at an average interval of 29.9 months. [4] Conversely, Lengeling et al. reported that 40 patients identified with "ulcerative ileitis" at ileocolonoscopy had no specific disease process development in a median follow-up of 3.2 years. [5] In this study, 23.5% of the patients were eventually diagnosed with CD on follow-up, and 41.2% of the patients achieved mucosal healing. The lower probability of achieving mucosal healing in this study could have been the result of the patients with different clinical symptoms, different follow-up lengths, and racial differences.

Aphthoid or small erosions have been considered one of the earliest manifestations of CD. Two previous studies showed that 44% (4/9) and 50% (5/10) of patients with aphthous-type CD later developed typical CD. [11,12] More recent studies have shown that the disease outcomes of ITILs are related to the clinical symptoms of patients. A study by Goldstein et al. reported that all 8 patients (29%) with ITILs who had developed CD on follow-up presented with abdominal pain, mucus-rich, blood-tinged stools; irregular bowel function with intermittent constipation and diarrhea; and low-level systemic malaise. [7] Recently, a study by Courville et al. reported that 10 of 15 (66.7%) symptomatic patients, and 0 of 14 asymptomatic patients had developed CD at the most recent follow-up. [10] Our findings are similar in those patients undergoing colonoscopy for symptoms; eight of 31 (26%) symptomatic patients and zero of three asymptomatic patients had developed CD during the follow-up. We conducted a logistic regression analysis and found that only abdominal pain was significantly associated with developing CD. Further analysis showed that the cumulative proportion of CD in the abdominal pain group after 3 years was statistically higher than that in the non-abdominal pain group.

Should patients with ITILs be treated? Two studies reported that isolated terminal ileal ulcerations completely resolved without any treatment on follow-up colonoscopy in 66.7% of asymptomatic patients (four of six patients and 62 of 93 patients, respectively). [4,10] In this present study, two of the three (66.7%) asymptomatic patients completely resolved without inflammatory bowel disease-related treatment. We conducted a logistic regression analysis and found that only abdominal pain was significantly associated with mucosal healing. Further analysis showed that the cumulative proportion of mucosal healing in the non-abdominal pain group was statistically higher than that in the abdominal pain group. Our findings suggest that these patients in the non-abdominal pain group do not warrant any inflammatory bowel disease-related treatment, and a wait and watch approach seems to be the most prudent at the present time.

A study by Courville et al. reported that the endoscopic and histopathological findings in patients with asymptomatic ileitis closely mimicked those observed in CD, but these patients did not progress to overt CD on long-term follow-up. [10] A recent study by Chang et al. reported that the proportion of patients with ulcerations <5 mm in diameter was not significantly different between the 60 patients showing isolated terminal ileal ulcerations resolution without treatment and the 31 patients with continued isolated terminal ileal ulcerations on follow-up. [4] Similar to these reports, we found that the numbers of lesions on the initial colonoscopy exams were not related to the ITIL disease outcomes. Similarly, the initial histologic findings were not related to the ITIL disease outcomes. Thus, the endoscopic or histopathological findings may not be useful in predicting the disease outcomes in patients with ITILs.

Irregular bowel movements, pain or bloating may coexist in a considerable number of IBD patients, which were present in 35.4–46% of CD patients and 37.5% (3/8) in this study. [13,14] There is uncertainty as to the aetiology of these apparent functional symptoms in IBD patients. Genetic factors, disordered gut permeability, psychosocial stress, or a persistent increase in TNF-α or mucosal pain receptor in colonic mucosa may contribute to these symptoms. [14–21] A previous study by Keohane et al. found that faecal calprotectin levels were helpful to identify CD patients with IBS-type symptoms. [22] Then, a study by Berrill et al. found a conflicting result. [23] However, a systematic diagnostic approach is required to assess IBD patients with IBS-type symptoms as sub-clinical inflammation may play a role in a proportion of cases. [23]

Calprotectin is an abundant calcium-binding protein that is derived predominantly from neutrophils and, to a lesser extent, from monocytes and reactive macrophages. [24] The presence of calprotectin in faeces is directly proportional to neutrophil migration towards the intestinal tract. [25–27] Two studies by Tibble and Carroccio et al. found that approximately half of patients with active celiac disease had elevated fecal calprotectin concentrations. [28,29] Another study by Berni et al examined a total of 38 children with celiac disease. They found that those patients with active celiac disease had elevated fecal calprotectin concentrations compared with healthy control subjects and that there was a trend toward normal values after 4 weeks of an exclusion diet. [30] However, the specificity for the diagnosis of ITILs should be low, as several diseases such IBD, microscopic colitis, allergic colitis, colorectal neoplasia, gastrointestinal infection and chronic diarrhea can also increase faecal calprotectin. [29,31–34] High concentration of calprotectin in faeces is a strong argument to carry out a colonoscopy in order to rule out the presence of IBD or other organic pathologies. Maybe faecal calprotectin is useful during the follow-up on ITILs.

In conclusion, the results of this study suggest that the ITIL disease outcomes are related to the clinical symptoms. ITILs are likely to develop into CD in patients with abdominal pain but are likely to resolve in patients without abdominal pain. It should be noted that all patients underwent gastroscopy and double contrast small bowel radiography instead of MRI, or videocapsule to evaluate their upper gastrointestinal and small intestinal mucosa, so subtle small bowel lesions may be missed diagnosis in these patients. Our study is limited by the small number of patients. Larger prospective studies are needed to confirm these initial findings. It remains unclear whether ITILs should be treated with 5-aminosalicylates or corticosteroids in patients with abdominal pain. Thus, further randomized, double-blind, placebo-controlled studies in large cohorts of subjects are needed to verify this question.

Author Contributions

Conceived and designed the experiments: ZF HW CY. Performed the experiments: ZF ZW XF. Analyzed the data: ZF HW. Contributed reagents/materials/analysis tools: ZF ZC CY. Wrote the paper: ZF ZC.

References

1. McHugh JB, Appelman HD, McKenna BJ (2007) The diagnostic value of endoscopic terminal ileum biopsies. Am J Gastroenterol 102:1084–1089.
2. Geboes K, Ectors N, D'Haens G, Rutgeerts P (1998) Is ileoscopy with biopsy worthwhile in patients presenting with symptoms of inflammatory bowel disease? Am J Gastroenterol 93:201–206.
3. Geboes K (2007) The strategy for biopsies of the terminal ileum should be evidence based. Am J Gastroenterol 102:1090–1092.
4. Chang HS, Lee D, Kim JC, Song HK, Lee HJ, et al. (2010) Isolated terminal ileal ulcerations in asymptomatic individuals: natural course and clinical significance. Gastrointest Endosc 72:1226–1232.
5. Lengeling RW, Mitros FA, Brennan JA, Schulze KS (2003) Ulcerative ileitis encountered at ileo-colonoscopy: likely role of nonsteroidal agents. Clin Gastroenterol Hepatol 1:160–169.
6. Greaves ML, Pochapin M (2006) Asymptomatic ileitis: past, present, and future. J Clin Gastroenterol 40:281–285.
7. Goldstein NS (2006) Isolated ileal erosions in patients with mildly altered bowel habits. A follow-up study of 28 patients. Am J Clin Pathol 125:838–846.
8. O'Donnell LJD, Virjee J, Heaton KW (1990) Detection of pseudodiarrhea by simple clinical assessment of intestinal transit rate. BMJ 300: 439–440.
9. Longstreth GF, Thompson WG, Chey WD, Houghton LA, Mearin F, Spiller RC (2006) Functional bowel disorders. Gastroenterology 130:1480–1491.
10. Courville EL, Siegel CA, Vay T, Wilcox AR, Suriawinata AA, Srivastava A (2009) Isolated asymptomatic ileitis does not progress to overt Crohn disease on long-term follow-up despite features of chronicity in ileal biopsies. Am J Surg Pathol 33:1341–1347.
11. Hizawa K, Iida M, Kohrogi N, Kuroki F, Yao T, et al. (1994) Crohn disease: early recognition and progress of aphthous lesions. Radiology 190:451–454.
12. Matsumoto T, Iida M, Nakamura S, Hizawa K, Yao T, Fujishima M (2000) Crohn's disease of aphthous type: serial changes in intestinal lesions. Br J Radiol 73:1046–1051.
13. Halpin SJ, Ford AC (2012) Prevalence of symptoms meeting criteria for irritable bowel syndrome in inflammatory bowel disease: systematic review and meta-analysis. Am J Gastroenterol 107:1474–1482.
14. Vivinus-Nébot M, Frin-Mathy G, Bzioueche H, Dainese R, Bernard G, et al. (2013) Functional bowel symptoms in quiescent inflammatory bowel diseases: role of epithelial barrier disruption and low-grade inflammation. Gut [Epub ahead of print]
15. Zucchelli M, Camilleri M, Andreasson AN, Bresso F, Dlugosz A, et al. (2011) Association of TNFSF15 polymorphism with irritable bowel syndrome. Gut 60:1671–1677.
16. Villani AC, Lemire M, Thabane M, Belisle A, Geneau G, et al. (2010) Genetic risk factors for post-infectious irritable bowel syndrome following a waterborne outbreak of gastroenteritis. Gastroenterology 138:1502–1513.
17. Porter CK, Gloor K, Cash BD, Riddle MS (2011) Risk of functional gastrointestinal disorders in U.S. military following self-reported diarrhea and vomiting during deployment. Dig Dis Sci 56:3262–3269.
18. Zhou Q, Zhang B, Verne GN (2009) Intestinal membrane permeability and hypersensitivity in the irritable bowel syndrome. Pain 146:41–46.
19. Singh S, Graff LA, Bernstein CN (2009) Do NSAIDs, antibiotics, infections, or stress trigger flares in IBD? Am J Gastroenterol 104:1298–1313.
20. Spiller R, Garsed K (2009) Postinfectious irritable bowel syndrome. Gastroenterology 136:1979–1988.
21. Akbar A, Yiangou Y, Facer P, Brydon WG, Walters JR, et al. (2010) Expression of the TRPV1 receptor differs in quiescent inflammatory bowel disease with or without abdominal pain. Gut 59:767–774.
22. Keohane J, O'Mahony C, O'Mahony L, O'Mahony S, Quigley EM, Shanahan F (2010) Irritable bowel syndrome-type symptoms in patients with inflammatory bowel disease: a real association or reflection of occult inflammation? Am J Gastroenterol 105:1788, 1789–1794.
23. Berrill JW, Green JT, Hood K, Campbell AK (2013) Symptoms of irritable bowel syndrome in patients with inflammatory bowel disease: examining the role of sub-clinical inflammation and the impact on clinical assessment of disease activity. Aliment Pharmacol Ther 38:44–51.
24. Bjerke K, Halstensen TS, Jahnsen F, Pulford K, Brandtzaeg P (1993) Distribution of macrophages and granulocytes expressing L1 protein (calprotectin) in human Peyer's patches compared with normal ileal lamina propria and mesenteric lymph nodes. Gut 34:1357–1363.
25. Vermeire S, Van Assche G, Rutgeerts P (2006) Laboratory markers in IBD: useful, magic, or unnecessary toys? Gut 55:426–431.
26. Vermeire S, Van Assche G, Rutgeerts P (2004) C-reactive protein as a marker for inflammatory bowel disease. Inflamm Bowel Dis 10:661–665.
27. Vermeire S, Van Assche G, Rutgeerts P (2005) The role of C-reactive protein as an inflammatory marker in gastrointestinal diseases. Nat Clin Pract Gastroenterol Hepatol 2:580–586.
28. Tibble JA, Sigthorsson G, Foster R, Forgacs I, Bjarnason I (2002) Use of surrogate markers of inflammation and Rome criteria to distinguish organic from nonorganic intestinal disease. Gastroenterology 123:450–460.
29. Carroccio A, Iacono G, Cottone M, Di Prima L, Cartabellotta Fe, et al. (2003) Diagnostic accuracy of fecal calprotectin assay in distinguishing organic causes of chronic diarrhea from irritable bowel syndrome: a prospective study in adults and children. Clin Chem 49(6 Pt 1):861–867.
30. Berni Canani R, Rapacciuolo L, Romano MT, Tanturri de Horatio L, Terrin G, et al. (2004) Diagnostic value of faecal calprotectin in paediatric gastroenterology clinical practice. Dig Liver Dis 36:467–470.
31. Tibble J, Teahon K, Thjodleifsson B, Roseth A, Sigthorsson G, et al. (2000) A simple method for assessing intestinal inflammation in Crohn's disease. Gut 47:506–513.

Use of Antibiotics within the IMCI Guidelines in Outpatient Settings in Papua New Guinean Children: An Observational and Effectiveness Study

Nicolas Senn[1,2,3,4*], Patricia Rarau[1], Mary Salib[1], Doris Manong[1], Peter Siba[1], Stephen Rogerson[4], Ivo Mueller[1,5,6❡], Blaise Genton[2,3❡]

1 Vector Born Unit, PNG Institute of Medical Research, Madang (MAD), Papua New Guinea, **2** Health Intervention Unit, Swiss Tropical and Public Health Institute, Basel (BS), Switzerland, **3** University of Basel, Basel (BS), Switzerland, **4** Department of Medicine, University of Melbourne, Melbourne, Australia, **5** Dept. of Infections & Immunity, Walter & Eliza Hall Institute of Medical Research, Melbourne, Australia, **6** Centre de Recerca en Salut Internacional de Barcelona (CRESIB), Barcelona, Spain

Abstract

Introduction: There is a need to investigate the effectiveness and appropriateness of antibiotics prescription within the Integrated Management of Childhood Illness (IMCI) strategy in the context of routine outpatient clinics.

Methods: Making use of a passive case detection system established for a malaria prevention trial in outpatient clinics in Papua New Guinea, the appropriateness and effectiveness of the use of antibiotics within the IMCI was assessed in 1605 young children. Main outcomes were prescription of antibiotics and re-attendances within 14 days for mild pneumonia, mild diarrhoea and uncomplicated malaria whether they were managed with or without antibiotics (proxy of effectiveness). Appropriateness was assessed for both mild and severe cases, while effectiveness was assessed only for mild diseases.

Results: A total of 6975 illness episodes out of 8944 fulfilled inclusion criteria (no previous attendance <14 days+full medical records). Clinical incidence rates (episodes/child/year; 95% CI) were 0.85 (0.81–0.90) for pneumonia, 0.62 (0.58–0.66) for malaria and 0.72 (0.65–0.93) for diarrhoea. Fifty three percent of 6975 sick children were treated with antibiotics, 11% were not treated with antibiotics when they should have been and in 29% antibiotics were prescribed when they should not have been. Re-attendance rates within 14 days following clinical diagnosis of mild pneumonia were 9% (126/1401) when managed with antibiotics compared to 8% (56/701) when managed without (adjusted Hazard Ratio (aHR) = 1.00 (0.57–1.76), p = 0.98). Rates for mild diarrhoea were 8% (73/874) and 9% (79/866) respectively (aHR = 0.8 (0.42–1.57), p = 0.53).

Conclusion: Non-adherence to IMCI recommendations for prescription of antibiotics is common in routine settings in Papua New Guinea. Although recommended, the use of antibiotics in young children with mild pneumonia as defined by IMCI criteria did not impact on their outcome. Better tools and new strategies for the identification of bacterial infections that require antibiotics are urgently needed.

Editor: Delmiro Fernandez-Reyes, National Institute of Medical Research, United Kingdom

Funding: Nicolas Senn is supported by an academic "bridge-relève" scholarship provided by the Leenaards Foundation (Lausanne, Switzerland). The funders had no role in study design, data collection and analysis, decision to publish, or preparation of the manuscript.

Competing Interests: The authors can otherwise confirm that the fact that Ivo Mueller (co-author).

* E-mail: nicolas.senn@gmail.com

❡ These authors contributed equally to this work.

Introduction

Worldwide, the leading causes of death in children under five years (excluding perinatal mortality) are pneumonia, diarrhoea and malaria. These three diseases are responsible for an estimated 5 million deaths yearly, over 90% of which occur in Africa and other developing countries with limited resources. [1] [2] At a community level and in outpatient settings, the few available studies show that pneumonia, diarrhoea and malaria are similarly responsible for a high burden of morbidity in developing countries [3,4,5,6,7].

For decades, a high importance was given to malaria as a cause of fever, which has led to an overestimation of its burden and at the same time an underestimation of other diseases. [8,9] Nowadays, case management strategy of sick children under five years in developing countries is usually based on clinical presentation of diseases (syndromes) rather than on aetiologies, as recommended by the World Health Organization (WHO), which developed the Integrated Management of Childhood Illness (IMCI) guidelines for this purpose. [10] The syndromic approach has some limitations such as the potential overlap of signs and symptoms between different diseases. [11,12,13] It remains unclear whether this overlap of signs/symptoms is because children are commonly infected with multiple pathogens, or because distinct diseases present with the same clinical picture [11,12].

Although the IMCI strategy has been used for more than 20 years, few studies have investigated its effectiveness and appropriateness. Specifically, there is limited information on how well health workers comply with IMCI guidelines in routine practice, and on the impact of IMCI recommendations on health outcomes. [14,15] Although most experts agree that the introduction of IMCI has improved the quality of care at limited cost, [16] IMCI has however some limitations such as the absence of objective diagnostic tools or no consideration of the local epidemiology. All may result in low specificity of IMCI algorithms, especially to identify bacterial infections that require antibiotics. [3,15,16,17,18,19,20] Therefore, many children might receive unnecessary antibiotics. Furthermore, it still remains debated how many children who receive antibiotics prescribed according to IMCI recommendations benefit from them. For example, a study from Pakistan demonstrated that children with mild pneumonia did not benefit from antibiotics. [21] This study was conducted in controlled conditions with defined inclusion and exclusion criteria. No study investigated the accuracy of diagnosis and the impact of appropriate treatment on health outcomes in routine practice.

Papua New Guinea (PNG) has a high burden of malaria in coastal areas, while pneumonia is the leading cause of admission in children under five years nationally. [22,23,24] Case management of sick children is almost exclusively syndrome-based using IMCI guidelines. In outpatient settings, few diagnostic tools are available and until 2011 microscopy or RDTs were rarely available in health facilities to confirm malaria infections. Thus, presumptive treatments with antimalarials and/or antibiotics are prescribed to cover common diseases such as pneumonia, malaria or otitis media. In PNG, as in many places, no data are available on the performance of the IMCI strategy in outpatient settings.

As part of a trial on malaria prevention, a passive case detection system was set up to record illness episodes in all study participants aged 3 to 27 months. All illness episodes were managed in accordance with the PNG IMCI guidelines, except for malaria, where treatment was guided by RDT instead of using presumptive diagnosis. [25] This study provides therefore a unique opportunity to investigate the appropriateness and effectiveness of antibiotics prescribed within IMCI.

Methods

This work was carried out alongside a 3-arm trial of Intermittent Preventive Treatment for malaria in infants (IPTi) that included 1605 children 3–27 months old from June 2006 to June 2010 (www.ClinicalTrials.gov: NCT00285662) [26].

Study Sites and Population

The study took place in two regions of PNG: Mugil (Madang Province) with 1125 study participants and in the Wosera (East Sepik Province) with 480 study participants. Each study site included approximately 20 villages, serviced by four major health centres: Mugil and Alexishafen in Madang area, and Kunjingini and Kaugia in Wosera. Several aid posts were also used for the morbidity surveillance. All IPTi preventive treatments were given at time of routine vaccination at 3, 6 and 9 months or of Vitamin A supplementation at 12 months following the PNG national expanded programme of immunization.

The study was carried out in accordance with Good Clinical Practice (GCP) and monitored by an independent external monitor. The study was approved by the PNG Medical Research Advisory Committee (MRAC number 05.20). Parents or carers were asked to fill a written consent form prior to enrolment of their child in the trial.

Children enrolled in the trial were randomly allocated to receive placebo or two different antimalarial drug regimes [sulphadoxine/pyrimethamine (single dose) with either 3 days of amodiaquine (SP-AQ3) or 3 days of artesunate (SP-AS3)]. The primary objective of the trial was the determination of the protective effect of the two IPTi regimens on malaria episodes.

Morbidity Surveillance

Throughout the trial, a passive case detection system was maintained at the four study health centres' outpatient clinics as well as at four aid posts to assure a continuous morbidity surveillance of study participants. This means that parents of study participants were asked to attend the study clinics free of charge for clinical management whenever their child was sick. They were seen by study nurses, often in collaboration with the health centre's staff. No active follow-up of study participants was performed for acute diseases (such as regular home visits). In that perspective, this approach is more likely to reflect routine practice in PNG and thus avoid overestimation of the burden of diseases. The passive surveillance records collected were used to perform the present analysis.

Each illness episode was assessed by study staff using a standard case report form. Main signs and symptoms were systematically recorded using tick boxes. In case of history of fever in the past 48 hours or an axillary temperature >37.5°C, a RDT for malaria (ICT Combo®, South Africa) was performed and haemoglobin (Hb) level measured using a portable Hemocue 201® machine (Angelholm, Sweden). Malaria treatment decision was based on the RDT result, and only children with a positive result were treated with artemether/lumefantrine, irrespective of the species. The children with moderate to severe anaemia (Hb<8 g/dl) received iron supplementation at the dose of 5 mg/Kg of ferrous sulphate for 6 weeks. Pulse oximetry was implemented in December 2007 in Mugil study clinic (Madang site) and used systematically to assess sick study participants from that date onwards. It was recommended to clinical staff that they should consider admitting the child if oxygen saturation dropped below 94%. All other illnesses were treated according to the standard treatment guidelines of PNG, which is based on IMCI. [27] Children were also assessed for danger signs or symptoms and referred to the health centre for admission when necessary. If children attended the health centre when study staff were not on duty, they received care from the regular health centre nursing staff. As they did not have the capacity to perform RDTs or other blood tests, treatment was delivered on presumptive diagnosis only. On site, study nurses recorded their presumptive diagnosis and provided treatment. All records were cross-checked by the study clinicians who confirmed the likely diagnosis. Both study nurses and clinicians could record as many as 3 different diagnoses for each episode.

A severe disease was defined as an illness episode with potential life-threatening features such as respiratory distress (nasal flaring or chest indrawing), impaired consciousness or severe pallor. At least one danger sign or symptom needed to be present for an episode to be classified as severe disease. A child with criteria for severe disease was not necessarily admitted for the following reasons: parents refused admission; health staff decided not to admit the child according to their personal judgment or because they did not identified properly danger signs and symptoms.

Study Staff

The medical staff was composed of about 20 nurses and community health workers (CHW). They were specifically trained for malaria and anaemia management in line with the trial's requirements (diagnosis and treatment). [26] For all other diseases (e.g. pneumonia, diarrhoea or otitis media), they were asked to follow the national recommendations. No specific training was provided for IMCI, except a broad refresher training of one day per year on the basic management of sick children, including measurement of respiratory rate, evaluation of danger signs and key features of IMCI. Therefore, the care provided for non-malarial illness episodes was very close to what is usually performed in government health facilities, except that there was no shortage of drugs and consumables.

Laboratory Procedures

A finger prick blood sample was used to perform a rapid diagnostic test (RDT) for malaria on site (to guide malaria treatment) and to record haemoglobin concentration. A blood slide was prepared for expert microscopy that was performed elsewhere.

Coding of Diagnosis and Treatments

Using records of signs and symptoms (tick boxes) of the passive case detection forms, objective diagnoses were generated by computer according to IMCI definitions of diseases (e.g. mild pneumonia = cough and/or difficulties in breathing+respiratory rate >50 if <1 year or respiratory rate >40 if >1 year without sign/symptom of severity). For the present study, three diseases were explored with different levels of severity according to IMCI: 1) mild and moderate-to-severe pneumonia, 2) mild and severe diarrhoea and 3) uncomplicated and severe malaria. **Table 1** displays the detailed definitions of the different syndromes based on IMCI criteria. We use the terminology of the PNG-specific IMCI guidelines that was in use at the time of the study. **Table 1** includes the correspondence with the WHO-IMCI classification.

Ten distinct treatment categories were created: 1) artemether/lumefantrine, 2) iron+folic acid, 3) albendazole, 4) amoxicillin, 5) co-trimoxazole, 6) paracetamol, 7) tinidazole, 8) other antibiotics (erythromycin, benzylpenicillin im, chloramphenicol and ceftriaxone iv/im), 9) other antimalarial drugs (artemether, quinine, amodiaquine, sulphadoxine/pyrimethamine, chloroquine, 10) other drugs.

Study Procedure

Illness episodes were included in the study if they fulfilled the following inclusion criteria:

- IPTi study participant
- No illness episode in the past 14 days (to avoid counting the same episode twice)
- Full clinical records (signs and symptoms available)

The appropriateness of the prescription of antibiotics by health staff was assessed for main diagnoses according to the IMCI recommendations, including both severe and mild disease episodes.

The effectiveness of antibiotics was investigated for mild diseases only, by calculating the rate of re-attendance within 14 days and the outcome upon re-attendance (death, severe illness or mild disease) for specific syndromes depending whether they were treated with antibiotics or not. Severe cases were excluded from this analysis for several reasons: i) severe cases (i.e. with danger signs) had to be admitted according to recommendations and managed systematically with intravenous antimalarial and antibiotics irrespective of the symptoms and signs; ii) the low prevalence of severe cases, which are almost all treated with antibiotics, prevent the investigation of the effectiveness because of the absence of a valid control group; iii) re-attendance rates was used as a proxy for effectiveness, but this is not a valid measure for assessing effectiveness in severe cases, as they should be all admitted in the first place and would therefore not re-attend; iv) there is no debate yet on the benefit of treating all severe cases with antibiotics.

This analysis was possible as syndromes were not necessarily correctly identified by health staff and therefore some children did not receive antibiotics when they should have.

Statistical Analysis

All data were double entered using FoxPro software. Data analyses were performed using STATA software (version 12.0). More than one diagnosis was possible for each illness episode. Incidence rates were calculated using a negative binomial regression model. Cox regression model was used to calculate hazard ratios for the impact of antibiotics on pneumonia, diarrhoea and malaria (excluding severe diseases). The model was adjusted for potential confounders (markers of severity of respiratory infections): respiratory rate (continuous), temperature (continuous) and pulse oximetry (continuous). Kaplan-Meier survival curves were also calculated and displayed as time to first re-attendance over a 14-day observation period following an initial pneumonia, malaria or diarrhoea. All rates are displayed with a confidence interval of 95%. Differences between rates were assessed using a chi square test.

Results

Baseline Characteristics

Out of 1605 children 1512 (94%) presented at least 1 illness episode (Madang = 1053 and Maprik = 459). The morbidity surveillance recorded a total of 8943 illness episodes (Madang = 5977 and Maprik = 2966). Three hundred seventy one severe illnesses and 13 deaths occurred during the study. Overall, 2903 illness episodes occurred in the placebo group, compared to 3038 in the SP-AQ group and 3002 in the SP-AS arm.

Inclusion criteria were fulfilled for 6975 illness episodes (no visit in the previous 14 days and full medical records available). **Table 2** displays the danger signs and symptoms, clinical and laboratory features. As shown, 80% of the illness episodes presented with fever/history of fever and 76% had cough. No significant difference was observed between the different IPTi treatment groups (data not shown).

Description of Main Diseases According to IMCI Criteria and their Incidence Rates

Out of the 6975 illness episodes, 76.5% (5335) were ARI, including 44.7% (3116) URTI, 30.1% (2102) mild pneumonia and 1.7% (117) severe pneumonia. 25.6% (1788) had diarrhoea, including 24.9% (1740) mild diarrhoea and 0.7% (48) severe diarrhoea. 25.1% (1750) had malaria, including 23.6% (1643) uncomplicated malaria and 1.5% (107) severe malaria. 10.2% (710) could not be classified in one of these syndromes. In this category, there were mainly children with running nose as single symptom (which cannot be classified as URTI according to IMCI), skin infections and fever without any other accompanying symptom.

The incidence rates (IR, episode/child/year) were 0.85 (95% CI, 0.81–0.90) for mild pneumonia, 0.72 (95% CI, 0.65–0.93) for

Table 1. Definition of diseases (including the use of RDT for malaria).

	Criteria	Standard treatment	WHO IMCI terminology
Respiratory infections			
Acute Respiratory Infection (ARI)	Cough and/or difficulties in breathing		**ARI**
Upper Respiratory Tract Infection (URTI)	Cough and/or difficulties in breathing AND RR<50 (<1 Y) RR<40 (>1 y) AND No respiratory distress (chest indrawing, cyanosis, nasal flaring)	Paracetamol	**no pneumonia/cough and cold**
All pneumonia	Cough and/or difficulties in breathing AND RR>50 (<1 Y) RR>40 (>1 y)		**n/a**
mild pneumonia	Cough and/or difficulties in breathing AND RR>50 (<1 Y) RR>40 (>1 y) AND No respiratory distress (chest indrawing, cyanosis, nasal flaring)	Amoxicillin 5 days	**non-severe pneumonia**
Severe pneumonia	Cough and/or difficulties in breathing AND RR>50 (<1 Y) RR>40 (>1 y) AND Respiratory distress (chest indrawing, cyanosis, nasal flaring)	Benzylpenicillin im or chloramphenicol im 10 days, admit	**severe and very severe pneumonia**
Diarrhoea			
All diarrhoea	Diarrhoea and/or vomit		**n/a**
Mild diarrhoea	Diarrhoea and/or vomit AND No dehydration (slow skin pinch, sunken eyes)	more hydration+breast feed	**No or some dehydration**
Severe diarrhoea	Diarrhoea and/or vomit AND dehydration (slow skin pinch, sunken eyes)	ORS or iv fluid +/− admit	**severe dehydration**
Malaria			
All malaria	Fever and/or history of fever in past 48 h AND positive RDT (any species)		**n/a**
Uncomplicated malaria	Fever and/or history of fever in past 48 h AND positive RDT (any species AND No danger sign	Artemether/ lumefantrine for 3 days	**n/a**
Severe malaria	Fever and/or history of fever in past 48 h AND positive RDT (any species) AND At least one danger sign	Artemether im+ sulfadoxine/ Pyrimethamine+admit	**n/a**

mild diarrhoea and 0.62 (95% CI, 0.58–0.66) for uncomplicated malaria. No differences were found in the incidence of non-malarial illnesses between the placebo and IPTi intervention arms. Indeed, incidence rates for all pneumonia in children 3–15 months old were very similar in all arms with 0.97 (95% CI, 0.89–1.06) in the placebo group, 1.00 (95% CI, 0.92–1.09) in the SP-AQ3 group and 0.98 (95% CI, 0.90–1.07) in the SP-AR3 group, p-values for incidence rate ratios (IRR) were 0.63 and 0.87 respectively. For diarrhoea (severe included), the incidence rates from 3–15 months were similar in all arms with: 0.94 (95% CI, 0.86–1.02) for placebo, 0.92 (95% CI, 0.84–1.0) for SP-AQ3 and 0.89 (95% CI, 0.81–0.99) for SP-AS3, p-values for IRR were 0.85 and 0.51 respectively. By contrast, the IPTi has proven to be effective on malaria as described elsewhere. Main results showed that the incidence of clinical malaria between the first dose at 3 months and 15 months was 0.85 per year-at-risk overall and 0.22 and 0.68 for P. falciparum and P. vivax, respectively. In the intention-to-treat analyses, the protective efficacy against all cases of malaria was 29% ([95% CI, 0.10, 0.43], p = <0.001) in the SP-AQ3 group and 12% ([95% CI, −0.11, 0.30], p = 0.12) in the SP-AS3 group [26].

Use of Antibiotics and Appropriateness of Prescription

Out of the 6975 illness episodes, 53.6% (3741) were treated with antibiotics (at least one of amoxicillin, co-trimoxazole, erythromycin or i.m. penicillin or ceftriaxone) and 25.1% (1750) received antimalarial drugs (97.6% of whom had a positive RDT result). Among the children who were treated for mild pneumonia with antibiotics, 69% received amoxicillin only, 9% received co-trimoxazole only, 16% received other antibiotics and 6% received a combination of amoxicillin and other antibiotics.

The overall appropriateness of antibiotics use was evaluated in 6969 illness episodes for which clear recommendations exist in the IMCI whether to prescribe or not antibiotics. According to these data, 40% of children were not treated appropriately, of whom 11% did not receive antibiotics when they should have and 29% received antibiotics when they should not have. (**Figure 1**).

Among the 2102 children with an objective diagnosis of mild pneumonia, 66.7% (1401) received (appropriately) antibiotics. Of 532 children who presented with criteria for both mild pneumonia and uncomplicated malaria (based on positive RDT), only 40% (213) were prescribed antibiotics. In contrast, when they had criteria for pneumonia only (without malaria), 75.7% (1188/1569) were prescribed antibiotics ($p<0.001$). Among 117 children with a diagnosis of severe pneumonia, 96.6% (113) received antibiotics, of whom 75.2% (88) were treated with parenteral antibiotics as per WHO guidelines and 49.6% (58) were admitted.

Effectiveness of Antibiotics for Mild Pneumonia, Uncomplicated Malaria and Mild Diarrhoea

Re-attendance rate within 14 days following an objective diagnosis of mild pneumonia (IMCI criteria) was 9% when treated with antibiotics compared to 8% when they did not receive any antibiotics, unadjusted Hazard Ratio (HR) was 1.09 (95% CI 0.80–1.49, p = 0.59). For uncomplicated malaria, re-attendance rates were 4% when they received antibiotics vs 6% when they did not [HR 0.66 (95% CI 0.39–1.10, p = 0.11)]. For diarrhoea,

Table 2. Clinical and paraclinical features of 6975 illness episodes.

	%	(N)
Danger signs		
Unable to eat	0.6	44
Vomit everything	0.5	38
Unconscious/drowsy	1.4	95
Respiratory distress	1.7	117
Fits	0.8	58
Inability to sit up	0.2	12
Neck stifness	0.1	8
Severe Dehydration	0.7	49
Pale with heart rate >160 or oedema	0.2	17
Main signs, symptoms		
Fever (temp>37.5°/hist of fev)	80.3	5603
Palor	2.7	185
Cough	76.4	5332
Difficulties in breathing	14.9	1037
Running nose	46.2	3207
Diarrhoea	21.1	1474
Abdominal pain	2.7	191
Vomit	10.2	713
Ear pain	0.6	44
Skin rash	0.3	13
Skin abscess	1	67
Pus out of the ear	2.6	183
Respiratory rate >50	19.9	1390
Laboratory findings		
Pulse O2<94%	3.4	54*
Pulse O2<93%	2.7	42*
Mean Hb level (g/L)	9.6	–
Hb <8 g/L	11.1	626**

*only 1582 records with pulse oxymetry measured.
**only 5644 records with Hb measured.

re-attendance rates were 8% when they received antibiotics and 9% when they did not [HR 0.85 (95% CI 0.61–1.16, p = 0.3)]. When adjusting for potential confounders including severity parameters (respiratory rate, pulse oximetry and fever), the adjusted HR (aHR) for mild pneumonia was 1.00 (95% CI, 0.57–1.76, p = 0.98), for mild malaria 0.70 (0.31–1.59, p = 0.39) and for mild diarrhoea 0.81(0.42–1.566, p = 0.53). **Figure 2** displays the re-attendance rates and outcomes within 14 days following the initial consultation for mild pneumonia, uncomplicated malaria and mild diarrhoea according to the prescription of antibiotics. **Figures 3a, 3b, 3c** displays the Kaplan-Meyer survival curves for these three diseases whether they were managed with or without antibiotics. There was no significant difference between the curves with or without antibiotics for all three diseases.

Discussion

The aim of this prospective study was to explore the appropriateness and effectiveness of prescription of antibiotics in routine outpatient settings of Papua New Guinea in the frame of the IMCI recommendations.

Overtreatment with Antibiotics

A high rate of antibiotic prescription was observed in the cohort, with 54% of cases treated (including mild and severe cases) when a maximum of 36% should have received antibiotics according to IMCI criteria, This is high compared to other settings, where it is usually reported that approximately 20% of patients require antibiotics when the diagnosis is made by highly skilled clinicians. [7,15] This high rate of prescription may be due to difficulties in accurately recognizing or measuring signs and symptoms by health staff. For example, it is frequently observed that respiratory rate is not properly assessed and therefore tachypnoea often overestimated. In our setting, despite the official recommendation of counting over 1 minute, most respiratory rates were even numbers suggesting that health workers are not counting according to standard operating procedures. (Senn & Rarau, personal communication) This is especially worrying as tachypnoea is a cornerstone for the diagnosis of pneumonia and hence for the prescription of

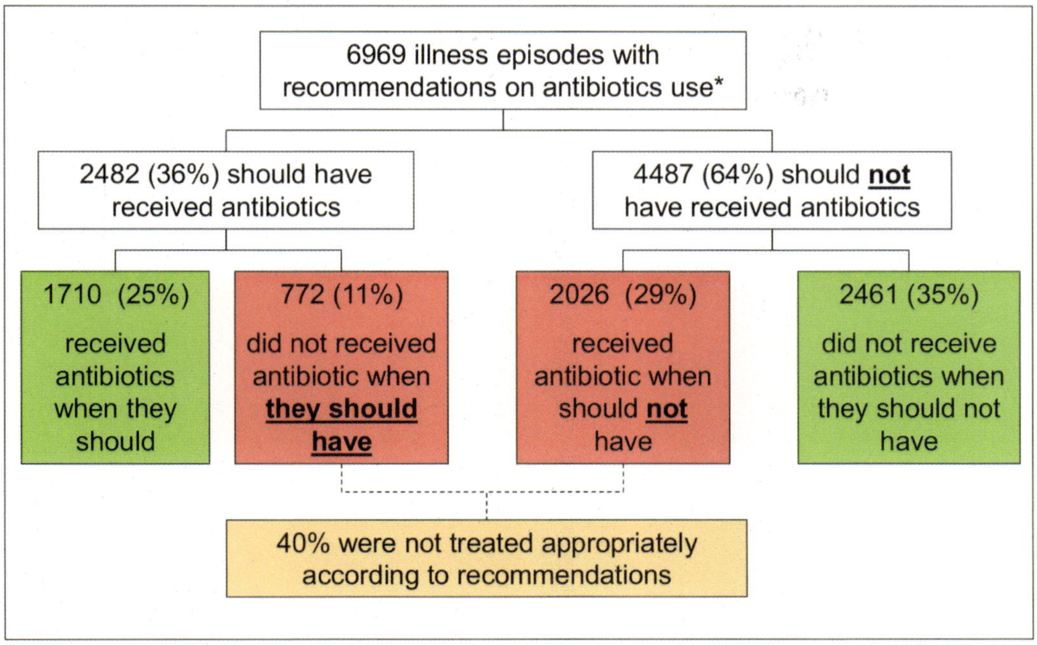

* Syndromes for which antibiotics are recommended: LRTI, otitis, severe diseases and skin infections

Figure 1. Appropriateness of antibiotics' use according to the IMCI recommendations.

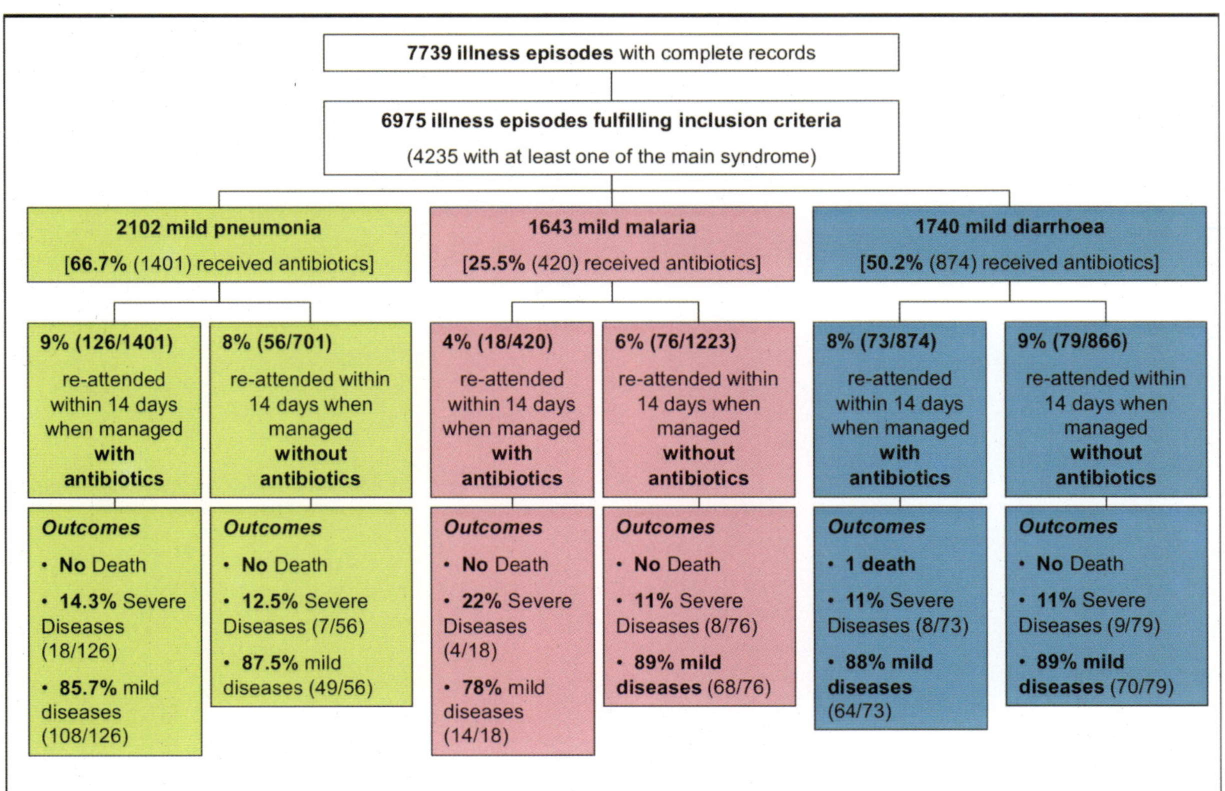

Figure 2. Re-attendance rates within 14 days and outcomes for the most common mild syndromes according to the prescription of antibiotics.

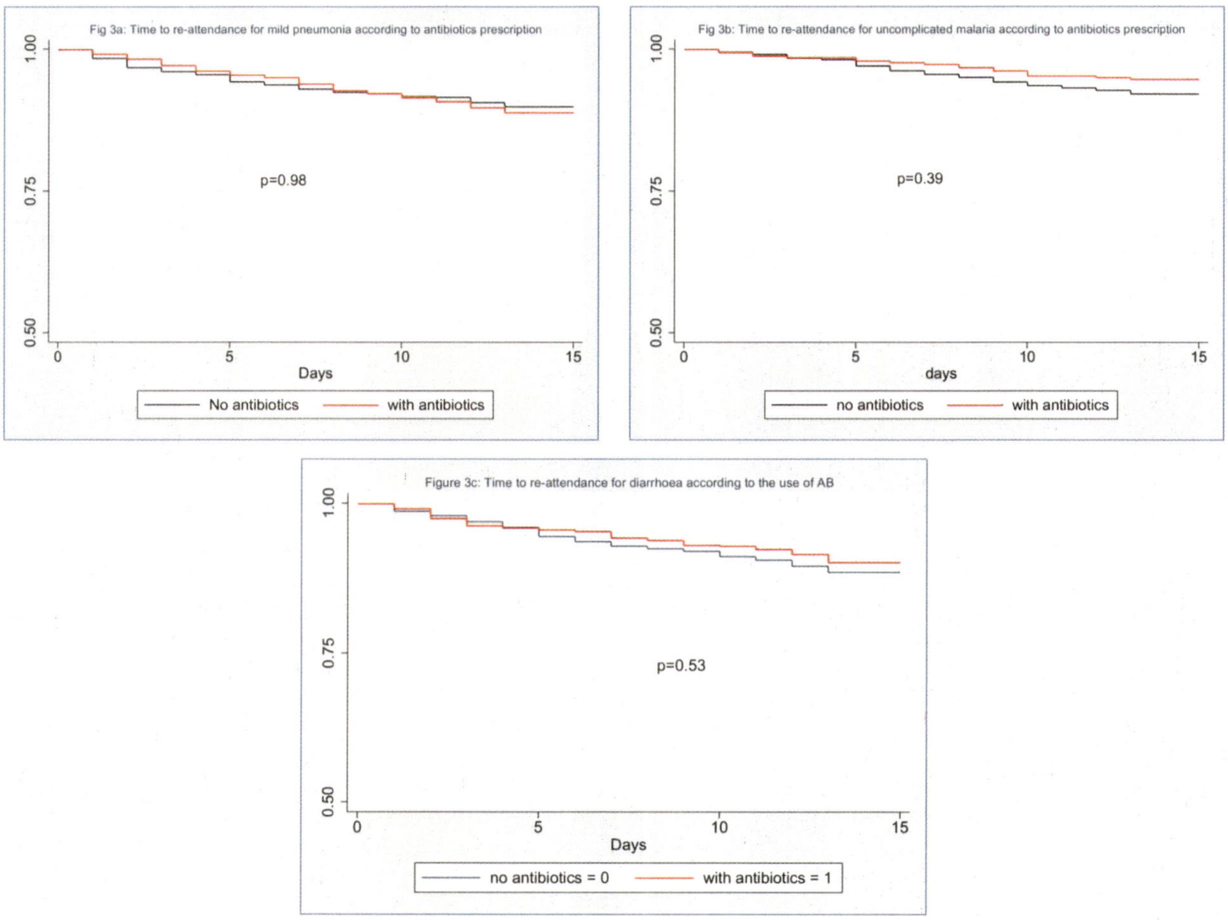

Figure 3. Kaplan–Meier estimates of the proportion of patients with mild pneumonia (3a), mild malaria (3b) or gastroenteritis (3c) re-attending the clinics within 14 days whether they received antibiotics (red line) or not (blue line).

antibiotics. Improving skills and eventually finding new tools for the accurate determination of the respiratory rate would be an important step towards more rational use of antibiotics.

Appropriateness of Antibiotics Prescription

A poor compliance to guidelines was observed as 40% of patients were not treated according to the recommendations (29% received antibiotics when they should not have and 11% did not receive antibiotics when they should have). Apart from the inaccurate clinical judgment of health staff, other factors might influence their decision. In our study, we observed that the prescription of antibiotics was strongly influenced by the result of the RDT for malaria in feverish patients. Indeed, we observed that in children presenting with criteria for mild pneumonia (who should receive antibiotics), only 40% were treated when the RDT was positive, compared to 76% when the test was negative. On one hand, it is reassuring to observe that clinicians are influenced in their clinical judgment and treatment attitude by an objective test. On the other hand, considering only one diagnosis may have potential serious consequences for children, as it might leave children with bacterial infections untreated. This may be the downside of the introduction of RDT in routine clinics. Indeed, improving the diagnosis of malaria may have adverse effects for the management of other diseases, which is in line with findings by Bisoffi et al. in Africa [28]. This will need to be addressed when redesigning guidelines.

It is finally reassuring to observe that almost all children (97%) with criteria for a severe pneumonia received antibiotics.

Effectiveness of Antibiotics

One might worry that such a high rate of non-compliance to standard IMCI recommendations might leave a lot of children with potential bacterial pneumonia untreated and might re-attend with a more severe clinical presentation associated with poor outcomes. However, our data indicate that it is in fact not the case. Indeed, the rate of re-attendance following a visit for mild pneumonia, which can be considered as a proxy of the effectiveness of the antibiotics, was similar, irrespective of antibiotic prescription (9% when they received antibiotics and 8% if they did not, adjusted hazard ratio of 1.0). This is well in line with recent findings in Pakistan where the use of amoxicillin was not found to provide any benefit for non-severe pneumonia as defined by WHO. [21] More generally and from a policy perspective, IMCI guidelines are not only aiming at reducing under five mortality by providing efficient strategies to treat acute severe cases but also to prevent the worsening of mild diseases. In that perspective, it was postulated that the broad prescription of antibiotics should mitigate the risk of poor outcomes. Our study looked specifically at that aspect in an outpatient setting and provides solid evidence to demonstrate that treating broadly mild diseases with antibiotics does not help prevent severe diseases. Recently, WHO and UNICEF, aware of the lack of specificity of the current IMCI guidelines, revised their recommendations and proposed a new classification of respiratory infections, notably merging non-severe and severe pneumonia into "pneumonia" and "severe pneumonia" being reserved for children with danger signs. The results of the present study validate and support this revision.

The absence of difference in the re-attendance rates is probably due to the fact that the vast majority of mild pneumonia episodes have a viral aetiology rather than bacterial, highlighting the lack of specificity of the clinical criteria to identify bacterial pneumonia. This was confirmed by a microbiological investigation made on nasal swabs in a sub-sample of these children. The rapid antigen diagnostic tests for viral pathogens showed that more than half of children with mild clinical pneumonia were positive for at least one of the four most common respiratory viruses: Influenza A&B, *Adenovirus* and Respiratory Syncytial Virus (Rarau et al. personal communication). Similar findings have also been published in other countries. [7] The fact that mortality was very low and most pneumonias were treated with amoxicillin (instead of co-trimoxazole), speaks against the hypothesis that similar outcomes between antibiotics users and non-users were due to the high prevalence of resistant pathogens [29].

The diagnosis of pneumonia is more complex than that of malaria as no reliable and easy-to-use tests are available to identify respiratory infections that require antibiotics. It has been recognized that pneumonia is often associated with virus detection and that there is a complex and poorly understood interplay between viruses and bacteria in the development of pneumonia. [30] Considering the dramatically high burden of respiratory illnesses, especially in very young children, the development of more accurate diagnostic strategies able to identify children with pneumonia requiring antibiotics should be on the top list of priorities. [7] The potential benefits of the use of RDT to document viral pathogens such as RSV or *Influenza* need to be investigated. Beyond the aetiology of respiratory infections, it would be also valuable to develop tests able to identify children with potentially severe (invasive) diseases, which require specific supportive care. In that regard, inflammatory markers such as procalcitonin (PCT) can be valuable tools. Recent reviews by Schuetz et al. [31,32] have shown that PCT-guided prescription of antibiotics for ARI was safe and reduce substantially the consumption of antibiotics. They also noted that evidence is lacking on usefulness of PCT in settings outside Europe. C - reactive protein (CRP) can be also another valuable biomarker but results of randomized trials and meta-analysis are more conflicting. [33,34,35,36] Finally, more experimental tools such as analysis of exhaled gases could be also considered [37]. New recommendations that integrate clinical assessment and biomarkers for the identification of cases that require antibiotics need to be seriously considered. However, further pragmatic research is needed to explore the most efficient, safe and cost-effective approach in children in resource-limited countries.

Similarly to what was observed with mild pneumonia, antibiotics did not provide any benefit for diarrhoea or malaria in our cohort, which supports the current WHO recommendations of not treating mild gastroenteritis and uncomplicated malaria with antibiotics.

Limitations of the Study

The main limitation of this study is that the clinical management of malaria episodes was performed in ideal conditions because it was conducted alongside a malaria prevention trial (i.e. treatment of only RDT positive cases). While RDT-based malaria treatment was not part of the PNG malaria treatment guidelines when the study was conducted, there was rapid roll-out and rapid up-take of RDTs [38] and the situation in our study therefore increasingly resembles the situation in almost all malaria endemic countries including PNG. On the other hand, for all other diseases, the recommendations made to the study nurses were identical to the national standard treatment protocols. Another limitation is the lack of randomization for the use of antibiotics, which might have led to selection biases. However, even when we adjusted for potential confounders of disease severity (such as respiratory rate or pulse oximetry), no significant difference was observed whether illness episodes were treated with antibiotics or not.

Conclusions

This study shows that adherence to IMCI recommendations for prescription of antibiotics was poor in routine outpatient settings of Papua New Guinea and was strongly influenced by RDT results for malaria, independently of the clinical presentation. However, the management of mild pneumonia with antibiotics based on IMCI guidelines did not change health outcome in terms of re-attendance and complications when compared to no antibiotics. This absence of effectiveness of antibiotics is certainly due to the lack of specificity of the present recommendations to differentiate children with true bacterial diseases and those with viral infections. It is urgently needed to develop better strategies to improve the identification of pneumonia and other syndromes that require antibiotics or more intensive clinical care.

Acknowledgments

We would like to warmly thank all study nurses of the IPTi trial who looked after the data collection as well as after the study participants. We would like also to thank all the laboratory staff of the PNG IMR who looked at some many slides and analysis.

Finally our deep gratitude goes to all the study participants and their parents for agreeing to participate to this study. We also would like to thank Dr Amanda Ross, who is a post-doctoral biostatistician at the Swiss TPH, for her guidance to perform the survival analysis.

Author Contributions

Conceived and designed the experiments: NS BG IM. Performed the experiments: NS PR DM MS. Analyzed the data: NS IM. Wrote the paper: NS BG IM SR. Facilitated the laboratory and field work: PS PNG IMR.

References

1. Bryce J, Boschi-Pinto C, Shibuya K, Black RE (2005) WHO estimates of the causes of death in children. Lancet 365: 1147–1152.
2. Lozano R, Naghavi M, Foreman K, Lim S, Shibuya K, et al. (2012) Global and regional mortality from 235 causes of death for 20 age groups in 1990 and 2010: a systematic analysis for the Global Burden of Disease Study 2010. Lancet 380: 2095–2128.
3. Animut A, Mekonnen Y, Shimelis D, Ephraim E (2009) Febrile illnesses of different etiology among outpatients in four health centers in Northwestern Ethiopia. Jpn J Infect Dis 62: 107–110.
4. Deressa W, Ali A, Berhane Y (2007) Household and socioeconomic factors associated with childhood febrile illnesses and treatment seeking behaviour in an area of epidemic malaria in rural Ethiopia. Trans R Soc Trop Med Hyg 101: 939–947.
5. Roca A, Quinto L, Saute F, Thompson R, Aponte JJ, et al. (2006) Community incidences of respiratory infections in an actively followed cohort of children <1 year of age in Manhica, a rural area of southern Mozambique. Trop Med Int Health 11: 373–380.

6. Velema JP, Alihonou EM, Gandaho T, Hounye FH (1991) Childhood mortality among users and non-users of primary health care in a rural west African community. Int J Epidemiol 20: 474–479.
7. Feikin DR, Olack B, Bigogo GM, Audi A, Cosmas L, et al. (2011) The Burden of Common Infectious Disease Syndromes at the Clinic and Household Level from Population-Based Surveillance in Rural and Urban Kenya. PLoS One 6: e16085.
8. Gwer S, Newton CR, Berkley JA (2007) Over-diagnosis and co-morbidity of severe malaria in African children: a guide for clinicians. Am J Trop Med Hyg 77: 6–13.
9. Reyburn H, Mbatia R, Drakeley C, Carneiro I, Mwakasungula E, et al. (2004) Overdiagnosis of malaria in patients with severe febrile illness in Tanzania: a prospective study. BMJ 329: 1212.
10. WHO (2007) Integrated management of childhood illnesses: World Health Organization.
11. Kallander K, Nsungwa-Sabiiti J, Peterson S (2004) Symptom overlap for malaria and pneumonia–policy implications for home management strategies. Acta Trop 90: 211–214.
12. O'Dempsey TJ, McArdle TF, Laurence BE, Lamont AC, Todd JE, et al. (1993) Overlap in the clinical features of pneumonia and malaria in African children. Trans R Soc Trop Med Hyg 87: 662–665.
13. Bassat Q, Machevo S, O'Callaghan-Gordo C, Sigauque B, Morais L, et al. (2011) Distinguishing malaria from severe pneumonia among hospitalized children who fulfilled integrated management of childhood illness criteria for both diseases: a hospital-based study in Mozambique. Am J Trop Med Hyg 85: 626–634.
14. Armstrong Schellenberg J, Bryce J, de Savigny D, Lambrechts T, Mbuya C, et al. (2004) The effect of Integrated Management of Childhood Illness on observed quality of care of under-fives in rural Tanzania. Health Policy Plan 19: 1–10.
15. Horwood C, Vermaak K, Rollins N, Haskins L, Nkosi P, et al. (2009) An evaluation of the quality of IMCI assessments among IMCI trained health workers in South Africa. PLoS One 4: e5937.
16. Armstrong Schellenberg J, Bryce J, de Savigny D, Lambrechts T, Mbuya C, et al. (2004) The effect of Integrated Management of Childhood Illness on observed quality of care of under-fives in rural Tanzania. Health Policy Plan 19: 1–10.
17. Shah D, Sachdev HP (1999) Evaluation of the WHO/UNICEF algorithm for integrated management of childhood illness between the age of two months to five years. Indian Pediatr 36: 767–777.
18. Horwood C, Voce A, Vermaak K, Rollins N, Qazi S (2009) Experiences of training and implementation of integrated management of childhood illness (IMCI) in South Africa: a qualitative evaluation of the IMCI case management training course. BMC Pediatr 9: 62.
19. El Arifeen S, Blum LS, Hoque DM, Chowdhury EK, Khan R, et al. (2004) Integrated Management of Childhood Illness (IMCI) in Bangladesh: early findings from a cluster-randomised study. Lancet 364: 1595–1602.
20. Factor SH, Schillinger JA, Kalter HD, Saha S, Begum H, et al. (2001) Diagnosis and management of febrile children using the WHO/UNICEF guidelines for IMCI in Dhaka, Bangladesh. Bull World Health Organ 79: 1096–1105.
21. Hazir T, Nisar YB, Abbasi S, Ashraf YP, Khurshid J, et al. (2011) Comparison of oral amoxicillin with placebo for the treatment of world health organization-defined nonsevere pneumonia in children aged 2–59 months: a multicenter, double-blind, randomized, placebo-controlled trial in pakistan. Clin Infect Dis 52: 293–300.
22. WHO (2005) Country Health Information Profile PNG. WHO.
23. Shann F, Gratten M, Germer S, Linnemann V, Hazlett D, et al. (1984) Aetiology of pneumonia in children in Goroka Hospital, Papua New Guinea. Lancet 2: 537–541.
24. Duke T, Michael A, Mgone J, Frank D, Wal T, et al. (2002) Aetiology of child mortality in Goroka, Papua New Guinea: a prospective two year study. Bull World Health Organ 80: 16–25.
25. Senn N, Rarau P, Manong D, Salib M, Siba P, et al. (2011) Rapid Diagnostic Test-Based Management of Malaria: An Effectiveness Study in Papua New Guinean Infants With Plasmodium falciparum and Plasmodium vivax Malaria. Clin Infect Dis 23: 23.
26. Senn N, Rarau P, Stanisic DI, Robinson L, Barnadas C, et al. (2012) Intermittent Preventive Treatment for Malaria in Papua New Guinean Infants Exposed to Plasmodium falciparum and P. vivax: A Randomized Controlled Trial. PLoS Med 9: e1001195.
27. Paediatric Society of Papua New Guinea (2005) Standard Treatment for the common illnesses of children in Papua New Guinea.
28. Bisoffi Z, Sirima SB, Meheus F, Lodesani C, Gobbi F, et al. (2011) Strict adherence to malaria rapid test results might lead to a neglect of other dangerous diseases: a cost benefit analysis from Burkina Faso. Malar J 10: 1475–2875.
29. Manning L, Laman M, Greenhill AR, Michael A, Siba P, et al. (2011) Increasing chloramphenicol resistance in Streptococcus pneumoniae isolates from Papua New Guinean children with acute bacterial meningitis. Antimicrobial agents and chemotherapy 55: 4454–4456.
30. Hament JM, Kimpen JL, Fleer A, Wolfs TF (1999) Respiratory viral infection predisposing for bacterial disease: a concise review. FEMS Immunol Med Microbiol 26: 189–195.
31. Schuetz P, Albrich W, Mueller B (2011) Procalcitonin for diagnosis of infection and guide to antibiotic decisions: past, present and future. BMC medicine 9: 107.
32. Schuetz P, Muller B, Christ-Crain M, Stolz D, Tamm M, et al. (2012) Procalcitonin to initiate or discontinue antibiotics in acute respiratory tract infections. The Cochrane database of systematic reviews 9: CD007498.
33. Falk G, Fahey T (2009) C-reactive protein and community-acquired pneumonia in ambulatory care: systematic review of diagnostic accuracy studies. Family practice 26: 10–21.
34. Flood RG, Badik J, Aronoff SC (2008) The utility of serum C-reactive protein in differentiating bacterial from nonbacterial pneumonia in children: a meta-analysis of 1230 children. The Pediatric infectious disease journal 27: 95–99.
35. Carrol ED, Mankhambo LA, Jeffers G, Parker D, Guiver M, et al. (2009) The diagnostic and prognostic accuracy of five markers of serious bacterial infection in Malawian children with signs of severe infection. PLoS One 4: e6621.
36. Diez-Padrisa N, Bassat Q, Morais L, O'Callaghan-Gordo C, Machevo S, et al. (2012) Procalcitonin and C-reactive protein as predictors of blood culture positivity among hospitalised children with severe pneumonia in Mozambique. Tropical Medicine & International Health 17: 1100–1107.
37. Schmidt HJ, Bhandari V, Bhandari A, Davies J, Marshall BC, et al. (2010) The future in paediatric respirology. Respirology 15: 733–741.
38. WHO (2012) World Malaria Report. Available: http://www.who.int/malaria/publications/world_malaria_report_2012/report/en/index.html ed.

17

Intestinal Parasitic Infections in HIV-Infected Patients, Lao People's Democratic Republic

Phimpha Paboriboune[1,2], Niranh Phoumindr[3], Elisabeth Borel[4], Khamphang Sourinphoumy[5], Saykham Phaxayaseng[6], Elodie Luangkhot[7], Bouachanh Sengphilom[3], Yathmany Vansilalom[3], Peter Odermatt[8], Eric Delaporte[2], Jean- François Etard[2], Meja Rabodonirina[4,7]*

1 Centre d'Infectiologie Christophe Mérieux du Laos, Ministry of Health, Vientiane, Lao People's Democratic Republic, **2** UMI 233, Institut de Recherche pour le Développement – Université Montpellier 1, Montpellier, France, **3** Department of Parasitology, University of Health Sciences, Vientiane, Lao People's Democratic Republic, **4** Faculté de Médecine Lyon-Sud Charles Mérieux, Université Lyon 1, Lyon, France, **5** Department of Infectious Diseases, Provincial Hospital, Savannakhet, Lao People's Democratic Republic, **6** Department of Infectious Diseases, Setthathirath Hospital, Vientiane, Lao People's Democratic Republic, **7** Service de Parasitologie, Hospices Civils de Lyon, Lyon, France, **8** Department of Epidemiology and Public Health, Swiss Tropical and Public Health Institute, Basel, Switzerland

Abstract

Background: HIV infection is an emerging problem in Laos. We conducted the first prospective study on intestinal parasites, including opportunistic protozoa, in newly diagnosed HIV infected patients, with or without diarrhea. The aims were to describe the spectrum of infections, to determine their prevalence and to assess their associations with diarrhea, CD4 cell count, place of residence and living conditions.

Methodology: One to three stool samples over consecutive days were obtained from 137 patients. The Kato thick smear method, formalin-ethyl concentration and specific stains for coccidia and microsporidia diagnosis were performed on 260 stool samples. Baseline characteristics regarding relevant demographics, place of residence and living conditions, clinical features including diarrhea, were collected using a standardized questionnaire.

Principal Findings: The 137 patients were young (median age: 36 years) and severely immunocompromised (83.9% at WHO stage 3 or 4, median CD4 cell count: 41/mm^3). Diarrhea was present in 43.0% of patients. Parasite infection was found in 78.8% of patients, infection with at least two species in 49.6%. Prevalence rates of protozoan and helminth infections were similar (54.7% and 58.4% respectively). *Blastocystis* sp. was the most frequent protozoa (26.3%). *Cryptosporidium* sp., *Cytoisospora belli* and microsporidia, found at low prevalence rates (6.6%, 4.4%, 2.9%, respectively), were described for the first time in Laos. *Cryptosporidium* sp. was associated with persistent diarrhea. *Strongyloides stercoralis* was the most prevalent helminth following *Opisthorchis viverrini* (20.4% and 47.5% respectively). The most immunocompromised patients, as assessed by a CD4 count $\leq$ 50 cells/mm^3, were more likely to be infected with intestinal parasites.

Conclusions/Significance: HIV infection was mainly diagnosed at an advanced stage of immunosuppression in Lao patients. Intestinal parasite infections were highly prevalent regardless of their diarrheal status. Opportunistic infections were reported. Improving the laboratory diagnosis of intestinal parasite infections and the knowledge on their local risk factors is warranted.

Editor: William A. Paxton, Institute of Infection and Global Health, United Kingdom

Funding: This investigation was funded by the association Ensemble Contre le Sida (https://www.sidaction.org/, project no. AI19-2/01454 2ème Appel d'Offres SIDACTION 2008) and by the Conseil Régional Rhône-Alpes (http://www.rhonealpes.fr/, Appels d'Offres Coopérations et Mobilités Internationales Rhône-Alpes project no. 08.03.391, no. 09.03.357, no. 10.03.343). PP was supported by the Fondation Mérieux (http://www.fondation-merieux.org/). The funders had no role in study design, data collection and analysis, decision to publish, or preparation of the manuscript.

Competing Interests: The authors have declared that no competing interests exist.

* E-mail: meja.rabodonirina@chu-lyon.fr

Introduction

Diarrhea is a major cause of morbidity in HIV-infected patients. Moreover, it is recognized as an independent marker of poor prognosis [1]. In previous studies from industrialized countries, infectious causes were demonstrated to be prevalent among the etiologies of diarrhea, especially parasites [1]. There is a paucity of microbiological data from emerging and developing countries because of the lack of equipment, reagents and/or trained laboratory staff [2]. Nevertheless, the identification and characterization of infectious agents are important at two levels: (i) for patient management by confirming or ruling out a clinical diagnosis, thereby allowing an appropriate treatment, (ii) for public healthcare policy by determining the true prevalence of a pathogen in a country or region and yielding epidemiological risk factors for specific infections.

Lao People's Democratic Republic (Lao PDR, Laos) is a landlocked country in the Mekong region of Southeast Asia, surrounded by countries with high HIV prevalence such as Thailand. The first case of HIV infection was identified in Laos in

1990 and antiretroviral therapy (ART) was provided for the first time in 2003 in the Savannakhet Regional Hospital by Médecins Sans Frontières [3]. Laos is considered to be a low-level HIV epidemic country with an estimated prevalence of 0.3% and an estimated 12,000 people living with HIV/AIDS in 2012 [4]. The development of the National AIDS Response led in 2012 to the treatment with ART of 2,212 patients in seven centers [4].

Parasitological analysis in Lao hospital laboratories is performed using direct examination of fresh unconcentrated stools and the Kato thick smear technique [5], allowing the diagnosis of helminth infections which are frequent in the general population of Laos [6,7,8,9,10,11]. Little information is available on intestinal protozoan infections. *Blastocystis*, an emerging pathogen, was recently reported for the first time in the general population [9]. Regarding opportunistic infections, information on major intestinal parasite infections among HIV patients such as *Cryptosporidium* and microsporidia has not been reported to date due to rare diagnostic performance.

To fill this gap, we conducted a cross-sectional study in two referral hospitals for HIV/AIDS care. The purpose was to assess the diversity and prevalence of intestinal parasitic infections in antiretroviral-naïve HIV-infected patients, and to determine their association with diarrhea, CD4 cell counts, place of residence and living conditions.

Methods

Ethics statement

The study protocol, including the consent procedure, was reviewed and approved by the Ethical Committee of the University of Health Sciences (Ministry of Public Health, Laos, reference no. 009/08). Patients were included in the study on a voluntary basis. After an information sheet had been read aloud, a written consent form was signed and obtained from the patients (or parents in the case of minors less than 16 years of age). This research followed the principles expressed in the Declaration of Helsinki. All infections diagnosed were treated using a standard treatment protocol.

Study sites and population

The study was carried out from October 2009 to September 2010 in two public hospitals of Laos: Setthathirath Hospital in Vientiane (Vientiane Capital) and Savannakhet Regional Hospital (Savannakhet province, Southern part of Laos). These hospitals are two of the seven HIV care and treatment centers of the country. Patients admitted for the care of a newly diagnosed HIV-infection were included before any treatment, including ART, was started. Each patient underwent a standard clinical assessment and a questionnaire was completed. The CD4 cell count was assessed and up to three stool samples were collected and analyzed.

Data collection

Baseline characteristics regarding relevant demographics, place of residence and living conditions (province of Laos, urban/rural housing, access to drinking water and in-house toilets, animal contact), clinical features (fever, weight loss, anorexia, diarrhea, nausea, vomiting, abdominal pain, and pulmonary, neurological and mucocutaneous symptoms) were collected at inclusion by the physician using a standardized questionnaire. According to World Health Organization definitions, diarrhea was defined as the passage of three or more loose or liquid stools per day [12]. It was considered acute when it lasted less than two weeks and persistent when it lasted 14 days or longer [12]. The immunological status of the patients related to HIV disease was assessed using the 2007 - revised World Health Organization HIV clinical staging and disease classification system [13].

Laboratory examination

Serological diagnosis of HIV infection was made using two rapid screening tests: Determine HIV 1/2 (Inverness Medical, Tokyo, Japan) and Uni-Gold HIV (Trinity Biotech, Bray, Ireland). In the case of discordant results, the diagnosis was confirmed by the ELISA test Vironostika HIV Uniform II plus O (BioMérieux, Marcy-l'Etoile, France). HIV viral load testing was not prescribed to patients with a newly diagnosed HIV infection because of limited availability of the technique. The CD4 lymphocyte count was determined by flow cytometry (Cyflow SL and Cyflow Counter, Partec GmbH, Munster, Germany).

Laboratory investigations for opportunistic infections were limited to direct diagnosis of mycobacterial infections and cryptococcosis using Ziehl-Neelsen stain on sputum samples and India ink test or antigen detection in cerebrospinal fluid samples, respectively.

Stool sample analysis

All patients were asked to provide three stool samples from three consecutive days. Each fresh stool specimen was processed as follows: the technicians of the hospital laboratories performed direct microscopic examination and examination of a Kato thick smear [5]. The sample was then preserved in 10% formalin and forwarded to the parasitological department of the Faculty of Medicine, University of Heath Sciences (Vientiane, Laos). The formalin-preserved samples were subjected to two techniques: formalin-ethyl concentration technique for protozoa and helminths diagnosis [14] and modified acid-fast staining for coccidia diagnosis (*Cryptosporidium* spp., *Cyclospora cayetanensis*, *Cytoisospora belli*, *Sarcocystis hominis*) [15]. The diagnoses were made with the assistance of parasitologists from the University of Lyon (France).

Two smears from formalin-preserved samples were also prepared for microsporidia diagnosis. They were sent to the University of Lyon where the diagnosis was made using the Weber trichrome stain [16] and the fluorescent stain with Uvitex 2B (Uvibio, LDBio Diagnostics, Lyon, France) [17].

Patients were considered infected with a parasite species if at least one of their stool samples was positive.

Statistical analysis

EpiData freeware, version 3.1 (EpiData Association, Odense, Denmark) was used for data entry. Analyses were performed using STATA software, version 11 (StataCorp., College Station, Texas, USA). Descriptive statistics were carried out. Frequencies were calculated for categorical variables. Proportions were compared using Fisher's exact test. Odds ratio (OR) and 95% confidence intervals (CI) were calculated by using a bi-variable logistic regression. Tests were considered significant at P value≤0.05. Factors potentially associated with intestinal parasite infections were diarrhea, CD4 cell count, place of residence and living conditions.

Results

Study population

A total of 140 HIV-positive patients met the criteria for inclusion in the study and gave their consent. Amongst them, 137 patients had complete data records (the CD4 cell count lacked for three patients) and were included in the final analysis. The median age was 36 years (interquartile range [IQR]: 28–41). Males accounted for 53.5% of patients. Sixty seven patients (48.9%)

came from the Northern provinces: Luang Namtha, Luang Prabang, Xaiyabury, Vientiane capital, Vientiane province, Xieng Kouang. The others came from the Southern provinces: Bolikhamxay, Savannakhet, Khammuane, Champasack, Saravane. Seventy four patients (54.0%) lived in rural areas. The proportion of patients living in rural areas was higher in Southern provinces than in Northern provinces (53 (75.7%) vs. 21 (31.3%), OR = 6.8, 95% CI = 2.9–15.8). One hundred patients (73.0%) had access to clean drinking water, 103 (75.2%) had in-house toilets and 48 (35.0%) reported animal contact, namely poultry (31.4%), pigs (18.2%) and bovine species (16.8%).

The patients were severely immunocompromised, as assessed by WHO clinical staging criteria (115 patients (83.9%) at stage 3 or 4) and by CD4 cell count (median: 41 cells/mm^3, [IQR]: 14–94 cells/mm^3). The proportion of patients at the advanced stages 3 or 4 was significantly higher in Southern provinces than in Northern provinces: 67 (95.7%) vs. 48 (71.6%), OR = 8.8, 95% CI = 2.3–34.1). Laboratory diagnosis of tuberculosis was performed in 49 patients (35.8%), leading to the identification of 10 cases of pulmonary tuberculosis (7.3% of all the patients). Eleven cases of cryptococcal meningitis (8.0% of all the patients) were diagnosed in the 44 patients (32.1%) who underwent laboratory investigations for cryptococcosis.

Fifty nine patients (43.0%) presented with diarrhea, of whom 20 (14.6%) had persistent diarrhea. The median duration of the diarrheal episodes was 14 days ([IQR]: 5–30). The median number of stools per day was four ([IQR]: 4–5). Table 1 summarizes demographic, clinical and laboratory characteristics of the patients, with or without diarrhea. Compared to patients without diarrhea, patients with diarrhea presented more often with other symptoms: fever (OR = 4.2, 95% CI = 1.5–11.4), anorexia (OR = 2.7, 95% CI = 1.1–7.1), reported weight loss (OR = 2.6, 95% CI = 1.1–6.3), abdominal pain (OR = 5.3, 95% CI = 2.3–12.0), oral candidiasis (OR = 2.2, 95% CI = 1.1–4.5). Diarrheal patients were also diagnosed at a more advanced stage of HIV infection (stages 3–4 *vs.* stages 1–2: OR = 4.1, 95% CI = 1.3–13.4). No demographic characteristic or a CD4 cell count ≤ 50/mm^3 was found to be associated with diarrhea. Amongst environmental conditions, living in the Southern provinces was associated with diarrhea compared to living in the Northern provinces (36 (61.0%) vs. 23 (39.0%), OR = 2.0, 95% CI = 1.0–4.2).

Intestinal parasitic infections

Two hundred and sixty stool specimens were obtained and analyzed. Thirty two patients (23.3%) gave three stool samples, 59 (43.1%) gave two samples and 46 (33.6%) gave one sample. Table 2 presents the parasite species diagnosed with regard to the region of residence. At least one parasite species was identified in the majority of patients (78.8%), two or more species in 68 patients (49.6%). Seventy five patients (54.7%) were infected with at least one protozoan species. *Blastocystis* spp., diagnosed in 36 patients (26.3%), was the most common protozoa, followed by *Entamoeba histolytica/dispar* (12.4%) and *Giardia intestinalis* (8.8%). Classical opportunistic agents (*Cryptosporidium* spp., *Cytoisospora belli*, *Cyclospora cayetanensis* and microsporidia) were present, but were less frequent (6.6%, 4.4%, 2.2% and 2.9% respectively). Eighty patients (58.4%) were infected with at least one helminth species. The most common helminths were *Opisthorchis viverrini* and *Strongyloides stercoralis*, detected in 65 (47.5%) and 28 patients (20.4%) respectively. No *Schistosoma mekongi* infection or cestode infections were diagnosed. The prevalence rates of helminthiases generally and of strongyloidiasis in particular, were higher in Southern provinces than in Northern provinces (67.1% vs. 49.2%, *P* = 0.03, and 28.5% vs. 11.9%, *P* = 0.01%, respectively). Environmental factors associated with infection with some parasite species were identified: helminth infections were more frequent in individuals who did not have in-house toilets compared to patients who had in-house toilets (79.4% vs. 51.5%, *P* <0.01) and *S. stercoralis* was more frequent in patients living in rural areas compared to patients living in cities (28.4% vs. 11.1%, *P* = 0.01).

Table 1. Demographic, clinical and laboratory characteristics of HIV-infected patients with regard to diarrhea, Laos (n = 137).

	Total (%)	Diarrhea, n = 59 (%)	OR (95% CI)
Demographic features			
Age group (years)			
< 35 y	77 (56.2)	34 (57.3)	1.1 (0.6–2.2)
≥ 35 y	60 (43.8)	25 (42.4)	1.00
Sex			
Male	73 (53.3)	35 (59.3)	1.5 (0.8–3.1)
Female	64 (46.7)	24 (40.7)	1.00
Clinical features			
Fever			
Yes	106 (77.4)	53 (89.8)	4.2 (1.5–11.4)
No	31 (22.6)	6 (10.2)	1.00
Anorexia			
Yes	109 (79.6)	52 (88.1)	2.7 (1.1–7.1)
No	28 (20.4)	77 (11.9)	1.00
Reported weight loss			
Yes	103 (75.2)	50 (84.8)	2.6 (1.1–6.3)
No	34 (24.8)	9 (15.2)	1.00
Abdominal pain			
Yes	50 (36.5)	34 (57.6)	5.3 (2.3–12.0)
No	87 (63.5)	25 (42.4)	1.00
Nausea and/or vomiting			
Yes	30 (21.9)	12 (20.3)	0.9 (0.4–1.9)
No	107 (78.1)	47 (79.7)	1.00
Oral candidiasis			
Yes	53 (38.7)	29 (49.2)	2.2 (1.1–4.5)
No	84 (61.3)	30 (50.8)	1.00
Pulmonary signs			
Yes	60 (43.8)	30 (50.9)	1.7 (0.8–3.3)
No	77 (56.2)	29 (49.1)	1.00
Neurological signs			
Yes	18 (13.1)	66 (10.2)	0.6 (0.2–1.8)
No	119 (86.9)	53 (89.8)	1.00
WHO clinical stages			
Stage 3–4	115 (83.9)	55 (93.2)	4.1 (1.3–13.4)
Stage 1–2	22 (16.1)	44 (6.8)	1.00
Laboratory features			
CD4 (cells/mm^3)			
≤ 50	80 (58.4)	34 (57.6)	0.9 (0.5–1.9)
> 50	57 (41.6)	25 (42.4)	1.00

OR, Odds Ratio.
CI, confidence interval.

Table 2. Intestinal parasitic infections in HIV-infected patients by region of residence (Southern or Northern provinces), Laos (n = 137).

	Total (%)	South, n = 70 (%)	North, n = 67 (%)	*P*-value
Parasites				
Any parasite	108 (78.8)	57 (81.4)	51 (76.1)	0.44
At least 2 parasite species	68 (49.6)	39 (55.7)	29 (43.3)	0.14
Any protozoa	75 (54.7)	35 (50.0)	40 (59.7)	0.25
Cryptosporidium spp.	9 (6.6)	2 (2.9)	7 (10.5)	0.09
Cytoisospora belli	6 (4.4)	3 (4.3)	3 (4.5)	0.95
Cyclospora cayetanensis	3 (2.2)	1 (1.4)	2 (3.0)	0.61
Giardia intestinalis	12 (8.8)	8 (11.4)	4 (6.0)	0.36
Entamoeba histolytica/dispar	17 (12.4)	11 (15.7)	6 (9.0)	0.30
Entamoeba coli	1 (0.7)	0	1 (1.5)	n.a.
Entamoeba hartmanii	5 (3.7)	1 (1.4)	4 (6.0)	0.20
Blastocystis spp.	36 (26.3)	16 (22.9)	20 (29.9)	0.35
Microsporidia	4 (2.9)	2 (2.9)	2 (3.0)	0.96
Any helminth	80 (58.4)	47 (67.1)	33 (49.2)	0.03
Opisthorchis viverrini	65 (47.5)	37 (52.9)	28 (41.8)	0.19
Large trematode	1 (0.7)	1 (1.4)	0	n.a.
Strongyloides stercoralis	28 (20.4)	20 (28.5)	8 (11.9)	0.01
Hookworm	19 (13.9)	10 (14.3)	9 (13.4)	0.88
Trichuris trichiura	3 (2.2)	2 (2.9)	1 (1.5)	0.58
Ascaris lumbricoides	1 (0.7)	0	1 (1.5)	n.a.

P-value of Fisher exact test.
n.a., not applicable.

Table 3 shows the results from analyses regarding association between intestinal parasites and acute or persistent diarrhea. Compared to acute diarrhea, persistent diarrhea was significantly associated with *Cryptosporidium* sp. infection (20.0% vs. 2.5%, $P = 0.04$).

Table 4 summarizes significant associations between different intestinal parasite species and CD4 cell count. CD4 count ≤ 50 cells/mm^3 showed significant positive associations with infection with any parasite (OR = 3.5, 95% CI = 1.4–8.6), with three parasite species (OR = 2.9, 95% CI = 1.1–7.5), with any protozoa (OR = 2.4, 95% CI = 1.2–4.9), with any helminth (OR = 2.0, 95% CI = 1.0–3.9) and with O. *viverrini* (OR = 2.1, 95% CI = 1.0–4.3).

Discussion

Although the HIV prevalence in Laos is estimated to be at the low level of 0. 3%, the absolute number of people living with HIV/AIDS is increasing every year: the estimated number of 3,300 in 2001 reached 12,000 in 2012 [4]. Optimal patient care requires the development of laboratory diagnosis of infections and knowledge on the local epidemiology of infections, both of which are currently limited. We conducted the first laboratory-documented study on endemic and opportunistic intestinal parasites in HIV-infected patients, with or without diarrhea. In particular, we used for the first time in Laos specific methods for the detection of microsporidia, *Cryptosporidium* and other coccidia in stool samples.

Clinical and immunological status of the population

This cross-sectional study was carried out in the first two implemented and most important ART centers of the country, one located in the capital Vientiane (Setthathirath Hospital) and the other in a Southern province (Savannakhet Hospital). In this population, HIV infection was diagnosed in young (median age: 36 years) and severely immunocompromised patients, as assessed by WHO clinical staging criteria (83.9% of patients classified as stage 3 or 4) and low median CD4 cell count (41 cells/mm^3). Three factors may explain the late diagnosis of HIV infection. Firstly, the majority of patients (54.0%) lived in rural areas, especially in Southern provinces where information about HIV infection may not be widespread. Secondly, HIV screening tests are not available in all the district hospitals and health centers, which means that patients are required to travel to the diagnostic centers. Finally, Lao people use traditional medicine first and go to hospitals only if traditional methods fail [18]. Our results support previous data on severely immunocompromised patients at HIV diagnosis in Laos [3,4] and confirm the urgent need for suitable care of patients who are at high risk of opportunistic infections. The low prevalence of pulmonary tuberculosis and cryptococcal meningitis reported here (7.3% and 8.0% respectively) is most likely an underestimation. Due to the low diagnostic rate of the microbiological tools routinely used in these hospitals and their limited availability (less than 40% of the patients underwent laboratory investigations for opportunistic infections), it is very likely that some diagnoses were missed.

Diarrhea and parasite infections

Nearly half of the patients presented with diarrhea, of which one third presented with persistent diarrhea of more than two weeks duration. This proportion of diarrheal HIV patients is closer to that reported in industrialized countries before the highly active

Table 3. Association of intestinal parasites with acute and persistent diarrhea in HIV-infected patients, Laos (n = 59).

Parasites	Diarrhea (%)	Acute diarrhea, n = 39 (%)	Persistent diarrhea, n = 20 (%)	*P*-value
Any parasite	44 (74.6)	28 (71.8)	16 (80.0)	0.55
At least 2 parasite species	29 (49.1)	16 (41.0)	13 (65.0)	0.08
Any protozoa	31 (52.5)	18 (46.2)	13 (65.0)	0.27
Cryptosporidium spp.	5 (8.5)	1 (2.6)	4 (20.0)	0.04
Cytoisospora belli	3 (5.1)	2 (5.1)	1 (5.0)	1.00
Cyclospora cayetanensis	1 (1.7)	0	1 (5.0)	n.a.
Giardia intestinalis	5 (8.5)	4 (10.3)	1 (5.0)	0.65
Blastocystis spp.	19 (32.2)	10 (25.6)	9 (45.0)	0.15
Microsporidia	1 (1.7)	0	1 (5.0)	n.a.
Any helminth	32 (54.2)	21 (53.9)	11 (55.0)	1.00
Strongyloides stercoralis	9 (15.3)	6 (15.4)	3 (15.0)	1.00

P-value of Fisher exact test.
n.a., not applicable.

antiretroviral therapy era (40 to 80%) [19] than to the proportion that is usually observed in developing countries (up to 95%) [20,21]. This may be related to under-reporting of diarrhea by physicians or by the patients themselves. The clinical picture was more severe and compatible with more advanced WHO stages of HIV infection in diarrheal patients compared to non-diarrheal ones. However, we found no correlation between diarrhea and immunological failure as assessed by CD4 cell counts. No demographic characteristic or environmental condition (place of residence, living conditions) was found to be associated with diarrhea, except living in the Southern provinces. This might be due to the fact that our study sample was relatively small and therefore, small risk differences could not be detected.

Table 4. Association of intestinal parasites with CD4 cell count in HIV-infected patients, Laos (n = 137).

Parasites	Total (%)	CD4 ≤50/mm^3, n = 80 (%)	OR (95% CI)
Any parasite	108 (78.3)	70 (87.5)	3.5 (1.4–8.6)
Three parasite species	30 (21.9)	23 (28.7)	2.9 (1.1–7.5)
Any protozoa	75 (54.7)	51 (63.8)	2.4 (1.2–4.9)
Cryptosporidium spp.	9 (6.6)	8 (10.0)	6.2 (0.7–53.2)
Cytoisospora belli	6 (4.4)	3 (3.8)	0.7 (0.1–3.6)
Cyclospora cayetanensis	3 (2.2)	1 (1.3)	0.3 (0.03–4.0)
Giardia intestinalis	12 (8.8)	9 (11.3)	2.3 (0.6–9.0)
Blastocystis spp.	36 (26.3)	22 (27.5)	1.2 (0.5–2.5)
Microsporidia	4 (2.9)	3 (3.8)	2.0 (0.2–21.8)
Any helminth	80 (58.4)	52 (65.0)	1.9 (1.0–3.9)
Strongyloides stercoralis	28 (20.4)	18 (22.5)	1.4 (0.6–3.2)
Opisthorchis viverrini	65 (47.5)	44 (55.0)	2.1 (1.0–4.3)

OR, Odds ratio.
CI, Confidence interval.

Parasitological analyses of stool specimens revealed high prevalence rates of parasitism (78.8%), multiparasitism (presence of at least two different parasite species: 49.6%), protozoan infection (54.7%) and helminth infection (58.4%). Such findings in HIV-infected patients were not reported from neighboring countries in Southeast Asia [22,23,24,25,26,27,28,29]. Comparing prevalence rates of parasitic infections in HIV-infected patients amongst different countries or regions requires caution. The observed variations may be due to the different study designs and laboratory techniques used. On the other hand, they may reflect true differences in epidemiological features and specific risk factors from each country or region. Concerning the high prevalence of parasitism, multiparasitism and helminth infections, our results from HIV patients are in agreement with those of previous studies on the general population of Laos [6,7,9,10,11].

We investigated the association between intestinal infection,CD4 cell count and diarrhea. Compared to patients with CD4 cell count >50 cells/mm^3, patients with CD4 count ≤ 50 cells/mm^3 were more likely to be affected by intestinal parasitism (with any parasite, protozoa or helminth or *O. viverrini*) and multiparasitism with more than two species. Persistent diarrhea and cryptosporidiosis was the unique association observed between diarrhea and parasite infection.

Protozoa infections

With the Kato smear method being the unique diagnostic technique, protozoan infections are under-diagnosed in Laos. Virtually all results reported from the general population concern helminth infections [6,7,9,10,11]. Considering the recent emergence of HIV infection, improving biological diagnosis and knowledge about intestinal protozoan infections is crucial. We found that protozoan infections, affecting half of the population, were almost as prevalent as helminth infections. *Cryptosporidium* sp. and microsporidia are described here for the first time in Laos, with low prevalence rates of 6.6% and 2.9% respectively. The prevalence rates of cryptosporidiosis and microsporidiosis in HIV-infected population varied widely in previous studies from industrialized and developing countries, including neighboring countries of Laos. Prevalence of cryptosporidiosis varied from 0 to 100% with a median of 32%, and that of microsporidiosis from 5 to 50% with an overall prevalence of 15% [22,23,24,25,26,

27,28,29,30,31,32,33,34,35,36,37,38]. The presence or absence of diarrhea was not always specified in these studies. In Lao patients, persistent diarrhea was clearly linked to cryptosporidiosis as already reported in HIV-infected patients from various countries around the world [32,34,37]. Other opportunistic coccidia, *Cytoisospora belli* and *Cyclospora cayetanensis*, were found in our patients, with or without diarrhea. To our knowledge, *C. belli* has not been described before in Laos. To date, *C. cayetanensis* was mentioned in only one study, in which it was found to be responsible for 0.1% of diarrheal cases [39]. HIV status of the patient was not specified. The prevalence rates of *C. belli* and *C. cayetanensis* infections in our patients (4.4% and 2.2%, respectively) were close to those reported in HIV-infected patients in two neighboring countries, Thailand and Cambodia [22,24,25,26,28,35,40]. Studies on coccidia and microsporidia infections should be performed on the general population of Laos to confirm their low prevalence rates and to investigate their specific epidemiological features.

A striking finding in this study was the high frequency of the emergent pathogen, *Blastocystis* (26.3%). A high prevalence of *Blastocystis* in HIV-positive patients was also reported in China (19.2%) [27], contrary to Thailand where a prevalence of approximately 2% was found [23,25,26,28]. *Blastocystis* was recently described for the first time in Laos, with a prevalence of 13.6% in the general population of the Champasack province [9]. *Blastocystis* appeared to be the most prevalent protozoa both in general and in HIV populations from Laos, but the rate of *Blastocystis* carriage seemed to be higher in HIV-positive patients, a finding already reported elsewhere [37,41]. Clinical features were not specified in the participants of the Champasack study [9]. No association between *Blastocystis* and diarrhea or other digestive symptoms was found in our HIV patients, as reported in many previous studies in immunocompetent or immunocompromised patients [37,41]. The role of *Blastocystis* in gastrointestinal disease, which may be related to specific subtypes and parasite burden [42,43,44], is still controversial. However, it seems currently wise to consider *Blastocystis* as a pathogen in immunocompromised persons, such as HIV-infected patients, and to treat the infection [37,41].

Data from Laos on *G. intestinalis* and *E. histolytica/dispar* infections as for other protozoan infections, is scarce. Their prevalence rates in the general population seemed lower than those in the HIV-positive population : less than 0.5% [9,45] *vs.* 12.4% for *E. histolytica/dispar* infection, and around 4.5% [8,9] *vs.* 8.8% for *G. intestinalis* infection. Neither acute nor persistent diarrhea was associated in our study with *E. histolytica/dispar* or *G. intestinalis* carriage. In fact, none of these two infections is currently considered as opportunistic, even though HIV infection was reported to increase the risk of developing invasive amoebiasis and symptomatic *G. intestinalis* infection with progressive immunosuppression following reduced CD4 cell counts [37,46].

Helminth infections

As expected, helminth infections were highly frequent in the Lao HIV-positive population. Living in the Southern provinces appeared to be associated with helminth infections, which were also associated with the absence of in-house toilets. Inadequate sanitation, recognized as a determinant factor for parasitic infections, was reported to be a major problem in Laos [9]. Such a frequency of HIV-helminth co-infection and moreover, of HIV-multiparasitism association, requires particular attention in Lao patients. The immune modulation by helminths combined with the progressive immunodeficiency by HIV may have deleterious effects on both HIV acquisition and disease progression and on increased susceptibility to parasitic infections [27,47,48].

No helminth species was associated with diarrhea in the HIV-infected patients of the study, even *S. stercoralis*. Strongyloidiasis was associated with living in rural areas and was more frequent in Southern provinces than in Northern provinces. The overall prevalence was high (20.4%). Lower prevalence rates were found in the general population from Laos [6,7,8,9,10,11] as well as in HIV-infected patients from neighboring countries [22,24,25, 27,28,29,49]. With the increasing use of antiretroviral drugs in developing countries, the problem of possible immune reconstitution inflammatory syndrome (IRIS) to *S. stercoralis* infection has recently emerged [50,51]. Considering the high prevalence of strongyloidiasis and the frequent advanced stage of immunosuppression at HIV infection diagnosis in Laos, the risk of developing *Strongyloides* IRIS should be carefully assessed and prevented when initiating ART.

Small flukes were the most prevalent helminths in the HIV population (47.5%), as already reported in the general population [6,7,10]. *O.viverrini* eggs and those of minute intestinal flukes belonging to the Heterophyidae, Lecithodendriidae and Echinostomatidae families were not differentiated. This procedure requires adult worm recovery or molecular identification [6,7,10,52]. Since the highest *O. viverrini* prevalence rates have been reported from Southern provinces along the Mekong River [52,53], we can postulate that our samples originating from Bolikhmaxay, Savannakhet, Khammuane, Champasack and Saravane provinces, were mainly infected with *O. viverrini.* Opisthorchiasis is recognized as a major health problem in Laos because of high prevalence and associated chronic hepatobiliary abnormalities and cholangiocarcinoma [52,53]. The estimated prevalence of cholangiocarcinoma in people living in endemic areas was 5% [52,53]. The high frequency of HIV – *O. viverrini* co-infection raises the question of a potentially increasing occurrence of cholangiocarcinoma in surviving Lao AIDS patients treated with ART. The increased risk of non-AIDS-defining cancer in HIV-infected persons compared to the general population has already been pointed out in developed countries in the ART era [54,55]. The occurrence of several other cancer types might be due to the combination of HIV-induced immunosuppression and oncogenic infection [56,57]. *O. viverrini* is considered as a type 1 carcinogen by the International Agency for Research on Cancer, World Health Organization [53].

Limitations of the study

There were some limitations to this study. Firstly, the possibility that the patients had treated themselves with antibiotics or antiparasitic treatments prior to the hospitalization could not be precluded: sulfamethoxazole-trimethoprime, metronidazole, mebendazole, albendazole and praziquantel are available without prescription in Laos. Secondly, 23.3% of the patients gave three stool samples: the analysis of only one or two stool samples might lead to missed parasitological diagnoses. Thirdly, the techniques used have a relatively low sensitivity for the detection of some parasite species and might also have led to a certain underdiagnosis.

Conclusions

Parasitism and multiparasitism were common in patients at HIV diagnosis in Lao PDR, as previously reported in the general population. Novel features were found in the HIV-infected patients, with or without diarrhea. Firstly, protozoa infections were almost as prevalent as helminth infections, the more frequent being *Blastocystis* sp. infection. Secondly, coccidia (*Cryptosporidium* sp., *C. belli*, *C. cayetanensis*) and microsporidia were observed, and *Cryptosporidium* sp. was associated with persistent diarrhea. Finally, *S. stercoralis* was the most prevalent helminth following *O. viverrini*. The most immunocompromised patients, as assessed by a CD4 count $\leq$ 50 cells/mm^3, were more likely to be infected with parasites, protozoa, helminths and *O. viverrini*. Since HIV infection is currently diagnosed at an advanced stage of immunosuppression in Laos, our findings highlight the importance of laboratory diagnosis of intestinal parasitic infections including protozoa, and the need for adequate care and treatment. Further studies are required: i) to assess the prevalence and specific risk factors of intestinal protozoan infections in the general population of Laos, ii) to genetically characterize protozoan isolates, iii) to confirm and complete our clinical and epidemiological data on parasitic infections in HIV-positive patients from all the centers of the country and to search for bacteria and viruses in the stools of diarrheal patients.

Acknowledgments

We are grateful to Ms. Kayalath Khammoune and Mr. Singvongsay Somphavanh for their technical assistance in Savannakhet and Setthathirath Hospitals laboratories. We acknowledge MoH/CHAS and the Health authorities of the provinces and hospitals for allowing us to carry out the study. We would also thank the Fondation Mérieux for its support, LDBio Diagnostics for kindly providing us with Uvibio reagent and Marina Vincent for reviewing the English text. Special thanks to Dr Eric Bénéfice and Ms. Amala Phanalasy from the Institut de Recherche pour le Développement in Lao PDR, for their precious administrative help.

Author Contributions

Conceived and designed the experiments: PP NP EB ED JFE MR. Performed the experiments: PP NP EB KS SP EL BS YV MR. Analyzed the data: PP EB PO JFE MR. Contributed reagents/materials/analysis tools: PP NP BS YV PO JFE MR. Wrote the paper: PP EB PO JFE MR. Critically revisited the article: NP KS SP EL BS YV ED.

References

1. Lewthwaite P, Gill GV, Hart CA, Beeching NJ (2005) Gastrointestinal parasites in the immunocompromised. Curr Opin Infect Dis 18: 427–435.
2. Urdea M, Penny LA, Olmsted SS, Giovanni MY, Kaspar P, et al. (2006) Requirements for high impact diagnostics in the developing world. Nature 444 Suppl 1: 73–79.
3. Bastard M, Soulinphumy K, Phimmasone P, Saadani AH, Ciaffi L, et al. (2013) Women experience a better long-term immune recovery and a better survival on HAART in Lao People's Democratic Republic. BMC Infect Dis 13: 27.
4. UNAIDS (2013) UNAIDS report on the global AIDS epidemic 2013. Available: http://www.unaids.org/en/media/unaids/contentassets/documents/epidemiology/2013/gr2013/UNAIDS_Global_Report_2013_en.pdf. Accessed 2013 Sep 24.
5. Kato K, Miura M (1954) Comparative examinations. Jpn J Parasitology 3: 35.
6. Chai JY, Han ET, Guk SM, Shin EH, Sohn WM, et al. (2007) High prevalence of liver and intestinal fluke infections among residents of Savannakhet Province in Laos. Korean J Parasitol 45: 213–218.
7. Chai JY, Han ET, Shin EH, Sohn WM, Yong TS, et al. (2009) High prevalence of *Haplorchis taichui*, *Phaneropsolus molenkampi*, and other helminth infections among people in Khammouane province, Lao PDR. Korean J Parasitol 47: 243–247.
8. Kounnavong S, Vonglokham M, Houamboun K, Odermatt P, Boupha B (2011) Soil-transmitted helminth infections and risk factors in preschool children in southern rural Lao People's Democratic Republic. Trans R Soc Trop Med Hyg 105: 160–166.
9. Sayasone S, Mak TK, Vanmany M, Rasphone O, Vounatsou P, et al. (2011) Helminth and intestinal protozoa infections, multiparasitism and risk factors in Champasack province, Lao People's Democratic Republic. PLoS Negl Trop Dis 5: e1037.
10. Sayasone S, Vonghajack Y, Vanmany M, Rasphone O, Tesana S, et al. (2009) Diversity of human intestinal helminthiasis in Lao PDR. Trans R Soc Trop Med Hyg 103: 247–254.
11. Vannachone B, Kobayashi J, Nambanya S, Manivong K, Inthakone S, et al. (1998) An epidemiological survey on intestinal parasite infection in Khammouane Province, Lao PDR, with special reference to *Strongyloides* infection. Southeast Asian J Trop Med Public Health 29: 717–722.
12. WHO (2009) Health topics. Diarrhea. General information. Diarrheal disease. Fact sheet N°330. Available: http://www.who.int/mediacenter/factsheets/fs330/en/index.html. Accessed 2009 Aug.
13. WHO (2007) WHO case definitions of HIV for surveillance and revised clinical staging and immunological classification of HIV-related disease in adults and children. Available: http://www.who.int/hiv/pub/guidelines/HIVstaging150307.pdf. Accessed 2007 Mar 15.
14. Ridley DS, Hawgood BC (1956) The value of formol-ether concentration of faecal cysts and ova. J Clin Pathol 9: 74–76.
15. Henricksen SA, Pohlenz JFL (1981) Staining of *Cryptosporidia* by a modified Ziehl Neelsen technique. Acta Vet Scand 22: 594–596.
16. Weber R, Bryan RT, Owen RL, Wilcox CM, Gorelkin L, et al. (1992) Improved light-microscopical detection of microsporidia spores in stool and duodenal aspirates. The Enteric Opportunistic Infections Working Group. N Engl J Med 326: 161–166.
17. Van Gool T, Snijders F, Reiss P, Eeftnck Schattenkerk JKM, Van Den Bergh Weerman MA, et al. (1993) Diagnosis of intestinal and disseminated microsporidial infections in patients with HIV by a new rapid fluorescence technique. J Clin Pathol 46: 694–699.
18. Sydara K, Gneunphonsavath S, Wahlstrom R, Freudenthal S, Houamboun K, et al. (2005) Use of traditional medicine in Lao PDR. Complement Ther Med 13: 199–205.
19. Feasey NA, Healey P, Gordon MA (2011) Review article: the aetiology, investigation and management of diarrhea in the HIV-positive patient. Aliment Pharmacol Ther 34: 587–603.
20. Carcamo C, Hooton T, Wener MH, Weiss NS, Gilman R, et al. (2005) Etiologies and manifestations of persistent diarrhea in adults with HIV-1 infection: a case-control study in Lima, Peru. J Infect Dis 191: 11–19.
21. Thom K, Forrest G (2006) Gastrointestinal infections in immunocompromised hosts. Curr Opin Gastroenterol 22: 18–23.
22. Chhin S, Harwell JI, Bell JD, Rozycki G, Ellman T, et al. (2006) Etiology of chronic diarrhea in antiretroviral-naive patients with HIV infection admitted to Norodom Sihanouk Hospital, Phnom Penh, Cambodia. Clin Infect Dis 43: 925–932.
23. Chokephaibulkit K, Wanachiwanawin D, Tosasuk K, Pavitpok J, Vanprapar N, et al. (2001) Intestinal parasitic infections among human immunodeficiency virus-infected and -uninfected children hospitalized with diarrhea in Bangkok, Thailand. Southeast Asian J Trop Med Public Health 32: 770–775.
24. Manatsathit S, Tansupasawasdikul S, Wanachiwanawin D, Setawarin S, Suwanagool P, et al. (1996) Causes of chronic diarrhea in patients with AIDS in Thailand: a prospective clinical and microbiological study. J Gastroenterol 31: 533–537.
25. Pinlaor S, Mootsikapun P, Pinlaor P, Pipitgool V, Tuangnadee R (2005) Detection of opportunistic and non-opportunistic intestinal parasites and liver flukes in HIV-positive and HIV-negative subjects. Southeast Asian J Trop Med Public Health 36: 841–845.
26. Saksirisampant W, Prownebon J, Saksirisampant P, Mungthin M, Siripatanapipong S, et al. (2009) Intestinal parasitic infections: prevalences in HIV/AIDS patients in a Thai AIDS-care center. Ann Trop Med Parasitol 103: 573–581.
27. Tian LG, Chen JX, Wang TP, Cheng GJ, Steinmann P, et al. (2012) Co-infection of HIV and intestinal parasites in rural area of China. Parasit Vectors 5: 36.
28. Waywa D, Kongkriengdaj S, Chaidatch S, Tiengrim S, Kowadisaiburana B, et al. (2001) Protozoan enteric infection in AIDS related diarrhea in Thailand. Southeast Asian J Trop Med Public Health 32 Suppl 2: 151–155.
29. Wiwanitkit V (2001) Intestinal parasitic infections in Thai HIV-infected patients with different immunity status. BMC Gastroenterol 1: 3.
30. Didier ES, Weiss LM (2006) Microsporidiosis: current status. Curr Opin Infect Dis 19: 485–492.
31. Espern A, Morio F, Miegeville M, Illa H, Abdoulaye M, et al. (2007) Molecular study of microsporidiosis due to *Enterocytozoon bieneusi* and *Encephalitozoon intestinalis* among human immunodeficiency virus-infected patients from two geographical areas: Niamey, Niger, and Hanoi, Vietnam. J Clin Microbiol 45: 2999–3002.
32. Hunter PR, Nichols G (2002) Epidemiology and clinical features of *Cryptosporidium* infection in immunocompromised patients. Clin Microbiol Rev 15: 145–154.
33. Leelayoova S, Vithayasai N, Watanaveeradej V, Chotpitayasunondh T, Therapong V, et al. (2001) Intestinal microsporidiosis in HIV-infected children with acute and chronic diarrhea. Southeast Asian J Trop Med Public Health 32: 33–37.
34. O'Connor R M, Shaffie R, Kang G, Ward HD (2011) Cryptosporidiosis in patients with HIV/AIDS. AIDS 25: 549–560.
35. Punpoowong B, Viriyavejakul P, Riganti M, Pongponaratn E, Chaisri U, et al. (1998) Opportunistic protozoa in stool samples from HIV-infected patients. Southeast Asian J Trop Med Public Health 29: 31–34.
36. Srisuphanunt M, Saksirisampant W, Karanis P (2011) Prevalence and genotyping of *Cryptosporidium* isolated from HIV/AIDS patients in urban areas of Thailand. Ann Trop Med Parasitol 105: 463–468.

37. Stark D, Barratt JL, van Hal S, Marriott D, Harkness J, et al. (2009) Clinical significance of enteric protozoa in the immunosuppressed human population. Clin Microbiol Rev 22: 634–650.
38. Wanachiwanawin D, Manatsathit S, Lertlaituan P, Thakerngpol K, Suwanagool P (1998) Intestinal microsporidiosis in HIV infected patients with chronic diarrhea in Thailand. Southeast Asian J Trop Med Public Health 29: 767–771.
39. Kimura K, Rai SK, Rai G, Insisiengmay S, Kawabata M, et al. (2005) Study on *Cyclospora cayetanensis* associated with diarrheal disease in Nepal and Lao PDR. Southeast Asian J Trop Med Public Health 36: 1371–1376.
40. Chariyalertsak S, Sirisanthana T, Saengwonloey O, Nelson KE (2001) Clinical presentation and risk behaviors of patients with acquired immunodeficiency syndrome in Thailand, 1994–1998: regional variation and temporal trends. Clin Infect Dis 32: 955–962.
41. Tan KS (2008) New insights on classification, identification, and clinical relevance of *Blastocystis* spp. Clin Microbiol Rev 21: 639–665.
42. Coyle CM, Varughese J, Weiss LM, Tanowitz HB (2012) *Blastocystis*: to treat or not to treat. Clin Infect Dis 54: 105–110.
43. Scanlan PD (2012) *Blastocystis*: past pitfalls and future perspectives. Trends Parasitol 28: 327–334.
44. Stensvold CR, Alfellani M, Clark CG (2012) Levels of genetic diversity vary dramatically between *Blastocystis* subtypes. Infect Genet Evol 12: 263–273.
45. Phetsouvanh R, Midorikawa Y, Nakamura S (1999) The seasonal variation in the microbial agents implicated in the etiology of diarrheal diseases among children in Lao People's Democratic Republic. Southeast Asian J Trop Med Public Health 30: 319–323.
46. Dib HH, Lu SQ, Wen SF (2008) Prevalence of *Giardia lamblia* with or without diarrhea in South East, South East Asia and the Far East. Parasitol Res 103: 239–251.
47. Brown M, Mawa PA, Kaleebu P, Elliott AM (2006) Helminths and HIV infection: epidemiological observations on immunological hypotheses. Parasite Immunol 28: 613–623.
48. Webb EL, Ekii AO, Pala P (2012) Epidemiology and immunology of helminth-HIV interactions. Curr Opin HIV AIDS 7: 245–253.
49. Vaiyavatjamai P, Boitano JJ, Techasintana P, Tungtrongchitr A (2008) Immunocompromised group differences in the presentation of intestinal strongyloidiasis. Jpn J Infect Dis 61: 5–8.
50. Lawn SD, Wilkinson RJ (2006) Immune reconstitution disease associated with parasitic infections following antiretroviral treatment. Parasite Immunol 28: 625–633.
51. Taylor CL, Ustianowski AP (2008) Immune reconstitution syndrome to *Strongyloides stercoralis* infection. AIDS 22: 998.
52. Sripa B, Bethony JM, Sithithaworn P, Kaewkes S, Mairiang E, et al. (2011) Opisthorchiasis and *Opisthorchis*-associated cholangiocarcinoma in Thailand and Laos. Acta Trop 120 Suppl 1: S158–168.
53. Sithithaworn P, Andrews RH, Nguyen VD, Wongsaroj T, Sinuon M, et al. (2012) The current status of opisthorchiasis and clonorchiasis in the Mekong Basin. Parasitol Int 61: 10–16.
54. Antiretroviral Therapy Cohort (2010) Causes of death in HIV-1-infected patients treated with antiretroviral therapy, 1996–2006: collaborative analysis of 13 HIV cohort studies. Clin Infect Dis 50: 1387–1396.
55. Simard EP, Pfeiffer RM, Engels EA (2012) Mortality due to cancer among people with AIDS: a novel approach using registry-linkage data and population attributable risk methods. AIDS 26: 1311–1318.
56. Grulich AE, Li Y, McDonald A, Correll PK, Law MG, et al. (2002) Rates of non-AIDS-defining cancers in people with HIV infection before and after AIDS diagnosis. AIDS 16: 1155–1161.
57. Shiels MS, Engels EA (2012) Increased risk of histologically defined cancer subtypes in human immunodeficiency virus-infected individuals: clues for possible immunosuppression-related or infectious etiology. Cancer 118: 4869–4876.

18

Shared Sanitation versus Individual Household Latrines: A Systematic Review of Health Outcomes

Marieke Heijnen[1], Oliver Cumming[1], Rachel Peletz[1], Gabrielle Ka-Seen Chan[1], Joe Brown[3], Kelly Baker[2], Thomas Clasen[1,2]*

1 Faculty of Infectious and Tropical Diseases, London School of Hygiene & Tropical Medicine, London, United Kingdom, 2 Department of Environmental Health, Rollins School of Public Health, Emory University, Atlanta, Georgia, United States of America, 3 School of Civil and Environmental Engineering, Georgia Institute of Technology, Atlanta, Georgia, United States of America

Abstract

Background: More than 761 million people rely on shared sanitation facilities. These have historically been excluded from international sanitation targets, regardless of the service level, due to concerns about acceptability, hygiene and access. In connection with a proposed change in such policy, we undertook this review to identify and summarize existing evidence that compares health outcomes associated with shared sanitation versus individual household latrines.

Methods and Findings: Shared sanitation included any type of facilities intended for the containment of human faeces and used by more than one household, but excluded public facilities. Health outcomes included diarrhoea, helminth infections, enteric fevers, other faecal-oral diseases, trachoma and adverse maternal or birth outcomes. Studies were included regardless of design, location, language or publication status. Studies were assessed for methodological quality using the STROBE guidelines. Twenty-two studies conducted in 21 countries met the inclusion criteria. Studies show a pattern of increased risk of adverse health outcomes associated with shared sanitation compared to individual household latrines. A meta-analysis of 12 studies reporting on diarrhoea found increased odds of disease associated with reliance on shared sanitation (odds ratio (OR) 1.44, 95% CI: 1.18–1.76).

Conclusion: Evidence to date does not support a change of existing policy of excluding shared sanitation from the definition of improved sanitation used in international monitoring and targets. However, such evidence is limited, does not adequately address likely confounding, and does not identify potentially important distinctions among types of shared facilities. As reliance on shared sanitation is increasing, further research is necessary to determine the circumstances, if any, under which shared sanitation can offer a safe, appropriate and acceptable alternative to individual household latrines.

Editor: Hamid Reza Baradaran, Iran University of Medical Sciences, Iran (Islamic Republic of)

Funding: Funding for this research has been provided by UNICEF and the SHARE research consortium supported by the UK Department for International Development. The funders had no role in study design, data collection and analysis, decision to publish, or preparation of the manuscript.

Competing Interests: The authors have declared that no competing interests exist.

* E-mail: tclasen@emory.edu

Introduction

Unsanitary disposal of human excreta, together with unsafe drinking water and poor hygiene conditions, is a leading cause of morbidity and mortality in low-income countries [1,2]. Much of this disease burden consists of diarrhoeal disease, a leading killer of young children. In addition, inadequate sanitation is implicated in schistosomiasis, helminth infections, enteric fevers and trachoma [3]. Lack of access to sanitation also has significant non-health consequences, particularly for women and girls, including lack of security and privacy, decreased school attendance and basic human dignity [4].

An estimated 2.5 billion people lack access to improved sanitation facilities [5]. In developing regions where people are most vulnerable to infection, only one in every three people has access to improved sanitation [5]. At the current pace, the Millennium Development Goal (MDG) sanitation target—to halve the proportion of people with access to basic sanitation by 2015—is set to miss the target by half a billion people [5].

The MDG target, which is expressed in terms of 'basic sanitation', was deemed to be context specific and to include 'the lowest-cost option for securing sustainable access to safe, hygienic, and convenient facilities and services for excreta and sullage disposal that provide privacy and dignity, while at the same time ensuring a clean and healthful living environment both at home and in the neighbourhood of users' [6]. However, the Joint Monitoring Programme for Water Supply and Sanitation (JMP), which monitors progress toward the target, defines "improved sanitation" in terms of service levels. This includes a private flush or pour-flush toilet or latrine connected to a piped sewer system or septic system, a simple pit latrine with a slab, a ventilated improved pit latrine or a composing toilet. Any other flush or pour-flush latrine, an open pit latrine, bucket latrine, a hanging latrine, or open defecation is "unimproved" and not scored toward the MDG target [5].

Significantly, public and other "shared facilities"—those used by two or more households—are excluded from the definition of

Table 1. Electronic databases searched.

Database		Last search date	Number of results
OvidSP (Ovid Technologies 2013)	EMBASE	October 7th, 2013	4248
	MEDLINE	October 7th, 2013	2976
	CAB Abstracts,	October 12th, 2013	6586
	Global Health,	October 7th, 2013	5660
	HMIC,	October 7th, 2013	74
	Social Policy & Practice	October 7th, 2013	42
Virtual Health Library	DESASTRES	October 3rd, 2013	332
	LEYES	October 3rd, 2013	29
	LILACS	October 3rd, 2013	36
	MedCarib	October 3rd, 2013	28
	REPIDISCA	October 3rd, 2013	73
Individually searched databases	Africa wide	October 4th, 2013	3495
	Cochrane	October 3rd, 2013	16
	IMEMR	October 4th 2013	10
	CEHA	October 4th, 2013	2
	HISA	October 4th, 2013	5
	WPRIM	October 4th, 2013	4
Chinese language databases	WANFANG	October 23rd, 2013	915
	CNKI	Ocotber 23rd, 2013	946

"improved sanitation" regardless of the service level [7]. The reason stems from concerns that shared facilities are unacceptable, both in terms of cleanliness (toilets may not be hygienic and fully separate human waste from contact with users) and accessibility (facilities may not be available at night or during periods of high demand) [5].

Nevertheless, shared facilities represent a large and growing proportion of sanitation options available in low-income countries. Nearly a fifth of the population of sub-Saharan Africa (18%) and Eastern Asia (19%) reports using shared sanitation; the practice is particularly common in Ghana (59%), Congo, and Gabon (both 34%) [5]. Globally, the number of users has increased by 437 million since 1990 – increasing from 6 per cent of the global population to 11 per cent in 21 years. In many countries, particularly in crowded urban areas, shared sanitation is the only viable option for those wishing to avoid open defecation; in rural areas, families often keep costs down by sharing latrines between one or more households with family ties [8]. In addition, shared sanitation might provide the opportunity for individuals to move away from open defecation and take the first step on the sanitation ladder.

Perhaps as a result, the JMP is considering a revision to its policy that would include shared sanitation as "improved" – and thus scored toward the post-MDG targets – if the facilities meet the required level of service and are shared among no more than 5 families or 30 persons, whichever is fewer [5]. This proposed change is based on advice from an expert committee [9].

We undertook this review to examine the evidence comparing the impact of shared sanitation versus individual household latrines (IHLs) on health outcomes.

Methods

The review was undertaken in accordance with a protocol, a copy of which is available on request.

Eligibility criteria

Studies were eligible for inclusion if they compared health outcomes of populations relying on shared sanitation with those relying on IHLs. In some cases the latrine type was inferred from the study report. For purposes of this review, shared sanitation included any type of facilities intended for the containment of human faeces and used primarily from home; this excludes "public" sanitation facilities designed primarily for use by householders when they are away from the home, such as schools, markets, train or bus stations, city streets, health facilities, governmental buildings or other public places. Health outcomes included diarrhoea, helminth infections, enteric fevers, other faecal-oral diseases, trachoma and adverse maternal or birth outcomes. Studies were included regardless of study design, location, language or publication status.

Information sources

Our search was performed through September 2013. We employed keywords for health related outcomes. The full lists of key search terms are listed in Table S2.

We performed an electronic search of 19 databases, including 2 Chinese language databases. An overview of the databases is shown in Table 1. Where possible, the same key search terms were used to search the grey literature sources for relevant literature. Conference proceedings from the following institutions were searched for relevant abstracts: WEDC (Loughborough University), IRC International Water and Sanitation Centre, and the German Agency for International Cooperation (GIZ). In addition, governmental agencies, non-governmental organisations (NGOs), universities and others involved in funding, implementing or investigating sanitation were contacted to solicit other studies that met the review's inclusion criteria. In all cases, references lists of studies were also reviewed for additional possible studies.

Study selection

Two authors independently examined the full text of potentially relevant articles using the standard protocol developed by the authors. For Chinese-language search results, a third author undertook the same process individually.

Data collection process

Relevant data, including a brief description of the study (study design, setting and year), details of the study population, specifications of the sanitation facilities and the outcome measures investigated were extracted independently from all eligible studies by two authors. If an article lacked necessary information, we contacted the authors or publishers to attempt to secure it.

Assessment for methodological quality

Each study included in the review was assessed for methodological quality. For observational studies, the STROBE (Strengthening of the Reporting of Observational studies in Epidemiology) statement was used as a guideline to extract data on the risks of bias. While the protocol for the review contemplated assessing studies with a specified intervention group using the Cochrane EPOC (Effective Practice and Organisation of Care) criteria, no such studies met the review's inclusion criteria.

Synthesis of results

We pooled studies reporting on diarrhoea and conducted a meta-analysis based on a random effects model. No further synthesis of results was undertaken to due to the limited number of studies reporting on other health outcomes.

Results

Study selection

Execution of the search strategy resulted in 25477 titles and abstracts. In addition, 169 unpublished documents were retrieved. These titles and abstracts were screened and the full text articles of 202 documents were obtained for further assessment. Of these studies, 22 documents met the review's inclusion criteria. A detailed overview is provided in Figure 1. Reasons for exclusion of documents are provided in Table S5.

Study characteristics

General diarrhoea was the outcome of interest in six studies [10–15], with two studies focusing specifically on watery diarrhoea [16,17] and another on bloody diarrhoea [18]. While other studies included all ages, Baker et al. [14], Chakraborty et al. [13], and Sobel et al. [12] limited the studies to diarrhoea in children under the age of 5 years. A variety of intestinal parasites were investigated in seven studies [11,19–24]. Other health outcome measures included *S.typhi* and *S. paratyphi* A [25], poliomyelitis [26], trachoma [27], *Shigella dysenteriae* type I [28], perinatal death and antenatal foetal death [29], preterm birth and low birth weight [30], and hospital admissions [31]. One study investigated diarrhoea specifically in an HIV-positive population [15].

Participants and settings. Most studies took place in urban settings, though one conducted a comparative urban-rural investigation [23]. Except for one study among an aboriginal population in Australia [31], all studies were conducted in low- and middle- income settings. Three studies were conducted in Kenya [16–18] and two in India [10,13], Bangladesh [11,21], and in Egypt [20,22]; and one in each of Brazil [12], Zambia [28], the Democratic Republic of Congo [24], Nigeria [30], Malawi [23], Zimbabwe [19], Taiwan [26], Jamaica [29], Ghana [32], Nepal [25], South Africa [15] and Tanzania [27]. One study was conducted in multiple countries [14]. Two studies, Shultz et al. and Mahamud et al., were conducted in long-established refugee camps [16,17].

The study population varied considerably, from only women in the studies on maternal and new born health [29,30], to only men in a study in Egypt [20]. Seven studies focused specifically on children, with ages ranging from children under the age of 5 [13,14,22], children under the age of three [10], children aged 1–5 [12,27] and children aged 3–14 years old [23]. As many of the health outcomes vary considerably with age, socio-economic class, population density and other covariates, the comparability of these results must be viewed with the significant differences in study populations and settings in mind.

Types of shared sanitation. The types of latrines assessed and reported on also varied considerably (Table 2). In most cases, the common facilities were shared with other families [14,18,23,31]; only Montgomery et al. provided information on the number of families sharing [27]. Shultz et al. looked at three or more households sharing a latrine (without a clearly specified comparison group) [16]. In some instances IHL was compared to 'sharing with at least one other family' [12,22,26]. Olusanya et al. [30] compared shared latrines with IHLs, though with no further details of the type of shared latrine. Similarly, Karkey et al. compared household latrines use versus community latrines [25], whereas Moshabela et al. report sharing sanitation facilities with an average of two other households [15].

In several cases, the type of shared sanitation was not well defined, with the authors using terms such as "communal" [13,21] to distinguish them from IHLs. Moreover, potentially important information such as ownership, management or approximate numbers of users was often omitted.

Ghosh [10] and Tuttle [28] looked at the sharing of a common latrine, and Golding [29] considered the sharing of toilets; in these cases, however, it was not clear that the comparison was an IHL. Tshikuka et al. investigated the number of persons per toilet as well as the number of people practicing open defecation [24]. Chandiwana et al. looked at the number of persons per latrine, without specifying a comparison group [19]. In these two cases where the number of people per toilet was reported, it was not clear whether this was actually counted, or if an average of households or persons per latrine was calculated.

Some studies included multiple comparisons, for example, Khan reported on communal latrines versus private or compound shared latrines [11] whereas Curtale looked at different settings, including rural IHLs and some sharing of family latrines in urban areas [20].

Study designs. All studies included in the review followed an observational study design. These were either cross-sectional, case control or cohort studies (Table 2).

Summary measures. The large variety of studies included resulted in different study measures (Table 2). Odds ratios were reported in 14 studies and for the remainder of studies only the percentages or differences in means were reported.

Assessment of methodological quality

The Supplementary Material provides detailed information on the methodological assessments (Table S3). Only one of the included studies reported a sample size calculation [23]. Similarly, only one study reported the interview response rate [27]. Seven studies reported using some form of random sampling [13,15,17,20,23–25], though only four of these clearly described the randomisation method [15,17,23,25]. Eight of the 11 included case control studies report matching of the cases and controls

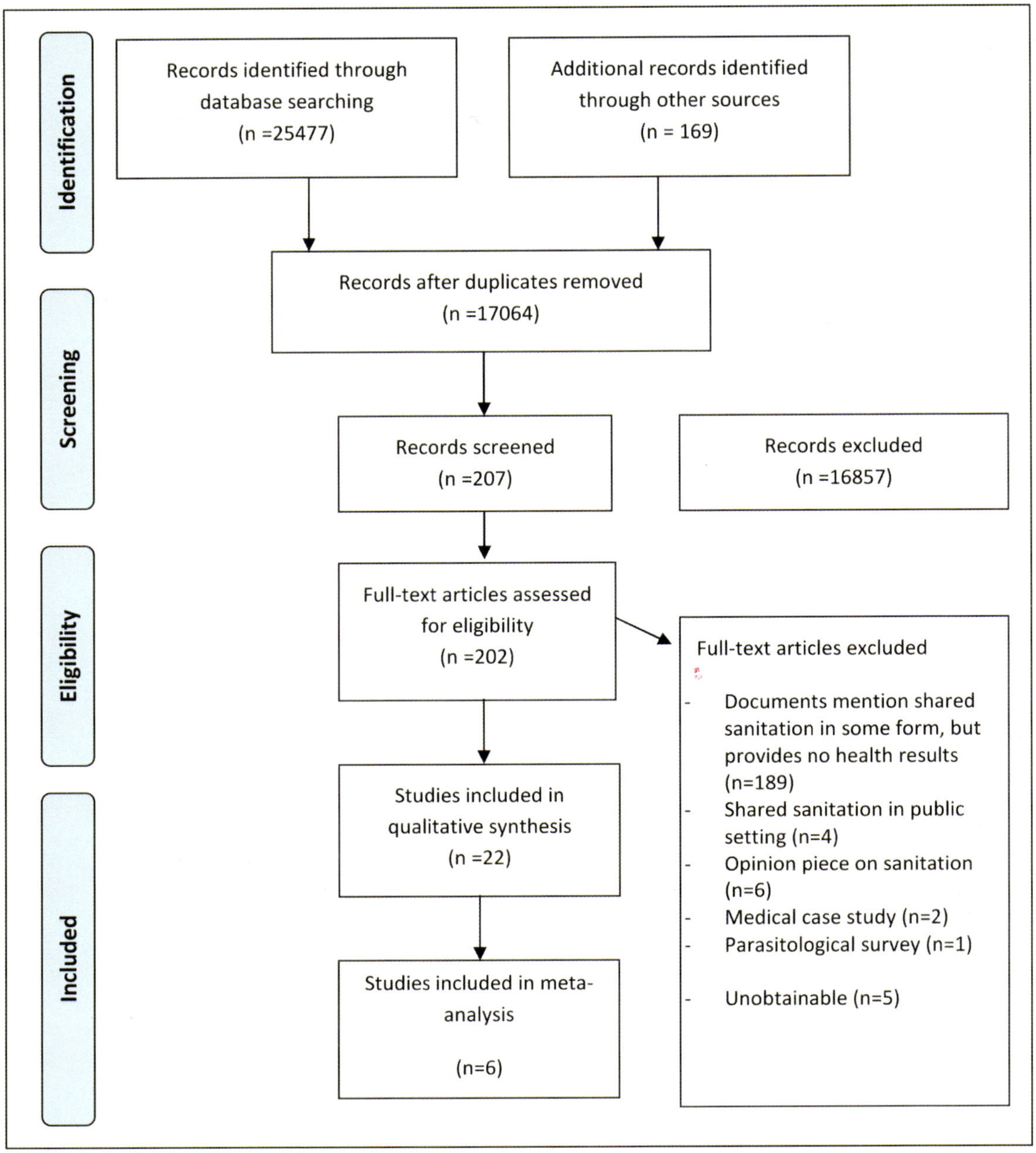

Figure 1. PRIMSA Flow Chart.

(matched [12,14,16–18,25,27,28], while three used unmatched cases and controls [10,15,26].)

Among the nine studies reporting on diarrhoea, only Baker et al. and Shultz et al. used clinically confirmed cases. All others relied on self-reported diarrhoea and failed to report on the recall period, both potential sources of bias [33].

Outcomes

Twenty-two studies reported on health outcomes associated with shared sanitation. These are summarized in Table 3.

Diarrhoeal disease. Nine studies investigated diarrhoeal disease as an outcome measure (Table 3). In all but two [13,15], sharing a latrine was found to be associated with an increased risk of diarrhoeal disease. Shultz et al. found that sharing a latrine with at least three households was associated with an increased risk of watery diarrhoea (Matched OR 2.17 [95% CI 1.01–4.68] [16]. Sobel et al. found that sharing a toilet with another household was a risk factor for acute diarrhoea cases presented at hospital (OR 1.48 [95% CI 1.07–2.04]) [12]. Similarly Tuttle et al. reported that households with shigella cases were more likely to share latrines than control households (Matched OR 3.3 [95% CI 1.1–10.2]) [28]. Initial results from a multi-country study by Baker et al. showed increased odds of moderate and severe diarrhoea when latrines are shared (matched OR 1.2 [95% CI 1.1–1.3]) [14]. A significant association between shared latrines and the incidence of diarrhoea is also reported by Ghosh et al. ($p = 0.008$) though no odds ratios or confidence intervals are presented [10]. Brooks et al. report an increased risk of bloody diarrhoea if other families are allowed to use the latrine (OR 2.40 [95% CI 1.19–4.48]), though no data is provided on the number of families sharing latrines [18].

Table 2. Summary of data extracted from included studies.

Author	Study design	Type of Shared Sanitation	Type of Comparison Sanitation	Main outcomes	Summary measures
Brooks 2003	Case control	'allowing other families to use the compound latrine'	Latrine for private use only	Risk factors for bloody diarrhoea	Matched Odds Ratio (95% CI)
Chakraborty 1983	Cross sectional	Community latrines in slum	Private latrine connected to sewer	Episodes of diarrhoea	Mean
Chandiwana 1989	Cross sectional	Shared latrines	No comparison	Prevalence and intensity of hookworm and roundworm	Prevalence, correlations
Curtale 1998	Cross sectional	Family latrine not shared with others	Latrine shared with others	Prevalence and intensity of intestinal helminth infection	Prevalence
Ghosh 1994	Case control	Sharing latrine	Private latrine*	Diarrhoeal disease	Percentages
Golding 1994	Cross sectional	Toilet used by others outside of family	Toilet only used by family	Perinatal death, antepartum fetal death	Adjusted OR (95% CI)
Hall 1994	Cross sectional	Shared and community latrine	Private latrine	*Strongyloides stercoralis* infection	Odds ratio (95% CI)
Khan 1987	Cross sectional	Communal latrines in peri urban slums	Open pit latrines in peri urban slums	Diarrhoea cases and intestinal parasite prevalence†	Prevalence
Kim-Farley 1984	Case control	Toilet shared >1 family	Private latrines*	Poliomyelitis	Odds ratio (95% CI)
Mahfouz 1997	Cross sectional	Sharing toilets with other family	Sole use of household latrine*	Prevalence of intestinal parasites and protozoa	Adjusted OR (95% CI)
Montgomery 2010	Case control	Shared latrines	Private latrines	Trachoma	Adjusted OR (95% CI)
Munoz 1992	Cohort	Communal toilet	Private toilet	Hospital admissions	Percentages, factor scores
Olusanya 2010	Cross sectional	Shared sanitation	Private sanitation	Preterm and low birthweight	Unadjusted OR (95% CI)
Phiri 2001	Cross sectional	Shared latrine	Private latrine*	Prevalence of helminths	Adjusted OR (95% CI)
Shultz 2009	Case control	Three or more households sharing same latrine	Not specified	Watery diarrhoea	Matched OR (95% CI)
Sobel 2004	Case control	Shared latrine with other household	Private latrine*	Acute diarrhoeal disease	Matched OR (95% CI)
Tshikuka 1994	Cross sectional	Sharing a toilet with others	Private latrine*	*Ascaris lumbricoides* infection	Means, Beta coefficient
Tuttle 1995	Case control	Shared latrine	Private latrine*	*Shigella dysenteriae* type1	Matched OR (95% CI)
Baker 2011	Case control (abstract)	Shared sanitation	Private latrine	Risk of diarrhoea	Matched OR (95% CI)
Moshabela 2012	Case control	Sharing latrine with an average of 2 households	Private latrine*	Diarrhoeal disease	Prevalence
Karkey, 2013	C ase control	Community latrine	Household latrine	Enteric infection (*S. typhi* or *S. paratyphi* A.)	Adjusted OR (95% CI)
Mahamud 2012	Case control	Communal latrine	Compound latrine	Diarrhoea and Cholera	Odds ratio (95% CI)

*Latrine type inferred from study report.
†Study mentions measurement of incidence. As this is a cross sectional study, it is interpreted as prevalence.

Chakraborty et al. found no difference in the incidence of diarrhoea between children living in the slum, where public latrines are available, and children living in a housing project, where each family had their own latrine [13]. It must be noted however, that the study population is children under 5 years, and the study also reports that few of these young children use latrines, irrespective of where they live. Similarly, Moshabela et al. found no difference between diarrhoeal disease for those reporting sharing sanitation facilities with other households (25.3% of cases and 23.7% of controls shared sanitation facilities, $p = 0.76$). All the subjects in this study were HIV positive individuals [15].

The studies reporting an effect on diarrhoea have been pooled in a meta-analysis using a random effects model (Figure 2). This yielded a pooled odds ratio (OR) of 1.44 (95%CI: 1.18–1.76), suggesting increased risk associated with shared sanitation. The pooled estimate is characterized by substantial heterogeneity ($I^2 = 77.9\%$). Some of the studies contributing data to our pooled analysis (Figure 2) on the effect of shared sanitation on diarrhoea is

Table 3. Summary of health outcomes.

Author	Study design	Main outcomes	Outcome measure
Diarrhoea			
Brooks 2003	Case control	Risk factors for bloody diarrhoea	OR 2.40 (95% CI 1.19–4.48)
Chakraborty 1983	Cross sectional	Episodes of diarrhoea	On average, there were 1.6 episodes of diarrhoea in the slum, versus 1.4 in the housing project
Khan 1987	Cross sectional	Diarrhoea cases and intestinal parasite prevalence	On average, there were 0.81 episodes of diarrhoea in the area with communal latrines, versus 0.7 in the area with open pit latrines (p<0.01). No CI.
Baker 2011	Case control (abstract)	Risk of severe to moderate diarrhoea	OR 1.20 (95% CI 1.1–1.3)
Shultz 2009	Case control	Watery diarrhoea	OR 2.17 (95% CI 1.01–4.68)
Sobel 2004	Case control	Acute diarrhoeal disease	OR 1.48 (95% CI 1.07–2.04)
Ghosh 1994	Case control	Diarrhoeal disease	P = 0.008 No CI.
Moshabela 2012	Case control	Diarrhoeal disease	25.3% of cases and 23.7% of controls (p = 0.76)reported sharing sanitation
Mahamud 2012	Case control	Watery diarrhoea/cholera	OR 3.33 (95% CI 1.34–8.30)
Helminths			
Chandiwana 1989	Cross sectional	Prevalence and intensity of hookworm and roundworm	Correlations between number of households and hookworm r = 0.72, (P<0.1), roundworm r = −0.009, (P<0.1)
Curtale 1998	Cross sectional	Prevalence and intensity of intestinal helminth infection	Sharing latrines and the absence of piped water in the house were associated with a significantly higher intensity of infection for *A. Lumbricoides* (p<0.001) and *T. Trichiura* (p<0.05)
Hall 1994	Cross sectional	*Strongyloides stercoralis* infection	OR 2.72 (95% CI 1.57–4.72)
Mahfouz 1997	Cross sectional	Prevalence of intestinal parasites and protozoa	Intestinal helminths: OR 1.95 (95% CI 1.38–2.75) Protozoa: OR 1.65 (95% CI 1.06–2.58)
Phiri 2001	Cross sectional	Prevalence of helminths	
Tshikuka 1994	Cross sectional	*Ascaris lumbricoides* infection	Nr of persons/toilet Beta 0.45 (P<0.01, SE 0.02)
Other health outcomes			
Tuttle 1995	Case control	*Shigella dysenteriae* type1	OR 3.3 (95% CI 1.1–10.2)
Karkey 2013	Case control	*S. typhi* and *S. paratyphi A*	aOR 4.92 (1.2–19.5) for *S. paratyphi* A aOR 7.26 (1.4–37.2) for *S.typhi*
Montgomery 2010	Case control	Trachoma	OR 0.95 (95% CI 0.55–1.67)
Munoz 1992	Cohort	Hospital admissions	'communal sanitation' was a significant variable in the factor analysis (p<0.01)
Olusanya 2010	Cross sectional	Preterm and low birthweight	Prematurity aOR 1.36 (95% CI 1.07–1.48) Low birth weight aOR 1.27 (95% CI 0.98–1.65)
Kim-Farley 1984	Case control	Poliomyelitis	OR 4.0 (95% CI 1.9–8.3)
Golding 1994	Cross sectional	Perinatal death, antepartum fetal death	Antepartum fetal death aOR 1.62 (95% CI 1.28–2.03) Perinatal death aOR 1.41 (95% CI 1.21–1.64)

drawn from preliminary, yet-to-be published results from seven countries included in the Global Enterics Multi-Centre Study (GEMS) [14]. However, the GEMS study design as well as the general methods for collection of water and sanitation exposure data and the definition for moderate and severe diarrhoea used to screen and enrol case and controls has been published [34,35]. The study used a case-control design where cases were based on clinical diagnoses of moderate to severe diarrhoea in children <5 years. As shown in Figure 2, initial results, adjusting for wealth and faeces visible in the facility, show that shared sanitation was a statistically significant risk factor in two countries (Pakistan, Mali) and was trending toward increased risk in three other countries (Gambia, Mozambique and Kenya). Interestingly, shared sanitation trended in the opposite direction, appearing protective in Bangladesh. This study reports that even though there is site variability, there is an overall trend among most sites. Except for Bangladesh, cases are more likely to live in a household that shares a latrine. The pooled odds ratio from the seven GEMS studies yields an OR of 1.26 (95% CI 1.01–1.57) compared to OR 2.01 (95% CI 1.44–2.81) for the five published studies (Figure S2).

Helminths and protozoan parasites. Six studies reported associations between shared sanitation facilities and helminth infections, of which only one study reported no association (Table 3). Tshikuka et al. found that the number of persons per toilet was statistically associated with *Ascaris lumbricoides* infection intensity [24]. However, it is not clear whether the persons per latrine were counted or calculated as an average. Mahfouz et al. found that sharing toilets with another family increased the risk of intestinal helminths (*A.lumbricoides, Trichuris trichiura, Hymenolepis nana, Oxyuris, Ancylostoma duodenale, Schistosoma mansoni*) (adjusted OR 1.95[95% CI 1.38–2.75]) and from protozoan parasites [*Giardia lamblia, Entamoeba histolytica*] (adjusted OR 1.65 [95% CI 1.06–2.58]) [22].

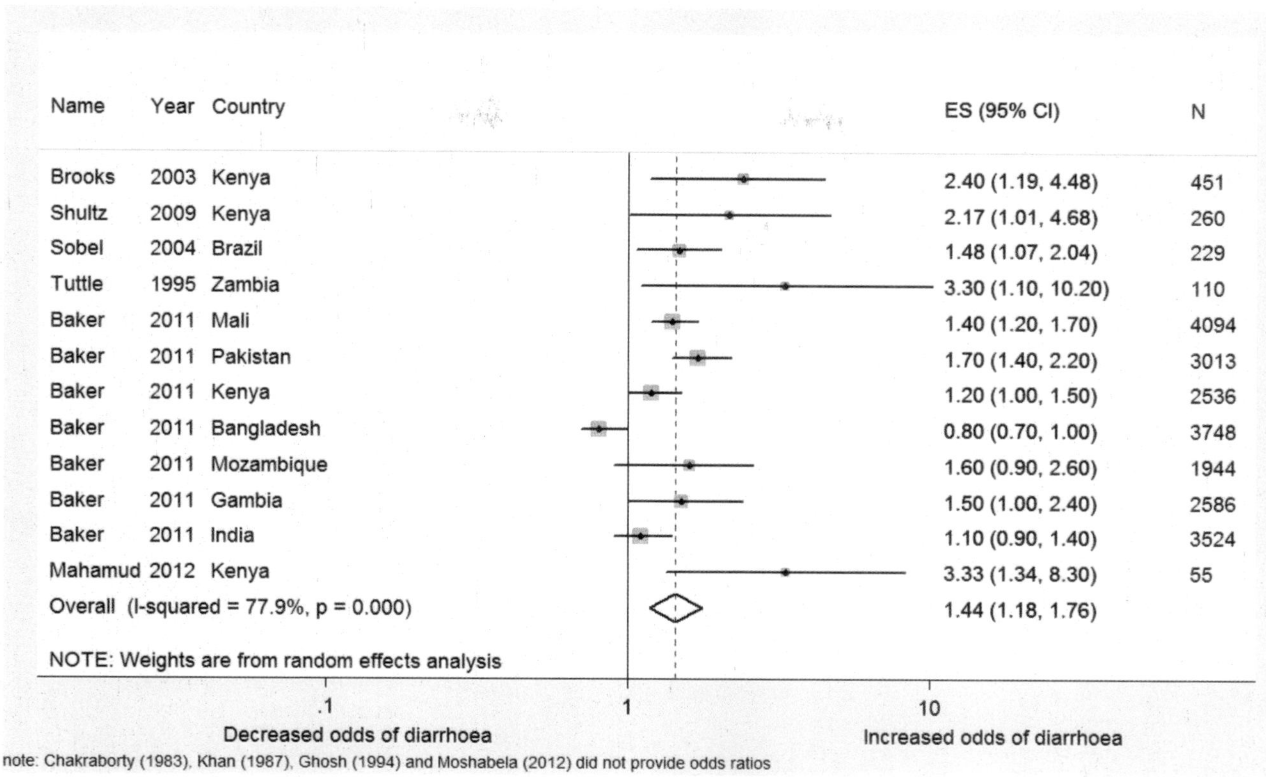

Figure 2. Meta-analysis for the use of shared sanitation and diarrhoea. Image produced using Stata (Statacorp LP, TX USA). CI: Confidence Interval. ES: Effect size (Odds Ratio).

Hall et al. found that for adults, using a community latrine rather than a private latrine was statistically significant risk factor for *S. stercoralis* infection (adjusted OR 2.72 [95% CI 1.57–4.72) [21]. On the other hand, they found that using a latrine shared between neighbours versus a private latrine showed no significant association. Similarly, for children the risk of *S. stercoralis* infection was increased when using communal latrines (adjusted OR 2.43 [95% CI 1.35–4.38]), whereas no such association could be found for shared latrines. No information was provided on the number of people or households using either the shared or the communal latrines.

In a study in Egypt, sharing latrine with other families and the absence of piped water inside the house were associated with a significantly higher intensity of infection for *A. lumbricoides* ($p<0.001$) and for *T. trichiura* ($p<0.05$) but not *for S. mansoni* [20]. No separate data were presented for shared latrines and no information was provided on the number of households sharing. Lastly, Phiri et al. found no statistically significant risk associated with *A. lumbricoides*, hookworm, *T. Trichiura*, or *S. stercoralis* infection and shared latrine facilities [23].

Other health outcomes. A study by Montgomery et al. found that shared latrines provided as much protection as private latrines in regard to the risk of trachoma (adjusted OR 0.95 [95% CI 0.55–1.67]) [27]. Also, the number of households sharing did not significantly alter the risk.

Kim-Farley et al. investigated a poliomyelitis outbreak in Taiwan using a case control design [26]. It was shown that more cases than controls shared toilets with other families (OR 4.0 [95% CI 1.9–8.3]). However, this was a univariate analysis, not controlled for other exposures.

Karkey et al. investigate enteric infection with either *S. typhi* or *S. paratyphi* A and found that communal latrine use (versus individual household latrines) was protective (adjusted OR 4.92 [95% CI 1.2–19.5] for *S. paratyphi* A and adjusted OR 7.26 [95% CI 1.4–37.2] for *S. typhi*). In this study, 92.2 per cent of the cases used a household latrine versus 77.9 per cent of the controls [25].

Several studies reported on adverse birth outcomes. Olusanya et al. investigated preterm birth and low birth weight risk factors [30]. Living in a house with shared sanitation facilities was found to be a risk factor for prematurity (adjusted OR 1.26 [95% CI 1.07–1.48]), whereas there was only a weak association with low birth weight (adjusted OR 1.27 [95% CI 0.98–1.65]). Golding and colleagues found an increased risk of perinatal death among women who had to share toilet facilities with people other than members of their family [29]. This was associated especially with antepartum fetal deaths (adjusted OR 1.62 [95% CI 1.28–2.03]) and perinatal death (adjusted OR 1.41 [95% CI 1.21–1.64]). In rural aboriginal communities in Australia, Munoz et al. reported that communal toilets were associated with an increased risk of hospital admissions for children [31]. However, the authors acknowledged that many community characteristics were strongly associated with differences in admission rates between communities thus limiting the potential for causal interferences.

Discussion

In general, the evidence suggests that those relying on shared sanitation facilities compared to IHLs are at increased risk of adverse health outcomes, including diarrhoeal disease, helminth infection, poliomyelitis, as well as prematurity, antepartum fetal death and perinatal death. The evidence on diarrhoeal disease and on helminth infection reflects a consistent pattern across most studies and study sites, while the evidence on poliomyelitis and adverse birth outcomes was generated from single studies. On the other hand, research found no increased risk of trachoma associated with reliance on shared sanitation.

Although most of the studies reviewed suggest a pattern of shared sanitation and adverse health outcomes, the quality of these studies varies and the actual strength of evidence is weak, and should be interpreted with caution. This is due to at least four major limitations.

First, as noted, many of the studies included in the review are of uncertain methodological quality. Fewer than a third of the studies reported using random selection of the study sites or population, presenting the potential for selection bias. The type of sanitation facilities being compared was not blinded to the study population or assessors. This and the fact that many studies relied on reported outcomes raises questions of reporting bias. Many of the studies fail to report on case definitions, participant eligibility and selection procedures, methods for assessing outcomes, potential sources of bias, etc. There are also statistical shortcomings, such as the failure to adjust for clustering and the treatment of populations as multiple rather than single units. Moreover, many studies reflect methodological problems common in assessments of environmental health interventions [36] and in the assessment of faecal-oral diseases such as diarrhoea [37].

Second, few of the studies report on possible factors other than the type of sanitation facilities that could be important confounders or effect modifiers. Most obvious of these, perhaps, is actual latrine use. There is evidence, for example, that a variety of factors such a distance, waiting time and cost can significantly impact the use of shared sanitation facilities [38,39]. Other factors that may vary between shared sanitation facilities and IHLs include latrine maintenance, distance to and quantity/quality of water supplies, the presence and use of hand washing facilities and soap, the manner in which users dispose of child faeces, and the way in which the waste is subsequently removed from the facilities and ultimately disposed of in the setting. Additionally, the population density, socio-economic status, gender or other equity issues of the users of shared facilities versus IHL may differ, aspects which are infrequently reported on in the studies specifying shared sanitation.

Third, there are substantial differences among the studies that limit their comparability. This includes differences in study design, settings, study populations and ambient conditions. It also includes fundamental differences (and in many cases, uncertainty) in the actual types of shared sanitation and the types of IHLs being compared. There are also important differences in outcomes, the manner in which they were assessed and in the methods for their analysis.

Finally, and perhaps most important, the studies undertaken to date allow only for only a weak causal inference between shared sanitation and adverse health outcomes. None of the studies identified in the review followed an experimental design. While many studies adjusted for known confounders, others did not. As observational studies, all are at risk of unknown confounders. We cannot rule out the possibility that that reliance on shared sanitation is simply a proxy for more direct causes of adverse health outcomes.

There is a need for rigorous studies in multiple study settings in order to determine the extent to which reliance on shared sanitation is causally associated with adverse health outcomes. There is also a need to identify the factors that may mitigate or otherwise modify any increased health risk associated with shared sanitation. Studies have found evidence that shared sanitation may be more poorly maintained, more costly, less accessible and less frequently used than IHLs [38–41]. These and other factors are likely to vary considerably depending on population density, the ratio of latrines per household or person, the quality of construction and upkeep, and the manner in which the latrines are managed. Future research, using both qualitative and quantitative methods, may help identify the circumstances in which shared sanitation might be a safe and effective alternative for increasing populations that do not have access to IHLs or where household-levels sanitation solutions are not possible or appropriate. Pending this research, policymakers and public health professionals should exercise caution in taking steps that may encourage the promotion of shared sanitation.

Supporting Information

Checklist S1

Figure S1 Sub group forest plot-Published data only. Image produced using Stata (Statacorp LP, TX USA). CI: Confidence Interval. ES: Effect size (Odds Ratio).

Figure S2 Sub group forest plot-Unpublished data only. Image produced using Stata (Statacorp LP, TX USA). CI: Confidence Interval. ES: Effect size (Odds Ratio).

Protocol S1

Table S1 Key search terms.

Table S2 Search strategy as performed in OVID databases.

Table S3 Methodological quality.

Table S4 Extracted data.

Table S5 Excluded documents.

Author Contributions

Conceived and designed the experiments: MH TC. Performed the experiments: MH OC RP GC JB KB. Analyzed the data: MH OC GC RP JB KB. Wrote the paper: MH TC.

References

1. Prüss-Üstün A, Bos R, Gore F, Bartram J (2008) Safer water, Better health-Costs, benefits and sustainability of interventions to protect and promote health. Geneva.
2. Lim SS, Vos T, Flaxman AD, Danaei G, Shibuya K, et al. (2012) A comparative risk assessment of burden of disease and injury attributable to 67 risk factors and risk factor clusters in 21 regions, 1990–2010: a systematic analysis for the Global Burden of Disease Study 2010. Lancet 380 2224–2260.
3. Bartram J, Cairncross S (2010) Hygiene, Sanitation, and Water: Forgotten Foundations of Health. PLoS Medicine 7:11.
4. Amnesty International (2010) Kenya: Insecurity and indignity: Women's experience in the slums of Nairobi, Kenya.
5. Joint Monitoring Programme (2013) Progress on Drinking Water and Sanitation: 2013 Update. WHO/UNICEF.
6. United Nations Millennium Project (2005) Health, Dignity, and Development. What Will it Take? Task Force on Water and Sanitation.

7. Joint Monitoring Programme (2010) Progress on Sanitation and Drinking Water: 2010 Update.
8. Joint Monitoring Programme (2012) Progress on Drinking Water and Sanitation: 2012 Update. UNICEF/WHO.
9. Joint Monitoring Programme (2012) Proposal for consolidated drinking water, sanitation and hygiene targets, indicators and definitions. the Hague, the Netherlands. 3–5 December.
10. Ghosh S, Sengupta PG, Mandal SK, Manna B, Sikder SN, et al. (1994) Maternal behaviour and feeding practices as determinants of childhood diarrhoea: some observations amongst rural Bengalee mothers. Indian Journal of Public Health 38:2 77–80.
11. Khan MU (1987) Limitation of communal latrines in changing the prevalence of parasites and diarrhoeal attack rate in Dhaka Peri-urban slums. Environmental Pollution 47:3 187–194.
12. Sobel J, Gomes TA, Ramos RT, Hoekstra M, Rodrigue D, et al. (2004) Pathogen-Specific Risk Factors and Protective Factors for Acute Diarrheal Illness in Children Aged 12–59 Months in Sao Paulo, Brazil. Clinical Infectious Diseases 38 1545–1551.
13. Chakraborty A, Das J (1983) Comparative study of incidence of diarrhea among children in two different environmental situations in Calcutta. Indian Pediatrics 20:12 907–913.
14. Baker K, O'Reilly CE, Mintz ED, Farag T, Nasrin D, et al. The risk of moderate and severe diarrhea in children less than 5 years old is increased among families who share a sanitation facility; Conference proceedings-American Society Tropical Medicine Hygiene; 2011.
15. Moshabela M, MacPherson P, Ezard N, Frean E, Mashimbye L, et al. (2012) Clinical and social determinants of diarrhoeal disease in a rural HIV/AIDS clinic, South Africa: A case-control study. International Journal of STD and AIDS 23:5 346–350.
16. Shultz A, Omollo JO, Burke H, Qassim M, Ochieng JB, et al. (2009) Cholera outbreak in Kenyan refugee camp: risk factors for illness and importance of sanitation. American Journal of Tropical Medicine & Hygiene 80:4 640–645.
17. Mahamud AS, Ahmed JA, Nyoka R, Auko E, Kahi V, et al. (2012) Epidemic cholera in Kakuma Refugee Camp, Kenya, 2009: The importance of sanitation and soap. Journal of Infection in Developing Countries 6:3 234–241.
18. Brooks JT, Shapiro RL, Kumar L, Wells JG, Phillips-Howard PA, et al. (2003) Epidemiology of sporadic bloody diarrhea in rural Western Kenya. American Journal of Tropical Medicine and Hygiene 68:6 671–677.
19. Chandiwana SK, Bradley M, Chombo F (1989) Hookworm and roundworm infections in farm-worker communities in the large-scale agricultural sector in Zimbabwe. Journal of Tropical Medicine and Hygiene 92:5 338–344.
20. Curtale F, Shamy MY, Zaki A, Abdel-Fattah M, Rocchi G (1998) Different patterns of intestinal helminth infection among young workers in urban and rural areas of Alexandria Governorate, Egypt. Parassitologia 40:3 251–254.
21. Hall A, Conway DJ, Anwar KS, Rahman ML (1994) Strongyloides stercoralis in an urban slum community in Bangladesh: factors independently associated with infection. Transactions of the Royal Society of Tropical Medicine and Hygiene 88:5 527–530.
22. Mahfouz AAR, El-Morshedy H, Farghaly A, Khalil A (1997) Ecological determinants of intestinal parasitic infections among pre-school children in an urban squatter settlement of Egypt. Journal of Tropical Pediatrics 43:6 341–344.
23. Phiri K, Whitty CJM, Graham SM, SSembatya Lule G (2000) Urban/rural differences in prevalence and risk factors for intestinal helminth infection in southern Malawi. Annals of Tropical Medicine and Parasitology 94:4 381–387.
24. Tshikuka JG, Scott ME, Gray-Donald K (1995) Ascaris lumbricoides infection and environmental risk factors in an urban African setting. Annals of Tropical Medicine and Parasitology 89:5 505–514.
25. Karkey A, Thompson CN, Tran Vu Thieu N, Dongol S, Le Thi Phuong T, et al. (2013) Differential Epidemiology of Salmonella Typhi and Paratyphi A in Kathmandu, Nepal: A Matched Case Control Investigation in a Highly Endemic Enteric Fever Setting. PLoS Neglected Tropical Diseases 7:8.
26. Kim-Farley RJ, Rutherford G, Lichfield P, Hsu ST, Orenstein WA, et al. (1984) Outbreak of paralytic poliomyelitis, Taiwan. Lancet 2:8415 1322–1324.
27. Montgomery MA, Desai MM, Elimelech M (2010) Comparing the effectiveness of shared versus private latrines in preventing trachoma in rural Tanzania. American Journal of Tropical Medicine and Hygiene 82:4 693–695.
28. Tuttle J, Ries AA, Chimba RM, Perera CU, Bean NH, et al. (1995) Antimicrobial-resistant epidemic Shigella dysenteriae type 1 in Zambia: modes of transmission. The Journal of infectious diseases 171:2 371–375.
29. Golding J, Greenwood R, McCaw-Binns A, Thomas P (1994) Associations between social and environmental factors and perinatal mortality in Jamaica. Paediatric and Perinatal Epidemiology 8:Suppl 1 17–39.
30. Olusanya BO, Ofovwe GE (2010) Predictors of preterm births and low birthweight in an inner-city hospital in sub-Saharan Africa. Maternal and Child Health Journal 14:6 978–986.
31. Munoz E, Powers JR, Nienhuys TG, Mathews JD (1992) Social and environmental factors in 10 Aboriginal communities in the Northern Territory: Relationship to hospital admissions of children. Medical Journal of Australia 156:8 529–533.
32. Fobil J, May J, Kraemer A (2010) Assessing the relationship between socioeconomic conditions and urban environmental quality in Accra, Ghana. International Journal of Environmental Research and Public Health.
33. Schmidt WP, Boisson S, Genser B, Baretto ML, Baisely K, et al. (2010) Weight-for-age z-score as a proxy marker for diarrhoea in epidemiological studies. Journal of Epidemiology and Community Health 64:12 1074–1079.
34. Kotloff K, Blackwelder W, Nasrin D, Nataro JP, Farag TH, et al. (2012) The Global Enteric Multicenter Study (GEMS) of Diarrheal Disease in Infants and Young Children in Developing Countries: Epidemiologic and Clinical Methods of the Case/Control Study. Clinical Infectious Diseases 55:Supplement 4 S232–245.
35. Levine MM, Kotloff KL, Nataro JP, Muhsen K (2012) The Global Enteric Multicenter Study (GEMS): impetus, rationale, and genesis. Clinical Infectious Diseases 55:Supplement 4 S215–224.
36. Blum D, Feachem RG (1983) Measuring the impact of water supply and sanitation investments on diarrhoeal diseases: problems in methodology. International Journal of Epidemiology 12 357–365.
37. Schmidt WP, Arnold BF, Boisson S, Genser B, Luby SP, et al. (2011) Epidemiological methods in diarrhoea studies – an update. International Journal of Epidemiology 40:6 1678–1692.
38. Biran A, Jenkins MW, Dabrase P, Bhagwat I (2011) Patterns and determinants of communal latrine usage in urban poverty pockets in Bhopal, India. Tropical Medicine and International Health 16:7 854–862.
39. Tiimub BM, Forson MA, Obiri-Danso K, Rahaman IA (2009) Pointed gaps in the provision, quality, patronage and management of toilet facilities in Bawku East District; 34th WEDC International Conference; Addis Ababa, Ethiopia.
40. Mukherjee N, Robiarto A, Saputra E, Wartono D (2012) Achieving and Sustaining Open Defecation Free Communities: Learning from East Java; WSP; Water and sanitation program.
41. Oduro-Kwarteng S, Awuah E, Nyarko KB (2009) Shifting from public shared toilets to home toilets in urban settlements: implications of household demand in Kumasi, Ghana; 34th WEDC International Conference; Addis Ababa, Ethiopia.

19

The Recognition of and Care Seeking Behaviour for Childhood Illness in Developing Countries

Pascal Geldsetzer[1]*, Thomas Christie Williams[2], Amir Kirolos[2], Sarah Mitchell[2], Louise Alison Ratcliffe[2], Maya Kate Kohli-Lynch[2], Esther Jill Laura Bischoff[2], Sophie Cameron[2], Harry Campbell[2]

1 Department of Global Health & Population, Harvard School of Public Health, Boston, Massachusetts, United States of America, **2** Public Health Sciences Section, Division of Community Health Sciences, University of Edinburgh, Edinburgh, United Kingdom

Abstract

Background: Pneumonia, diarrhoea, and malaria are among the leading causes of death in children. These deaths are largely preventable if appropriate care is sought early. This review aimed to determine the percentage of caregivers in low- and middle-income countries (LMICs) with a child less than 5 years who were able to recognise illness in their child and subsequently sought care from different types of healthcare providers.

Methods and Findings: We conducted a systematic literature review of studies that reported recognition of, and/or care seeking for episodes of diarrhoea, pneumonia or malaria in LMICs. The review is registered with PROSPERO (registration number: CRD42011001654). Ninety-one studies met the inclusion criteria. Eighteen studies reported data on caregiver recognition of disease and seventy-seven studies on care seeking. The median sensitivity of recognition of diarrhoea, malaria and pneumonia was low (36.0%, 37.4%, and 45.8%, respectively). A median of 73.0% of caregivers sought care outside the home. Care seeking from community health workers (median: 5.4% for diarrhoea, 4.2% for pneumonia, and 1.3% for malaria) and the use of oral rehydration therapy (median: 34%) was low.

Conclusions: Given the importance of this topic to child survival programmes there are few published studies. Recognition of diarrhoea, malaria and pneumonia by caregivers is generally poor and represents a key factor to address in attempts to improve health care utilisation. In addition, considering that oral rehydration therapy has been widely recommended for over forty years, its use remains disappointingly low. Similarly, the reported levels of care seeking from community health workers in the included studies are low even though global action plans to address these illnesses promote community case management. Giving greater priority to research on care seeking could provide crucial evidence to inform child mortality programmes.

Editor: Malcolm G. Semple, University of Liverpool, United Kingdom

Funding: Funding was provided by the Centre for Population Health Sciences, University of Edinburgh. The funders had no role in study design, data collection and analysis, decision to publish, or preparation of the manuscript.

Competing Interests: The authors have declared that no competing interests exist.

* E-mail: pag395@mail.harvard.edu

Introduction

In 2012 it was estimated that 6.6 million children under the age of five died worldwide [1], eighty-two per cent of which in Sub-Saharan Africa and Southern Asia. Thirty-three per cent of these deaths were due to pneumonia (17%), diarrhoea (9%) and malaria (7%).

Morbidity and mortality from these diseases can be reduced considerably if care is sought early. Thus, the ability of caregivers to recognise and seek appropriate care for these common childhood illnesses is instrumental in reducing child deaths in low-and middle-income countries (LMICs) and in reaching the Millennium Development Goal 4 target of reducing child mortality by two thirds by 2015 [2].

Recognising the importance of care seeking, the World Health Organisation (WHO) and UNICEF highlighted activities to improve family and community health practices (including disease recognition and care seeking) as one of the three central components of the Integrated Management of Childhood Illness (IMCI) strategy [3]. The IMCI strategy has been introduced in the majority of LMICs with moderate to high child mortality and has been shown to be effective in a number of settings [4].

The importance of caregivers' ability to recognise and seek appropriate care for their children is also one of the recommended key activities in the WHO's and UNICEF's Global Action Plan for the Control of Pneumonia and Diarrhoea [5]. In addition, a research priority setting exercise conducted by WHO using the Child Health and Nutrition Research Initiative (CHNRI) methodology identified the investigation of barriers to healthcare seeking and healthcare access as the highest primary research priority for reducing mortality from childhood pneumonia worldwide [6].

Herbert et al. have recently performed a systematic review of the percentage of caregivers who seek care for neonatal illness from different categories of healthcare providers [7]. However, there has not been a review of the literature on the recognition of, and care seeking behaviour for, the three main infectious causes of childhood mortality worldwide: pneumonia, diarrhoea and malaria. This review aims to estimate the percentage of caregivers in LMICs with a child of less than 5 years who were able to recognise signs of pneumonia, diarrhoea and malaria in their child and subsequently sought care from different types of health care providers.

Methods

Search Strategy

We reviewed published data on childhood pneumonia, diarrhoeal disease and malaria over the period from 1966 to November 2012. Searches were conducted of the following electronic databases: Medline [8], Embase [9], WHOLIS [10], Web of Knowledge (previously Web of Science) [11], LILACs [12], PAHO [13] and IndMED [14]. The databases were searched using key words and medical subject headings (MESH) for: pneumonia, diarrhoea, malaria, caregiver, recognition, danger signs, and care seeking. The searches were limited to published literature in children less than 5 years with abstracts in English. Otherwise, no restrictions were placed on publication language or type. See Table S1 for a complete list of search terms, formatted for Ovid Medline and Embase, and Table S2 for the study's PRISMA checklist. The review is registered with PROSPERO (registration number: CRD42012003216) [15].

The titles and abstracts of retrieved studies were reviewed for relevance using the inclusion criteria detailed below. The full-text versions of potentially relevant articles were then analysed according to the inclusion criteria. Reference lists of all included studies were checked for additional references [16]. All citations were imported into an electronic database (Mendeley).

Inclusion/Exclusion Criteria

Studies were included if: 1) the study presented original data, 2) the study was carried out in a LMIC, 3) the sample size was ≥50 participants, and 4) the study provided data on illness-recognition or care seeking for children <5 years of age. In addition, for recognition of disease, the study had to present quantitative data on the sensitivity and specificity of caregivers' ability to recognise a disease or certain clinical features of the disease in their child. For care seeking, the study had to present quantitative data on the percentage of caregivers who sought healthcare for their child.

We excluded qualitative studies that described determinants of care seeking rather than enumerating care seeking events. Some publications described care seeking for two or three disease entities. If care seeking data were given separately for each disease entity they were included in the review.

Definitions

Recognition of illness. For malaria, caregivers' abilities to recognise a fever was compared to a thermometer measurement of axillary temperature, and their ability to recognise pallor to a haemoglobin measurement or haematocrit. Caregivers' ability to recognise malaria was compared to a diagnosis made with a positive blood film, with (2 studies) or without (1 study) a raised temperature.

For dehydration during diarrhoeal disease, the ability of the caregiver to recognise features of dehydration was compared to a diagnosis made by a physician. For diarrhoea, the caregiver's ability to describe diarrhoea was compared with a diagnosis using specified criteria. In two studies this was the WHO diagnostic criteria of at least three loose or liquid stools in a 24 hour period, and one study used a definition of at least 3 stools in 12 hours of daylight.

For pneumonia, the ability of caregivers to recognise rapid breathing and chest indrawing was compared to an assessment made by the study researchers. In all cases the WHO definition of pneumonia based on rapid breathing was used. This defines rapid breathing as a rate >60 breaths per minute in a child aged <2 months, >50 breaths per minute in a child aged <1 year, and > 40 breaths per minute in a child over 1 year of age. The data was analysed separately for studies that employed open questioning (caregivers were asked to describe features of their child's illness) and closed questioning (caregivers were asked whether the child had rapid breathing or chest indrawing).

Care seeking. Care seeking was defined as any care sought outside the home for an unwell child with a suspected episode of diarrhoea, malaria or pneumonia. A caregiver was defined as the individual who sought, or would have sought care for a sick child. In most cases this was a family member, most frequently the mother. For pneumonia, three studies specified acute respiratory infections (ARI) rather than acute lower respiratory tract infections (ALRI) and did not offer further qualifications. The remainder used the term "severe ARI" or reported signs suggesting pneumonia.

The following definitions of healthcare providers were adopted: 'all health facilities' included all government and private healthcare providers, pharmacies and traditional healers; 'appropriate providers' included all government and trained private health practitioners, but not traditional healers, pharmacies and unqualified medical practitioners; 'all government providers' also included non-governmental organisations (NGOs), which provided a free service, and was further subdivided into hospitals, health centres/clinics, and community health workers; 'private facility' included private hospitals and private health centres and clinics; 'pharmacy' referred to public and private pharmacies, chemists and drug vendors; and 'traditional healer' referred to practitioners of alternative medicine. Caregivers sought 'no treatment' when they neither gave home care nor sought external care. Oral rehydration therapy (ORT) for diarrhoea included oral rehydration solution (ORS) and sugar salt solution (SSS) as well as treatment given at home and that prescribed by care providers. If figures were provided only for ORT given at home, and did not include that supplied by care providers, the data was excluded from the analysis.

Data Extraction and Assessment of the Studies

Data were extracted from studies and entered into Microsoft Excel spreadsheets. For intervention studies, only data from the control arm of the study or baseline data were included in the analysis. In addition to the data for illness recognition and care seeking, the following variables were extracted for each study: study location and geographical setting, date of data collection, total number of participants in the study, number of participants with an illness or suspected illness, sampling method, study design (including prospective or retrospective data collection), recall period, and the study's definition of the disease entity and of recognition of the disease and/or care seeking for the disease.

If the sensitivity, specificity, and positive and negative predictive value of caregiver recognition of malaria, diarrhoea, pneumonia or features of the diseases were given, these data were extracted. Otherwise they were calculated from the published data, where possible. For care seeking, the proportion of caregivers that sought care and where they sought care was tabulated. In some studies data were given for both hypothetical and actual health care seeking behaviour. In these studies data on actual care seeking behaviour was used. In cases where only data on hypothetical care seeking behaviour was reported, this data was used. When care seeking from multiple providers was reported, then the first or preferred choice was extracted. Where possible, we calculated the percentage of care seeking from 'any health facility' and 'any appropriate health facility' if they were not stated in the study. Due to the wide variation in study designs, a meta-analysis was not possible. Instead, the median and range were calculated for care seeking within each category.

Results

Results of the Literature Search

The searches retrieved 16,637 studies for diarrhoea, 11,867 for malaria, and 23,542 for pneumonia, (Figure 1). After analysis of the full text, application of the inclusion criteria, and a reference search, 91 studies were included in the analysis (Table 1). 89 of these studies were in English; two were in French. 18 studies looked at recognition of disease, and 77 at care seeking behaviour (three studies contained data on both recognition of, and care seeking for the disease). Studies were excluded most commonly for being conducted in a high-income country, including children aged 5 years or older or not specifying the age of included children, having a sample size of less than 50 participants, collecting only qualitative data, and not presenting data for separate disease entities.

For each illness category, there were more studies with data on care seeking than for recognition of illness. The largest number of studies was found for diarrhoeal disease, and the fewest for pneumonia (38 and 27 studies respectively).

Study Characteristics

The majority (75/91) of selected studies were carried out within a single country. One study presented data on care seeking for diarrhoea in 6 countries in Africa, Asia and Latin America [17] and one study on care seeking for malaria in 6 African countries [18]. The majority of the studies were carried out in Africa (13/18 for recognition of disease, 50/77 for care seeking, 60/91 in total) and Asia (5/18 for recognition of disease, 24/77 for care seeking, 29/91 in total). Few studies were found for Latin America (none for recognition of disease, 6/77 for care seeking).

For recognition of disease (Table 2), 10 of 18 studies were undertaken between 1990 and 1999. Seven studies reported recognition of features of pneumonia, six of diarrhoea, and five of malaria. For care seeking behaviour (Table 3), there was an increase in the number of studies published over time: 9 before 1990, 23 between 1990 and 1999, and 43 between 2000 and 2009. Most studies on care seeking behaviour (48/77) had fewer than 1000 participants; 11 had over 5000 participants. The majority of studies (71/77) examined care seeking for children under the age of 5 years. In terms of study design (Table 4), most studies were retrospective (54/77) and a significant proportion (17/77) examined hypothetical decisions made by caregivers rather than actual care seeking behaviour; these will be referred to as "simulated case studies".

42/77 studies on care seeking used clinical criteria to define diarrhoea, malaria or pneumonia, 26/77 used caregiver descriptions of illness, and 9/77 did not give any definition of disease. Most studies (59/77) defined care seeking as seeking care from defined health care providers; the remainder defined it as seeking

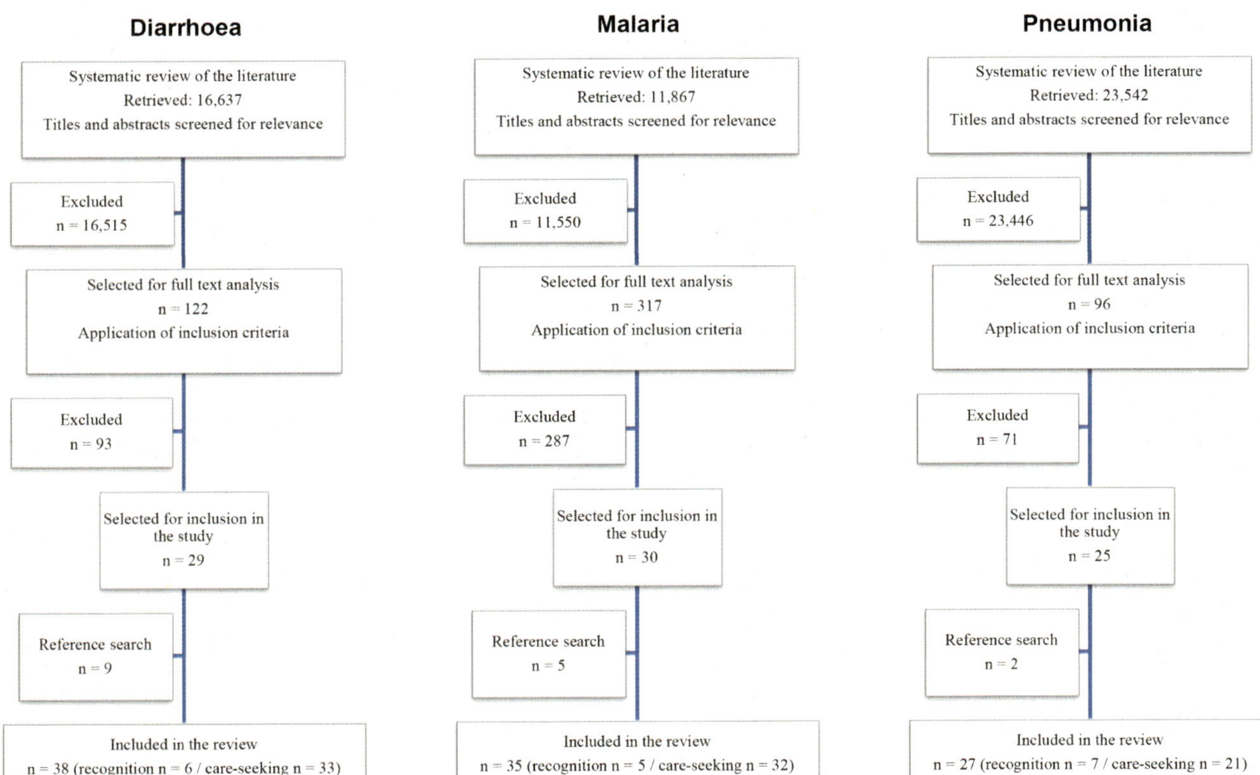

Figure 1. Summary of the literature searches.

Table 1. Studies retrieved from literature search.

Illness category	Total number of articles retrieved	Selected for full text review	Included in the review[1]	With data on recognition of illness	With data on care seeking for illness
Diarrhoea	16,637	122	38	6	33
Malaria	11,867	317	35	5	32
Pneumonia	23,542	96	27	7	21
Total			91[2]	18	77[2]

[1]This number includes studies found through searching the references of already included studies.
[2]Five studies examined two diseases, two studies examined all three diseases and three studies contained data on both recognition of disease and care seeking.

care outside the home. Approximately half of the studies were undertaken in rural locations (40/77).

Recognition of Childhood Illness

Definitions of disease varied between studies, as described in the methods. Three studies reported sensitivities and specificities for the overall caregiver recognition of malaria and diarrhoea. Only one study [19] looked at caregiver recognition of pneumonia, while six studies looked at recognition of rapid breathing and chest indrawing (Table 5). Median sensitivities were 37.4% for the recognition of malaria, 36.0% for diarrhoea, and 45.8% for pneumonia. The specificity of caregiver recognition of disease was highest for diarrhoea (96.0%) and lowest for malaria (58.0%); the specificity for recognition of pneumonia was 67.1%. The positive predictive value of a caregiver diagnosis of illness was highest for diarrhoea (67.7%) and lowest for pneumonia (28.9%).

The median sensitivity of recognition of anaemia by caregivers was low (22.4%), but the sensitivity of recognition of fever was higher (64.7%). Caregivers' sensitivity of detection of rapid breathing was markedly increased on closed compared to open questioning (69.8% vs 22.0%), as was recognition of chest indrawing (68.0% vs 17.0%). However closed questioning led to a fall in the specificity (97.6% vs. 71.5% for rapid breathing, 97.2% vs. 64.0% for chest indrawing). The sensitivity of caregiver recognition of features of moderate to severe dehydration was high: 88.0% for weakness, 85.0% for thirst, 75.5% for a sunken fontanelle, 74.0% for sunken eyes, and 71.0% for dry mouth. Caregivers were less able to recognise decreased urine production (sensitivity: 21.0%) or the absence of tears (sensitivity: 16.0%).

Care Seeking for Childhood Illness

In 2012, the countries with the highest number of child deaths, in descending order, were India, Nigeria, the Democratic Republic of the Congo (DRC), Pakistan and China [1]. Table 6 shows the number of studies on care seeking that were carried out in each of these five countries. 6 and 11 studies were carried out in India and Nigeria, respectively. However, only 2 of the included studies were carried out in each the DRC, Pakistan and China. We did not identify any studies from Nigeria, China or the DRC that investigated care seeking for pneumonia. Our literature search may however have missed articles in Chinese or French without an English abstract.

Table 7 summarises the studies on care seeking behaviour for all three diseases for all continents. More detailed data for each

Table 2. Characteristics of studies on recognition of illness.

		Diarrhoea *(n = 6)*	Malaria *(n = 5)*	Pneumonia *(n = 7)*	Total *(n = 18)*
Location	Africa	4	5	4	13
	Asia	2	0	3	5
	Latin America	0	0	0	0
Date of data collection[1]	1989 or earlier	4	0	1	5
	1990–1999	1	4	5	10
	2000–2009	0	1	1	2
	2010–2012	1	0	0	1
Age of participants	<1 years	0	0	2	2
	<2 years	2	1	0	3
	<3 years	3	0	0	3
	<5 years	1	4	5	10
Sample size	50–100	1	0	0	1
	101–500	3	3	4	10
	501–1000	0	1	1	2
	1001–5000	1	1	1	3
	>5000	1	0	1	2

[1]This is the mid-year of data collection. If the date of data collection was not stated, year of publication was used instead.

Table 3. Characteristics of studies on care seeking behavior.

		Diarrhoea *(n = 33)*	Malaria *(n = 32)*	Pneumonia *(n = 21)*	Total[1] *(n = 77)*
Location	Africa	17	31	8	49
	Asia	15	1	10	24
	Latin America	3	0	3	6
Date of data collection	Before 1990	6	3	1	9
	1990–1999	9	6	9	23
	2000–2009	17	21	11	42
	2010–2012	1	2	0	3
Age of participants	<2 years	0	1	0	1
	<3 years	2	2	1	5
	<5 years	31	29	20	71
Sample size	50–100	2	4	2	7
	101–500	7	12	9	28
	501–1000	5	6	2	13
	1001–5000	11	8	6	18
	>5000	8	2	2	11

[1]Five studies examined two diseases, two studies examined all three diseases and one study was carried out in three continents (Africa, Asia and Latin America).

Table 4. Features of studies on care seeking behavior.

Study design		Definitions		Study setting
Prospective, retrospective or simulated case study[1]	**Recall period**	**Definition of disease**	**Definition of care seeking**	
Total n = 77				
Prospective: 6	≤2 weeks: 33	Clinical criteria: 42	Seeking care outside the home: 18	Rural: 39
Retrospective: 54	>2 weeks: 16	Caregiver description: 26	Seeking care from defined providers: 59	Urban: 16
Simulated case study: 17	Not stated: 5	Not defined: 9		Rural/urban[2]: 19
	Not retrospective: 23			Not specified: 3
Diarrhoea n = 33				
Prospective: 3	≤2 weeks: 21	Clinical criteria: 20	Seeking care outside the home: 17	Rural: 12
Retrospective: 27 Simulated case study: 3	>2 weeks: 5	Caregiver description: 4	Seeking care from defined providers: 16	Urban: 11
	Not stated: 1	Not defined: 9		Rural/urban[2]: 9
	Not retrospective: 6			Not specified: 1
Malaria n = 32				
Prospective: 3	≤2 weeks: 14	Clinical criteria: 9	Seeking care outside the home: 4	Rural: 17
Retrospective: 23	>2 weeks: 7	Caregiver description: 22	Seeking care from defined providers: 28	Urban: 4
Simulated case study: 6	Not stated: 2	Not defined: 1		Rural/urban[2]: 9
	Not retrospective: 9			Not specified: 2
Pneumonia n = 21				
Prospective: 0	≤2 weeks: 7	Clinical criteria: 19	Seeking care outside the home: 3	Rural: 15
Retrospective: 13	>2 weeks: 4	Caregiver description: 2	Seeking care from defined providers: 18	Urban: 5
Simulated case study: 8	Not stated: 2	Not defined: 0		Rural/urban[2]: 1
	Not retrospective: 8			Not specified: 0

[1]Simulated case studies presented caregivers with a scenario of an illness in their child and asked whether and where he/she would seek care.
[2]Rural/urban refers to studies that were carried out in both urban and rural areas.

Table 5. Caregivers' recognition of diarrhoea, malaria, pneumonia and clinical features of these diseases.

		Median % and range			
Condition	**Feature recognized by caregivers**	**Sensitivity**	**Specificity**	**Positive predictive value**	**Negative predictive value**
Diarrhoea	Diarrhoea [30,84,85]	36.0 (14.3–54.6)	96.0 (94.7–97.1)	67.7 (61.1–70.6)	86.6 (55.4–96.3)
	Thirst [86–88]	85.0 (73.0–89.0)	29.0 (10.0–30.0)	-	-
	Dry mouth [86–88]	71.0 (67.0–74.0)	35.0 (30.0–44.0)	-	-
	Weakness [86–88]	88.0 (67.0–95.0)	20.0 (13.0–50.0)	-	-
	Sunken eyes [86–88]	74.0 (64.0–94.0)	49.0 (36.0–60.0)	-	-
	Decreased urine production [86–88]	21.0 (11.0–35.0)	80.0 (70.0–87.0)	-	-
	Sunken fontanelle [87,88]	75.5 (71.0–80.0)	24.5 (20.0–29.0)	-	-
	No tears [86]	16.0	80.0	-	-
Malaria	Malaria [52,89,90]	37.4 (32.0–40.0)	58.0 (55.0–92.0)	36.8 (13.8–61.2)	83.6 (34.3–90.2)
	Anaemia[1] [89,91]	22.4 (4.1–46.8)	81.5 (95.6–67.5)	15.9 (10.4–21.4)	86.2 (78.5–94.0)
	Fever[2] [91,92]	64.7 (53.3–76.2)	87.1 (80.4–87.1)	45.1	90.7 (85.1–96.4)
Pneumonia	Moderate pneumonia[3] [19]	45.8	67.1	28.9	80.9
	Rapid breathing (open questioning[4]) [31,93–95]	22.0 (15.6–78.0)	97.6 (84.0–100.0)	100.0	37.2
	Rapid breathing (closed questioning[5]) [93,95–97]	69.8 (48.7–78.0)	71.5 (34.0–90.0)	77.0 (73.1–93.2)	59.0 (52.0–61.6)
	Recognition of chest indrawing (open questioning) [31,93,95]	17.0 (7.5–35.3)	97.2 (93.0–100.0)	100.0	41.9
	Recognition of chest indrawing (closed questioning) [93,95,97]	68.0 (56.7–69.0)	64.0 (49.0–100.0)	89.5 (79.0–100.0)	56.8 (53.0–60.6)

[1]Defined as a haemoglobin concentration of $<$7 gram per decilitre or haematocrit $<$25%.
[2]Defined as an axillary temperature $\geq$37.5°C.
[3]Defined as the presence of a cough and a raised respiratory rate.
[4]Open questioning: the caregiver was asked to describe features of the child's illness.
[5]Closed questioning: the caregiver was asked whether the child suffered from rapid breathing or chest indrawing.

continent is provided in Table 8 (Africa), Table 9 (Asia) and Table 10 (Latin America). Table 11 shows the same data separated by each disease entity.

A median of 73.0% (range: 5.3%–100.0%) of caregivers sought care from a healthcare provider when their child was suffering from diarrhoea, malaria or pneumonia and a median of 44.9% (range: 6.1%–100.0%) sought care from appropriate providers. Care seeking was highest for pneumonia with a median of 91.3% of caregivers seeking care from any provider, and lowest for diarrhoea with 68.5% (Table 7). Seeking no care was commonest for diarrhoea (21.3%) and least common for malaria (8.1%). Appropriate care was sought most frequently for pneumonia (84.0%), and least frequently for malaria (42.5%). Government facilities were attended more frequently than private facilities for all diseases, except for pneumonia in Asia (only one study [20] provided data for care seeking from private care providers for pneumonia in Asia). Care seeking from community health workers (CHWs) was low: 5.4% for diarrhoea, 4.2% for pneumonia, and 1.3% for malaria. Caregivers sought care from pharmacies and drug vendors most frequently in cases of malaria (30.8%), and least frequently for pneumonia (15.2%). Traditional healers were consulted most frequently for pneumonia (21.4%). ORT was used by caregivers in 34.0% (range: 13.4%–68.1%) of cases of diarrhoea.

Table 6. Number of studies on care seeking behaviour, by the 5 countries with the highest number of under-five deaths[1].

Country	Number of studies
India [20,27,42,98–100]	6
Nigeria[17,18,25,34,36,58,59,62,101–103]	11
Democratic Republic of the Congo [17,18]	2
Pakistan [48,53]	2
China [28,104]	2

[1]The five countries with the highest number of under-five deaths were taken from the annual report by the UN Interagency Group for Child Mortality Estimation [1].

It was difficult to compare care seeking in Latin America to Asia or Africa, as only 6 studies were carried out in Latin America. Comparing Africa and Asia (see Table 11), carers were less likely to seek care for diarrhoea in Africa (67.3%) than in Asia (78.7%) but more likely to seek care for pneumonia (98.0% versus 80.0%). Care seeking from private care providers was more common in Asia than in Africa for both diarrhoea (29.3% versus 11.7%) and pneumonia (49.0% versus 20.0%). In both continents, carers were more likely to give no treatment for diarrhoea than for pneumonia. Rates of ORT use were low both in Africa (40.5%) and Asia (34.0%). For pneumonia and malaria, none of the included studies reported data on care seeking from pharmacies and traditional healers in Asia.

Table 7. The median percentage of caregivers who sought healthcare, by disease (all continents)[1].

		Appropriate health facilities									
			Government facilities								
	All health facilities	All appropriate facilities[2]	Gov. Hospital[3]	Health centre or clinic	CHW	All gov. facilities	Private facilities	Pharmacy or drug vendor	Trad. healer	Home care	No care
Diarrhoea [17,20–23,27–30,36–41, 46–48,54,59–66,69,98,104–107]	68.5 (14.9–96.0)	44.5 (7.3–87.0)	8.0 (2.0–18.0)	21.2 (0.3–80.0)	5.4 (5.0–21.0)	30.8 (7.3–85.0)	22.0 (1.0–68.8)	16.7 (4.9–55.7)	6.3 (1.4–20.7)	32.1 (4.0–68.0) ORT: 34.0 (13.4–68.1)	21.3 (6.0–39.4)
Malaria [18,21,22,24–26,32–34,44,45, 49,50,52,58,68,89,100–103,105,107–116]	72.6 (6.1–100.0)	42.4 (6.1–98.4)	9.1 (1.2–20.0)	21.0 (5.5–71.0)	1.3 (0–40.2)	21.3 (10.8–81.5)	7.2 (1.9–28.6)	30.8 (1.6–49.7)	3.5 (1.2–60.0)	38.7 (4.5–88.0)	8.1 (0.0–51.7)
Pneumonia [4,19–22,29,38,42,43,51,53, 55–57,79,99,117–121]	91.3 (5.3–100)	84.0 (20.9–100.0)	46.0 (19.6–60.0)	32.8 (18.0–56.3)	4.2 (2.0–18.0)	50.0 (20.9–100.0)	24.0 (6.7–49.9)	15.2 (2.5–27.6)	21.4 (3.1–64.4)	20.0 (2.8–94.6)	11.0 (0.9–11.5)

[1]The range is shown in brackets if there are two or more data points. The definition of each category of healthcare is stated in the methods. The values do not add up to 100% because of the varying categorisation of healthcare providers in the included studies and because some studies recorded more than one care seeking event.
[2]Appropriate health facilities included all government and trained private health practitioners, but not traditional healers, pharmacies and unqualified medical practitioners.
[3]Abbreviations: Gov. = Governmental; CHW = Community Health Worker; Trad. Healer = Traditional Healer; ORT = Oral Rehydration Therapy.

Table 8. The median percentage of caregivers who sought healthcare, by disease (Africa)[1].

		Appropriate health facilities									
			Government facilities								
	All health facilities	All appropriate facilities[2]	Gov. Hospital[3]	Health centre or clinic	CHW	All gov. facilities	Private facilities	Pharmacy or drug vendor	Trad. healer	Home care	No care
Diarrhoea[17,21,22,29,30,36,37, 41,46,47,60,62,63,65,66,105,107]	67.3 (14.9–86.0)	39.0 (7.3–68.9)	8.8 (5.3–17.4)	28.0 (2.0–42.5)	5.4 (5.0–21.0)	18.7 (7.3–66.2)	11.7 (1.0–37.6)	22.2 (10.5–45.0)	7.0 (2.2–20.7)	32.4 (14.0–60.7) ORT: 40.5 (13.4–68.1)	30.8 (6.0–39.4)
Malaria [18], [22], [23], [25–27], [33–35], [45], [46], [50], [51], [53], [59], [69], [91], [102–104], [106], [108–117]	72.1 (6.1–100.0)	41.6 (6.1–98.4)	9.1 (1.2–20.0)	21.0 (5.5–71.0)	1.3 (0–40.2)	29.5 (10.8–72.3)	7.2 (1.9–28.6)	30.8 (1.6–49.7)	3.5 (1.2–60.0)	38.7 (4.5–88.0)	8.1 (0.0–51.7)
Pneumonia [22], [23], [30], [44], [52], [119–121]	98.0 (62.9–100.0)	86.0 (27.2–100.0)	46.0 (19.6–51.5)	35.6 (20.0–56.3)	3.1 (2.0–4.2)	57.0 (35.6–100.0)	20.0 (6.7–24.0)	16.6 (2.5–27.6)	21.4 (3.1–64.4)	-	0.0

[1]The range is shown in brackets if there are two or more data points. The definition of each category of healthcare is stated in the methods. The values do not add up to 100% because of the varying categorisation of healthcare providers in the included studies and because some studies recorded more than one care seeking event.
[2]Appropriate health facilities included all government and trained private health practitioners, but not traditional healers, pharmacies and unqualified medical practitioners.
[3]Abbreviations: Gov = Governmental; CHW = Community Health Worker; Trad. Healer = Traditional Healer; ORT = Oral Rehydration Therapy; - = no data available.

Table 9. The median percentage of caregivers who sought healthcare, by disease (Asia)[1].

	Appropriate health facilities										
			Government facilities								
	All health facilities	All appropriate facilities[2]	Gov. Hospital[3]	Health centre or clinic	CHW	All gov. facilities	Private facilities	Pharmacy or drug vendor	Trad. healer	Home care	No care
Diarrhoea[17], [21], [28], [29], [39], [41], [49], [55], [60], [62], [65], [70], [99], [105], [107]	78.7 (32.0–96.0)	65.0 (25.4–87.0)	7.1 (2.0–18.0)	25.1 (0.3–80.0)	-	32.2 (15.0–85.0)	29.3 (5.5–68.8)	10.5 (4.0–55.7)	3.0 (1.4–5.0)	19.8 (4.0–68.0) ORT: 34.0 (29.0–46.0)	20.0 (8.75–21.3)
Malaria [101]	81.5	81.5	-	-	1.2	81.5	-	-	-	-	-
Pneumonia [4], [19], [21], [39], [43], [54], [57], [80], [100], [122]	80.0 (5.3–92.5)	68.8 (20.9–92.5)	60.0	32.5 (18.0–47.0)	-	33.5 (20.9–60.0)	49.0	-	-	25.6 (2.8–94.6)	6.2 (0.9–11.5)

[1]The range is shown in brackets if there are two or more data points. The definition of each category of healthcare is stated in the methods. The values do not add up to 100% because of the varying categorisation of healthcare providers in the included studies and because some studies recorded more than one care seeking event.
[2]Appropriate health facilities included all government and trained private health practitioners, but not traditional healers, pharmacies and unqualified medical practitioners.
[3]Abbreviations: Gov = Governmental; CHW = Community Health Worker; Trad. Healer = Traditional Healer; ORT = Oral Rehydration Therapy; - = no data available.

Table 10. The median percentage of caregivers who sought healthcare, by disease (Latin America)[1].

	Appropriate health facilities										
			Government facilities								
	All health facilities	All appropriate facilities[2]	Gov. Hospital[3]	Health centre or clinic	CHW	All gov. facilities	Private facilities	Pharmacy or drug vendor	Trad. healer	Home care	No care
Diarrhoea [17], [24], [40]	40.5 (22.0–59.0)	46.0 (33.0–59.0)	8.0	10.0	-	18.0	-	-	-	41.0 ORT: 23.2	20.0
Malaria	-	-	-	-	-	-	-	-	-	-	-
Pneumonia [56], [58], [118]	87.5 (83.5–91.6)	89.0 (83.5–94.6)	30.9	30.0	-	60.9	46.6	13.4 (11.6–15.2)	3.3	5.5	11.0

[1]The range is shown in brackets if there are two or more data points. The definition of each category of healthcare is stated in the methods. The values do not add up to 100% because of the varying categorisation of healthcare providers in the included studies and because some studies recorded more than one care seeking event.
[2]Appropriate health facilities included all government and trained private health practitioners, but not traditional healers, pharmacies and unqualified medical practitioners.
[3]Abbreviations: Gov = Governmental; CHW = Community Health Worker; Trad. Healer = Traditional Healer; ORT = Oral Rehydration Therapy; - = no data available.

Table 11. The median percentage of caregivers who sought healthcare, by disease and continent[1].

		Appropriate health facilities									
			Government facilities								
	All health facilities	All appropriate facilities[2]	Gov. Hospital[3]	Health centre or clinic	CHW	All gov. facilities	Private facilities	Pharmacy or drug vendor	Trad. healer	Home care	No care
Diarrhoea											
Africa[17], [22], [23], [30], [31], [37], [38], [42], [47], [48], [61], [63], [64], [66], [67], [106], [108]	67.3 (14.9–86.0)	39.0 (7.3–68.9)	8.8 (5.3–17.4)	28.0 (2.0–42.5)	5.4 (5.0–21.0)	18.7 (7.3–66.2)	11.7 (1.0–37.6)	22.2 (10.5–45.0)	7.0 (2.2–20.7)	32.4 (14.0–60.7) ORT: 40.5 (13.4–68.1)	30.8 (6.0–39.4)
Asia [17], [21], [28], [29], [39], [41], [49], [55], [60], [62], [65], [70], [99], [105], [107]	78.7 (32.0–96.0)	65.0 (25.4–87.0)	7.1 (2.0–18.0)	25.1 (0.3–80.0)	-	32.2 (15.0–85.0)	29.3 (5.5–68.8)	10.5 (4.0–55.7)	3.0 (1.4–5.0)	19.8 (4.0–68.0) ORT: 34.0 (29.0–46.0)	20.0 (8.75–21.3)
Latin America [17], [24], [40]	40.5 (22.0–59.0)	46.0 (33.0–59.0)	8.0	10.0	-	18.0	-	-	-	41.0 ORT: 23.2	20.0
Pneumonia											
Africa [22], [23], [30], [44], [52], [119–121]	98.0 (62.9–100.0)	86.0 (27.2–100.0)	46.0 (19.6–51.5)	35.6 (20.0–56.3)	3.1 (2.0–4.2)	57.0 (35.6–100.0)	20.0 (6.7–24.0)	16.6 (2.5–27.6)	21.4 (3.1–64.4)	-	0.0
Asia [4], [19], [21], [39], [43], [54], [57], [80], [100], [122]	80.0 (5.3–92.5)	68.8 (20.9–92.5)	60.0	32.5 (18.0–47.0)	-	33.5 (20.9–60.0)	49.0	-	-	25.6 (2.8–94.6)	6.2 (0.9–11.5)
Latin America [56], [58], [118]	87.5 (83.5–91.6)	89.0 (83.5–94.6)	30.9	30.0	-	60.9	46.6	13.4 (11.6–15.2)	3.3	5.5	11.0
Malaria											
Africa [18], [22], [23], [25–27], [33–35], [45], [46], [50], [51], [53], [59], [69], [91], [102–104], [106], [108–117]	72.1 (6.1–100.0)	41.6 (6.1–98.4)	9.1 (1.2–20.0)	21.0 (5.5–71.0)	1.3 (0.0–40.2)	29.5 (10.8–72.3)	7.25 (1.9–28.6)	30.8 (1.6–49.7)	3.5 (1.2–60.0)	38.7 (4.5–88.0)	8.1 (0.0–51.7)
Asia [101]	81.5	81.5	-	-	1.2	81.5	-	-	-	-	-
Latin America	-	-	-	-	-	-	-	-	-	-	-

[1]The range is shown in brackets if there are two or more data points. The definition of each category of healthcare is stated in the methods. The values do not add up to 100% because of the varying categorisation of healthcare providers in the included studies and because some studies recorded more than one care seeking event.
[2]Appropriate health facilities included all government and trained private health practitioners, but not traditional healers, pharmacies and unqualified medical practitioners.
[3]Abbreviations: Gov = Governmental; CHW = Community Health Worker; Trad. Healer = Traditional Healer; ORT = Oral Rehydration Therapy; - = no data available.

Factors Influencing Care Seeking for Childhood Illness

Identifying studies which contained data on factors that influence care seeking was not a primary aim of this review. However, many of the studies included in the review presented data on influencing factors. This section summarises these studies' findings.

Geography. 18 studies examined the association between geographical factors and care seeking behaviour. Six studies [21–26] found that caregivers in urban areas were more likely to seek care than those in rural locations, and eight studies [26–33] showed that rates of care seeking were inversely related to the distance to the closest health facility. In addition, two studies [30,34] showed that caregivers were more likely to seek traditional care if they were further away from a health facility.

Severity of illness. Twelve studies examined the association between illness severity and care seeking behaviour. Six studies [35–39] found that the more severe caregivers perceived the child's illness to be, the more likely they were to seek care. The same association was present when severity of illness was defined by clinical criteria [37–42]. Of studies reporting data on fatal illness, a study on care seeking for pneumonia [43] found that rates of care seeking from appropriate providers had been high in children who died from the illness (100%). However, another two studies [44,45] on fatal illness showed that care was sought initially from an appropriate provider in only 49.0% and 44.7% of cases, respectively.

Socioeconomic status and cost of health care. Eighteen studies examined links between socioeconomic status, the cost of care, and care seeking behaviour. Three studies [38,46,47] found no association between socioeconomic status and rates of care seeking behaviour. Four studies [22,48–50] found a positive correlation between socioeconomic status and rates of care seeking. One study [28] reported a positive association between the level of maternal education and appropriate care seeking. Participants in six studies [21,27,33,44,51,52] cited cost as a reason for not seeking care for children with illness. However, two studies [29,53] commented on the low rates of appropriate care seeking despite health care being free of charge at the point of care in the study locations. One study [54] found that wealthier caregivers were more likely to attend hospitals than health centres when their child was ill, and another [55] reported that they were more likely to seek care from private providers.

Gender. Seven studies examined whether the gender of the child influenced care seeking. Four studies in Kenya, Ethiopia, Pakistan and Sri Lanka [21,38,50,53] found no significant difference in care seeking rates between male and female children. Two studies carried out in Indonesia and Burkina Faso [30,54], however, found that carers were more likely to seek care for boys than girls. One study looking at cases of fatal malaria [45] showed that carers were more likely to take boys to traditional healers than girls.

Two studies commented that attending a healthcare provider had frequently been delayed because mothers had wanted to consult the head of the household before seeking care [55,56].

Discussion

Treatments for childhood diarrhoea, malaria and pneumonia are usually very effective if care is sought in time. The challenge, therefore, is to implement on-going programmes, which educate caregivers to recognise when to seek care and which facilitate appropriate care seeking behaviour.

Caregiver Recognition of Illness and Importance of Local Context

We found a paucity of studies with data on the sensitivity and specificity of caregiver recognition of disease, and furthermore a decrease in the number of these studies over time. The studies that were available showed that caregivers' sensitivity for recognition of diarrhoea, malaria and pneumonia was low, with median sensitivities of 26.0%, 37.4% and 45.8% respectively. The positive predictive value of a caregiver diagnosis of an illness was highest for diarrhoea (67.7%) and lowest for pneumonia (28.9%). Definitions of disease varied between the studies, making comparison difficult. Furthermore, the sensitivity and specificity of caregiver recognition of disease depended on how caregivers were questioned. For pneumonia, for example, asking closed rather than open questions led to a significant increase in sensitivity but a corresponding decrease in specificity.

More high-quality studies on the recognition of childhood illness are needed to allow for the design of health education and communication strategies that are informed by what diseases and clinical features caregivers already recognise and which ones they do not. Several of the included studies suggest that health education programmes can improve caregiver recognition of childhood illness and appropriate care seeking. A cross-sectional study in Peru [57] found that mothers who reported to have been exposed to a national pneumonia educational campaign on television were more likely to select rapid breathing and chest retraction as signs of pneumonia in a questionnaire. In addition, a before-and-after evaluation [58] of community information activities and a training of trainers for leaders of women groups in Nigeria found significant improvements in knowledge of the symptoms of malaria and its treatment, increased rates of appropriate care seeking for severely ill children, and reductions in rates of consultations with traditional healers for severely ill children (from 60% to 6.7% of cases). In addition, the IMCI strategy can be effective in improving appropriate care seeking. A cluster randomised trial of IMCI in Bangladesh [4] demonstrated the effectiveness of the facility-based component of IMCI in improving appropriate care-seeking for childhood illness. In this study, rates of appropriate care seeking for childhood illness were 20% in IMCI areas compared to 8% in control areas after three years. The subsequent employment of village health workers in IMCI areas further increased appropriate care seeking to 24% after 1.5 years compared to 5% in control areas.

Whilst education programmes can be effective, they must also be maintained over time. The included studies with data on the use of ORT for diarrhoea showed a fairly constant level of ORT use over time: a median of 31.0% (23.2%–46.0%) before 1990, 34.8% (15.7%–55.1%) from 1990 to 1999, and 36.3% (13.4%–68.1%) from 2000 to 2010 [20–23,37,48,59–66]. The authors of one of the studies included in this review [66] commented that there had been no recent campaigns to encourage ORT use in the study areas in Kenya. They suggested that the previous generation of caregivers may in fact be more informed than the current one about the benefit of ORT use in diarrhoeal disease. Overall, the levels of ORT use (a median of 34.0% across all studies) are disappointingly low given that ORT was introduced and then recommended by the WHO more than 40 years ago, and that programmes have been promoting ORT for many years.

An evaluation of the IMCI strategy noted that global strategies must be accompanied by country level implementation guidelines [67]. Knowledge of local context is important to understand some of the factors that influence care seeking behaviour. We found that in most studies there was an inverse association between distance to a health care facility and the likelihood of seeking care.

However, associations with other factors (such as socioeconomic status and gender) were more culturally or geographically dependent with results varying across studies. Despite cost being cited as a reason not to seek care by participants in some studies, several studies found a low uptake of government services even though these were free at the point of access [29,40,53,55,68,69].

Use of Data on Childhood Illness Reported by Caregivers in Disease Burden Estimations

In general, the sensitivity and specificity of caregiver recognition of malaria, pneumonia and diarrhoea was low (medians of 36% sensitivity and 96% specificity for diarrhoea; 46% sensitivity and 67% specificity for pneumonia; 37% sensitivity and 58% specificity for malaria). This strongly suggests that survey data based on these reports should not be used for disease burden estimations. It further suggests that reported diarrhoeal illness (but not pneumonia or malarial illness in a child) is of sufficiently high specificity to be a reasonably valid endpoint for evaluation of an intervention in a controlled trial.

Low Utilisation of Community-based Health Workers

A recent review has highlighted the effectiveness of community-based interventions and platforms in improving breastfeeding rates, managing neonatal infections and childhood pneumonia and improving levels of care seeking [70,71]. Community-based packaged interventions delivered through CHWs have been shown to improve immunization uptake and levels of care seeking for childhood illnesses [70,72–74] and reduce levels of inappropriate use of antibiotics for diarrhoea and mortality and treatment failure rates for pneumonia [70,71]. In this review we found very low levels of care seeking from CHWs, with a median of only 1.3% of caregivers utilising them for malaria, 4.2% for pneumonia, and 5.4% for diarrhoea. This low level of utilisation of CHWs is consistent with the recent multi-country IMCI evaluation, which reported that implementation of the community arm of IMCI has been disappointing and that interventions to improve care seeking had not been introduced [7]. This is of particular concern as community case management is now a major UNICEF and WHO strategy. Reasons given by caregivers for not using CHWs included perceived low status within the communities they worked in [60] and a lack of supplies and medications [33]. However, most of the included studies did not elaborate on reasons for low uptake of their services and reasons may include supply-side as well as demand-side factors.

Private Practitioners

Several of the included studies found a fairly high rate of consultation with private providers in the presence of free governmental care [18,53,55,69]. Caregivers were more likely to seek care from private facilities in Asia than Africa. This is perhaps not surprising, given that the proportion of private healthcare providers is generally larger in Asia [75]. Participants gave a variety of reasons for seeking care from private rather than public providers. These included convenience (both in terms of geography and opening times), prompt care and more courteous service. These findings are supported by a recent review, which found that the public sector appeared frequently to lack timeliness and hospitality towards patients [76]. We found in this review that participants in some studies stated they felt they obtained higher quality care from the private sector, and there was an increased likelihood of receiving what they perceived to be appropriate treatment (e.g. injections for pneumonia and antibiotics or anti-motility agents for diarrhoea).

Given the high proportion of people in LMICs seeking care from private providers, it has been suggested that one way to improve health outcomes is to invest in the private health care sector [77,78] although recognising that there are significant challenges [77]. Indeed, three studies [18,38,53] in our review reported lower standards of care in the private sector.

Traditional Healers and Pharmacies

Another source from which caregivers sought help were traditional healers. They were consulted most frequently in Africa for pneumonia, with a median of 20.8% seeking care. Reasons given for consulting traditional healers included cost [44], ease of access [30,34], and perceived severity [60] or mildness of disease [29]. In general, they were associated with poorer health outcomes: seeking care from traditional healers in one study was associated with higher mortality [60] whilst another study found high rates of consultation with traditional healers among children who died [79]. Consultations with traditional healers were found in one study to result in delayed presentation to appropriate providers [56] and this is the most likely reason for poorer health outcomes.

This review also found high rates of care seeking from pharmacies and drug vendors. The highest rates (median: 30.8%) were for malaria in Africa. Given that rates of care seeking from pharmacies, drug vendors and traditional healers are high, the authors of several studies advocated working with these providers to increase uptake of appropriate treatments for diarrhoea [66,80], malaria [44] and pneumonia [56]. A recent cluster-randomised controlled trial shows that such an approach can be successful. It evaluated the delivery of subsidised artemisinin-based combination therapy (ACT) to private retailers and found an increase of 40.2% in the number of children who received ACT on the day of fever or the following day in the intervention group compared to an increase of 14.6% in the control group ($p<0.0001$) [81].

The studies in this review demonstrate the importance of private care providers, pharmacies and traditional healers, in addition to government facilities, in providing care to children with diarrhoea, pneumonia and malaria. The studies also highlight the low uptake of care provided by community health workers and persistently low rates of ORT use. On the whole, there are few published studies on this important topic, with widely varying definitions of both disease and care seeking. There are also important geographical gaps in the published literature. Data on care seeking is available in the DHS (Demographic and Health Survey) [82] and MICS (Multiple Indicator Cluster Survey) [83] datasets and we would recommend that they were published in journal summary analyses. These would make the data more widely available, foster peer review, and encourage wider discussion of the findings and issues. Stepping up research efforts into interventions that aim to increase the ability of caregivers to recognise and seek appropriate care for childhood illness will be instrumental for designing evidence-based programmes and thus, further reducing childhood mortality in LMICs.

Limitations of the Review

It is unlikely that this review has identified all relevant studies because we did not search the grey literature, the search strategy was carried out using English search terms only, and studies without an English abstract were not reviewed for inclusion in the review. The variations in study designs (e.g. prospective and retrospective designs), illness definitions and healthcare provider categories between studies affected the comparability of the studies' results and also made a meta-analysis unfeasible. In particular, we decided to include studies reporting data on both hypothetical and actual care seeking behaviour because of the relatively low number of identified publications. There may, however, be considerable differences in care seeking rates reported in a hypothetical versus an actual illness scenario. Similarly, while education about illness and access to care is likely to have changed in many settings over the years, we did not exclude studies based on the year of data collection as this would have further reduced the already small number of publications identified for this review. A further weakness of the included studies arises from the fact that there is considerable overlap in the clinical presentation between the three diseases included in this review as well as other childhood illnesses. It is, therefore, likely that a proportion of participants in the included studies were misdiagnosed. Finally, given the wide variation in care seeking rates between studies and the significant geographical gaps in the literature, care should be taken in generalising this review's findings to particular settings.

Acknowledgments

We would like to thank Sheila Fisken, librarian at the University of Edinburgh, for her help in reviewing our search strategies.

Author Contributions

Conceived and designed the experiments: PG LAR HC. Performed the experiments: PG TCW AK SM LAR MKK EJLB SC. Analyzed the data: PG TCW AK SM LAR MKK EJLB SC HC. Wrote the paper: PG TCW.

References

1. UNICEF WHO, The World Bank, United Nations (2012) Levels and Trends in Child Mortality: Report 2012 website. Available: http://www.childmortality.org/files_v9/download/Levels and Trends in Child Mortality Report 2012.pdf. Accessed 2013 Jan 23.
2. United Nations (n.d.) Millennium Development Goals website. Available: http://www.un.org/millenniumgoals/childhealth.shtml. Accessed 2013 Jan 23.
3. WHO (n.d.) Integrated Management of Childhood Illness (IMCI) website. Available: http://www.who.int/child_adolescent_health/topics/prevention_care/child/imci/en/index.html. Accessed 2013 Jan 23.
4. Arifeen SE, Hoque DME, Akter T, Rahman M, Hoque ME, et al. (2009) Effect of the Integrated Management of Childhood Illness strategy on childhood mortality and nutrition in a rural area in Bangladesh: a cluster randomised trial. Lancet 374: 393–403.
5. UNICEF (2003) Communities and families - Improving knowledge of caregivers website. Available: http://www.unicef.org/communities/index_improvingknowledge.html. Accessed 2013 Jan 23.
6. Rudan I, El Arifeen S, Bhutta ZA, Black RE, Brooks A, et al. (2011) Setting research priorities to reduce global mortality from childhood pneumonia by 2015. PLoS Med 8: e1001099. Available: http://dx.plos.org/10.1371/journal.pmed.1001099. Accessed 2013 Jan 23.
7. Herbert HK, Lee ACC, Chandran A, Rudan I, Baqui AH (2012) Care seeking for neonatal illness in low- and middle-income countries: a systematic review. PLoS Med 9: e1001183. Available: http://www.plosmedicine.org/article/info%3Adoi%2F10.1371%2Fjournal.pmed.1001183 Accessed 2013 Jan 23.
8. US National Library of Medicine (n.d) PubMed website. Available: http://www.ncbi.nlm.nih.gov/pubmed. Accessed 2013 Jan 23.
9. Embase (n.d) website. Available: http://www.embase.com. Accessed 2013 Jan 23.
10. WHOLIS (n.d) website. Available: http://www.who.int/library/databases/en. Accessed 2013 Jan 23.
11. Web of Knowledge (previously Web of Science) (n.d) website. Available: http://wok.mimas.ac.uk. Accessed 2013 Jan 23.
12. LILACS (Literature on the Health Sciences in Latin America and the Caribbean) (n.d.) website. Available: http://bases.bireme.br/cgibin/wxislind.exe/iah/online/?IsisScript = iah/iah.xis&base = LILACS&lang = i&form = F. Accessed 2013 Jan 23.
13. PAHO (Pan American Health Organization) (n.d.) website. Available: http://new.paho.org/hq/index.php?lang = en. Accessed 2013 Jan 23.
14. IndMED (n.d.) website. Available: http://indmed.nic.in/indmed.html. Accessed 2013 Jan 23.
15. Williams T, Geldsetzer P, Kirolos A (2012) A systematic literature review of the recognition of, and care-seeking behaviour for, childhood and neonatal illness in developing countries. Available: http://www.crd.york.ac.uk/PROSPERO/display_record.asp?ID = CRD42012003216. Accessed 2013 Jan 23.
16. Goodman LA (1961) Snowball Sampling. Ann Math Stat 32: 148–170.
17. Yoder PS, Hornik RC (1994) Perceptions of severity of diarrhoea and treatment choice: a comparative study of HealthCom sites. J Trop Med Hyg 97: 1–12.
18. Littrell M, Gatakaa H, Evance I, Poyer S, Njogu J, et al. (2011) Monitoring fever treatment behaviour and equitable access to effective medicines in the context of initiatives to improve ACT access: baseline results and implications for programming in six African countries. Malar J 10: 327. Available: http://www.malariajournal.com/content/10/1/327. Accessed 2013 Jan 23.
19. Tupasi TE, Miguel CA, Tallo VL, Bagasao TM, Natividad JN, et al. (1989) Child care practices of mothers: implications for intervention in acute respiratory infections. Ann Trop Paediatr 9: 82–88.
20. Gupta N, Jain SK, Chawla U, Hossain S, Venkatesh S (2007) An evaluation of diarrheal diseases and acute respiratory infections control programmes in a Delhi slum. Indian J Pediatr 74: 471–476.
21. Breiman RF, Olack B, Shultz A, Roder S, Kimani K, et al. (2011) Healthcare-use for major infectious disease syndromes in an informal settlement in Nairobi, Kenya. J Health Popul Nutr 29: 123–133.
22. Burton DC, Flannery B, Onyango B, Larson C, Alaii J, et al. (2011) Healthcare-seeking behaviour for common infectious disease-related illnesses in rural Kenya: a community-based house-to-house survey. J Health Popul Nutr 29: 61–70.
23. DeClerque J, Bailey P, Janowitz B, Dominik R, Fiallos C (1992) Management and treatment of diarrhea in Honduran children: factors associated with mothers' health care behaviors. Soc Sci Med 34: 687–695.
24. Holtz TH, Kachur SP, Marum LH, Mkandala C, Chizani N, et al. (n.d.) Care seeking behaviour and treatment of febrile illness in children aged less than five years: a household survey in Blantyre District, Malawi. Trans R Soc Trop Med Hyg 97: 491–497.
25. Oreagba AI, Onajole AT, Olayemi SO, Mabadeje AFB (2004) Knowledge of malaria amongst caregivers of young children in rural and urban communities in Southwest Nigeria. Trop J Pharm Res 3: 299–304.
26. Glik DC, Ward WB, Gordon A, Haba F (1989) Malaria treatment practices among mothers in Guinea. J Health Soc Behav 30: 421–435.
27. Sur D, Manna B, Deb AK, Deen JL, Danovaro-Holliday MC, et al. (2004) Factors associated with reported diarrhoea episodes and treatment-seeking in an urban slum of Kolkata, India. J Health Popul Nutr 22: 130–138.
28. Gao W, Dang S, Yan H, Wang D (2012) Care-seeking pattern for diarrhea among children under 36 months old in rural western China. PLoS One 7: e43103. Available: http://www.plosone.org/article/info%3Adoi%2F10.1371%2Fjournal.pone.0043103. Accessed 2013 Jan 23.
29. Bigogo G, Audi A, Aura B, Aol G, Breiman RF, et al. (2010) Health-seeking patterns among participants of population-based morbidity surveillance in rural western Kenya: implications for calculating disease rates. Int J Infect Dis 14: e967–73. Available: http://www.ijidonline.com/article/S1201-9712(10)02438-0/fulltext. Accessed 2012 Dec 9.
30. Wilson SE, Ouédraogo CT, Prince L, Ouédraogo A, Hess SY, et al. (2012) Caregiver recognition of childhood diarrhea, care seeking behaviors and home treatment practices in rural Burkina Faso: a cross-sectional survey. PLoS One 7: e33273. Available: http://www.plosone.org/article/info%3Adoi%2F10.1371%2Fjournal.pone.0033273. Accessed 2013 Jan 23.
31. Gombojav N, Manaseki-Holland S, Pollock J, Henderson AJ (2009) The effects of social variables on symptom recognition and medical care seeking behaviour for acute respiratory infections in infants in urban Mongolia. Arch Dis Child 94: 849–854.
32. Müller O, Traoré C, Becher H, Kouyaté B (2003) Malaria morbidity, treatment-seeking behaviour, and mortality in a cohort of young children in rural Burkina Faso. Trop Med Int Health 8: 290–296.
33. Baume C, Helitzer D, Kachur SP (2000) Patterns of care for childhood malaria in Zambia. Soc Sci Med 51: 1491–1503.
34. Uzochukwu BSC, Onwujekwe EO, Onoka CA, Ughasoro MD (2008) Rural-urban differences in maternal responses to childhood fever in South East Nigeria. PLoS One 3: e1788. Available: http://www.plosone.org/article/metrics/info%3Adoi%2F10.1371%2Fjournal.pone.0001788;jsessionid = 908D8D8D3E6C86A59C1A14639AE62321. Accessed 2012 Dec 18.
35. Yoder PS, Hornik RC (1994) Perceptions of severity of diarrhoea and treatment choice: a comparative study of HealthCom sites. J Trop Med Hyg 97: 1–12.

36. Babaniyi OA, Maciak BJ, Wambai Z (1994) Management of diarrhoea at the household level: a population-based survey in Suleja, Nigeria. East Afr Med J 71: 531–535.
37. Langsten R, Hill K (1995) Treatment of childhood diarrhea in rural Egypt. Soc Sci Med 40: 989–1001.
38. Amarasiri de Silva MW, Wijekoon A, Hornik R, Martines J (2001) Care seeking in Sri Lanka: one possible explanation for low childhood mortality. Soc Sci Med 53: 1363–1372.
39. Pérez-Cuevas R, Guiscafré H, Romero G, Rodríguez L, Gutiérrez G (1996) Mothers' health-seeking behaviour in acute diarrhoea in Tlaxcala, Mexico. J Diarrhoeal Dis Res 14: 260–268.
40. Vathanophas K, Indrasukhsri T, Bunyaratabandhu P, Suthienkul O, Varavithya W (1988) The study of knowledge, attitudes and practices of mothers concerning diarrhoea and oral rehydration salts in the Bangkok metropolis. J Med Assoc Thai 71: 177–182.
41. Page AL, Hustache S, Luquero FJ, Djibo A, Manzo ML, et al. (2011) Health care seeking behavior for diarrhea in children under 5 in rural Niger: results of a cross-sectional survey. BMC Public Health 11: 389. Available: http://www.biomedcentral.com/1471-2458/11/389. Accessed 2013 Jan 23.
42. Kapoor SK, Reddaiah VP, Murthy GV (n.d.) Knowledge, attitude and practices regarding acute respiratory infections. Indian J Pediatr 57: 533–535.
43. Sodemann M, Jakobsen MS, Mølbak K, Alvarenga IC, Aaby P (1997) High mortality despite good care-seeking behaviour: a community study of childhood deaths in Guinea-Bissau. Bull World Health Organ 75: 205–212.
44. Beiersmann C, Sanou A, Wladarsch E, De Allegri M, Kouyaté B, et al. (2007) Malaria in rural Burkina Faso: local illness concepts, patterns of traditional treatment and influence on health-seeking behaviour. Malar J 6: 106. Available: http://www.malariajournal.com/content/6/1/106. Accessed 2013 Jan 23.
45. De Savigny D, Mayombana C, Mwageni E, Masanja H, Minhaj A, et al. (2004) Care-seeking patterns for fatal malaria in Tanzania. Malar J 3: 27. Available: http://www.malariajournal.com/content/3/1/27. Accessed 2013 Jan 23.
46. Sodemann M, Jakobsen MS, Mølbak K, Martins C, Aaby P (1996) Maternal perception of cause, signs and severity of diarrhoea in a suburban west African community. Acta Paediatr 85: 1062–1069.
47. De Zoysa I, Carson D, Feachem R, Kirkwood B, Lindsay-Smith E, et al. (1984) Perceptions of childhood diarrhoea and its treatment in rural Zimbabwe. Soc Sci Med 19: 727–734.
48. Qureshi AF, Lobo MA (1994) Socio-anthropological determinants and home management in childhood diarrhoea in a squatter settlement of Karachi, Pakistan. J Trop Pediatr 40: 378–380.
49. Rutebemberwa E, Kallander K, Tomson G, Peterson S, Pariyo G (2009) Determinants of delay in care-seeking for febrile children in eastern Uganda. Trop Med Int Health 14: 472–479.
50. Deressa W, Ali A, Berhane Y (2007) Household and socioeconomic factors associated with childhood febrile illnesses and treatment seeking behaviour in an area of epidemic malaria in rural Ethiopia. Trans R Soc Trop Med Hyg 101: 939–947.
51. Amofah GK, Essegbey IT, Opoku SA, Oduro J (1995) Intended response of caretakers of pre-school children to acute respiratory infection in a rural district in Ghana. East Afr Med J 72: 619–622.
52. Théra MA, D'Alessandro U, Thiéro M, Ouedraogo A, Packou J, et al. (2000) Child malaria treatment practices among mothers in the district of Yanfolila, Sikasso region, Mali. Trop Med Int Health 5: 876–881.
53. Hussain R, Lobo MA, Inam B, Khan A, Qureshi AF, et al. (1997) Pneumonia perceptions and management: an ethnographic study in urban squatter settlements of Karachi, Pakistan. Soc Sci Med 45: 991–1004.
54. Simanjuntak CH, Punjabi NH, Wangsasaputra F, Nurdin D, Pulungsih SP, et al. (2004) Diarrhoea episodes and treatment-seeking behaviour in a slum area of North Jakarta, Indonesia. J Health Popul Nutr 22: 119–129.
55. Lindblade KA, Johnson AJ, Arvelo W, Zhang X, Jordan HT, et al. (2011) Low usage of government healthcare facilities for acute respiratory infections in guatemala: implications for influenza surveillance. BMC Public Health 11: 885. Available: http://www.biomedcentral.com/1471-2458/11/885. Accessed 2013 Jan 23.
56. McNee A, Khan N, Dawson S, Gunsalam J, Tallo VL, et al. (1995) Responding to cough: Boholano illness classification and resort to care in response to childhood ARI. Soc Sci Med 40: 1279–1289.
57. Gálvez CA, Modeste N, Lee JW, Betancourt H, Wilkins RL (2002) Peruvian mothers' knowledge and recognition of pneumonia in children under 5 years of age. Rev Panam Salud Publica 11: 99–108.
58. Okeke TA (2010) Improving malaria recognition, treatment and referral practices by training caretakers in rural Nigeria. J Biosoc Sci 42: 325–339.
59. Babaniyi OA (1991) Oral rehydration of children with diarrhoea in Nigeria: a 12-year review of impact on morbidity and mortality from diarrhoeal diseases and diarrhoeal treatment practices. J Trop Pediatr 37: 57–63.
60. Olango P, Aboud F (1990) Determinants of mothers' treatment of diarrhea in rural Ethiopia. Soc Sci Med 31: 1245–1249.
61. Ali M, Atkinson D, Underwood P (2000) Determinants of use rate of oral rehydration therapy for management of childhood diarrhoea in rural Bangladesh. J Health Popul Nutr 18: 103–108.
62. Ene-Obong HN, Iroegbu CU, Uwaegbute AC (2000) Perceived causes and management of diarrhoea in young children by market women in Enugu State, Nigeria. J Health Popul Nutr 18: 97–102.
63. Biritwum RB, Asante A, Amoo PK, Gyekye AA, Amissah CR, et al. (2004) Community-based cluster surveys on treatment preferences for diarrhoea, severe diarrhoea, and dysentery in children aged less than five years in two districts of Ghana. J Health Popul Nutr 22: 182–190.
64. Prohmmo A, Cook LA, Murdoch DR (2006) Childhood diarrhoea in a district in northeast Thailand: incidence and treatment choices. Asia Pac J Public Health 18: 26–32.
65. Othero DM, Orago ASS, Groenewegen T, Kaseje DO, Otengah PA (2008) Home management of diarrhea among underfives in a rural community in Kenya: household perceptions and practices. East Afr J Public Health 5: 142–146.
66. Olson CK, Blum LS, Patel KN, Oria PA, Feikin DR, et al. (2011) Community case management of childhood diarrhea in a setting with declining use of oral rehydration therapy: findings from cross-sectional studies among primary household caregivers, Kenya, 2007. Am J Trop Med Hyg 85: 1134–1140.
67. Bryce J, Victora CG, Habicht JP, Black RE, Scherpbier RW (2005) Programmatic pathways to child survival: results of a multi-country evaluation of Integrated Management of Childhood Illness. Health Policy Plan 20 Suppl 1: i5–i17.
68. Rutebemberwa E, Pariyo G, Peterson S, Tomson G, Kallander K (2009) Utilization of public or private health care providers by febrile children after user fee removal in Uganda. Malar J 8: 45. Available: http://www.malariajournal.com/content/8/1/45. Accessed 2013 Jan 23.
69. Kaljee L, Thiem VD, von Seidlein L, Genberg BL, Canh DG, et al. (2004) Healthcare use for diarrhoea and dysentery in actual and hypothetical cases, Nha Trang, Viet Nam. J Health Popul Nutr 22: 139–149.
70. Bhutta ZA, Das JK, Walker N, Rizvi A, Campbell H, et al. (2013) Interventions to address deaths from childhood pneumonia and diarrhoea equitably: what works and at what cost? Lancet 381: 1417–1429.
71. Theodoratou E, Al-Jilaihawi S, Woodward F, Ferguson J, Jhass A, et al. (2010) The effect of case management on childhood pneumonia mortality in developing countries. Int J Epidemiol 39 Suppl 1: i155–71.
72. Lassi ZS, Haider BA, Bhutta ZA (2010) Community-based intervention packages for reducing maternal and neonatal morbidity and mortality and improving neonatal outcomes. Cochrane Database Syst Rev: CD007754. Available: http://onlinelibrary.wiley.com/doi/10.1002/14651858.CD007754.pub2/abstract;jsessionid=FBA43D44D0B025B437820733C1073C6D.f04t02. Accessed 2013 Jan 23.
73. Lassi ZS, Haider BA, Bhutta ZA (2012) Community-based intervention packages for reducing maternal morbidity and mortality and improving neonatal outcomes 1. J Dev Eff 4: 151–187.
74. Global Health Workforce Alliance, WHO (2010) Global Experience of Community Health Workers for Delivery of Health Related Millennium Development Goals: A Systematic Review, Country Case Studies, and Recommendations for Integration into National Health Systems website. Available: http://www.who.int/workforcealliance/knowledge/resources/chwreport/en/. Accessed 2013 July 5.
75. Hanson K, Berman P (1998) Private health care provision in developing countries: a preliminary analysis of levels and composition. Health Policy Plan 13: 195–211.
76. Basu S, Andrews J, Kishore S, Panjabi R, Stuckler D (2012) Comparative performance of private and public healthcare systems in low- and middle-income countries: a systematic review. PLoS Med 9: e1001244. Available: http://dx.plos.org/10.1371/journal.pmed.1001244. Accessed 2012 Nov 2.
77. Patouillard E, Goodman CA, Hanson KG, Mills AJ (2007) Can working with the private for-profit sector improve utilization of quality health services by the poor? A systematic review of the literature. Int J Equity Health 6: 17. Available: http://www.equityhealthj.com/content/6/1/17. Accessed 2013 Jan 23.
78. Loevinsohn B, Harding A (2005) Buying results? Contracting for health service delivery in developing countries. Lancet 366: 676–681.
79. Sutrisna B, Reingold A, Kresno S, Harrison G, Utomo B (1993) Care-seeking for fatal illnesses in young children in Indramayu, west Java, Indonesia. Lancet 342: 787–789.
80. Ellis AA, Winch P, Daou Z, Gilroy KE, Swedberg E (2007) Home management of childhood diarrhoea in southern Mali–implications for the introduction of zinc treatment. Soc Sci Med 64: 701–712.
81. Kangwana BP, Kedenge SV, Noor AM, Alegana VA, Nyandigisi AJ, et al. (2011) The impact of retail-sector delivery of artemether-lumefantrine on malaria treatment of children under five in Kenya: a cluster randomized controlled trial. PLoS Med 8: e1000437. Available: http://www.plosmedicine.org/article/info%3Adoi%2F10.1371%2Fjournal.pmed.1000437. Accessed 2012 Nov 15.
82. US AID, The DHS Program (nd) MEASURE DHS - Quality information to plan, monitor and improve population, health, and nutrition programs website. Available: http://www.measuredhs.com/. Accessed 2013 July 10.
83. UNICEF (2012) UNICEF Statistics and Monitoring - Multiple Indicator Cluster Survey (MICS) website. Available: http://www.unicef.org/statistics/index_24302.html. Accessed 2013 July 10.
84. Cogswell ME, Oni GA, Stallings RY, Brown KH (1991) Sociodemographic and clinical factors affecting recognition of childhood diarrhea by mothers in Kwara State, Nigeria. Soc Sci Med 33: 1209–1216.
85. Thomas JC, Neumann CG, Frerichs RR (1989) The effect of misclassification of diarrhoea on estimates of its occurrence, the identification of risk factors, and the assessment of prevention efforts. J Diarrhoeal Dis Res 7: 63–69.

86. Mobley CC, Boerma JT, Titus S, Lohrke B, Shangula K, et al. (1996) Validation study of a verbal autopsy method for causes of childhood mortality in Namibia. J Trop Pediatr 42: 365–369.
87. Kalter HD, Gray RH, Black RE, Gultiano SA (1990) Validation of postmortem interviews to ascertain selected causes of death in children. Int J Epidemiol 19: 380–386.
88. Kalter HD, Gray RH, Black RE, Gultiano SA (1991) Validation of the diagnosis of childhood morbidity using maternal health interviews. Int J Epidemiol 20: 193–198.
89. Bailo Diallo A, De Serres G, Béavogui AH, Lapointe C, Viens P (2001) Home care of malaria-infected children of less than 5 years of age in a rural area of the Republic of Guinea. Bull World Health Organ 79: 28–32.
90. Lubanga RG, Norman S, Ewbank D, Karamagi C (1997) Maternal diagnosis and treatment of children's fever in an endemic malaria zone of Uganda: implications for the malaria control programme. Acta Trop 68: 53–64.
91. Yé Y, Traoré C, Meissner P, Coulibaly B, Becher H, et al. (2007) Ability of mothers to diagnose fever and anaemia in their young children, in a malaria-endemic region of West Africa. Ann Trop Med Parasitol 101: 297–303.
92. Desai MR, Phillips-Howard PA, Terlouw DJ, Wannemuehler KA, Odhacha A, et al. (2002) Recognition of pallor associated with severe anaemia by primary caregivers in western Kenya. Trop Med Int Health 7: 831–839.
93. Mull DS, Mull JD, Kundi MZ, Anjum M (1994) Mothers' perceptions of severe pneumonia in their own children: a controlled study in Pakistan. Soc Sci Med 38: 973–987.
94. Kambarami RA, Rusakaniko S, Mahomva LA (1996) Ability of caregivers to recognise signs of pneumonia in coughing children aged below five years. Cent Afr J Med 42: 291–294.
95. Harrison LH, Moursi S, Guinena AH, Gadomski AM, el-Ansary KS, et al. (1995) Maternal reporting of acute respiratory infection in Egypt. Int J Epidemiol 24: 1058–1063.
96. Campbell H, Byass P, Greenwood BM (1990) Acute lower respiratory infections in Gambian children: maternal perception of illness. Ann Trop Paediatr 10: 45–51.
97. Gadomski AM, Aref GH, Hassanien F, el Ghandour S, el-Mougi M, et al. (1993) Caretaker recognition of respiratory signs in children: correlation with physical examination findings, x-ray diagnosis and pulse oximetry. Int J Epidemiol 22: 1166–1173.
98. Shah MS, Ahmad A, Khalique N, Afzal S, Ansari MA, et al. (2012) Home-based management of acute diarrhoeal disease in an urban slum of Aligarh, India. J Infect Dev Ctries 6: 137–142.
99. Saini NK, Gaur DR, Saini V, Lal S (1992) Acute respiratory infections in children: a study of knowledge and practices of mothers in rural Haryana. J Commun Dis 24: 75–77.
100. Yadav SP (2010) A study of treatment seeking behaviour for malaria and its management in febrile children in rural part of desert, Rajasthan, India. J Vector Borne Dis 47: 235–242.
101. Oguonu T, Okafor HU, Obu HA (2005) Caregivers's knowledge, attitude and practice on childhood malaria and treatment in urban and rural communities in Enugu, south-east Nigeria. Public Health 119: 409–414.
102. Okeke TA, Okeibunor JC (2010) Rural-urban differences in health-seeking for the treatment of childhood malaria in south-east Nigeria. Health Policy 95: 62–68.
103. Akogun OB, John KK (2005) Illness-related practices for the management of childhood malaria among the Bwatiye people of north-eastern Nigeria. Malar J 4: 13. Available: http://www.malariajournal.com/content/4/1/13. Accessed 2013 Jan 23.
104. Wang X, von Seidlein L, Robertson SE, Ma JC, Han CQ, et al. (2004) A community-based cluster survey on preferences for treatment of diarrhoea and dysentery in Zhengding county, Hebei province, China. J Health Popul Nutr 22: 104–112.
105. Kaatano GM, Muro AIS, Medard M (2006) Caretaker's perceptions, attitudes and practices regarding childhood febrile illness and diarrhoeal diseases among riparian communities of Lake Victoria, Tanzania. Tanzan Health Res Bull 8: 155–161.
106. Samosornsuk S, Jitsanguansuk S, Sirima N, Sudjai S, Tapchaisri P, et al. (2004) Preferences for treatment of diarrhoea and dysentery in Kaengkhoi district, Saraburi province, Thailand. J Health Popul Nutr 22: 113–118.
107. Dabis F, Breman JG, Roisin AJ, Haba F (1989) Monitoring selective components of primary health care: methodology and community assessment of vaccination, diarrhoea, and malaria practices in Conakry, Guinea. ACSI-CCCD team. Bull World Health Organ 67: 675–684.
108. Njama D, Dorsey G, Guwatudde D, Kigonya K, Greenhouse B, et al. (2003) Urban malaria: primary caregivers' knowledge, attitudes, practices and predictors of malaria incidence in a cohort of Ugandan children. Trop Med Int Health 8: 685–692.
109. Foster D, Vilendrer S (2009) Two treatments, one disease: childhood malaria management in Tanga, Tanzania. Malar J 8: 240. Available: http://www.malariajournal.com/content/8/1/240. Accessed 2013 Jan 23.
110. Ringsted FM, Bygbjerg IC, Samuelsen H (2006) Early home-based recognition of anaemia via general danger signs, in young children, in a malaria endemic community in north-east Tanzania. Malar J 5: 111. Available: http://www.malariajournal.com/content/5/1/111. Accessed 2013 Jan 23.
111. Talani P, Samba G, Moyen G (2003) Management of children's fever at home in a rural area of Boko (Congo-Brazzaville)]. Sante Publique 15: 485–490.
112. Hamel MJ, Odhacha A, Roberts JM, Deming MS (2001) Malaria control in Bungoma District, Kenya: a survey of home treatment of children with fever, bednet use and attendance at antenatal clinics. Bull World Health Organ 79: 1014–1023.
113. Fourn L, Sakou G, Zohoun T (2001) [Utilization of health services by mothers of children with fever in the south of Benin]. Sante Publique 13: 161–168.
114. Mukanga D, Tibenderana JK, Peterson S, Pariyo GW, Kiguli J, et al. (2012) Access, acceptability and utilization of community health workers using diagnostics for case management of fever in Ugandan children: a cross-sectional study. Malar J 11: 121. Available: http://www.malariajournal.com/content/11/1/121. Accessed 2013 Jan 23.
115. Smith LA, Bruce J, Gueye L, Helou A, Diallo R, et al. (2010) From fever to anti-malarial: the treatment-seeking process in rural Senegal. Malar J 9: 333. Available: http://www.malariajournal.com/content/9/1/333. Accessed 2013 Jan 23.
116. Deming MS, Gayibor A, Murphy K, Jones TS, Karsa T (1989) Home treatment of febrile children with antimalarial drugs in Togo. Bull World Health Organ 67: 695–700.
117. Luque JS, Whiteford LM, Tobin GA (2008) Maternal recognition and health care-seeking behavior for acute respiratory infection in children in a rural Ecuadorian county. Matern Child Health J 12: 287–297.
118. Källander K, Hildenwall H, Waiswa P, Galiwango E, Peterson S, et al. (2008) Delayed care seeking for fatal pneumonia in children aged under five years in Uganda: a case-series study. Bull World Health Organ 86: 332–338.
119. Teka T, Dagnew M (1995) Health behaviour of rural mothers to acute respiratory infections in children in Gondar, Ethiopia. East Afr Med J 72: 623–625.
120. Simiyu DE, Wafula EM, Nduati RW (2003) Mothers' knowledge, attitudes and practices regarding acute respiratory infections in children in Baringo District, Kenya. East Afr Med J 80: 303–307.
121. Jordan HT, Prapasiri P, Areerat P, Anand S, Clague B, et al. (2009) A comparison of population-based pneumonia surveillance and health-seeking behavior in two provinces in rural Thailand. Int J Infect Dis 13: 355–361.

Early *Clostridium difficile* Infection during Allogeneic Hematopoietic Stem Cell Transplantation

Melissa A. Kinnebrew[4,5], Yeon Joo Lee[1], Robert R. Jenq[2,5], Lauren Lipuma[3], Eric R. Littmann[1], Asia Gobourne[3], Daniel No[3], Marcel van den Brink[2,3,4,5], Eric G. Pamer[1,3,4,5], Ying Taur[1,3,5]*

1 Infectious Diseases Service, Memorial Sloan Kettering Cancer Center, New York, New York, United States of America, **2** Adult Bone Marrow Transplant Service, Memorial Sloan Kettering Cancer Center, New York, New York, United States of America, **3** Lucille Castori Center for Microbes, Inflammation, and Cancer, Memorial Sloan Kettering Cancer Center, New York, New York, United States of America, **4** Immunology Program, Sloan-Kettering Institute, New York, New York, United States of America, **5** Weill Cornell Medical College, New York, New York, United States of America

Abstract

Clostridium difficile infection (CDI) is frequently diagnosed in recipients of allogeneic hematopoietic stem cell transplantation (allo-HSCT). We characterized early-transplant CDI and its associations, and analyzed serially-collected feces to determine intestinal carriage of toxigenic *C. difficile*. Fecal specimens were collected longitudinally from 94 patients during allo-HSCT hospitalization, from the start of pre-transplant conditioning until up to 35 days after stem cell infusion. Presence of *C. difficile* 16S rRNA and *tcdB* genes was determined. Clinical variables and specimen data were analyzed for association with development of CDI. Historical data from an additional 1144 allo-HSCT patients was also used. Fecal specimens from 37 patients (39%) were found to harbor *C. difficile*. Early-transplant CDI was diagnosed in 16 of 94 (17%) patients undergoing allo-HSCT; cases were generally mild and resembled non-CDI diarrhea associated with transplant conditioning. CDI was associated with preceding colonization with tcdB-positive *C. difficile* and conditioning regimen intensity. We found no associations between early-transplant CDI and graft-versus-host disease or CDI later in transplant. CDI occurs with high frequency during the early phase of allo-HSCT, where recipients are pre-colonized with toxigenic C. difficile. During this time, CDI incidence peaks during pre-transplant conditioning, and is correlated to intensity of the treatment. In this unique setting, high rates of CDI may be explained by prior colonization and chemotherapy; however, cases were generally mild and resembled non-infectious diarrhea due to conditioning, raising concerns of misdiagnosis. Further study of this unique population with more discriminating CDI diagnostic tests are warranted.

Editor: Vassiliki A. Boussiotis, Beth Israel Deaconess Medical Center, Harvard Medical School, United States of America

Funding: This work was supported by the National Institutes of Health [grant numbers 1K23 AI095398-01 to Y.T., 1RO1 AI42135 to E.G.P., and T32GM07739 to M.A.K.], the Lucille Castori Center for Microbes, Inflamation, and Cancer, and the Tow Foundation. The funders had no role in study design, data collection and analysis, decision to publish, or preparation of the manuscript.

Competing Interests: The authors have declared that no competing interests exist.

* E-mail: taury@mskcc.org

Introduction

Clostridium difficile infection (CDI) is a frequent cause of diarrhea in hospitalized patients, with disturbances of the intestinal microbiota following antibiotic administration as one of the major risk factors. Patients undergoing allogeneic hematopoietic stem cell transplantation (allo-HSCT) receive chemotherapy, radiation, and antibiotics, which represent significant risk factors for CDI. Previous studies demonstrated that approximately 15–30% of allo-HSCT recipients develop CDI during transplantation [1–5], greatly exceeding rates in most other patient populations.

Allo-HSCT patients have often been previously hospitalized, and each hospitalization increases exposure to *C. difficile*, providing a potential explanation for the high incidence of CDI. Although *C. difficile* can be acquired during hospitalization, prospective molecular typing of *C. difficile* isolates from hospitalized patients suggests that transmission may account for a minority of CDI cases, and that many patients who enter the hospital are colonized with *C. difficile* [6].

Previous studies have correlated CDI in allo-HSCT recipients with the development of graft-versus-host disease (GVHD). However, the rates of *C. difficile* colonization and the risk of CDI in colonized patients remain undefined in this population. Therefore, we examined the colonization status of patients over the course of early allo-HSCT, using a previously described cohort in which fecal specimens were collected throughout their transplant hospitalization. We also examined 13 years of observational data of allo-HSCT recipients cared for at our institution to supplement findings from our biospecimen cohort.

Methods

Biospecimen Protocol Group

Fecal specimens were collected from adult patients undergoing allo- HSCT at Memorial Sloan-Kettering Cancer Center. We developed a biospecimen collection protocol in which consenting patients underwent once weekly serial specimen collection during their transplant hospitalization, from up to 15 days pre-transplantation until up to 35 days post-transplantation. For each patient, specimen collection and study observation occurred within this 50-day window and while patients were still hospitalized for transplantation. For each subject we required that a minimum of one pre- and two post-transplant fecal specimens be collected for inclusion. Collection took place for patients with dates of transplantation from 4 September 2009 to 4 August 2011. This cohort of patients has been described in a previous report [7].

Analysis of Fecal Specimens: *tcdB*

Fecal specimens collected from the biospecimen group were frozen and stored at −80°C upon collection until processed. DNA was purified from the stool specimens using a phenol-chloroform extraction process as previously described [8,9]. DNA was purified further using QIAamp mini spin columns (Qiagen). Extracted DNA was analyzed by real-time PCR for the presence of *C. difficile* toxin B gene (*tcdB*). For the PCR reaction, 50 ng of extracted DNA was used as starting material along with 12.5 µL of Dynamo SYBR Green Master Mix (Thermo) and 400 nM of toxin B-specific primer sequences (Forward: GAAAGTCCAAGTT-TACGCTCAAT, Reverse: GCTGCACCTAAACTTACACCA) [10–12].

Each specimen was run in duplicate. Real-time PCR was performed by the Step One Plus Real-Time PCR (Applied Biosystems). The PCR parameters were as follows: 94°C for 3 min and 30 cycles of 94°C for 30 sec, 52°C for 30 sec, and 72°C for 1 min. Amplification of bacterial 16S rRNA gene using universal primers was performed in parallel to ensure the specimen was not contaminated with PCR inhibitors (Forward: GCCAG-CAGCCGCGGTAA and Reverse: AGGGTATCTAATCCT) [13,14]. Melting curves of each reaction were examined and compared to positive controls to identify specific amplification.

For quantitation of *C. difficile* in the stool, primers specific for the *C. difficile* 16S rRNA gene were used in the same protocol described above (Forward: TTGAGCGATTTACTTCGG-TAAAGA, Reverse: CCATCCTGTACTGGCTCACCT) [15]. Standard curves were prepared with known concentrations of a plasmid containing 1 copy of the *C. difficile* 16S rRNA gene.

Observational Group

To complement the results from data in the biospecimen group, we gathered a larger dataset containing historical clinical data from medical records of patients undergoing allo-HSCT at our institution from 1 January 1999 to 29 March 2012, spanning approximately 13 years. To avoid analysis of duplicate data, patients included in the biospecimen group were excluded from the observational data group.

Clinical Data

For both the biospecimen group and the observational group, clinical data were obtained for each patient through abstraction from electronic medical records. Data obtained included age, sex, underlying disease, conditioning regimen intensity [16], stem cell donor source, whether stem cell were ex-vivo T-cell depleted [17], antibiotics used during hospitalization (with start and stop dates), development of gastrointestinal graft-versus-host disease (GVHD) up to 100 days post-transplantation [18].

The diagnosis of CDI was based on a compatible clinical history with positive laboratory test, which was performed at the discretion of the transplant healthcare provider. Our microbiology laboratory only tested unformed stool for evidence of CDI. The severity of CDI cases was assessed using a three-tiered scoring system, described previously: low severity, medium severity, and severe disease [19].

The method of detection for toxin-producing *C. difficile* employed by our institution varied over the course of the study period. Prior to 29 August, 2008, a cell culture-based cytotoxicity assay (toxin and antitoxin reagents from TechLab, Wi-38 cell lines from Diagnostic Hybrids and Viromed Labs) was used. From 29 August, 2008 to 10 September, 2010, our hospital employed a two-step procedure involving detection of the GDH antigen (C. Diff Chek-60, Wampole Laboratories), followed by confirmatory cytotoxicity assay in GDH-positive specimens. On 10 September 2010, clinical CDI testing was switched to a PCR assay that detects *C. difficile* Toxin B (Xpert *C. difficile* assay, Cepheid GeneXpert), and continues to be used currently.

At our institution, routine antibiotic prophylaxis was given to patients undergoing allo-HSCT. Practice patterns varied slightly over the course of the study period, but were more formalized starting June 11, 2006. In general, intravenous vancomycin and ciprofloxacin were given to patients undergoing allo-HSCT with myeloablative or reduced intensity conditioning, from 2 days pre- to 7 days post-transplantation. Ciprofloxacin treatment could be longer, or for a non-myeloablative transplant, depending on anticipated time to engraftment. Our institution does not administer metronidazole for prevention of infection or GVHD.

Ethics Statement

Specimen collection and analysis of the biospecimen group was approved by the Memorial Sloan-Kettering Cancer Center Institutional Review Board (IRB# 09-067). All biosepcimen group subjects provided written consent for specimen collection and analysis. For analysis of data from subjects from the observational group, we obtained an existing-data waiver from the Memorial Sloan-Kettering Cancer Center Institutional Review Board.

Analytic Methods

Subjects within the biospecimen subset group were analyzed separately from the remaining observational cohort. Predictors of early transplant CDI were assessed using Cox proportional hazards regression, where predictors included clinical variables listed above, as well as preceding detection of *tcdB* for the biospecimen subset group. As secondary analyses, we also assessed the predictivity of early CDI onto the endpoints of late CDI and the development of gastrointestinal GVHD. We also assessed the risk factors for the presence of *tcdB* colonization in the first collected specimen, as an additional analysis.

Firth's penalized likelihood method was applied to all survival regression calculations, in order to avoid divergent parameter estimates due to monotone likelihood [20]. Since presence of *tcdB* and antibiotic administration were variables that changed over time, these predictors were coded and analyzed as time-dependent variables. In each of these analyses, predictors were analyzed separately in a univariate fashion; predictors with a univariate P-value less than or equal to 0.20 were analyzed in a multivariate model, to account for confounding influences. Survival plots for CDI were constructed using the Kaplan-Meier method. All analyses were performed using R version 3.01 (R Development Core Team, Vienna, Austria).

Results

Fecal specimens were collected from 105 consented patients; 11 were excluded due to insufficient sample collection, leaving a total of 94 patients for study in the biospecimen group. From these subjects, a total of 436 fecal specimens were collected (3 to 8 per patient). Clinical characteristics of these patients are described in Table 1. During the observation period, 16 (17%) subjects were diagnosed with CDI. Among the remaining 78 subjects not diagnosed with CDI, an additional 21 patients had detectable *tcdB* by PCR. The approximate threshold of detection was 200 colony-forming units per gram of stool. We confirmed the presence of *C. difficile* in these specimens by quantitative PCR specific for *C. difficile* 16S rRNA genes. In patients diagnosed with CDI, a greater proportion of patients received myeloablative conditioning compared with those not diagnosed with CDI. Most patients diagnosed with CDI received treatment with metronidazole. Based on CDI severity scoring [19], cases were considered mild or moderate (13 low severity, 3 medium severity), with no cases of severe CDI.

Within the observational data group, a total of 1144 subjects were included. CDI was diagnosed in 138 patients (12.1%), and showed similar clinical characteristics as the biospecimen group (Table S1). In both the biospecimen and observational groups, most cases of CDI occurred in the immediate peri-transplant period (i.e. within a few days of stem cell infusion), peaking just prior to stem cell infusion (Figure 1). This pattern of distribution over relative day of transplant was observed regardless of CDI testing method, though the overall CDI rate in this population increased over time (Figure S1).

Analysis of risk factors for CDI are listed in Table 2. Myeloablative conditioning increased the risk of CDI three-fold in comparison to regimens of lower intensity (Figure 2). These findings are consistent with recent studies describing CDI in patients following allo-HSCT [2,5]. In addition to conditioning, the observational group showed that an underlying diagnosis of leukemia and ex-vivo T-cell depletion were also associated with CDI, and beta-lactam administration was protective against subsequent CDI. Analysis of the biospecimen group demonstrated that preceding colonization with *tcdB*-positive *C. difficile* was highly predictive of subsequent diagnosis of CDI. On multivariate analysis, conditioning regimen, prior colonization in the biospecimen group, and beta-lactam administration in the observational group remained as independent predictors (Table S2 and S3). A follow-up analysis of predictors of toxigenic *C. difficile* colonization within the first collected specimen showed no significant associations (Table S4).

Selected patients diagnosed with CDI are shown in Figure 3 (plots of all patients are listed in Figure S2). *C. difficile* 16S was detectable in all *tcdB*-positive specimens. Conversely, there were

Table 1. Characteristics of Patients, Biospecimen Group (N = 94)[a].

Parameter	Diagnosed with CDI	Not Diagnosed with CDI		Total (Combined)
		tcdB+	*tcdB−*	
Age (years)[g]	50.5 (19–69)	57 (28–65)	54 (23–69)	53.5 (19–69)
Sex (female)	4 (25.0%)	10 (47.6%)	27 (47.4%)	41 (43.6%)
Underlying Disease				
Leukemia	11 (68.8%)	9 (42.9%)	24 (42.1%)	44 (46.8%)
Lymphoma	2 (12.5%)	6 (28.6%)	18 (31.6%)	26 (27.7%)
Multiple Myeloma	1 (6.2%)	3 (14.3%)	4 (7.0%)	8 (8.5%)
Myelodysplastic Syndrome	2 (12.5%)	1 (4.8%)	9 (15.8%)	12 (12.8%)
Other	0 (0.0%)	2 (9.5%)	2 (3.5%)	4 (4.3%)
Prior antibiotics (14 d)[f]	8 (50.0%)	7 (33.3%)	27 (47.4%)	42 (44.7%)
Conditioning Regimen Intensity				
Non-myeloablative	1 (6.2%)	5 (23.8%)	10 (17.5%)	16 (17.0%)
Reduced Intensity	2 (12.5%)	5 (23.8%)	14 (24.6%)	21 (22.3%)
Myeloablative	13 (81.2%)	11 (52.4%)	33 (57.9%)	57 (60.6%)
T-cell depleted graft	10 (62.5%)	10 (47.6%)	22 (38.6%)	42 (44.7%)
Stem cell source (cord vs. other)	3 (18.8%)	5 (23.8%)	15 (26.3%)	23 (24.5%)
Time to engraftment (≥14 d)[b]	3 (18.8%)	4 (19.0%)	17 (29.8%)	24 (25.5%)
Antibiotics[c,d]				
Vancomycin (IV)	15 (93.8%)	20 (95.2%)	50 (87.7%)	85 (90.4%)
Fluoroquinolone	3 (18.8%)	5 (23.8%)	25 (43.9%)	33 (35.1%)
Metronidazole	14 (87.5%)	3 (14.3%)	13 (22.8%)	30 (31.9%)
Beta-lactams[e]	13 (81.2%)	17 (81.0%)	52 (91.2%)	82 (87.2%)
Number of Specimens Collected[g]				
Pre-transplant	2 (1–2)	2 (1–2)	1 (1–3)	2 (1–3)
Post-transplant	3 (2–6)	3 (2–7)	3 (2–5)	3 (2–7)
Total	**16 (100.0%)**	**21 (100.0%)**	**57 (100.0%)**	**94 (100.0%)**

[a]Characteristics of patients in the observational group (N = 1144) can be found in Table S1.
[b]Engraftment was defined as an absolute neutrophil count greater than 500 cells/μL for three consecutive days.
[c]Assessed during inpatient allo-HSCT hospitalization, from beginning of pre-transplant up to 35 days post-transplant.
[d]Antibiotics are not mutually exclusive categories and thus does not sum to 100%.
[e]Beta-lactams include cephalosporins, beta-lactam/beta-lactamase combinations, and carbapenems.
[f]Prior antibiotics refer to antibiotics given prior to allo-HSCT and prior to observation time, within 14 days.
[g]Reported as median, with range in parentheses.

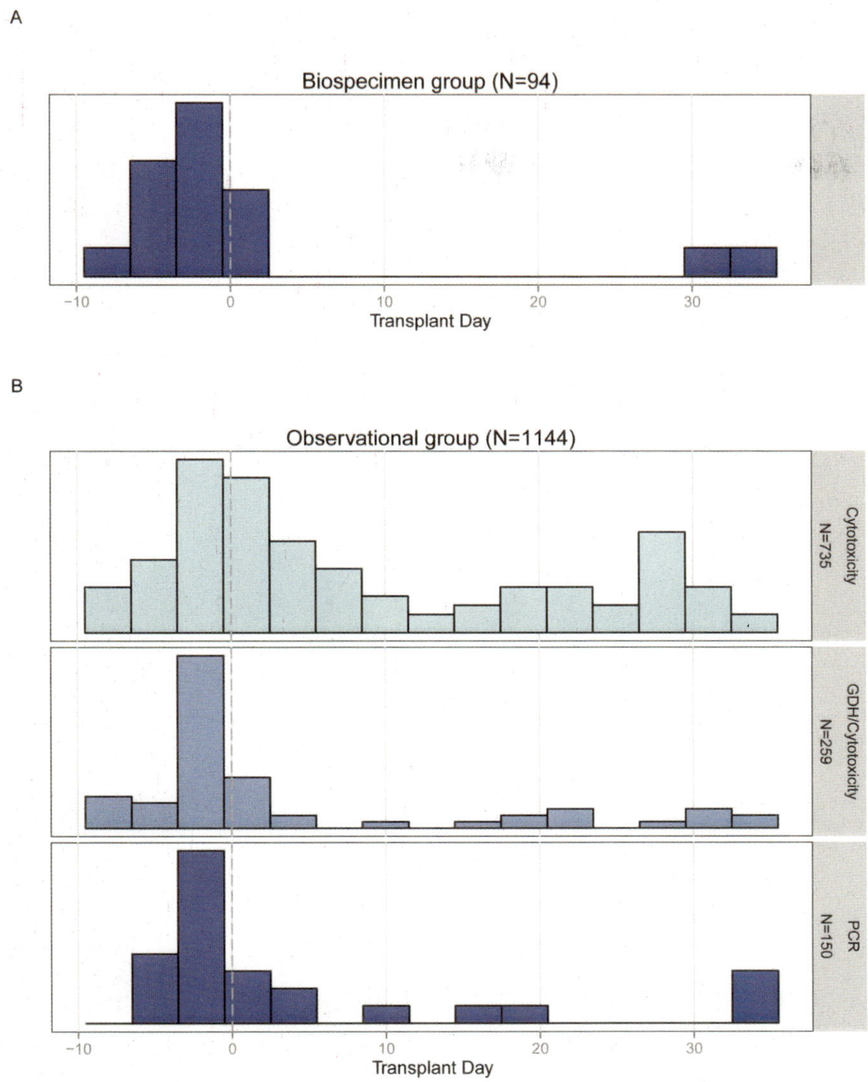

Figure 1. Histogram of early CDI cases by transplant day. Cases peaked approximately on or slightly prior to stem cell infusion. This pattern was evident in both subject groups and regardless of CDI testing method. *A*, Biospecimen group (N = 94). *B*, Observational group (N = 1144).

some specimens in which *C. difficile* 16S was detectable, but were *tcdB*-negative. These specimens may represent non-toxigenic strains of *C. difficile* or closely related species. Patients diagnosed with CDI often had preceding colonization by *tcdB*-positive *C. difficile*. In almost all cases, *tcdB* became undetectable upon initiation of treatment with metronidazole.

C. difficile colonization status over the course of transplant is shown for each patient in Figure 4. Colonization was detectable in 37 out of 94 patients (39%). In these patients, *tcdB* positivity was intermittent over the course of hospitalization, but was often detected near the start of hospitalization. Of these subjects, 16 (43%) were clinically diagnosed with CDI within the study period and treated. In two cases of CDI, prior fecal specimens were negative for *tcdB* colonization (3% of all previously non-colonized); three subjects did not have evaluable specimens prior to CDI diagnosis.

During times of treatment with metronidazole, *tcdB* was typically undetectable. Only two CDI cases were diagnosed beyond three days after stem cell infusion, while nine CDI cases occurred within 72 hours of stem cell infusion. 15 of 16 patients were diagnosed by PCR while one was diagnosed by cytotoxicity testing.

We analyzed early-transplant CDI with subsequent clinical endpoints within the biospecimen cohort; we found no detectable associations with gastrointestinal GVHD (HR 0.45, 95% CI 0.05–1.81) or CDI later in the course of transplantation (HR 2.44, 95% CI 0.71–7.16).

Discussion

CDI continues to be a significant concern in recipients of allo-HSCT. In this study we observed a high rate of CDI during conditioning and the first month following transplantation, occurring in 17% of our biospecimen group and 12.1% of our observational group. Similar CDI rates have been described for allo-HSCT recipients at other centers [1–5]. We found CDI to be mild to moderate in severity and temporally associated with allo-HSCT conditioning. We and others have observed that a large proportion of cases occur during the early allo-HSCT period, prior to stem cell engraftment when patients are neutropenic [1,2].

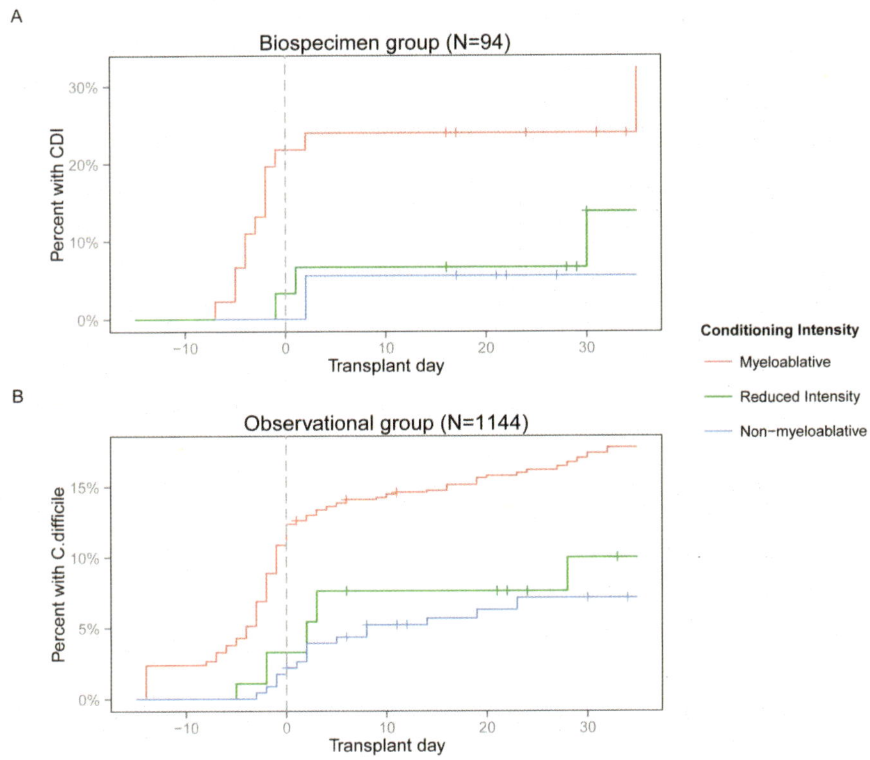

Figure 2. Kaplan-Meier plot of CDI during allo-HSCT. Patients receiving greater intensity conditioning regimens were more likely to develop CDI. *A*, Biospecimen group (N = 94). *B*, Observational group (N = 1144).

In this study we further characterized CDI during the first month following allo-HSCT by prospective fecal specimen analysis.

Clinically, we found that the diagnosis of early transplant CDI was common and patients appeared to respond rapidly to antibiotic therapy. Early allo-HSCT CDI correlated with high

Table 2. Univariate predictors of CDI in the biospecimen group and observational group, by Cox proportional hazards regression.

Predictor	Biospecimen group (N = 94)[a]		Observational Group (N = 1144)[b]	
	Haz ratio (95% CI)	**P**	**Haz ratio (95% CI)**	**P**
Age (years)	0.98 (0.94–1.02)	0.311	1.01 (0.99–1.02)	0.279
Sex (female)	0.41 (0.12–1.14)	0.089	1.02 (0.72–1.42)	0.928
Underlying Disease (leukemia vs. other)	2.44 (0.92–7.35)	0.075	1.42 (1.01–2.02)	0.044
Conditioning Regimen (myeloablative vs. other)	3.18 (1.14–10.63)	0.026	1.99 (1.30–3.17)	0.001
T-cell depleted graft	1.96 (0.72–5.51)	0.185	1.59 (1.14–2.24)	0.007
Stem cell source (cord vs. other)	0.49 (0.11–1.62)	0.263	1.31 (0.74–2.16)	0.331
Prior antibiotics (14 days)[f]	1.31 (0.50–3.45)	0.580		
Antibiotics[c]				
Vancomycin (IV)	3.16 (0.85–11.91)	0.085	0.79 (0.53–1.18)	0.242
Metronidazole	0.43 (0.00–3.63)	0.518	0.73 (0.41–1.24)	0.252
Fluoroquinolones[d]	0.28 (0.03–1.44)	0.139	0.90 (0.60–1.33)	0.605
Beta-lactam[e]	1.28 (0.40–3.78)	0.666	0.67 (0.45–1.00)	0.048
***tcdB* positivity**[c]	17.16 (6.40–51.97)	0.000		

[a]Multivariate analysis of the biospecimen group can be found in Table S2.
[b]Multivariate analysis of the observational group can be found in Table S3.
[c]Analyzed as a time-varying predictor.
[d]Fluoroquinolones consist of ciprofloxacin and levofloxacin.
[e]Beta-lactams include cephalosporins, beta-lactam/beta-lactamase combinations, and carbapenems.
[f]Prior antibiotics refer to antibiotics given prior to allo-HSCT and prior to observation time, within 14 days, and were not analyzed as time-varying predictors.

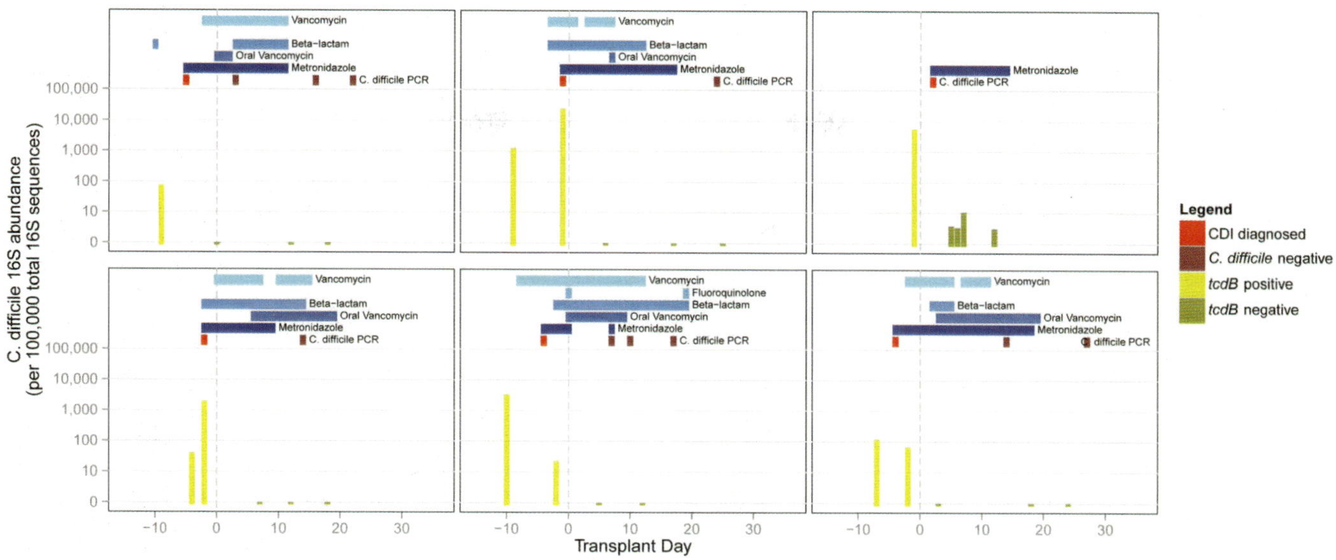

Figure 3. Intestinal composition of *C. difficile* in six selected cases of CDI. Observed abundance of C. difficile 16S is shown for each fecal specimen in the bargraph over the course of transplantation. The corresponding timing of CDI and antibiotic administration is shown at the top of each plot. Plots of all 94 patients in the biospecimen group can be found in Figure S1.

intensity chemotherapy regimens, but not with antibiotic administration. It is noteworthy that most cases of CDI occurred prior to hematopoietic stem cell infusion. This early in the course of transplantation, patients have not yet undergone hematopoietic stem cell infusion, and many have only received prophylactic antibiotics thus far. Though there can be exceptions, risk of bloodstream infection and the corresponding empiric treatment with broad-spectrum antibiotics generally come later, and peak several days after stem cell infusion. Therefore it could be that CDI in this setting arises largely as a result of chemotherapy and radiation that is given as part of the conditioning regimen, and less to antibiotic administration. Our observed association with conditioning regimen intensity would seem to support this. Several factors we examined, including stem cell characteristics and antibiotic administration, may have occurred largely after the peak of CDI. Though we performed a time-dependent analysis for some factors in order to avoid survival bias, this might explain why these factors were not significantly associated. We observed that T-cell depletion was a significant univariate risk factor in our observational cohort; this association is more likely related to associated pre-transplant confounders, rather than to T-cell depletion itself. Indeed, this became non-significant in the multivariate model. We repeated the analysis with observation time for CDI starting at the time of stem cell infusion, and did not find any additional significant predictors of CDI (results not shown).

Within our biospecimen cohort, we found that 39% of patients harbored toxigenic *Clostridium difficile* based on PCR detection of *tcdB*, revealing a high rate of colonization in these patients. Patients in this study who ultimately developed CDI were generally pre-colonized, whereas CDI in a previously non-colonized patient was rare. Though our study did not focus on pre-transplantation events, we did not detect any clear predictors of pre-colonization itself. A high colonization rate with toxigenic *C. difficile*, combined with disruption of intestinal microbiota and intestinal epithelial barriers by intense myeloablative conditioning may, at least in part, explain the high rates of CDI observed in this population.

Alternatively, however, it is possible that CDI is misdiagnosed during early stages of allo-HSCT. Most CDI diagnoses were made when diarrhea resulting from pre-transplant conditioning is common. In allo-HSCT patients diagnosed with CDI, diarrhea was usually mild and essentially indistinguishable from conditioning-related diarrhea. At our institution, diarrhea during transplantation is extremely common. Using this study's data as one estimate, fecal specimens were submitted for clinical testing in 95% (89/94) of patients in our biospecimen cohort and 84% (960/1144) of our observational cohort, suggesting a high rate of diarrhea. Other centers have also reported high rates of diarrhea [21]. False positivity, in the setting of a high colonization rate, combined with an inherent testing bias around the time of stem cell infusion, might explain the high frequency of CDI diagnoses during the early transplant period and could also explain the association of CDI with intense conditioning. Also consistent with this is the observation that CDI during early allo-HSCT was not predictive of subsequent CDI at later time points in the post-transplantation period.

If true, then it is possible that the CDI rate reported by our institution and other transplant centers is overestimated. The recent introduction of PCR assays to diagnose CDI may increase the risk for false positivity, since PCR does not distinguish between CDI and asymptomatic colonization [22]. Thus, *C. difficile* PCR assays may be particularly problematic in patient populations with high colonization rates and alternative causes of diarrhea. Improved methods for detection hold some promise to enhance the specificity of CDI diagnosis. For instance, use of a functional cytotoxicity assay [23] that detects and quantifies toxin (similar to the cytotoxicity assay) could demonstrate active toxin expression, presumably a better indicator of disease, rather than simply demonstrating the presence of the gene encoding the *C. difficile* toxin.

In this study, metronidazole treatment appeared to inhibit detectable toxigenic *C. difficile*. However, this may not reflect complete elimination, since our method of detection was not optimized to detect *C. difficile* spores. This form is resistant to antibiotics, and may very well be linked to the pathogenesis of recurrent CDI infections [24]. At our institution, early CDI was typically treated with metronidazole. Oral vancomycin and

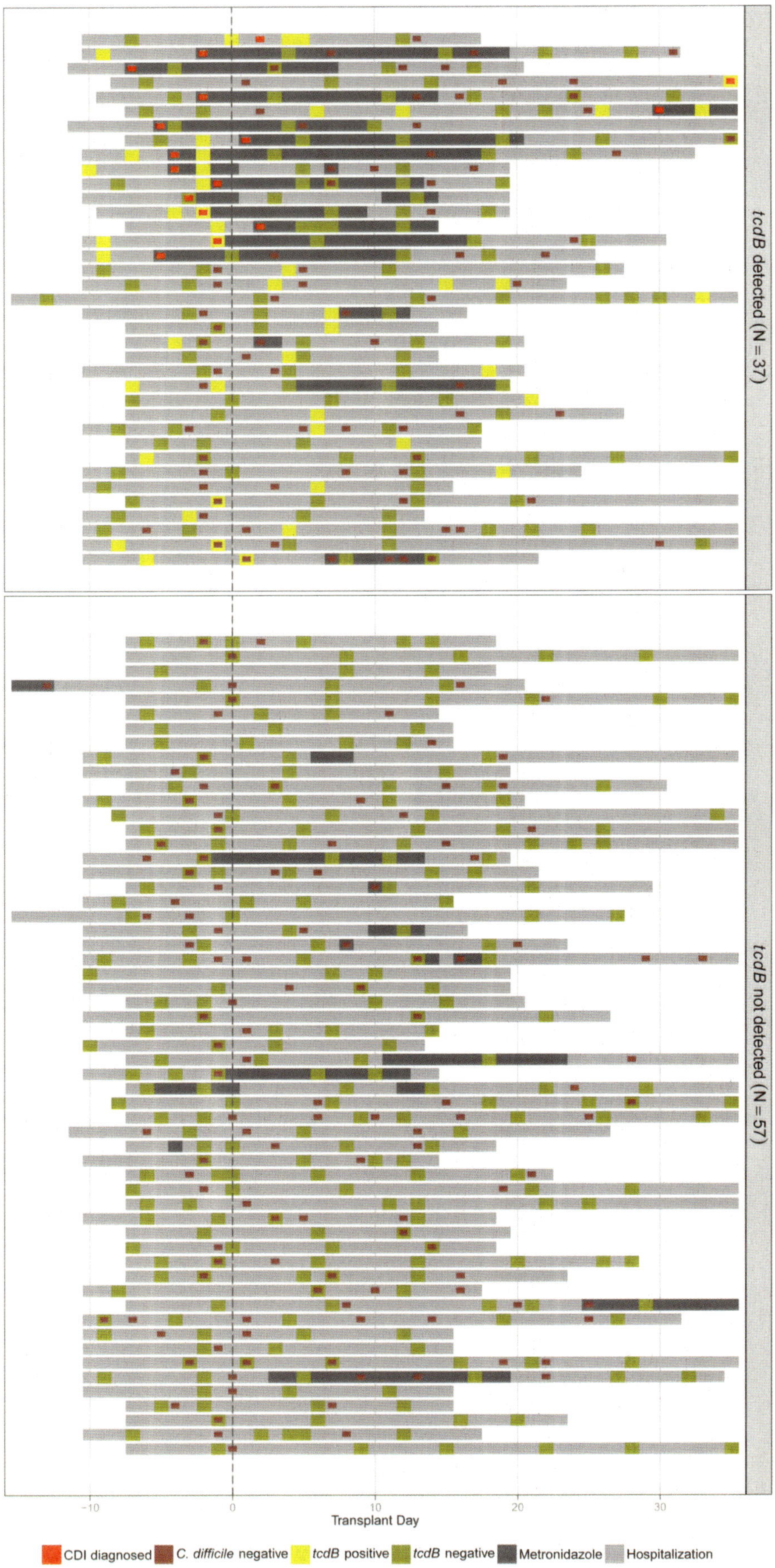
tcdB detected (N = 37)
tcdB not detected (N = 57)
-10
0
10
20
30
Transplant Day
CDI diagnosed
C. difficile negative
tcdB positive
tcdB negative
Metronidazole
Hospitalization

Figure 4. *C. difficile* colonization status in the biospecimen group subjects (N = 94) over the course of allo-HSCT. Each row represents one subject during hospitalization for allo-HSCT. Yellow squares represent results of *tcdB* testing of fecal specimens; red squares represent clinical testing for CDI. Dark shading shows metronidazole administration.

fidaxomycin are alternative agents which may be preferred agents for moderate-to-severe CDI or recurrences [25,26], but our study suggests that CDI during early allo-HSCT is generally mild and does not predispose to CDI later in the course of transplant. Therefore in this particular clinical scenario, metronidazole may be sufficiently efficacious compared with other *C. difficile* agents.

However, unnecessary treatment of *C. difficile*-colonized patients is not inconsequential. Metronidazole is associated with subsequent intestinal domination and bloodstream infection by vancomycin-resistant *Enterococcus* (VRE), independent of conditioning intensity [7]. Other studies have also demonstrated that metronidazole and other antibiotics with anti-anaerobic activity are potent promoters of dense intestinal VRE colonization [27–29]. Furthermore, prior studies demonstrated that colonization with toxigenic or non-toxigenic *C. difficile* with CDI can be protective [30–32]. Fidaxomicin has a narrower spectrum of activity and may be less likely to promote VRE colonization [33]; it could be that this treatment might be preferred for early transplant CDI, given the consequences of a perturbed microbiota in this population [7,34].

Several studies have correlated CDI with GVHD [2,4,5,35], raising the possibility that prevention of CDI might reduce the risk of GVHD. However, we did not detect an association between CDI during the first month following allo-HSCT and subsequent GVHD. There are several possible explanations for this disparity. For example, in the subset of patients undergoing T-cell depleted allo-HSCT, ex-vivo T-cell depletion of hematopoietic stem cell grafts prior to infusion results in a markedly lower incidence of GVHD, which might reduce statistical power and impair our ability to detect an association. Alternatively, there were some notable differences in analytic methodology. We analyzed CDI as a time-dependent predictor for GVHD as an endpoint, in order to obtain an unbiased estimate using only CDI occurring prior to onset of GVHD. Of the prior studies, only two performed survival analysis [2,5], and of those, only one utilized a time-dependent analysis, and in that study the predictor and endpoint were switched: preceding GVHD was examined as a risk factor for subsequent CDI [2]. Finally, yet another possibility is that, similar to the association with high intensity chemotherapy, the observed association between CDI and GVHD may be explained by an inherent bias in testing.

In conclusion, we find that CDI is frequently diagnosed during early allo-HSCT, particularly using PCR detection. Given the high frequency of diarrhea in patients receiving high-intensity allo-HSCT conditioning, the risk of false positivity is unknown but potentially significant. Thus, uncertainty as to the true CDI rate in allo-HSCT patients remains, and distinguishing CDI from diarrhea associated with pre-transplant conditioning or graft-versus-host disease continues to be a major clinical challenge. Given the high rate of colonization and intensive treatments with antibiotics, chemotherapy, and immunosuppressants, CDI should continue to remain a concern in recipients of allo-HSCT, but further study and application of better diagnostic strategies will be required to restrict CDI treatment to only those patients with *C. difficile* toxin-mediated colitis.

Supporting Information

Figure S1 Incidence of Clostridium difficile infection within observation period, in entire study cohort (biospecimen+observational group, N = 1238). Expressed as percentage of transplant recipients.

Figure S2 Intestinal composition of C. difficile in the biospecimen group (N = 94). Fecal specimens are barplotted over transplant day. The timing of C. difficile testing and antibiotic administration is shown at the top of each plot.

Table S1 Characteristics of Patients, Observational Group (N = 1144).

Table S2 Multivariate predictors of CDI in biospecimen group (N = 94).

Table S3 Multivariate predictors of CDI in observational group (N = 1144).

Table S4 Predictors of toxigenic *Clostridium difficile* colonization, by fecal detection of tcdB (N = 94).

Author Contributions

Conceived and designed the experiments: MAK EGP YT. Performed the experiments: MAK LL ERL AG DN. Analyzed the data: MAK EGP YT. Wrote the paper: MAK YJL RRJ LL ERL MvdB EGP YT.

References

1. Chopra T, Chandrasekar P, Salimnia H, Heilbrun LK, Smith D, et al. (2011) Recent epidemiology of *Clostridium difficile* infection during hematopoietic stem cell transplantation. Clinical Transplantation 25: E82–E87.
2. Willems L, Porcher R, Lafaurie M, Casin I, Robin M, et al. (2012) *Clostridium difficile* Infection after Allogeneic Hematopoietic Stem Cell Transplantation: Incidence, Risk Factors, and Outcome. Biology of Blood and Marrow Transplantation 18: 1295–1301.
3. Leung S, Metzger BS, Currie BP (2010) Incidence of *Clostridium difficile* infection in patients with acute leukemia and lymphoma after allogeneic hematopoietic stem cell transplantation. Infection Control and Hospital Epidemiology 31: 313–315.
4. Chakrabarti S, Lees A, Jones S, Milligan D (2000) *Clostridium difficile* infection in allogeneic stem cell transplant recipients is associated with severe graft-versus-host disease and non-relapse mortality. Bone marrow transplantation 26: 871–876.
5. Alonso CD, Treadway SB, Hanna DB, Huff CA, Neofytos D, et al. (2012) Epidemiology and Outcomes of *Clostridium difficile* Infections in Hematopoietic Stem Cell Transplant Recipients. Clinical infectious diseases 54: 1053–1063.
6. Walker AS, Eyre DW, Wyllie DH, Dingle KE, Harding RM, et al. (2012) Characterisation of *Clostridium difficile* Hospital Ward-Based Transmission Using Extensive Epidemiological Data and Molecular Typing. PLoS medicine 9: e1001172.
7. Taur Y, Xavier JB, Lipuma L, Ubeda C, Goldberg J, et al. (2012) Intestinal Domination and the Risk of Bacteremia in Patients Undergoing Allogeneic Hematopoietic Stem Cell Transplantation. Clinical Infectious Diseases 55: 905–914.
8. Turnbaugh PJ, Hamady M, Yatsunenko T, Cantarel BL, Duncan A, et al. (2008) A core gut microbiome in obese and lean twins. Nature 457: 480–484.
9. Ubeda C, Taur Y, Jenq RR, Equinda MJ, Son T, et al. (2010) Vancomycin-resistant *Enterococcus* domination of intestinal microbiota is enabled by antibiotic

treatment in mice and precedes bloodstream invasion in humans. The Journal of clinical investigation 120: 4332.
10. van den Berg RJ, Vaessen N, Endtz HP, Schülin T, van der Vorm ER, et al. (2007) Evaluation of real-time PCR and conventional diagnostic methods for the detection of *Clostridium difficile*-associated diarrhoea in a prospective multicentre study. Journal of medical microbiology 56: 36–42.
11. Berg R, Kuijper E, Coppenraet L, Claas E (2006) Rapid diagnosis of toxinogenic *Clostridium difficile* in faecal samples with internally controlled real-time PCR. Clinical microbiology and infection 12: 184–186.
12. Knetsch C, Bakker D, De Boer R, Sanders I, Hofs S, et al. (2011) Comparison of real-time PCR techniques to cytotoxigenic culture methods for diagnosing *Clostridium difficile* infection. Journal of clinical microbiology 49: 227–231.
13. Manichanh C, Reeder J, Gibert P, Varela E, Llopis M, et al. (2010) Reshaping the gut microbiome with bacterial transplantation and antibiotic intake. Genome research 20: 1411–1419.
14. Nossa CW, Oberdorf WE, Yang L, Aas JA, Paster BJ, et al. (2010) Design of 16S rRNA gene primers for 454 pyrosequencing of the human foregut microbiome. World journal of gastroenterology: WJG 16: 4135.
15. Naaber P, Štšepetova J, Smidt I, Rätsep M, Kõljalg S, et al. (2011) Quantification of *Clostridium difficile* in antibiotic-associated-diarrhea patients. Journal of clinical microbiology 49: 3656–3658.
16. Bacigalupo A, Ballen K, Rizzo D, Giralt S, Lazarus H, et al. (2009) Defining the intensity of conditioning regimens: working definitions. Biology of Blood and Marrow Transplantation 15: 1628–1633.
17. Jakubowski AA, Small TN, Kernan NA, Castro-Malaspina H, Collins N, et al. (2011) T Cell-Depleted Unrelated Donor Stem Cell Transplantation Provides Favorable Disease-Free Survival for Adults with Hematologic Malignancies. Biology of Blood and Marrow Transplantation 17: 1335–1342.
18. Rowlings P, Przepiorka D, Klein J, Gale R, Passweg J, et al. (1997) IBMTR Severity Index for grading acute graft-versus-host disease: retrospective comparison with Glucksberg grade. British journal of haematology 97: 855.
19. Kaltsas A, Simon M, Unruh LH, Son C, Wroblewski D, et al. (2012) Clinical and laboratory characteristics of *Clostridium difficile* infection in patients with discordant diagnostic test results. Journal of clinical microbiology 50: 1303–1307.
20. Heinze G, Schemper M (2001) A solution to the problem of monotone likelihood in Cox regression. Biometrics 57: 114–119.
21. Avery R, Pohlman B, Adal K, Bolwell B, Goldman M, et al. (2000) High prevalence of diarrhea but infrequency of documented *Clostridium difficile* in autologous peripheral blood progenitor cell transplant recipients. Bone marrow transplantation 25: 67–69.
22. Wilcox M (2012) Overcoming barriers to effective recognition and diagnosis of *Clostridium difficile* infection. Clinical Microbiology and Infection 18: 13–20.
23. Ryder AB, Huang Y, Li H, Zheng M, Wang X, et al. (2010) Assessment of *Clostridium difficile* infections by quantitative detection of tcdB toxin by use of a real-time cell analysis system. Journal of clinical microbiology 48: 4129–4134.
24. McFarland LV, Elmer GW, Surawicz CM (2002) Breaking the cycle: treatment strategies for 163 cases of recurrent *Clostridium difficile* disease. The American journal of gastroenterology 97: 1769–1775.
25. Cohen SH, Gerding DN, Johnson S, Kelly CP, Loo VG, et al. (2010) Clinical practice guidelines for *Clostridium difficile* infection in adults: 2010 update by the Society for Healthcare Epidemiology of America (SHEA) and the Infectious Diseases Society of America (IDSA). infection control and hospital epidemiology 31: 431–455.
26. Mullane KM, Miller MA, Weiss K, Lentnek A, Golan Y, et al. (2011) Efficacy of fidaxomicin versus vancomycin as therapy for *Clostridium difficile* infection in individuals taking concomitant antibiotics for other concurrent infections. Clinical infectious diseases 53: 440–447.
27. Pultz NJ, Stiefel U, Subramanyan S, Helfand MS, Donskey CJ (2005) Mechanisms by which anaerobic microbiota inhibit the establishment in mice of intestinal colonization by vancomycin-resistant *Enterococcus*. Journal of Infectious Diseases 191: 949–956.
28. Donskey CJ, Hanrahan JA, Hutton RA, Rice LB (1999) Effect of parenteral antibiotic administration on persistence of vancomycin-resistant *Enterococcus faecium* in the mouse gastrointestinal tract. Journal of Infectious Diseases 180: 384–390.
29. Donskey CJ, Chowdhry TK, Hecker MT, Hoyen CK, Hanrahan JA, et al. (2000) Effect of antibiotic therapy on the density of vancomycin-resistant enterococci in the stool of colonized patients. New England Journal of Medicine 343: 1925–1932.
30. Samore MH, DeGirolami PC, Tlucko A, Lichtenberg DA, Melvin ZA, et al. (1994) *Clostridium difficile* colonization and diarrhea at a tertiary care hospital. Clinical infectious diseases 18: 181–187.
31. Kyne L, Warny M, Qamar A, Kelly CP (2000) Asymptomatic carriage of *Clostridium difficile* and serum levels of IgG antibody against toxin A. New England Journal of Medicine 342: 390–397.
32. Shim JK, Johnson S, Samore MH, Bliss DZ, Gerding DN, et al. (1998) Primary symptomless colonisation by *Clostridium difficile* and decreased risk of subsequent diarrhoea. Lancet 351: 633.
33. Nerandzic MM, Mullane K, Miller MA, Babakhani F, Donskey CJ (2012) Reduced acquisition and overgrowth of vancomycin-resistant enterococci and *Candida* species in patients treated with fidaxomicin versus vancomycin for *Clostridium difficile* infection. Clinical infectious diseases 55: S121–S126.
34. Jenq RR, Ubeda C, Taur Y, Menezes CC, Khanin R, et al. (2012) Regulation of intestinal inflammation by microbiota following allogeneic bone marrow transplantation. The Journal of experimental medicine 209: 903–911.
35. Dubberke ER, Reske KA, Srivastava A, Sadhu J, Gatti R, et al. (2010) *Clostridium difficile*-associated disease in allogeneic hematopoietic stem-cell transplant recipients: risk associations, protective associations, and outcomes. Clinical transplantation 24: 192–198.

Cobalamin and Folate Status in 6 to 35 Months Old Children Presenting with Acute Diarrhea in Bhaktapur, Nepal

Manjeswori Ulak[1,2]*, Ram K. Chandyo[1,4], Ramesh K. Adhikari[3], Pushpa R. Sharma[3], Halvor Sommerfelt[1], Helga Refsum[5], Tor A. Strand[1,6]

1 Centre for International Health, University of Bergen, Norway, **2** Department of Child Health, Institute of Medicine, Kathmandu, Nepal, **3** Department of Pediatrics, Kathmandu Medical College, Nepal, **4** Community Medicine, Kathmandu Medical College, Nepal, **5** Department of Nutrition, Institute of Basic Medical Sciences, University of Oslo, Norway, **6** Medical Microbiology, Innlandet Hospital Trust, Lillehammer, Norway

Abstract

Background: Cobalamin and folate are essential micronutrients and are important in DNA and RNA synthesis, cell proliferation, growth, hematopoiesis, and cognitive function. However, data on cobalamin and folate status are lacking particularly from young children residing in low and middle income countries.

Objective: To measure cobalamin and folate status and identifies their predictors among 6 to 35 months old children presenting with acute diarrhea.

Design: This was a cross-sectional study in 823 children presenting with acute diarrhea. We measured plasma cobalamin, folate, methylmalonic acid and total homocysteine who sought treatment for acute diarrhea between June 1998 and August 2000.

Results: The mean (SD) plasma concentrations of cobalamin, folate, total homocysteine and methylmalonic acid were 206 (124) pmol/L, 55 (32) nmol/L, 11.4 (5.6) µmol/L and 0.79 (1.2) µmol/L, respectively. The prevalence of low plasma cobalamin (<150 pmol/L) was 41% but less than 2% (15) children had low folate concentration (<10 nmol/L). Plasma homocysteine and methylmalonic acid concentrations were negatively associated with cobalamin concentration but not associated with folate status. The prevalence of cobalamin deficiency was higher in breastfed than non-breastfed children (44% vs 24%; $p = <0.001$). The prevalence of hyperhomocysteinemia (>10 µmol/L) and elevated methylmalonic acid (>0.28 µmol/L) were 73% and 52%, respectively. In the regression analyses, the plasma cobalamin concentration was positively associated with age, and introduction of animal or formula milk.

Conclusions: Our study indicated that poor cobalamin status was common particularly among breastfed children. Folate deficiency was virtually none existent. Possible consequences of cobalamin deficiency in young children need to be explored.

Editor: Beverley-Ann Biggs, University of Melbourne, Australia

Funding: The study was funded by EU-INCO-DC (contract number IC18-CT96-0045: "Effect of zinc and vitamin A supplementation on diarrhoea and physical growth in children" and NUFU (project number PRO 52-53/96: "Institutional capacity and competence building in research and education for promotion of child health and nutrition in South Asia). The funders had no role in study design, data collection and analysis, decision to publish, or preparation of the manuscript.

Competing Interests: The authors have declared that no competing interests exist.

* E-mail: manjeswori@gmail.com

Introduction

Cobalamin and folate are essential nutrients for young children and is important for DNA and RNA synthesis, cell proliferation growth, hematopoiesis and cognitive function. Recent studies suggest that deficiencies of these nutrients are common in young children [1,2]. However, the status of cobalamin and folate in many low and middle-income countries (LMIC) including Nepal is still not known.

The main source of vitamin B12 is animal-derived foods, which are expensive and for cultural and religious reasons often not eaten at all [3]. The recommended daily allowances (RDA) of cobalamin for young children range form 0.5–0.9 µg/day [4] which is not possible to obtain from a strictly vegetarian or lacto-vegetarian diet [5,6]. On the other hand, folate is abundant in vegetarian based diets such as in lentils, beans and green vegetables [7].

Deficiencies of both folate and cobalamin can result in an increase in the total homocysteine (tHcy) concentration [8] which is associated with an increased risk for abortion, birth defects, low birth weight [9,10] and cardiovascular diseases [11]. Cobalamin deficiency also leads to an elevation in methylmalonic acid (MMA) concentration due to its role in the conversion of methylmalonyl CoA to succinyl CoA [7,8]. Early stages of cobalamin and folate deficiencies can be detected by analyzing MMA and tHcy

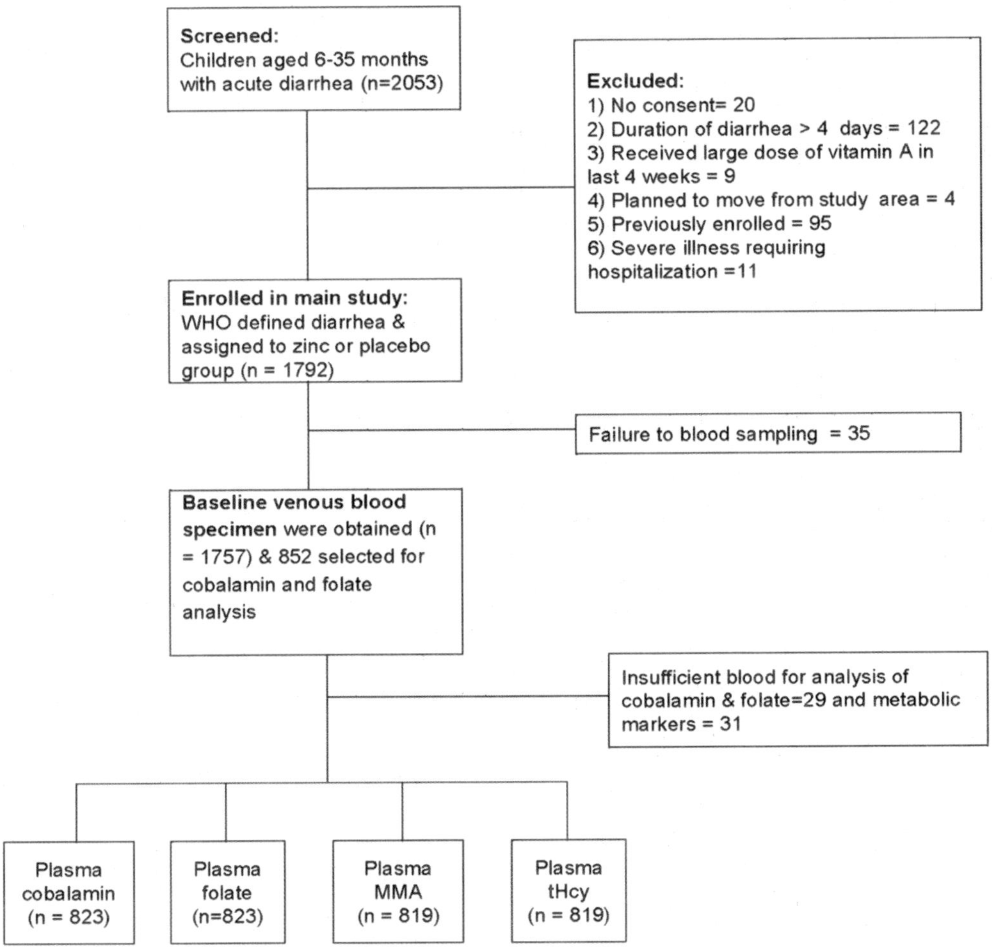

Figure 1. Flow chart of recruitment of children, blood sampling and analysis.

concentrations. Megaloblastic anemia occurs in both of these vitamin deficiencies but usually only when it is more pronounced. Cobalamin deficiency may also cause neuro-psychiatric disorders and result in cognitive impairment [12,13].

In an antenatal clinic based study from Kathmandu valley, 61% had elevated serum MMA, and 49% had low serum cobalamin concentration [14]. Similar findings were also observed among non-pregnant women of reproductive age in Bhaktapur [15] and in a study in southern Nepal [16]. The cobalamin status was found poor in infants whose mothers consumed a predominantly vegetarian diet, as maternal cobalamin status is reflected in the breast milk [17–19]. The common staple diet in Nepal particularly for young children is mostly vegetarian and seldom includes meat or meat products [20]. There are few population-based studies in LMIC that include tHcy and MMA to assess cobalamin and folate status. In this paper, we report cobalamin and folate status and its predictors in children 6–35 months of age with acute diarrhea residing in the peri-urban Bhaktapur community in Nepal. All children residing in the defined area, who had diarrhea, and in the right age range were eligible for participation.

Subjects and Methods

Study site and population

The study was conducted in Bhaktapur municipality and its surrounding suburbs, which is located 15 km east of the capital Kathmandu. Bhaktapur is situated about 1400 meter above sea level and there is a cold and dry winter from November to March, the summer months are generally hot and humid, and the autumn is relatively warm. The municipality has approximately 84,000 inhabitants; Bhaktapur is the most densely populated district in Nepal [21]. The local people mostly practice Hinduism or Buddhism and about 88% belong to the Newar ethnic group and are mainly engaged in work related to agriculture. In the study area, there are some migrants mainly belonging to the Tamang and Lama ethnic groups, most of them work in the carpet factories. Rice is the main staple food in this community and grown on their own land whereas consumption of lentils and green or dry vegetables varies with season. Although most of the people in the study are non-vegetarian, consumption of meat products is rare and depends on availability, which may be occasionally higher during festivals and ceremonies. The recruitment of study subjects was done in Siddhi Memorial Children's Hospital, which is a non-profit private organization providing 24-hour pediatric services in this community.

Study design

This was a cross-sectional study and included children 6 to 35 months with acute diarrhea, participating in a double blind randomized clinical trial, aimed to measure the effect of zinc administration during an episode of diarrhea [22]. The study was conducted from June 1998 to September 2000. Children were

Table 1. Variables assessed in the multivariable linear regression models measuring predictors for plasma folate, cobalamin, homocysteine, or methylmalonic acid in 823 Nepalese children 6 to 35 months of age.

Variables	Continuous	Categorical
Breastfeeding		yes/no
Age	months	Infants: yes/no
Age x breastfeeding interaction		Breastfeeding: yes/no
Gender		male/females
Living in joint families		yes/no
Members in the household	number	
Years of schooling, mother	Years	school: yes/no
Years of schooling, father	Years	school: yes/no
Weight for age Z score (WAZ)	Z scores	<-2 WAZ: yes/no
Weight for length Z score (WHZ)	Z scores	<-2 WHZ: yes/no
Height for age Z score (HAZ)	Z scores	<-2 HAZ: yes/no
Maternal age	Years	
Paternal age	Years	
Ownership of land		yes/no
Stool frequency	Number, past 24 hours	
Animal or formula milk use regularly		yes/no
Introduction of semi-solid or solid foods		yes/no
Season		three categories
Dehydration		yes/no

identified through weekly surveillance or spontaneous visits to our field clinic and were screened by a physician. Diarrhea was defined according to the WHO guidelines as a passage of three or more loose or watery stools in past 24 hours with a recent change in stool consistency. A total of 1,792 eligible children were enrolled in the main study and informed written consent was obtained from one of the parents. Baseline venous blood was collected from 1,758 children before initiation of the intervention. We randomly selected approximately half of the enrolled children (852) for analysis of folate and cobalamin status. The current analysis is based on 823 children from whom we had obtained sufficient amounts of blood to analyze plasma cobalamin, folate, MMA and tHcy concentrations. Exclusion criteria and selection of subjects for cobalamin and folate status are shown in **Figure 1.**

Data collection and blood sampling

All baseline and morbidity information was recorded on the day of enrollment. The children were weighed using a scale to the nearest 100 g (Salter, SECA, Germany) and length or height was measured using a locally made length board to the nearest ± 0.1 cm. A study physician collected blood from each child's cubital vein into heparinized polypropylene tubes (Monovette; Sarstedt, Numbrecht, Germany), mainly between 9 AM and 1 PM. The hemoglobin concentration was measured with a HemoCue® Hb 201^{+} hemoglobinometer (HemoCue AB, Ängelholm, Sweden) immediately after blood sampling according to the manufacture's instruction. The blood was then centrifuged at 760×g for 10 min in room temperature, and plasma was divided into polypropylene vials (Eppendorf, Hinz, Germany) and wrapped immediately by aluminum foil to prevent from light and stored at −40°C until transfer to Norway on dry ice for analysis. Then the specimens were stored at −70°C for 3–4 years and analyzed at the pharmacology laboratory, Oxford University, UK. After thawing, cobalamin and folate (n = 823) were analyzed by microbiological assays using a chloramphenicol-resistant strain of Lactobacillus casei and colistin sulfate-resistant strain of *Lactobacillus leichmannii*, respectively [23,24]. These assays were adapted to a microtiter plate format and carried out by a robotic workstation [25]. Plasma concentrations of MMA and tHcy (n = 819) were analyzed by a modified gas chromatography-mass spectrometry method based on ethylchloroformate derivatization [26].Total homocysteine was analyzed by using commercial kits from Abbott Laboratories [27].

Definitions

We used the WHO definitions of cobalamin and folate deficiency which is <150 pmol/L of plasma cobalamin and < 10 nmol/L of plasma folate [28]. We defined marginal cobalamin deficiency as being present when the concentration was between 150 to 200 pmol/L. There are no reference limits available tHcy and MMA in children. So we defined hyperhomocysteinemia when plasma tHcy concentration was >10 µmol/L and elevated methylmalonic acid when the plasma MMA concentration was > 0.28 µmol/L. Hemoglobin concentration was adjusted on altitude, as partial pressure of oxygen is decreased in the higher altitude. Thus, we added 0.3 g/dL to the standard cut off values of Hb for the 1400 meter altitude of the study area thus anemia was defined as having Hb concentration <11.3 g/dL [29].

Data entry and statistical analysis

All forms were checked manually by supervisors and physicians for completeness and consistency. The data was then double entered into Microsoft Visual FoxPro databases with computerized logic, range and consistency checks. Weight for age, length/height for age, and weight for length/height Z-scores were calculated using the most recent WHO growth charts [30]. Statistical analyses were undertaken using Stata®, version 10 (Stata

Table 2. General and clinical characteristics of 823 study children with acute diarrhea in Bhaktapur, Nepal.

Characteristics	Values[1]
Mean age of child in months, (SD)	15.7±7.6
Boys	465 (56)
Breastfed	673 (82)
Animals or formula milk fed	279 (34)
Semisolid or solid food	791 (96)
Living in joint family	457 (56)
Ownership of land	596 (72)
< -2 Z-score weight for age	210 (25)
< -2 Z-score length/height for age	282 (34)
< -2 Z-score weight for length/height	81 (10)
Mean age of mother in year	25 (4.6)
Mean schooling of mother in year, (SD)	2.6±3.4
Mean schooling of father in year, (SD)	6.7±3.6
History of fever in last 24 hour prior to enrollment	236 (29)
Body temperature >100°F	69 (8)
History of cough and or difficulty breathing in last 24 hour prior to enrollment	322 (39)
Mean duration of diarrhea before enrollment, days (SD)	3.1±1.1
Children with blood in stool in last 24 hour prior to enrollment	99 (12)
Children with dehydration according to WHO/IMCI	93 (11)
Mean plasma cobalamin (pmol/L) (SD)	206±125
Mean plasma folate (nmol/L) (SD)	55±32
Mean plasma total homocysteine (μmol/L) (SD)	11.4±5.6
Mean plasma methylmalonic acid (μmol/L) (SD)	0.79±1.2
Mean hemoglobin (g/dL)[2] (SD)	11.1±1.1
Anemia[3] (hemoglobin <11.3 g/dL)	352 (52)

[1]*Values are number (%) unless otherwise mentioned.* [2]*Hemoglobin was measured from 674 subjects.*
[3]*Altitute adjusted hemoglobin cut off value.*

Corp, College Station, TX). We presented mean, median or interquartile ranges (IQR) of cobalamin, folate, tHcy and MMA according to age group and breastfeeding status. We used chi square to test differences in prevalence between groups. Spearman rank correlation analyses was used to measure crude associations between plasma concentrations of cobalamin, folate, MMA and tHcy. A P value of <0.05 was considered to reflect statistical significance. Simple and multiple regression analyses were used to examine the associations between the dependent variables (cobalamin, folate, MMA and tHcy) and different independent variables. The variables listed in **Table 1** including breastfeeding status (yes or no), age, maternal and paternal age and education, weight for age, length/height for age and weight for length/height Z-scores, family size, ownership of land, loose or watery stool, stool frequency, dehydration and intake of milk and other foods etc. were included in the initial assessments. We used a stepwise process to select the variables for the final model using cut off of P value <0.15 as described elsewhere [31]. The interaction between various potential predictors on markers of cobalamin and folate status was also analyzed by inclusion of interaction terms in the multiple regression models. We also assessed the linearity between the continuous independent (listed in Table 1) and dependent variables in the regression models using generalized additive models in R (http://www.r-project.org) adjusting for the same variables as in the multiple linear regression models.

Ethical considerations

The study had ethical clearances from the Nepal Health Research Council, Kathmandu. The implementation of all aspects of the project was in agreement with the International Ethical Guidelines for Research Involving Human Subjects as stated in the latest version of the Helsinki Declaration. Informed written consent was obtained from at least one of each child's parents.

Results

The baseline characteristics of the study population are presented in **Table 2**. A total of 823 children were included for cobalamin and folate biomarker analyses; the mean age was 15.7 months and 465 (56%) were boys. Most of the children [673 (82%)] were breastfed at the time of enrollment and more than half were living in joint families [457 (55.5%)]. The prevalence of stunting, underweight, and wasting (<-2 Z score of length or height for age, weight for age and weight for length or height) were 34%, 25% and 10% respectively. About half (52%) of the 674 children in whom we measured hemoglobin concentration had anemia. The mean duration of diarrhea before enrollment was 3.1 days, 11% children had some signs of dehydration and 12% children had dysentery. Sixty-nine children (8.3%) had fever (axillary temperature >100°F) and 322 (39%) children had cough and/or difficult breathing.

Table 3. Plasma cobalamin, folate, methylmalonic acid and total homocysteine concentrations in different age groups according to breastfeeding status of the study children in Bhaktapur, Nepal.

	Breastfed			**Not breastfed**		
	Age (months)			**Age (months)**		
	06 to 11	**12 to 23**	**24 to 35**	**06 to 11**	**12 to 23**	**24 to 35**
	Cobalamin					
Median (pmol/L)	147	181	195	379	231	231
IQR (pmol/L)	103–239	119–264	128–253	314–399	159–349	148–306
Number	315	318	40	6	24	120
	Folate					
Median (nmol/L)	65.6	49	29.7	35.5	30.78	20.6
IQR (nmol/L)	46.6–93.0	35.2–70.2	16.5–47.0	11.8–48.8	17.8–43.2	13.6–32.7
Number	315	318	40	6	24	120
	Methylmalonic acid					
Median (μmol/L)	0.52	0.42	0.42	0.42	0.49	0.38
IQR (μmol/L)	0.3–1.0	0.2–0.8	0.2–0.7	0.3–0.6	0.3–0.6	0.3–0.6
Number	310	319	40	6	24	120
	Total homocysteine					
Median (μmol/L	12.4	10	9.6	7.2	7.4	7.3
IQR (μmol/L)	9.2 –15.7	7.5–13	7.4–13	5.3–8.2	5.8–9.2	6.0–9.4
Number	310	319	40	6	24	120

Plasma cobalamin, folate and their metabolic markers according to age group and breastfeeding status

The mean (SD) cobalamin, folate, total homocysteine and methylmalonic acid concentrations were 207 (125) pmol/L, 55 (32) nmol/L, 11.4 (5.6) μmol/L and 0.79 (1.2), μmol/L respectively. The median (interquartile range; IQR) cobalamin concentration was lower in breastfed (147; 103-239 pmol/L) than in non-breastfed children (379; 314–399 pmol/L) among 6–11 months old infants ($p = 0.003$). In the same age group, the median (IQR) folate was higher in breastfed (65.6; 46.6–93.0 nmol/L) than in non-breastfed (35.5; 22.8–48.8 nmol/L; $p = 0.005$) infants and it declined with increasing age. The median plasma MMA and tHcy concentrations were also higher among those who were breastfed than in those who were not (MMA of 0.52 vs 0.42 μmol/L, $p = 0.007$ and tHcy of 12.4 vs 7.2 μmol/L, $p = <0.001$) (**Table 3**).

Proportion who were cobalamin or folate deficient (Table 4)

Low cobalamin concentration (<150 pmol/L) was found in 40.7% (335) and 56% had plasma cobalamin <200 pmol/L. Forty four percent (299) of the breastfed and 24% (36) of the non-breastfed children had a cobalamin concentration <150 pmol/L. The mean tHcy and MMA concentrations were also higher in those with low cobalamin than in those with adequate plasma cobalamin concentration (13.2 vs 9.1 μmol/L, $p = <0.001$ and 1.0 vs 0.5 μmol/L, $p = <0.001$ respectively). None of the children had a plasma folate concentration <5 nmol/L and only 15 children (2%) had a folate concentration of <10 nmol/L. Most of the children (n = 14) with low folate were more than one years old. Only one (0.3%) child had both a cobalamin concentration < 150 pmol/L and a folate concentration <10 nmol/L.

The associations between plasma tHcy or MMA and cobalamin are depicted in **Figure 2 and 3.** The cobalamin concentration was negatively associated with MMA ($r = -0.35$, $p = <0.001$) and tHcy ($r = -0.47$, $p = <0.001$]. The graphs indicate that MMA and tHcy levels start to rise when the cobalamin concentration drops below 150–200 pmol/L.

Predictors for cobalamin and folate status

The results from the multiple linear regression analyses (**Table 5**) show that the plasma cobalamin concentration was significantly higher in non-breastfed children [adjusted mean difference 29.7 (95% CI: 0.27, 59.2) pmol/L] and positively associated with age [adjusted mean difference 2.0 (95% CI: 0.3, 3.4) pmol/L]. It was higher in children whose parents did not own land and in children who were dehydrated at enrollment. The concentration of plasma cobalamin was lower in those who did not consume animal or formula milk compared to those who did [adjusted mean difference −43.0 (95% CI: −60.8, −25.1) pmol/L]. The plasma folate concentration was negatively associated with age but in breastfed children only (p for interaction 0.002). The folate concentration was higher in those who did not consume animal or formula milk regularly [adjusted mean difference 8.6 (95% CI: 4.6, 12.5) nmol/L] and it was lower by −10.2 (95% CI: −16.1, −4.4) nmol/L in non-dehydrated children compared to those who were dehydrated. We also found a significantly higher plasma folate concentration during the spring season [adjusted mean difference 7.3 (95% CI: 3.3, 11.5) nmol/L] than in the summer. MMA concentration was negatively associated with age. Plasma tHcy was also negatively associated with age, however, only in breastfed children (p interaction <0.001) and it was lower in the spring than during the summer. Both cobalamin and folate and their metabolic markers were not significantly associated with anthropometric measurements or with clinical parameters listed in **Table 1**.

Table 4. Cobalamin and folate concentrations in the study children according to age, gender, breastfeeding status and their metabolic markers.[1]

Characteristics	Plasma cobalamin (pmol/L)				Plasma folate (nmol/L)		
	<150	150–200	>200	P value[2]	<10	>10	P value[2]
Total children	335 (40.7)	129 (15.7)	359 (43.6)		15 (1.8)	808 (98.2)	
Age							
6–11 months	163 (48.6)	43 (33.3)	115 (32.0)	<0.001	1 (6.7)	320 (39.6)	<0.001
12–35 months	172 (51.4)	86 (66.7)	244 (68.0)		14 (93.3)	488 (60.4)	
Gender							
Male	193 (57.6)	80 (62.0)	192 (53.5)	0.2	10 (66.7)	455 (56.3)	0.4
Female	142 (42.4)	49 (38.0)	167 (46.5)		5 (33.3)	353 (43.7)	
Breast feeding status							
Breastfed	299 (89.3)	107 (83.0)	267 (74.4)	<0.001	4 (26.7)	669 (82.8)	<0.001
Non-breastfed	36 (10.7)	22 (17.0)	92 (25.6)		11 (73.3)	139 (17.2)	
Plasma folate							
<10 nmol/L	1 (0.3)	2(1.5)	12(3.3)	0.01	–	–	
≥10 nmol/L	334 (99.7)	127(98.5)	347(96.7)		–	–	
Plasma cobalamin							
<150 pmol/L	–	–	–		1 (6.7)	334 (41.3)	0.007
≥150 pmol/L	–	–	–		14 (93.3)	474 (58.7)	
Plasma tHcy[3]	14.0±6.4	11.9±5.7	9.1±3.7	<0.001	9.7±4.5	11.4±5.7	
>10 μmol/L	240 (72.3)	62 (48.4)	127(35.5)	<0.001	8 (53.3)	384 (47.8)	0.6
<10 μmol/L	92(27.7)	66 (51.6)	231(64.5)		7(46.7)	419 (52.2)	
Plasma MMA[3]	1.0±1.5	0.7±1.2	0.5±0.6	<0.001	0.7±0.4	0.8±1.2	
>0.28 μmol/L	280 (84.7)	95 (74.2)	223 (62.3)	<0.001	13 (86.7)	585 (72.8)	0.2
<0.28 μmol/L	52 (15.3)	33 (25.8)	135 (37.7)		2 (13.3)	218 (27.2)	

[1]*Values are number (%) unless otherwise mentioned*
[2]*P values were obtained from Chi-square test or t-test*
[3]*Plasma tHcy and MMA were analysed from 819 subject.*

Discussion

We assessed cobalamin and folate status and identified their predictors in 6–35 months old Nepalese children with acute diarrhea. We found that poor cobalamin status was affecting almost one in every second child, which was more common in breastfed than in non-breast infants. Similar findings have been reported from studies conducted in India [2] and in other countries [32–34]. Infants who consumed animal or formula milk had higher plasma cobalamin concentrations than those who didn't, as was observed among Norwegian healthy children who were given animal milk [32]. This is most likely because the content of cobalamin in animal milk is 10 times higher than in breast milk [35]. Animal milk, particularly buffalo or cow's milk, or in the form of milk-tea (diluted with water) is given to infants in our community from 6–7 months of age [20] but the practice may vary according to culture and the socio-economic status of the family. Further, cobalamin status of newborns and infants are positively associated with the breast milk concentration [5]. Specker *et al.* also reported that the cobalamin concentration in breast milk was positively correlated with maternal serum cobalamin concentrations which were lower in strict vegetarian women than in women on omnivorous diets [17]. In the current study, we didn't collect blood samples from the mothers; neither did we collect any dietary information or details on exclusive breastfeeding. However, in a previous study among women from the same community, we found that 83% had poor cobalamin status, as reflected in high MMA and low cobalamin concentration in plasma, and that 69% of the women consumed <1 μg of cobalamin per day [15] which is ~50% of the RDA [4]. The poor cobalamin status observed in our study population is probably due to low cobalamin content in complementary food and/or poor cobalamin status of the mothers. Other contributing factors might be gastro-intestinal infections such as giardiasis which is common in developing countries and found in association with cobalamin deficiency [36].

The median plasma folate concentration in this study was 48.7 nmol/L which is approximately twice as high as in a study of a similar age group children in New Delhi [2] and it is interesting to note that none had plasma folate <5 nmol/L, the cut off which is frequently used to define folate deficiency [37] indicating that folate deficiency is not a problem in this population. In concordance with earlier findings [2,32,38], we also found higher plasma folate concentrations in breastfed and in children aged 6–11 months compared with older and non-breastfed children. In our study population, the low prevalence of folate deficiency may be due to the high proportion of breastfed children. The folate concentration is high in breast milk [39] which is, to a large extent, independent of folate status of the mother [40]. It may also be due to frequent consumption of foods like cereals, legumes and green leafy vegetables, which are rich sources of folate. We found that the mean plasma folate concentration was higher in the spring compared to in the summer season. This could be due to several factors, including that this season carries a relatively good availability of green leafy vegetables. In contrast to plasma

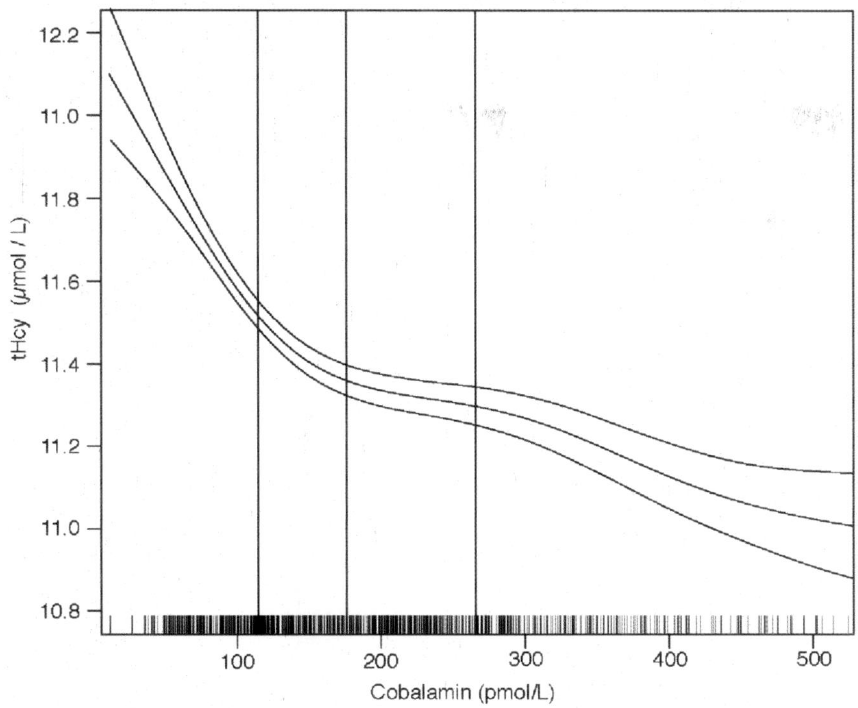

Figure 2. Association between plasma cobalamin and total homocysteine (tHcy) and methylmalonic acid (MMA) concentrations. The graphs were made by using generalized additive models in R. The upper and lower horizontal lines represent 95% CIs of regression line. The small bars on the x-axis show the distribution of individual observation and the vertical lines indicate the 25th, 50th and 75th percentiles of the plasma cobalamin.

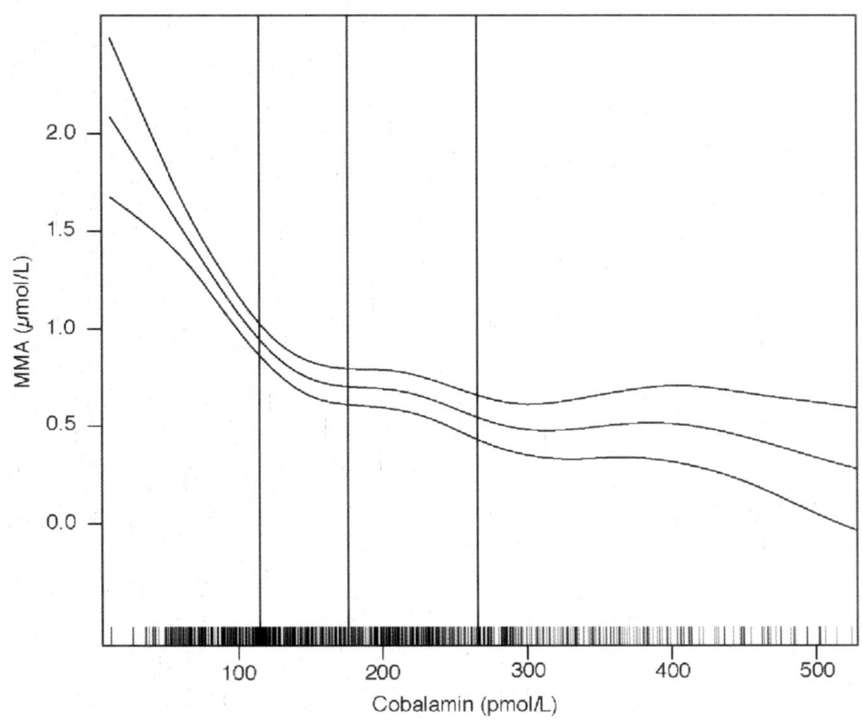

Figure 3. Association between plasma cobalamin and methylmalonic acid (MMA) concentrations. The graphs were made by using generalized additive models in R. The upper and lower horizontal lines represent 95% CIs of regression line. The small bars on the x-axis show the distribution of individual observation and the vertical lines indicate the 25th, 50th and 75th percentiles of the plasma cobalamin.

Table 5. Predictors for plasma cobalamin, folate, methylmalonic acid & total homocysteine concentrations among Nepalese children with acute diarrhea in Bhaktapur, Nepal.

Variables	Plasma cobalamin (pmol/L)			Plasma folate (nmol/L)			Methylmalonic acid (μmol/L)			Homocysteine (μmol/L)		
	Coeff*	95% CI	*P*-value	Coeff*	95% CI	*P*-value	Coeff*	95% CI	*P*-value	Coeff*	95% CI	*P*-value
Breastfeeding status												
Yes												
No	29.7	(0.27, 59.2)	0.04		Interaction						Interaction	
Age	2.0	(0.3, 3.4)	0.01		Interaction		−0.01	(−0.03, −0.001)	0.04		Interaction	
Age in breast fed				−1.96	(−2.3, −1.6)	<0.001				−0.24	(−0.31, −0.2)	<0.001
Age in non-breastfed				−0.61	(−1.4, 0.15)	0.12				0.04	(−0.11, 0.19)	0.6
Age and breastfeeding interaction				1.3	(0.5, 2.1)	0.002				0.27	(0.11, 0.43)	<0.001
Ownership of land												
Yes												
No	27.5	(9.0, 46.0)	0.003				0.21	(0.02, 0.4)	0.02	1.34	(0.5, 2.1)	0.001
Dehydration												
Yes												
No	−28.0	(−54.1, −1.9)	0.03	−10.2	(−16.1, −4.4)	0.001						
Use of animal or formula milk												
Yes												
No	−43.0	(−60.8, −25.2)	<0.001	8.6	(4.6, 12.5)	<0.001						
Seasons of enrollment												
Jun-Sept												
Oct-Jan				0.07	(−5.0, 4.8)	0.9	0	(−0.24, 0.18)	0.8	−1.92	(−2.8, −0.95)	<0.001
Feb-May				7.3	(3.1, 11.5)	0.001	−0.18	(−0.37, −0.004)	0.04	−1.19	(−2.0, −0.36)	0.005

** Adjusted regression coefficient and P values obtained from linear regression model adjusted for the variables included in this table, R square values of plasma cobalamin, folate, tHcy and MMA are 0.083, 0.30, 0.15 and 0.02, respectively.*

cobalamin concentration, which reflects cobalamin intake over a long period of time, the plasma folate levels reflect recent dietary intake. Red blood cell folate status is recommended to reflect folate intake in individuals over extended periods of time [41]. However, we believe that this will not affect the overall mean folate status but can lead to unnecessary variability of the folate status indicator. It is also possible that the high folate concentration is due to the "folate trap" mechanism where the plasma concentration of folate is high because of poor cobalamin status [42].

Strengths and Limitations

The main strength of the current study was its large sample size and that the data collection spanned over more than two years, including three hot and wet seasons. We also included measurements of the functional metabolic markers of cobalamin MMA and tHcy [43]. Our study included children with acute diarrhea, which is a selected child population. Incipient dehydration due to diarrhea at the time of blood collection may change the concentration of the biomarkers. In this study, 11% of the children had mild to moderately dehydration at the time of blood sampling, and we found that cobalamin and folate concentration were slightly higher in dehydrated children probably due to hemoconcentration. Also the use of non-fasting blood specimen may lead to under estimation of prevalence of folate deficiency. So the prevalence of cobalamin and folate deficiency among otherwise healthy children without dehydration might be even higher than our findings from children with acute diarrhea. Although, there were not any degradation of plasma MMA and tHcy, plasma folate concentration was degraded by 3% per year while storing at freeze [44]. Our plasma samples were stored for 3–4 years indicating that our estimate of plasma folate could be lower by 10–15% compared with the baseline values. We did not have all ages equally represented. Most of our study children were between 6–24 months old and breastfed (82%). The concentrations of these vitamins were associated with age, and our prevalence estimates might accordingly have been somewhat different if all ages were represented equally.

These limitations need to be kept in mind when drawing conclusions on the status of these vitamins in the general child population; however, we did not find any significant association of plasma cobalamin and folate with the duration and numbers of loose or watery stool. Nor did we observe any significant association with dysentery or vomiting episodes (data not shown). We did not obtain detailed information on dietary intake, exclusive breastfeeding pattern, the use of folic acid supplements by children and mother. Nor we were able to measure vitamin B6 which also can influence tHcy concentration [45]. Dietary intake may vary in different regions and in different ethnic groups. This information would have been useful for improving the interpretation of our findings.

Generalizability

Our findings are to a certain extent generalizable to young children in other low-income countries with similar socio-economic conditions, and where the food habits are comparable. The present study was clinic based and included children with acute diarrhea. Most of the people in this study were from the Newar ethnic group and were non-vegetarian although regular intake of meat and fish was not common. Therefore we are uncertain whether or not our findings of prevalence of cobalamin deficiency can be generalized to all children and other parts of Nepal where the dietary habits may differ [46]. However, we believe that cobalamin deficiency is more prevalent in other communities of Nepal where vegetarian based foods are predominantly consumed. In a previous study, women belonging to the Chhetri ethnic group had significantly higher tHcy, MMA and lower cobalamin compared to the Newars [14].

Conclusions

Cobalamin deficiency was common in children with acute diarrhea in this community, suggesting that this may represent a health problem. Breastfed infants had the highest prevalence of cobalamin deficiency. Future studies including healthy children need to be undertaken in order to expand on these findings and to explore consequences of poor and sub-optimal cobalamin status. If these finding are confirmed in other parts of Nepal, it may be justified to consider including cobalamin supplementation in a national strategy to improve nutritional status in children.

Acknowledgments

We thank all children and families who participated in the study. We are also grateful for the contribution of Prof. Hemang Dixit, Fakir Gami; Field supervisors Chandrawati Chitrakar, Narayan Regmi; data managers Samir K.C, Uma Regmi, and all field staff; founder Shyam Dhaubhadel and all staff of Siddhi Memorial Hospital for their cooperation; the staff of Laboratory for Clinical and Biochemistry, Haukeland Hospital, of Norway.

Author Contributions

Conceived and designed the experiments: MU RKC TAS HS RKA. Performed the experiments: MU RKC TAS PRS. Analyzed the data: MU TAS RKC. Contributed reagents/materials/analysis tools: TAS HR. Wrote the paper: MU RKS TAS HS RKA HR PRS.

References

1. Bjorke-Monsen AL, Ueland PM (2011) Cobalamin status in children. J Inherit Metab Dis 34: 111–119.
2. Taneja S, Bhandari N, Strand TA, Sommerfelt H, Refsum H, et al. (2007) Cobalamin and folate status in infants and young children in a low-to-middle income community in India. Am J Clin Nutr 86: 1302–1309.
3. Allen LH (2008) Causes of vitamin B12 and folate deficiency. Food Nutr Bull 29: S20-34; discussion S35–27.
4. IOM (1998) Institute of Medicine. Food and Nutrition Board. Dietary Reference Intakes: Thiamin, Riboflavin, Niacin, Vitamin B6, Folate, Vitamin B12, Pantothenic Acid, Biotin, and Choline. Washington, DC: National Academy Press.
5. Allen LH (1994) Nutritional supplementation for the pregnant woman. Clin Obstet Gynecol 37: 587–595.
6. Trumbo P, Yates AA, Schlicker S, Poos M (2001) Dietary reference intakes: vitamin A, vitamin K, arsenic, boron, chromium, copper, iodine, iron, manganese, molybdenum, nickel, silicon, vanadium, and zinc. J Am Diet Assoc 101: 294–301.
7. Snow CF (1999) Laboratory diagnosis of vitamin B12 and folate deficiency: a guide for the primary care physician. Arch Intern Med 159: 1289–1298.
8. Klee GG (2000) Cobalamin and Folate Evaluation: Measurement of Methylmalonic Acid and Homocysteine vs Vitamin B12 and Folate. Clinical Chemistry 46:8(B): 1277–1283.
9. Vollset SE, Refsum H, Irgens LM, Emblem BM, Tverdal A, et al. (2000) Plasma total homocysteine, pregnancy complications, and adverse pregnancy outcomes: the Hordaland Homocysteine study. Am J Clin Nutr 71: 962–968.
10. Yajnik CS, Deshpande SS, Panchanadikar AV, Naik SS, Deshpande JA, et al. (2005) Maternal total homocysteine concentration and neonatal size in India. Asia Pac J Clin Nutr 14: 179–181.
11. Wald DS, Law M, Morris JK (2002) Homocysteine and cardiovascular disease: evidence on causality from a meta-analysis. BMJ 325: 1202.
12. Lindenbaum J, Savage DG, Stabler SP, Allen RH (1990) Diagnosis of cobalamin deficiency: II. Relative sensitivities of serum cobalamin, methylmalonic acid, and total homocysteine concentrations. Am J Hematol 34: 99–107.
13. Chandra J (2010) Megaloblastic anemia: back in focus. Indian J Pediatr 77: 795–799.
14. Bondevik GT, Schneede J, Refsum H, Lie RT, Ulstein M, et al. (2001) Homocysteine and methylmalonic acid levels in pregnant Nepali women. Should cobalamin supplementation be considered? Eur J Clin Nutr 55: 856–864.
15. Chandyo RK (2002) Cobalamin and folate status among women of reproductive age in Bhaktapur, Nepal.
16. Jiang T, Christian P, Khatry SK, Wu L, West KP, Jr. (2005) Micronutrient deficiencies in early pregnancy are common, concurrent, and vary by season among rural Nepali pregnant women. J Nutr 135: 1106–1112.
17. Specker BL, Black A, Allen L, Morrow F (1990) Vitamin B-12: low milk concentrations are related to low serum concentrations in vegetarian women and to methylmalonic aciduria in their infants. Am J Clin Nutr 52: 1073–1076.
18. Baker H, Frank O, Deangelis B, Feingold S, Kaminetzky HA (1981) Role of placenta in maternal-fetal vitamin transfer in humans. Am J Obstet Gynecol 141: 792–796.
19. Allen LH (2005) Multiple micronutrients in pregnancy and lactation: an overview. Am J Clin Nutr 81: 1206S–1212S.
20. Ulak M, Chandyo RK, Mellander L, Shrestha PS, Strand TA (2012) Infant feeding practices in Bhaktapur, Nepal: A cross-sectional, health facility based survey. Int Breastfeed J 7: 1.
21. CBS (2011) National Population and Housing Census 2011,Central Bureau of Statistics (CBS). Government fof Nepal. National Planning Commission Secretariat.
22. Strand TA, Chandyo RK, Bahl R, Sharma PR, Adhikari RK, et al. (2002) Effectiveness and efficacy of zinc for the treatment of acute diarrhea in young children. Pediatrics 109: 898–903.
23. O'Broin S, Kelleher B (1992) Microbiological assay on microtitre plates of folate in serum and red cells. J Clin Pathol 45: 344–347.
24. Kelleher BP, Walshe KG, Scott JM, O'Broin SD (1987) Microbiological assay for vitamin B12 with use of a colistin-sulfate-resistant organism. Clin Chem 33: 52–54.
25. Molloy AM, Scott JM (1997) Microbiological assay for serum, plasma, and red cell folate using cryopreserved, microtiter plate method. Methods Enzymol 281: 43–53.
26. Husek P (1995) Simultaneous profile analysis of plasma amino and organic acids by capillary gas chromatography. J Chromatogr B Biomed Appl 669: 352–357.
27. Shipchandler MT, Moore EG (1995) Rapid, fully automated measurement of plasma homocyst(e)ine with the Abbott IMx analyzer. Clin Chem 41: 991–994.
28. Bryce J, Boschi-Pinto C, Shibuya K, Black RE (2005) WHO estimates of the causes of death in children. Lancet 365: 1147–1152.
29. USAID/INACG (2002) Adjusting Hemoglobin Values in Program Surveys.
30. De Onis M (2006) WHO child growth standards : length/height-for-age, weight-for-age, weight-for-length, weight -for-height and body mass index-for-age : methods and development. Geneva, World Health Organization.
31. Hosmer DW, S L (2000) Applied Logistic Regression. New York: John Wiley & Sons Inc.
32. Hay G, Johnston C, Whitelaw A, Trygg K, Refsum H (2008) Folate and cobalamin status in relation to breastfeeding and weaning in healthy infants. Am J Clin Nutr 88: 105–114.
33. Karademir F, Suleymanoglu S, Ersen A, Aydinoz S, Gultepe M, et al. (2007) Vitamin B12, folate, homocysteine and urinary methylmalonic acid levels in infants. J Int Med Res 35: 384–388.
34. Davis RE, Icke GC, Hilton JM, Orr E (1986) Serum thiamin, pyridoxal, cobalamin and folate concentrations in young infants. Acta Paediatr Scand 75: 402–407.
35. Rimestad AH, Borgejordet Å, Vesterhus KN (2001) Den store matvaretabellen. (The Norwegian food composition table.) 2nd ed. Oslo, Norway: National Nutrition Council, 2001 (in Norwegian).
36. Olivares JL, Fernandez R, Fleta J, Ruiz MY, Clavel A (2002) Vitamin B12 and folic acid in children with intestinal parasitic infection. J Am Coll Nutr 21: 109–113.
37. Clarke R, Grimley Evans J, Schneede J, Nexo E, Bates C, et al. (2004) Vitamin B12 and folate deficiency in later life. Age Ageing 33: 34–41.
38. Bjorke Monsen AL, Ueland PM (2003) Homocysteine and methylmalonic acid in diagnosis and risk assessment from infancy to adolescence. Am J Clin Nutr 78: 7–21.
39. Mackey AD, Picciano MF (1999) Maternal folate status during extended lactation and the effect of supplemental folic acid. Am J Clin Nutr 69: 285–292.
40. Murphy SP, Allen LH (2003) Nutritional importance of animal source foods. J Nutr 133: 3932S–3935S.

41. WHO. (2012) Serum and red blood cell folate concentrations for assessing folate status in populations. Vitamin and Mineral Nutrition Information System. Geneva, World Health Organization.
42. Scott JM, Weir DG (1981) The methyl folate trap. A physiological response in man to prevent methyl group deficiency in kwashiorkor (methionine deficiency) and an explanation for folic-acid induced exacerbation of subacute combined degeneration in pernicious anaemia. Lancet 2: 337–340.
43. Ueland PM, Refsum H, Stabler SP, Malinow MR, Andersson A, et al. (1993) Total homocysteine in plasma or serum: methods and clinical applications. Clin Chem 39: 1764–1779.
44. Hannisdal R, Gislefoss RE, Grimsrud TK, Hustad S, Morkrid L, et al. (2010) Analytical recovery of folate and its degradation products in human serum stored at -25 degrees C for up to 29 years. J Nutr 140: 522–526.
45. Bostom AG, Gohh RY, Bausserman L, Hakas D, Jacques PF, et al. (1999) Serum cystatin C as a determinant of fasting total homocysteine levels in renal transplant recipients with a normal serum creatinine. J Am Soc Nephrol 10: 164–166.
46. MOHP (2011) Ministry of Health and Population [Nepal], New ERA, and ICF International Inc. 2012. Nepal Demographic and Health Survey 2011. Kathmandu, Nepal: Ministry of Health and Population, New ERA, and ICF International, Calverton, Maryland.

Economic Outcomes of Maintenance Gefitinib for Locally Advanced/Metastatic Non-Small-Cell Lung Cancer with Unknown EGFR Mutations: A Semi-Markov Model Analysis

Xiaohui Zeng[1], Jianhe Li[2,3], Liubao Peng[2]*, Yunhua Wang[1], Chongqing Tan[2,3], Gannong Chen[4], Xiaomin Wan[2,3], Qiong Lu[2], Lidan Yi[2]

1 PET-CT Center, the Second Xiangya Hospital of Central South University, Changsha, Hunan, People's Republic of China, **2** Department of Pharmacy, the Second Xiangya Hospital of Central South University, Changsha, Hunan, People's Republic of China, **3** School of Pharmaceutical Sciences, Central South University, Changsha, Hunan, People's Republic of China, **4** Department of Surgery, the Second Xiangya Hospital of Central South University, Changsha, Hunan, People's Republic of China

Abstract

Background: Maintenance gefitinib significantly prolonged progression-free survival (PFS) compared with placebo in patients from eastern Asian with locally advanced/metastatic non-small-cell lung cancer (NSCLC) after four chemotherapeutic cycles (21 days per cycle) of first-line platinum-based combination chemotherapy without disease progression. The objective of the current study was to evaluate the cost-effectiveness of maintenance gefitinib therapy after four chemotherapeutic cycle's stand first-line platinum-based chemotherapy for patients with locally advanced or metastatic NSCLC with unknown EGFR mutations, from a Chinese health care system perspective.

Methods and Findings: A semi-Markov model was designed to evaluate cost-effectiveness of the maintenance gefitinib treatment. Two-parametric Weibull and Log-logistic distribution were fitted to PFS and overall survival curves independently. One-way and probabilistic sensitivity analyses were conducted to assess the stability of the model designed. The model base-case analysis suggested that maintenance gefitinib would increase benefits in a 1, 3, 6 or 10-year time horizon, with incremental $184,829, $19,214, $19,328, and $21,308 per quality-adjusted life-year (QALY) gained, respectively. The most sensitive influential variable in the cost-effectiveness analysis was utility of PFS plus rash, followed by utility of PFS plus diarrhoea, utility of progressed disease, price of gefitinib, cost of follow-up treatment in progressed survival state, and utility of PFS on oral therapy. The price of gefitinib is the most significant parameter that could reduce the incremental cost per QALY. Probabilistic sensitivity analysis indicated that the cost-effective probability of maintenance gefitinib was zero under the willingness-to-pay (WTP) threshold of $16,349 (3×per-capita gross domestic product of China). The sensitivity analyses all suggested that the model was robust.

Conclusions: Maintenance gefitinib following first-line platinum-based chemotherapy for patients with locally advanced/ metastatic NSCLC with unknown EGFR mutations is not cost-effective. Decreasing the price of gefitinib may be a preferential choice for meeting widely treatment demands in China.

Editor: Jörg D. Hoheisel, Deutsches Krebsforschungszentrum, Germany

Funding: This study was funded by National Natural Science Foundation of China (No.81173028) (URL: http://www.nsfc.gov.cn/Portal0/default152.htm). The funders had no role in study design, data collection and analysis, decision to publish, or preparation of the manuscript.

Competing Interests: The authors have declared that no competing interests exist.

* E-mail: pengliubao@126.com

Introduction

Lung cancer, the most commonly diagnosed form of cancer, is also the leading mortality cause of cancer in males [1]. Non-small-cell lung cancer (NSCLC) accounts for approximately 80% of all lung cancer cases, and the majority of patients with NSCLC have locally advanced/metastatic disease when they are diagnosed with carcinoma [2,3]. Platinum-based combination therapies are recommended as first-line chemotherapy for unselected patients with locally advanced/metastatic NSCLC [4,5]. However, the duration of them (4–6 chemotherapeutic cycles, 21 days per cycle) are limited by cumulative toxicities, and response rates (20%–35%) and median overall survival (7–12 months) are modest [6,7]. On the basis of previous investigations, efforts to improve treatment outcome have focused on the specific goal of prolonging tumour response, progression-free survival (PFS) and overall survival (OS) with well tolerated maintenance treatment in patients who have attained tumor control during first-line treatment [8–12]. Because of these trials and other findings, both erlotinib and pemetrexed (for patients with histologies other than squamous cell carcinoma), have been approved by clinical guidelines as a category 2A recommendation for switch maintenance therapy and also been approved by FDA, in patients without disease progression after 4–6 chemotherapeutic cycles of first-line therapy [4,13,14].

In *The Lancet Oncology* recently, Li Zhang et al, based on a double-blind randomised phase 3 trial, reported that maintenance gefitinib significantly prolonged PFS compared with placebo in patients from 27 centres across China with locally/metastatic NSCLC, which indicates that gefitinib should be considered as a maintenance treatment choice in eastern Asian patients [15]. Several economic studies were conducted of maintenance therapy [16–23]. Two analyses concluded that maintenance erlotinib is cost-effective versus best supportive care for locally advanced/metastatic NSCLC [16,17]. Except for the study by Greenhalgh et al [18], the 4 other studies of maintenance pemetrexed indicated that the new therapy was not cost-effective [19–22]. The evaluation from Zhu J et al, on the basis of the clinical trial, suggested that the maintenance gefitinib therapy was cost-effective for locally advanced/metastatic NSCLC patients with activating EGFR mutations [23]. However, it is unclear whether the new therapy is cost-effective in patients with unknown EGFR mutations after first-line platinum-based combination chemotherapy without disease progression.

The objective of the current study was to evaluate the long-term cost-effectiveness (10 year time horizon) of maintenance gefitinib therapy after four chemotherapeutic cycles of stand first-line platinum-based chemotherapy for locally advanced/metastatic NSCLC patients with unknown EGFR mutations, from a Chinese health care system perspective.

Materials and Methods

A previously constructed semi-Markov model was used to compare the long-tern impact of maintenance gefitinib treatment versus placebo after 4 chemotherapeutic cycles of first-line platinum-based chemotherapy for patients with locally advanced/metastatic NSCLC [22], on the basis of the double-blind randomised phase III trial from China by Li Zhang et al [15]. The model along with two-parametric Weibull and Log-logistic distribution were used for calculating the direct medical costs, life-years gained (LYGs) and quality-adjusted life-years (QALYs) gained of the practice presented in the trial [15]. Due to the perspective of the Chinese health care system, only direct medical costs related to the practice were estimated, including maintenance gefitinib therapy, treatment of major adverse events, routine follow-up treatment for patients without progression, follow-up treatment for progressive disease and terminal-phase cost. Costs in this study were estimated in US dollars (USD), corresponding to the 2011 consumer price index and assuming an average exchange rate of 1 USD to 6.45 Chinese Yuan (RMB). Utilities for the model were derived from the literature. The future costs and outcomes were discounted at 3% annually in compliance with the request of China Guidelines for Pharmacoeconomic Evaluations (version 8) [24].

Effectiveness data were stemmed from the multicentre, double-blind randomised clinical trial [15], which is the only phase III trial compared maintenance gefitinib treatment in patients with locally advanced/metastatic NSCLC according to our literature search. In brief, 296 patients with histological or cytological NSCLC in stage IIIb or IV between September 28, 2008 and August 11, 2009, who were 18 years or older and had a WHO performance status of 0–2 and more than 12 weeks life expectancy after completion of four chemotherapeutic cycle's first-line platinum-based chemotherapy without disease progression, were eligible for the maintenance gefitinib or placebo treatment (1:1 randomization ratio). Eligible patients continued to take either gefitinib (250 mg per day) or placebo orally until disease progression, intolerable toxicity, withdrawal of consent, serious non-compliance with protocol, or dose delay or interruption >14 days. In this report, there were 40 and 39 patients were deemed know EGFR mutation status in gefitinib group and placebo group, respectively. Therefore there were 108 patients and 109 patients with unknown EGFR mutation received maintenance gefitinib and placebo treatment separately. The primary endpoint of the trial was progression-free survival, and the survival analysis revealed that median PFS for patients with unknown EGFR mutation was 6.0 months in gefitinib group and 2.7 months in placebo group (HR 0.40 [95% CI 0.29–0.54]; p<0.0001). Median OS was not significantly different between the two groups (HR 0.84 [95% CI 0.62–1.14]; p = 0.26; median OS 18.7 months *vs* 16.9 months). The incidence of adverse events in gefitinib group was more frequent than that in placebo group (80% vs. 53%). The cumulative probabilities of serious adverse events were 7% and 3% in the maintenance gefitinib and placebo groups, respectively.

The model outcomes were presented as costs, LYGs and QALYs, from the perspective of the Chinese health care system. Sensitivity analyses of input parameters with the high/low values and various distributions were conducted to assess the stability of the model at a value of recommended willingness-to-pay (WTP) threshold of $16,349 (3×per-capita gross domestic product, GDP), based on the cost-effectiveness guidelines of Word Health Organization (WHO) [25].

Model Structure

The simplified model structure was shown in Figure 1, which comprised 3 mutually exclusive health states: PFS (entry state); progressed survival (PS state), and death. Patients move from one state to another during each Markov cycle length of 3 weeks (short enough to detect all clinically relevant events) until time horizon termination of 10-year (>95% patients died). Two-parametric Weibull survival and Log-logistic distribution analyses using R for Statistical Computing version 2.15.2 (R Foundation, Wien, Austria) were fitted to the PFS and OS curves respectively, on the basis of survival data extracted from the published Kaplan-Meier curves [15], by using GetData Graph Digitizer software (version 2.24). Table 1 shows the Weibull and Log-logistic distribution parameters of model estimated. The estimated Weibull parameters are used to measure the time-dependency transition probabilities from PFS to PS state, according to the following formula:

$$tp\,(t_u) = 1 - \exp\{\lambda(t-\mu)^{\gamma} - \lambda t^{\gamma}\}\ (\lambda > 0;\ \gamma > 0)$$

where the λ defines the scale of the distribution, the γ gives the shape, the u is the Markov cycle and t_u indicates that t is calculated as integer multiples of the cycle length of the model. The transition probabilities of death at current t due to the following formula:

$$tp\,(t_u) = 1 - \frac{1 + \exp(\theta)\,(t-\mu)^{\kappa}}{1 + \exp(\theta)\,t^{\kappa}}\ (\kappa > 0)$$

where the θ and κ are the theta and kappa from the estimated Log-logistic parameters, indications of the u and the t_u are the same as above.

Medical Costs and Utilities

Medical costs for each strategy (Table 2), from the perspective of Chinese health care system, were based on outlining current

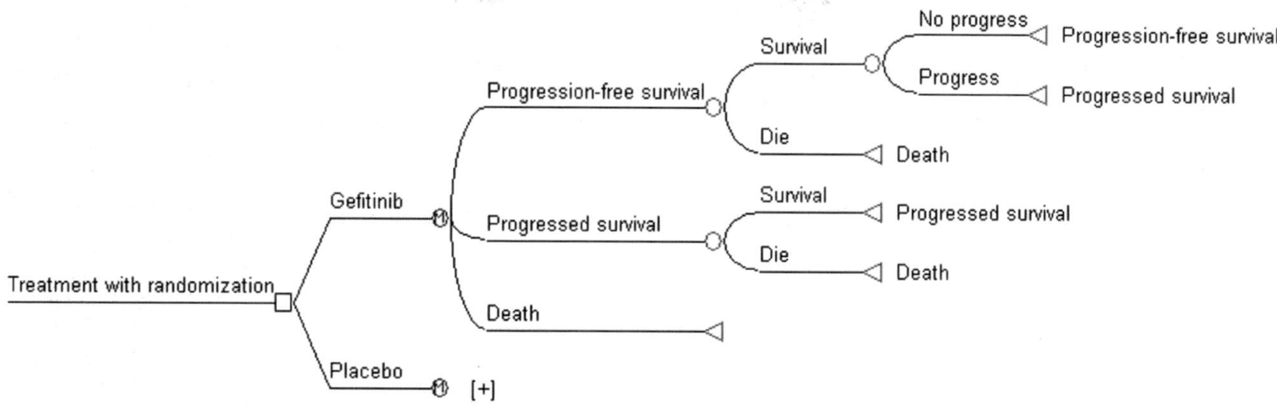

Figure 1. Markov model of locally advanced/metastatic non-small-cell lung cancer.

practice [15], which reflected the effectiveness of maintenance gefitinib treatment in Chinese patients with locally advanced/ metastatic NSCLC. Direct medical costs related to the practice were estimated, including maintenance gefitinib therapy, treatment of major adverse events, routine follow-up treatment for patients without progression, follow-up treatment in PS state and terminal-phase cost. Prices of gefitinib, follow-up treatment cost in PS state and terminal-phase cost were obtained from our previous study, in which we have calculated healthcare costs associated with the time- and health status-related treatment resources that advanced NSCLC may anticipate based on health expenditure data for 253 cases of advanced NSCLC registered at the Second Xiangya Hospital of Central South University in China between 2006 and 2010 [26]. The aggregate annual medical costs for patients in either PFS or PS state and monthly healthcare costs accumulated during the terminal 3 months, were estimated and evaluated using 95% confidence intervals through bootstrapping with the R software (version 2.14.0; R Foundation, Vienna, Austria) [26]. According to Gefitinib Patients Assistance Program of the pharmaceutical producer in China, NSCLC patients receive donations of gefitinib after six months treatment [23]. Therefore six months was applied to calculate the total cost of the maintenance drug. Routine follow-up treatment cost for patients without progression, including computed tomography scan, physician visit, and other examinations and drugs, was derived from the literature by Wu B et al [27]. Based on expert opinion, only diarrhoea and other grade 3/4 adverse events were considered to estimate the costs of treatment-associated toxicity. Therefore the unit costs of diarrhoea treated and liver protected were multiplied by published rates of corresponding events to populate the model analysis (we assumed patients with grade 3/4 alanine aminotransferase, aspartate aminotransferase or aminotransferases increased should receive treatment of liver protected). The unit costs of diarrhoea and liver protected were estimated according to local charges in China.

Health state utility values of the PFS and PS states presented in Table 2 were derived from the published literature by Nafees et al, who assessed quality of life using the visual analogue scale and standard gamble interview in 100 participants, on the basis of the health state descriptions which were developed after rounds of in-depth interviews with oncologists, oncology specialist nurses and psychometric experts [28]. According to the literature, diarrhoea and rash reported in the trial, were significantly associated with the utility values of PFS [15,28]. Therefore we calculated the utility value in PFS based on the published proportion of the adverse events (diarrhoea and rash) [15] and utility values of PFS on oral therapy (0.67), PFS plus rash (0.62), and PFS plus diarrhoea (0.61) [28]. The utility of PS state was 0.47 (range, 0.19–0.56) and was used in both arms.

Sensitivity Analysis

Each key parameter was fitted high/low values and specific pattern of distribution in our model (Table 2) to reflect substantial uncertainty of the input parameters using one-way and probabi-

Table 1. Weibull and Log-logistic parameters of model estimated for progression-free and overall survival curves, respectively.

Progression-free survival[a]	Scale, Mean (Range)	Shape, Mean (Range)	Adjusted R^2	Correlation Coefficient
Placebo arm	0.10443 (0.04509/0.16377)	1.29221 (0.99662/1.58780)	0.9729	−0.995165
Gefitinib arm	0.10231 (0.06622/0.13840)	0.83852 (0.71474/0.96230)	0.9782	−0.998386
Overall survival[b]	**Theta, Mean (Range)**	**Kappa, Mean (Range)**	**Adjusted R^2**	**Correlation Coefficient**
Placebo arm	−6.54311 (−7.16112/−5.92510)	2.09373 (1.89823/2.28923)	0.9855	−0.999986
Gefitinib arm	−5.04069 (−5.53622/−4.54516)	1.54139 (1.38359/1.69919)	0.9801	−0.999852

[a]R output for Weibull regression fitted to progression-free curves of locally advanced/metastatic non-small-cell lung cancer patients derived from the Phase III trial [15].
[b]R output for Log-logistic regression fitted to overall curves of locally advanced/metastatic non-small-cell lung cancer patients derived from the Phase III trial [15].

Table 2. Base cases, ranges and distributional assumptions of parameters.

Variables	Base case	Range	Distribution
Costs ($)			
Treatment costs			
Gefitinib per 250 mg [26]	81.0	64.8/81.0[a]	Fixed in PSA
Routine follow-up of patients per unit [27]	51.5	45.0/58.4	Lognormal
Follow-up treatment in PS state each year [26]	14,519	12,011/16,871	Lognormal
Terminal phase cost in last month [26]	3754	3274/4238	Lognormal
Adverse events			
Liver protected per unit[b]	57.78	32.07/96.22	Lognormal
Diarrhoea per unit[b]	1.48	0.89/2.08	Lognormal
Utility values			
Progression-free survival on oral therapy [28]	0.67	0.27/0.80	Beta
Progression-free survival plus rash [28]	0.62	0.25/0.74	Beta
Progression-free survival plus diarrhoea [28]	0.61	0.24/0.73	Beta
Progressed disease survival [28]	0.47	0.19/0.56	Beta
Discount rate (%) [24]	3	0/8	Fixed in PSA
Risk for adverse events			
Rash in gefitinib arm [15]	0.50	0.35/0.65[c]	Beta
Rash in placebo arm [15]	0.095	0.067/0.124[c]	Beta
Diarrhoea in gefitinib arm [15]	0.25	0.18/0.32[c]	Beta
Diarrhoea in placebo arm [15]	0.088	0.062/0.114[c]	Beta
ALT increased in gefitinib arm (grade 3,4) [15]	0.020	0.014/0.026[c]	Beta
AST increased in gefitinib arm (grade 3,4) [15]	0.007	0.0049/0.0091[c]	Beta
ATR increased in gefitinib arm (grade 3,4) [15]	0.014	0.0098/0.0182[c]	Beta

PSA = Probabilistic sensitivity analysis; ALT = Alanine aminotransferase;
AST = Aspartate aminotransferase; ATR = Aminotransferases.
[a]Price of gefitinib was reduced 20% and was fixed in probabilistic sensitivity analysis because it is a brand name drug.
[b]Estimated according to local charges in China.
[c]Varied by ±30%.

listic sensitivity analyses (PSA). Many ranges were derived from published reports [26–28]; price of gefitinib was reduced 20% and fixed in PSA because it is a brand name drug; costs of adverse events were estimated by local charges in China; probabilities of adverse events were varied by ±30%. Lognormal distributions were chosen for all input costs except gefitinib (fixed in PSA); beta distributions were chosen for utility values and probabilities of adverse events; bivariate normal distributions were adopted for the Weibull and Log-logistic parameters; discount rate with high/low values was fixed in PSA, in compliance with the request of China Guidelines for Pharmacoeconomic Evaluations (Version 8) [24]. The WTP threshold of 3×per-capita GDP ($16,349/QALY) was used. A tornado diagram and an incremental cost-effectiveness scatter plot were developed to depict the results of one-way sensitivity analyses (OSA) and PSA.

Results

Base Case Model Analysis

The Log-logistic and two parameters Weibull model matched the survival curves of the clinical trial by Zhang L et al [15] satisfactorily (Figure 2). The validity of the simulated survival curves tail beyond the observed time horizon of clinical trial was conducted by comparing the 5 years overall survival rate calculated from the current distribution models for placebo arm (5.7%) to the data from the Surveillance, Epidemiology and End Results (SEER) Program, which shows that 5-year survival rate of distant lung cancer patients is 3.9% [29], and the site of http://lungcancer.about.com/, which shows that 5-year survival rate of metastatic NSCLC is sadly less than 10%. Base case model analyses in different time horizon are displayed in Table 3, which suggested that maintenance gefitinib therapy after four chemotherapeutic cycles of stand first-line platinum-based chemotherapy for patients with locally advanced/metastatic NSCLC patients would increase the effectiveness in a 1-, 3-, 6-, or 10-year time horizon, with incremental QALYs gained of 0.0233, 0.1462, 0.2699 and 0.3496. Incremental costs per QALY for the new therapy compared with placebo were $184,828, $19,214, $19,328 and $21,308, respectively, at 1, 3, 6, and 10 years.

One-way Sensitivity Analysis

The results of one-way sensitivity analyses of key populated variables (displayed in Table 2) were depicted in a tornado diagram (Figure 3) to show the influence with regard to the incremental cost-effectiveness ratio (ICER), which means incremental cost per QALY gained in current study. The utility of PFS plus rash impacted utmost on the ICER. The other sensitive variables included utility of PFS plus diarrhoea, utility of progressed disease, price of gefitinib, cost of follow-up treatment in PS state, and utility of PFS on oral therapy. All of these variables

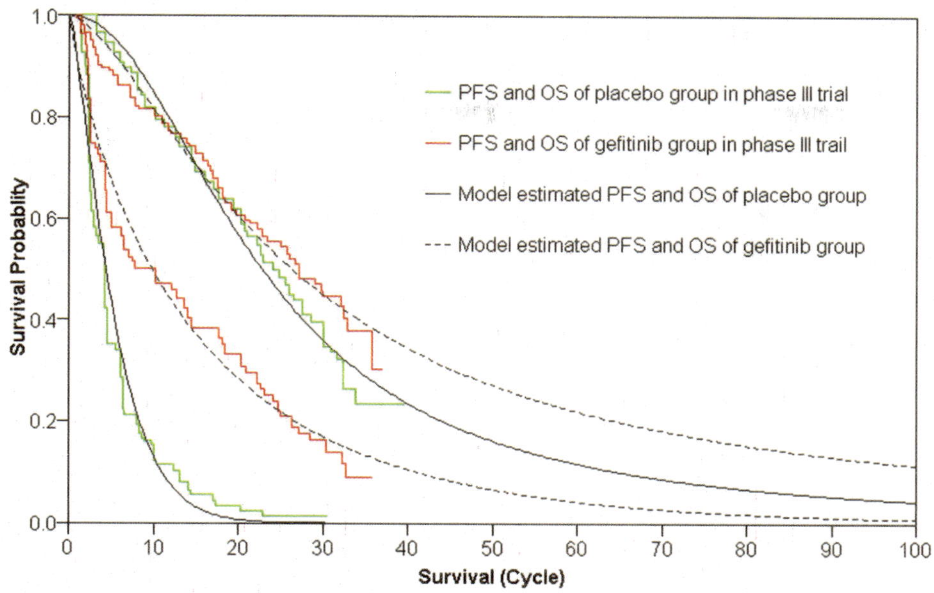

Figure 2. Survival curves in patients with maintenance gefitinib group or placebo group after first-line platinum-based combination chemotherapy of four cycles in locally advanced/metastatic non-small-cell lung cancer. The original curves from the clinical trial are shown, together with the Weibull and Log-logistic model estimated for progression-free survival and overall survival separately.

did not led to an ICER entrancing the WTP threshold of $16,349 per QALY (3×per-capita GDP of China). None of the other parameters significantly altered the ICER.

Probabilistic Sensitivity Analysis

Incremental cost-effectiveness scatter plot of 1000 simulations (Figure 4), showed a zero probability meeting the WTP threshold of $16,349/QALY. If the WTP was >$21,323 (per-capita GDP: $7,108), more 50% of locally advanced/metastatic NSCLC, with maintenance gefitinib therapy after four cycles of first-line platinum-based combination chemotherapy without disease progression, could achieve cost-effectiveness. Acceptability curves (Figure 5) suggested that the cost-effectiveness likelihood of maintenance gefitinib therapy increased with increasing thresholds of WTP, and about $17,700 to $26,300 was the sensitivity range. At WTPs >$26,300, almost all cases could achieve cost-effectiveness.

Table 3. Base-case model analyses of life-years gained (LYGs), quality-adjusted life-years (QALYs), costs and incremental cost per LYG/QALY of maintenance gefitinib therapy arm and placebo arm after four cycles of stand first-line platinum-based chemotherapy for patients with locally advanced/metastatic NSCLC, on the basis of 1000 simulation cases.

Arm	LYGs Gained	QALYs Gained	Cost ($)	Incremental cost ($)	
				Per LYG	Per QALY
1-year					
Placebo arm	0.865	0.465	9,082	–	–
Gefitinib arm	0.845	0.488	13,396		
Dominated	184,829				
3-year					
Placebo arm	1.516	0.772	18,866	–	–
Gefitinib arm	1.658	0.918	21,675	19,788	19,214
6-year					
Placebo arm	1.735	0.875	22,129	–	–
Gefitinib arm	2.112	1.144	27,345	13,816	19,328
10-year					
Placebo arm	1.814	0.912	23,302	–	–
Gefitinib arm	2.357	1.262	30,751	13,734	21,308

Discussion

Maintenance gefitinib therapy has been proven to prolong PFS significantly than placebo for patients with locally advanced/metastatic NSCLC after 4 chemotherapeutic cycles of first-line platinum-based combination chemotherapy without disease progression, based on a Chinese phase III trial across 27 centres [15]. However, its economic impact is necessary to be considered before it is widely used for the appropriate patients, especially for China, where the population is >1.3 billion and the health care resources are in serious shortage [30].

Resource allocation decisions in health care are rife based on results from economic assessments. However from Clinical trials, it is of difficulty to collect enough financial data for economic evaluation [27]. Thus, mathematical models that can estimate long-term cost-effectiveness of alternative strategies, is a helpful technique to support economic analyses of health care resource ulitization [26,27]. In current study, a semi-Markov model along with two-parametric Weibull and Log-logistic distribution were used for measuring the time-dependency transition probabilities and calculating the direct medical costs, LYGs and QALYs gained of the practice presented in the trial [15].

A cost-effectiveness evaluation was performed to analysis the economic impact of maintenance gefitinib therapy for patients with locally advanced/metastatic NSCLC with unknown EGFR mutations. Base case analyses of 1-, 3-, 6-, and 10-year time

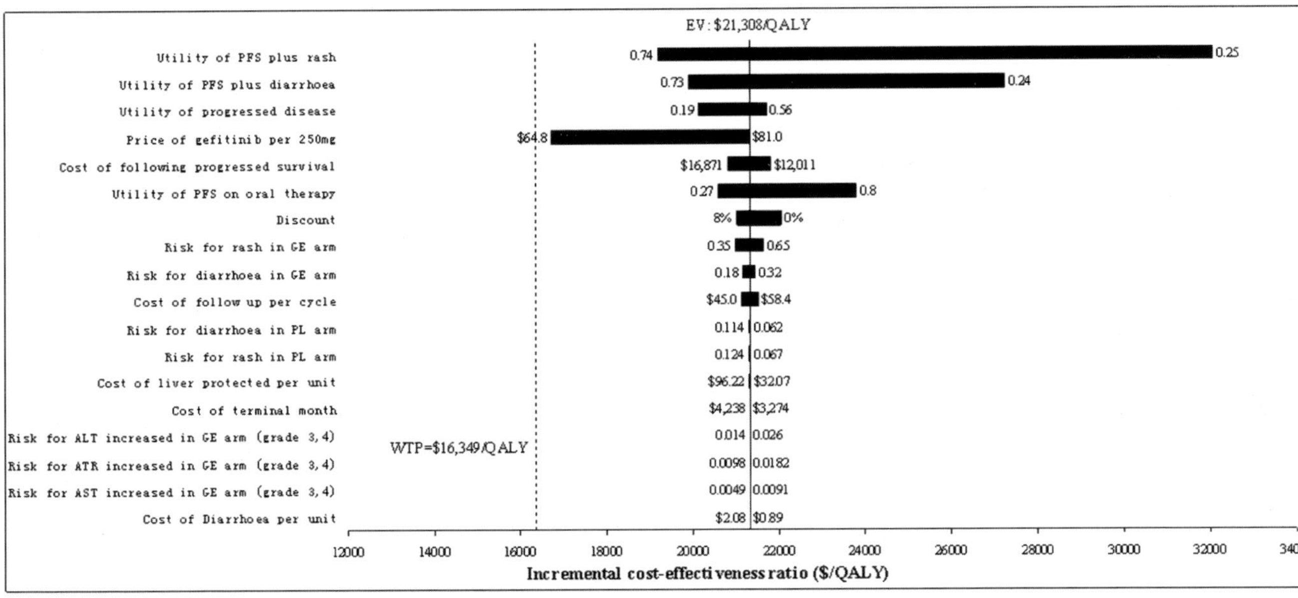

Figure 3. Tornado diagram for one-way sensitivity analysis revealing variables' influence on the incremental cost-effectiveness ratio. PFS = progression-free survival; GE = gefitinib; PL = placebo; QALY = quality-adjusted life-years.

horizon showed an unfavorable ICER of $184,829, $19,214, $19,328, and $21,308 per QALY gained, respectively. OSA and PSA all revealed that the model we applied was robust to the results. Monte Carlo simulations of 1,000 cases suggested that all ICERs for maintenance gefitinib therapy were higher than the recommended WTP threshold (3×per-capita GDP) of cost-effectiveness guidelines from Word Health Organization (WHO). There are 31 province-level administrative units in Chinese mainland, the per-capita GDP of which differs significantly. In 2011, for example, it ranged from $2,495 in Guizhou province to $13,392 in Tianjin city [31]. According to the recommended threshold of WHO [25], the WTP threshold, of different province-level administrative units, extended from $7,485 (3×$2,495) to $40,176 (3×$13,392) per QALY gained, which exceeded the

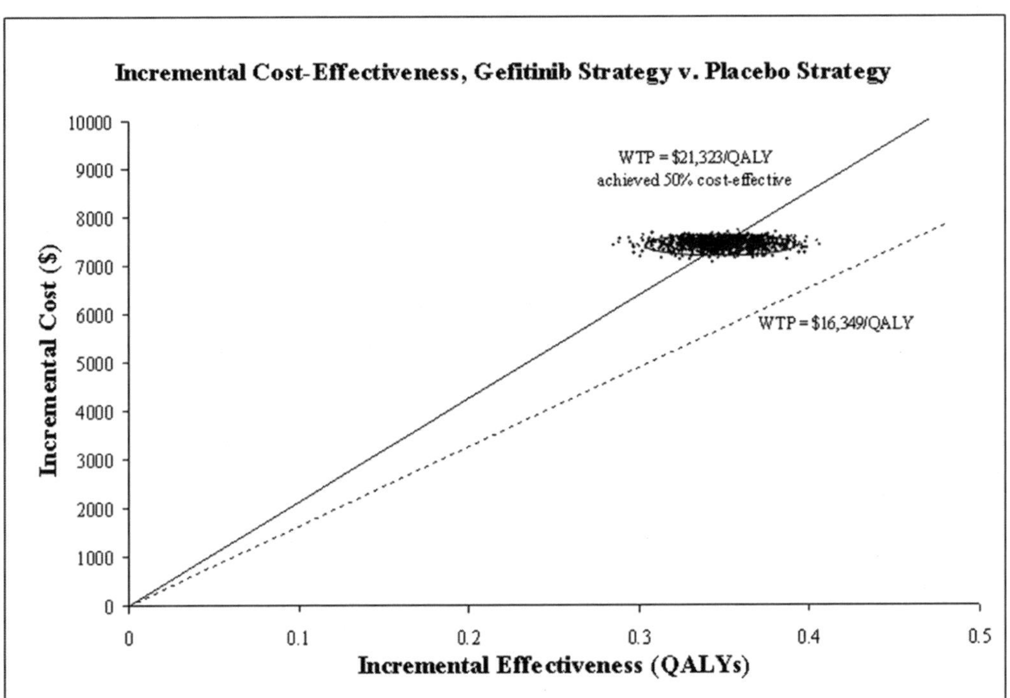

Figure 4. Probabilistic sensitivity analysis of 1000 cases study comparing maintenance gefitinib strategy and placebo strategy. WTP = willingness to pay; QALY = quality-adjusted life-years.

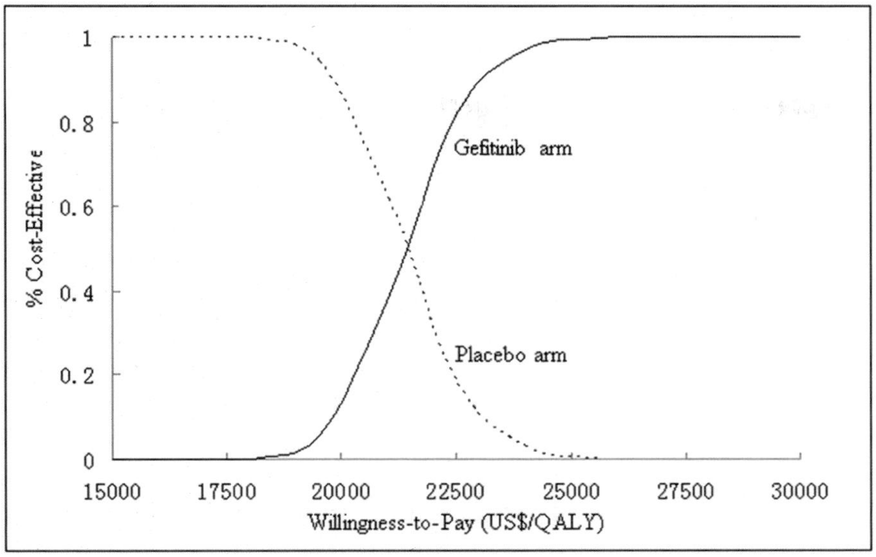

Figure 5. Acceptability curves of maintenance gefitinib arm and placebo arm. QALY = quality-adjusted life-years.

sensitivity range of the WTP (about $17,700 to $26,300) obtained from PSA of the current study. Obviously local government could take fully into account covering maintenance gefitinib treatment following first-line platinum-based chemotherapy for locally advanced/metastatic NSCLC with unknown EGFR mutations in accordance with local economic development level. Cost-effective probability for different economic level provinces, displayed in Table 4, could supply available information for local governments, when gefitinib is approved by local governments' finance before it has access to the directory of drugs for national basic medical insurance in China.

A number of different survival models, such as Weibull, Exponential, Log-logistic, Gompertz, et al, can be used to perform extrapolation according to the observed trial data [32]. It is therefore very vital to choose the justifiable extrapolation approach, to ensure the associated results of economic analysis confident to decision makers. In the current study, after the deviance information criterion test (reported by Jackson et al [33] to alternative models introduced by Latimer [32], we chose Weibull and Log-logistic for PFS and OS respectively, instead of Weibull for extrapolating both PFS and OS curves like the previous study undertaken by Zhu J et al [23]. In addition, a hazard ration (HR) of PFS was applied to derive the PFS curve for the gefitinib strategy in the previous study [23]. Latimer, however in the resent published paper, pointed out that the HR used may cause bias because of the requirement of the assumptions–that is, the HR was from a related model and was constant over time [34]. Obviously the bias should be considered, especially if the HR impacts the results markedly. Unfortunately, the HR of PFS was one of the two most influential parameters on the basis of one-way sensitivity analyses performed by Zhu J et al [23]. In view of the above cases, independent parametric models were fitted to both control and experimental groups in our study.

Utility of PFS played a great role in the results not only in the resent study [23] but also in the current study. Nafees et al [28] reviewed that all toxicities (diarrhoea, rash, nausea and vomiting, neutropenia, fatigue, and hair loss) were related to pulling utility down significantly. Of the toxicities, rash and diarrhoea were associated with maintenance gefitinib strategy as reported the clinical trial [15]. For higher accuracy, we weighted the utility of PFS according to the risks of the rash and diarrhoea, which were displayed in Table 2.

In particularly, one point revealed by one-way sensitivity analysis (Figure 3), should be highlighted that the price of gefitinib

Table 4. The cost-effective probabilities of gefitinib arm for 31 provinces of Chinese mainland.

Region	Per-capita GDP ($)	WTP (3×Per-capita GDP, $)	Cost-effective Probability
Mainland China	5,449.71	16,349	0
More affluent regions[a]	>8,767	>26,300	1.00
Guangdong	7,819	23,457	0.932
Liaoning	7,795	23,385	0.926
Fujian	7,344	22,032	0.717
Shandong	7,273	21,819	0.655
Less affluent regions[b]	<5,900	<17,700	0

[a]Consist of Tianjin, Shanghai, Beijing, Jiangsu, Zhejiang and Inner Mongolia.
[b]Consist of Jilin, Chongqing, Hubei, Hebei, Shanxi, Ningxia, Heilongjiang, Shangxi, Xinjiang, Hunan, Qinghai, Henan, Hainan, Jiangxi, Sichuan, Guangxi, Anhui, Tibet, Gansu, Yuannan and Guizhou.

would be the most significant parameter that could reduce the ICER. With the gefitinib price reduction of 20% discount, the ICER decreased to $16,731 per QALY gained, which is very close to the WTP threshold of $16,349 per QALY. Therefore if the price of gefitinib decreases >20%, maintenance gefitinib therapy after the standard chemotherapy in patients with locally advanced/metastatic NSCLC may be a cost-effectiveness strategy.

There are some limitations in the present study. First, using Weibull and Log-logistic distribution to extrapolate the survival curves beyond the time scope of the trial was an unavoidable limitation of this process. There is not enough survival data, provided by the short follow-ups of the clinical trial, to compare the long-term outcomes estimated by the model. Our results should be updated when long-term survival data are available. Another important limitation is that the utility weight parameters originated from the published literature that may not reflect Chinese patients' trait. It is an inevitable limitation of the current analysis because utilities data are not yet available for China. Fortunately, opinions from Chinese oncologists suggested that, quality of life of locally advanced or metastatic NSCLC patients in China should not be of significant difference from abroad patients. Finally, because there is no head-to-head clinical trial comparing maintenance gefitinib with other maintenance drugs (eg, erlotinib) after the standard chemotherapy of four chemotherapeutic cycles, we have not conducted a cost-effectiveness analysis of gefitinib in comparison with other maintenance therapies.

Although the current estimates were derived from just one study, which is also the only phase III trial compared maintenance gefitinib treatment in patients with locally advanced/metastatic NSCLC according to our literature search, we believe that the analysis of our study, based on a current Chinese phase III trial and the justifiable extrapolation approach, can provide important reference information for decision makers in China. First of all, the clinical study itself is a multicentre, double-blind, randomized controlled-trial (RCT), which represents the best evidence available and is deemed to be the most accepted scientific method of determining the benefit of a drug or a therapeutic procedure. Second, the analysis method applied in our study was reliable and widely used in economic evaluations, especially in the field of medical and health care. In addition, the Log-logistic and two parameters Weibull model matched the survival curves of the clinical trial satisfactorily (Figure 2), which shows that the model we constructed can mirror the effectiveness data of the trial commendably. And then, direct medical costs related to each strategy were estimated, including maintenance gefitinib therapy, treatment of major adverse events, routine follow-up treatment for patients without progression, follow-up treatment in PS state and terminal-phase cost. Although the costs originated from our previous study [26], the published literature [27] or estimates according to local charges based on expert opinion, all of them stemmed from a Chinese health care system perspective, as well as in view of patients with advanced NSCLC, which echoed the purpose of the current study. Last but not least, to reflect substantial uncertainty of the input parameters, the sensitivity analyses (including OSA and PSA) were conducted for each key parameter, and all sensitivity analyses revealed that the model we applied was robust to the results.

In conclusion, according to the recommended WTP threshold (3×per-capita GDP) of cost-effectiveness guidelines from WHO, maintenance gefitinib therapy after the standard chemotherapy of four chemotherapeutic cycles in locally advanced/metastatic NSCLC patients with unknown EGFR mutations is likely to be not cost-effective for Chinese mainland, from the Chinese health care system perspective. Local governments, with different economic level however, could take fully into account covering maintenance gefitinib treatment. Because for rich regions (the per-capita GDP> $8,767), the new strategy seems to be a reasonable option, and if the per-capita GDP ranges from $5,900 to $8,767, the maintenance therapy may be favourable in terms of the different cost-effective probabilities. Decreasing the price of gefitinib, the most significant parameter that could reduce the ICER, should be considered to as a preferential factor for meeting widely treatment demands in China.

Acknowledgments

Prof. L.B. Peng and J.H. Li are the guarantors for the overall content. The authors greatly thank many clinicians and the data managers who have recorded the initial data diligently of medicines over the years. In particular, they thank Ouyang Lihui, Wang Siying, Zhao Ziying and Qiu Zhenhua for their help in the data collection and valuable discussions and advices.

Author Contributions

Conceived and designed the experiments: JL LP. Performed the experiments: GC QL LY. Analyzed the data: XZ CT. Contributed reagents/materials/analysis tools: YW XW. Wrote the paper: XZ CT.

References

1. Jemal A, Bray F, Center MM, Ferlay J, Ward E, et al. (2011) Global cancer statistics. CA Cancer J Clin 61: 69–90.
2. Fathi AT, Brahmer JR. (2008) Chemotherapy for advanced stage non-small cell lung cancer. Semin Thorac Cardiovasc Surg 20: 210–216.
3. Govindan R, Page N, Morgensztern D, Read W, Tierney R, et al. (2006) Changing epidemiology of small-cell lung cancer in the United States over the last 30 years: analysis of the surveillance, epidemiologic, and end results database. J Clin Oncol 24: 4539–4544.
4. Nation Comprehensive Cancer Network (2013) Non–small cell lung cancer (version 2.2014). Available: http://www.nccn.org/professionals/physician_gls/pdf/nscl.pdf. Accessed 21 January 2014.
5. Azzoli CG, Baker JS, Temin S, Pao W, Aliff T, et al. (2009) American Society of Clinical Oncology Clinical Practice Guideline update on chemotherapy for stage IV non-small-cell lung cancer. J Clin Oncol 27: 6251–6266.
6. D'Addario G, Felip E (2009) Non-small-cell lung cancer: ESMO clinical recommendations for diagnosis, treatment and follow-up. Ann Oncol (Suppl 4): 68–70.
7. Bareschino MA, Schettino C, Rossi A, Maione P, Sacco PC, et al. (2011) Treatment of advanced non small cell lung cancer. J Thorac Dis 3: 122–133.
8. Brodowicz T, Krzakowski M, Zwitter M, Tzekova V, Ramlau R, et al. (2006) Cisplatin and gemcitabine first-line chemotherapy followed by maintenance gemcitabine or best supportive care in advanced non-small cell lung cancer: a phase III trial. Lung Cancer 52: 155–163.
9. Fidias PM, Dakhil SR, Lyss AP, Loesch DM, Waterhouse DM, et al. (2009) Phase III study of immediate compared with delayed docetaxel after front-line therapy with gemcitabine plus carboplatin in advanced non-small-cell lung cancer. J Clin Oncol 27: 591–598.
10. Ciuleanu T, Brodowicz T, Zielinski C, Kim JH, Krzakowski M, et al. (2009) Maintenance pemetrexed plus best supportive care versus placebo plus best supportive care for non-small-cell lung cancer: a randomised, double-blind, phase 3 study. Lancet 374: 1432–1440.
11. Cappuzzo F, Ciuleanu T, Stelmakh L, Cicenas S, Szczésna A, et al. (2010) Erlotinib as maintenance treatment in advanced non-small-cell lung cancer: a multicentre, randomised, placebo-controlled phase 3 study. Lancet Oncol 11: 521–529.
12. Paz-Ares L, de Marinis F, Dediu M, Thomas M, Pujol JL, et al. (2012) Maintenance therapy with pemetrexed plus best supportive care versus placebo plus best supportive care after induction therapy with pemetrexed plus cisplatin for advanced non-squamous non-small-cell lung cancer (PARAMOUNT): a double-blind, phase 3, randomized controlled trial. Lancet Oncol 13: 247–255.
13. Cohen MH, Johnson JR, Chattopadhyay S, Tang S, Justice R, et al. (2010) Approval summary: erlotinib maintenance therapy of advanced/metastatic non-small cell lung cancer (NSCLC). Oncologist 15: 1344–1351.
14. Cohen MH, Cortazar P, Justice R, Pazdur R (2010) Approval summary: pemetrexed maintenance therapy of advanced/metastatic nonsquamous, non-small cell lung cancer (NSCLC). Oncologist 15: 1352–1358.

15. Zhang L, Ma S, Song X, Han B, Cheng Y, et al. (2012) Gefitinib versus placebo as maintenance therapy in patients with locally advanced or metastatic non-small-cell lung cancer (INFORM; C-TONG 0804): a multicentre, double-blind randomised phase 3 trial. Lancet Oncol 13: 466–475.
16. Walleser S, Ray J, Bischoff H, Vergnenègre A, Rosery H, et al. (2012) Maintenance erlotinib in advanced non-small cell lung cancer: cost-effectiveness in EGFR wild-type across Europe. Clinicoecon Outcomes Res 4: 269–275.
17. Vergnenègre A, Ray JA, Chouaid C, Grossi F, Bischoff HG, et al. (2012) Cross-market cost-effectiveness analysis of erlotinib as first-line maintenance treatment for patients with stable non-small cell lung cancer. Clinicoecon Outcomes Res 4: 31–37.
18. Greenhalgh J, McLeod C, Bagust A, Boland A, Fleeman N, et al. (2010) Pemetrexed for the maintenance treatment of locally advanced or metastatic non-small cell lung cancer. Health Technol Assess 14: 33–39.
19. Klein R, Wielage R, Muehlenbein C, Liepa AM, Babineaux S, et al. (2010) Cost-effectiveness of pemetrexed as first-line maintenance therapy for advanced nonsquamous non-small cell lung cancer. J Thor Oncol 5: 1263–1272.
20. Tsuchiya T, Fukuda T, Furuiye M, Kawabuchi K (2011) Pharmacoeconomic analysis of consolidation therapy with pemetrexed after first-line chemotherapy for non-small cell lung cancer. Lung Cancer 74: 521–529.
21. Matter-Walstra K, Joerger M, Kühnel U, Szucs T, Pestalozzi B, et al. (2012) Cost-Effectiveness of Maintenance Pemetrexed in Patients with Advanced Nonsquamous-Cell Lung Cancer from the Perspective of the Swiss Health Care System. Value Health 15: 65–71.
22. Zeng XH, Peng LB, Li JH, Chen GN, Tan CQ, et al. (2013) Cost-Effectiveness of Continuation Maintenance Pemetrexed after cisplatin and pemetrexed chemotherapy for Advanced Non-squamous Non-small-cell Lung Cancer: estimates from the Chinese Perspective of Health Care System. Clin Ther 35: 54–65.
23. Zhu J, Li T, Wang XH, Ye M, Cai J, et al. (2013) Gene-guided Gefitinib switch maintenance therapy for patients with advanced EGFR mutation-positive Non-small cell lung cancer: an economic analysis. BMC Cancer 13: 39.
24. China Center for Health Economic Research. China Guidelines for Pharmacoeconomic Evaluations (Version 8) [in Chinese] (2010) Available: http://www.cpa.org.cn/Article/UploadFiles/201011/20101125090 52247.pdf.Accessed 21 January 2014.
25. WHO. Cost-effectiveness thresholds. Available: http://www.who.int/choice/costs/CER_thresholds/en/. Accessed 21 January 2014.
26. Zeng XH, Karnon J, Wang SY, Wu B, Wan XM, et al. (2012) The cost of treating advanced non-small cell lung cancer: estimates from the Chinese experience. PLoS ONE 7: e48323.
27. Wu B, Chen H, Shen J, Ye M (2011) Cost-effectiveness of adding rh-endostatin to first-line chemotherapy in patients with advanced non-small-cell lung cancer in China. Clin Ther 33: 1446–1455.
28. Nafees B, Stafford M, Gavriel S, Bhalla S, Watkins J (2008) Health state utilities for non small cell lung cancer. Health Qual Life Out 6: 84.
29. National Cancer Institute (2013) SEER Stat Fact Sheets: Lung and Bronchus Cancer. Available: http://seer.cancer.gov/statfacts/html/lungb.html. Accessed 21 January 2014.
30. Liu Q, Wang B, Kong Y, Cheng KK (2011) China's primary health-care reform. Lancet 377: 2064–2066.
31. National Bureau of Statistics of China (2012) China statistical yearbook 2012. Available: http://www.stats.gov.cn/english/. Accessed 21 January 2014.
32. Latimer N (2011) NICE DSU Technical Support Document 14: Undertaking survival analysis for economic evaluations alongside clinical trials–extrapolation with patient-level data. Available: http://www.nicedsu.org.uk. Accessed 21 January 2014.
33. Jackson CH, Sharples LD, Thompson SG (2010) Survival models in health economic evaluations: Balancing fit and parsimony to improve prediction. Int J Biostat 6: 34.
34. Latimer NR (2013) Survival analysis for economic evaluations alongside clinical trials–extrapolation with patient-level data: inconsistencies, limitations, and a practical guide. Med Decis Making 33: 743–754.

Effects of β-Lactam Antibiotics and Fluoroquinolones on Human Gut Microbiota in Relation to *Clostridium difficile* Associated Diarrhea

Henrik Knecht[1]❡, Sven C. Neulinger[2]❡, Femke Anouska Heinsen[1], Carolin Knecht[3], Anke Schilhabel[2], Ruth A. Schmitz[2], Alexandra Zimmermann[1], Vitor Martins dos Santos[4,5], Manuel Ferrer[6], Philip C. Rosenstiel[1], Stefan Schreiber[1,7], Anette K. Friedrichs[1,7]¶, Stephan J. Ott[1,7]*¶

1 Institute of Clinical Molecular Biology (IKMB), Christian-Albrechts-University (CAU), Kiel, Germany, **2** Institute for General Microbiology (IFAM), Christian-Albrechts-University (CAU), Kiel, Germany, **3** Institute of Medical Informatics and Statistics (IMIS), Christian-Albrechts-University (CAU), Kiel, Germany, **4** Systems and Synthetic Biology, Wageningen University, Wageningen, The Netherlands, **5** LifeGlimmer GmbH, Berlin, Germany, **6** Laboratory of Enzyme Discovery, CSIC - Institute of Catalysis, Madrid, Spain, **7** Department of Internal Medicine I, University Hospital Schleswig-Holstein (UKSH), Kiel, Germany

Abstract

Clostridium difficile infections are an emerging health problem in the modern hospital environment. Severe alterations of the gut microbiome with loss of resistance to colonization against *C. difficile* are thought to be the major trigger, but there is no clear concept of how *C. difficile* infection evolves and which microbiological factors are involved. We sequenced 16S rRNA amplicons generated from DNA and RNA/cDNA of fecal samples from three groups of individuals by FLX technology: (i) healthy controls (no antibiotic therapy); (ii) individuals receiving antibiotic therapy (Ampicillin/Sulbactam, cephalosporins, and fluoroquinolones with subsequent development of *C. difficile* infection or (iii) individuals receiving antibiotic therapy without *C. difficile* infection. We compared the effects of the three different antibiotic classes on the intestinal microbiome and the effects of alterations of the gut microbiome on *C. difficile* infection at the DNA (total microbiota) and rRNA (potentially active) levels. A comparison of antibiotic classes showed significant differences at DNA level, but not at RNA level. Among individuals that developed or did not develop a *C. difficile* infection under antibiotics we found no significant differences. We identified single species that were up- or down regulated in individuals receiving antibiotics who developed the infection compared to non-infected individuals. We found no significant differences in the global composition of the transcriptionally active gut microbiome associated with *C. difficile* infections. We suggest that up- and down regulation of specific bacterial species may be involved in colonization resistance against *C. difficile* providing a potential therapeutic approach through specific manipulation of the intestinal microbiome.

Editor: Stefan Bereswill, Charité-University Medicine Berlin, Germany

Funding: This work was supported by the ERANET Project PathoGenoMics program grant number 0315441A. The funders had no role in study design, data collection and analysis, decision to publish, or preparation of the manuscript.

Competing Interests: LifeGlimmer GmbH is Start-up Company founded in 2012 by Prof. V. A. Pires Martins dos Santos, who is one of the co-authors of the manuscript. Prof. V. A. Pires Martins dos Santos primarily works at the University of Wageningen, The Netherlands. The shareholder status of the company has not compromised the objectivity or validity of the research, analyses, or interpretations in the paper.

* E-mail: s.ott@mucosa.de

❡ These authors contributed equally to this work.

¶ These authors share senior authorship.

Introduction

Clostridium difficile-associated diarrhea (CDAD) is caused by *C. difficile* toxins A and B and represents a serious burden for the clinical environment and the health care system [1]. Although the natural intestinal microbiota of healthy individuals can prevent colonization by *C. difficile* [2,3], the incidence of *C. difficile* infections has increased in the last decade [4]. Although approximately 5% of the adult population is colonized by *C. difficile* without showing any symptoms of diarrhea, the colonization rate increases up to 20% in hospitalized individuals [5]. Other factors such as advanced age, parenteral nutrition, renal insufficiency, previous hospitalizations, treatment with proton pump inhibitors and previous antibiotic (AB) treatment increase the risk of developing CDAD [6–8]. Several studies have shown an association between AB treatments such as Ampicillin, cephalosporins and fluoroquinolones and an increased risk of developing CDAD [9,10]. AB treatment can lead to AB-induced dysbiosis of the host-associated microbiome, with the potential absence of important gut microbial commensal species and an indirect break of mutualistic interactions [11,12]. This dysbiosis may result in the unlimited expansion of *C. difficile* [13,14]. Only a few studies have investigated the effect of AB on the dynamic changes of the intestinal microbiome in relation to the development of CDAD in humans. In additions to an increase of *C. difficile*, shifts within Bacteroidetes, *C. coccoides*, *Eubacterium rectale*, *Ruminococcus gnavus* and

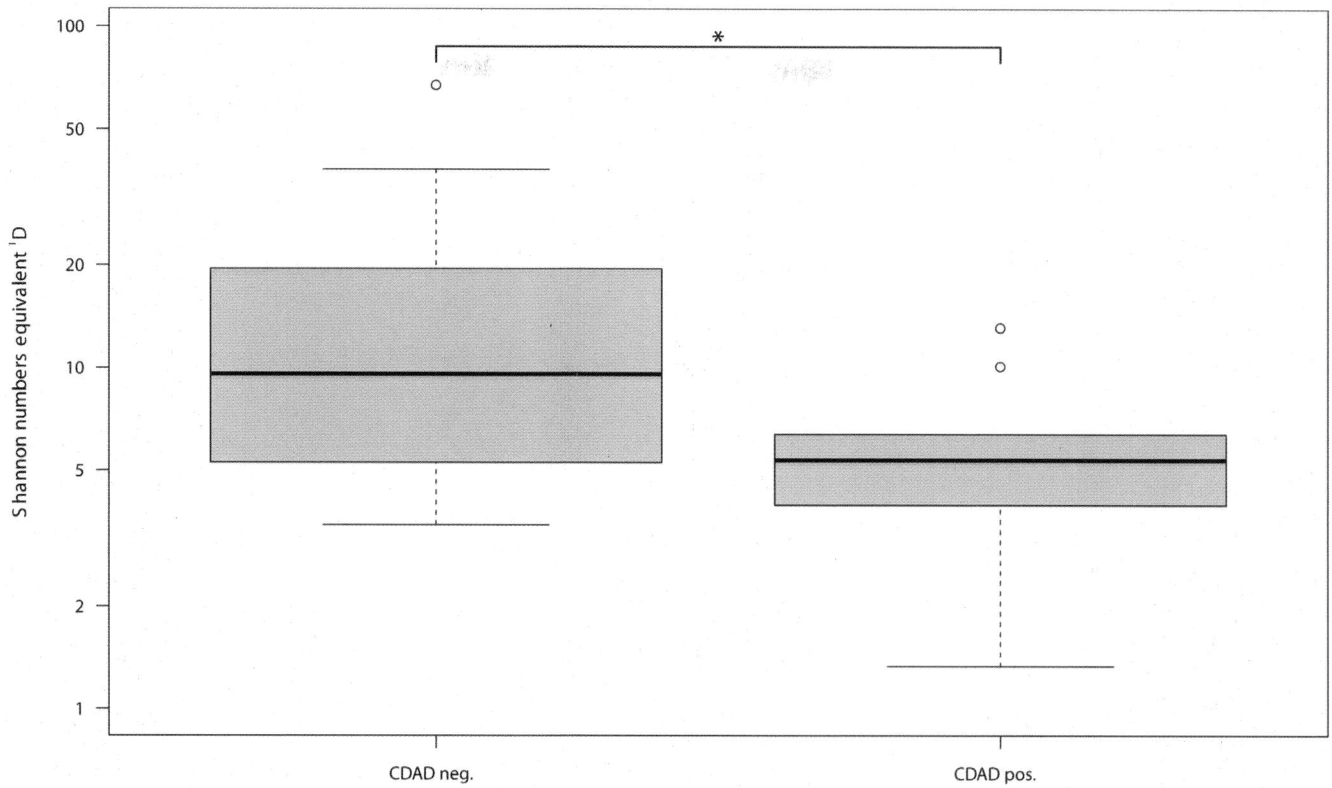

Figure 1. Distribution of Shannon number equivalents at DNA level concerning CDAD positive and CDAD negative individuals.

C. nexile have been shown [15]. A marked decrease in the microbial alpha diversity (the variety of organisms inhabiting a defined habitat) is likely responsible for facilitating intestinal colonization with *C. difficile* as has been observed by temperature gradient gel electrophoresis (TGGE) and bacterial clone libraries [14–16]. Manges *et al.* illustrated that low levels of Bacteroidetes are significantly associated with CDAD [14] and other data suggest that the absence of Bacteroidetes results in chronically relapsing *C. difficile* diarrhea [17]. A study investigating *C. difficile*-colonized infants revealed that low Firmicutes and Bacteroidetes ratios and an increase in facultative anaerobes facilitate colonization with *C. difficile* [18]. No previous studies have highlighted the specific role of the species present in the gut microbiota (indicated by the amounts of the 16S rRNA genes generated from DNA) and particularly the metabolically active species (indicated by the amounts of the 16S rRNA amplicons generated from cDNA) in individuals with CDAD due to antibiotic therapy [19].

We hypothesize that the gut microbial composition of individuals who develop CDAD is different from that of CDAD-negative individuals, in terms of the total and the active microbiota as determined by alpha and beta diversity measures. We further postulate that the alteration of the gut microbial composition is similar for different ABs (fluoroquinolones, cephalosporins and Ampicillin/Sulbactam).

Results

We compared the total microbiota and the microbiota with protein synthesis potential (potentially active) [19] of individuals developing CDAD to those not developing CDAD during the course of AB treatment with cephalosporins or Ampicillin/Sulbactam ($n=5$ each). This investigation was conducted by analysis of the V1–V2 variable regions of the bacterial 16S rRNA gene amplified from DNA or cDNA generated from RNA. We also investigated alterations of the gut microbiota composition induced by AB treatment with different AB classes, including fluoroquinolones, cephalosporins and Ampicillin/Sulbactam ($n=5$ each). Control cases ($n=18$) who did not receive antibiotic therapy were also included in the study.

Pyrosequencing yielded 524,582 sequences across all samples after preprocessing and a quality check. Sequences have been deposited in MG-RAST (http://metagenomics.anl.gov) under accession numbers 4546490.3 to 4546560.3. Random subsampling produced 96,387 sequences (1,083 reads for each sample) for further analysis. The sequences were binned at the 97% similarity level into a total of 4,991 operational taxonomic units (OTUs), with 2,763 and 3,175 OTUs at the DNA and RNA levels, respectively, with an avg. length of 355 bp in both cases.

Alpha diversity

As illustrated in Figure 1 and 2, significant differences in bacterial alpha diversity at the DNA ($P_{C.\ difficile\ DNA}=0.05$) but not at the RNA level ($P_{C.\ difficile\ RNA}=0.86$) were found between individuals with CDAD and the individuals without CDAD during AB therapy. Differences between the effects of Ampicillin/Sulbactam and cephalosporin treatments were not significant at either level ($P_{AB\ DNA}=0.90$, $P_{AB\ RNA}=0.20$). Consequentially, these antibiotics were treated as one group, named the ß-lactams (Ampicillin/Sulbactam/cephalosporins) in comparison to the fluoroquinolones and controls. Pair-wise differences regarding the bacterial alpha diversity of the healthy individuals and individuals treated with the ß-lactam antibiotics or fluoroquinolones were not statistically significant at the DNA level. At the RNA level the difference between healthy controls and individuals

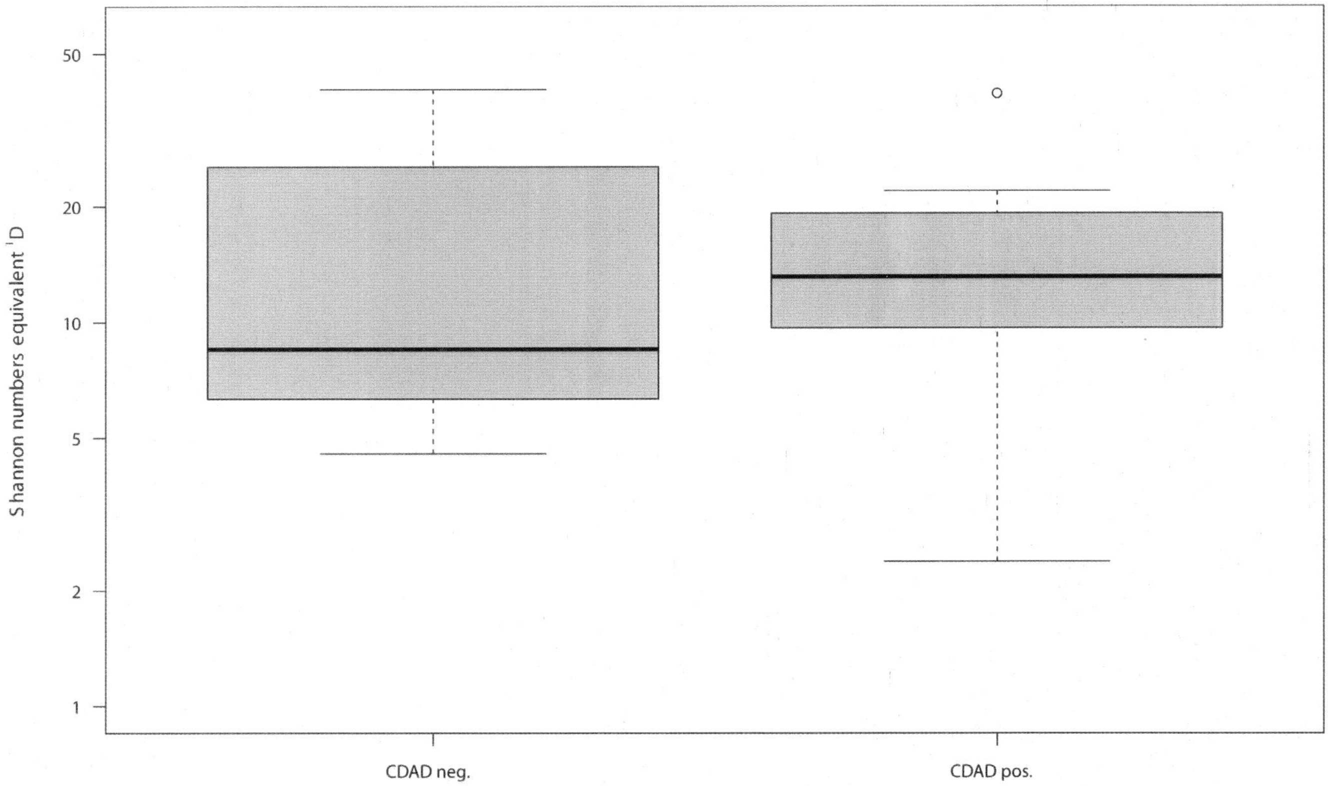

Figure 2. Distribution of Shannon number equivalents at RNA level concerning CDAD positive and CDAD negative individuals.

treated with ß-lactam antibiotics reached statistical significance (Figure S1) ($P_{Contr\text{-}ß\text{-}lactam\ RNA} = 0.01$).

Beta diversity

Redundancy analyses (RDA) with subsequent pair-wise comparisons were used to assess the differences in total and potentially active OTUs of the gut microbial community in the individuals with and without CDAD development during AB treatment. No significant difference was found in total and potentially active gut microbiota of individuals with CDAD compared to individuals without CDAD.

Individuals treated with Ampicillin/Sulbactam or cephalosporins showed no significant differences in total and potentially active gut microbiota. These groups were further treated as one group (cephalosporins/Ampicillin/Sulbactam (ß-lactam)). Graphical representations of the RDA models are shown in Figure 3 (DNA) and 4 (RNA). The gut microbiota of individuals treated with ß-lactam were significantly different from those treated with fluoroquinolones at the DNA level ($P_{DNA} < 0.01$), but not at the RNA level ($P_{RNA} = 0.26$). Healthy controls harbored gut microbiota significantly different compared to those of individuals treated with either ß-lactam antibiotics or fluoroquinolones at both levels ($P_{ß\text{-}Lactam\ DNA} < 0.01$, $P_{fluoroquinolones\ DNA} < 0.01$, $P_{ß\text{-}Lactam\ RNA} < 0.01$, $P_{fluoroquinolones\ RNA} < 0.01$).

Bacterial distribution in fecal samples (OTU-independent)

As shown in Figures S2 and S3, fluctuations among the relative amounts of bacterial phyla and families were observed at the DNA and RNA levels. Firmicutes were the dominant phylum in all control and AB samples.

Compared to controls, treatment with ß-lactam antibiotics resulted in a decrease in Firmicutes and increase of Bacteroidetes at the DNA and RNA levels. This decrease did not occur with fluoroquinolone treatment. The relative amount of Proteobacteria increased at DNA level (mean increase from $0{,}65\%_{DNA\text{-}controls}$ to $15\%_{DNA\text{-}ß\text{-}lactam}$, $1{,}85\%_{DNA\text{-}fluoroquinolones}$) and RNA level (mean increase from $12{,}48\%_{RNA\text{-}controls}$ to $22{,}5\%_{RNA\text{-}ß\text{-}lactam}$, $17{,}24\%_{RNA\text{-}fluoroquinolones}$) due to treatment with ß-lactam antibiotics and fluoroquinolones in all individuals. At the bacterial family level AB treatments resulted in an increase of Enterobacteriaceae (mean increase from $0{,}38\%_{DNA\text{-}controls}$ to $15\%_{DNA\text{-}ß\text{-}lactam}$, $1{,}7\%_{DNA\text{-}fluoroquinolones}$) at DNA but not at RNA level. Furthermore, a marked decrease of Lachnospiraceae, compared to controls, at RNA level (mean decrease from $23\%_{RNA\text{-}controls}$ to $6{,}6\%_{RNA\text{-}ß\text{-}lactam}$, $15\%_{RNA\text{-}fluoroquinolones}$) was observed. Thereby, reduction of Lachnospiraceae in individuals with CDAD (mean decrease from $23\%_{RNA\text{-}controls}$ to $4{,}4\%_{RNA\text{-}ß}$-lactam and $17\%_{DNA\text{-}controls}$ to $4\%_{DNA\text{-}ß\text{-}lactam}$) differed from individuals without CDAD (mean decrease from $23\%_{RNA\text{-}controls}$ to $9\%_{RNA\text{-}ß\text{-}lactam}$ and $17\%_{DNA\text{-}controls}$ to $11\%_{DNA\text{-}ß\text{-}lactam}$).

Indicator taxa

Indicator OTUs (in analogy to indicator taxa) are OTUs predominant in a certain sample type while only irregularly found in a comparison sample type. Because no significant difference in gut microbial composition was observed among individuals treated with different ABs at the RNA level (fluoroquinolones compared to ß-lactam antibiotics), an indicator analysis was performed by comparing all AB samples treated as one group to the healthy controls at the RNA level. Indicator OTUs listed in Tables S1a–c were responsible for differences between controls and individuals treated with ß-lactam antibiotics and fluoroquinolones at DNA level (Table S1a) and between controls and ABs at the RNA level (Table S1b). Eighteen and 20 indicator OTUs were identified at

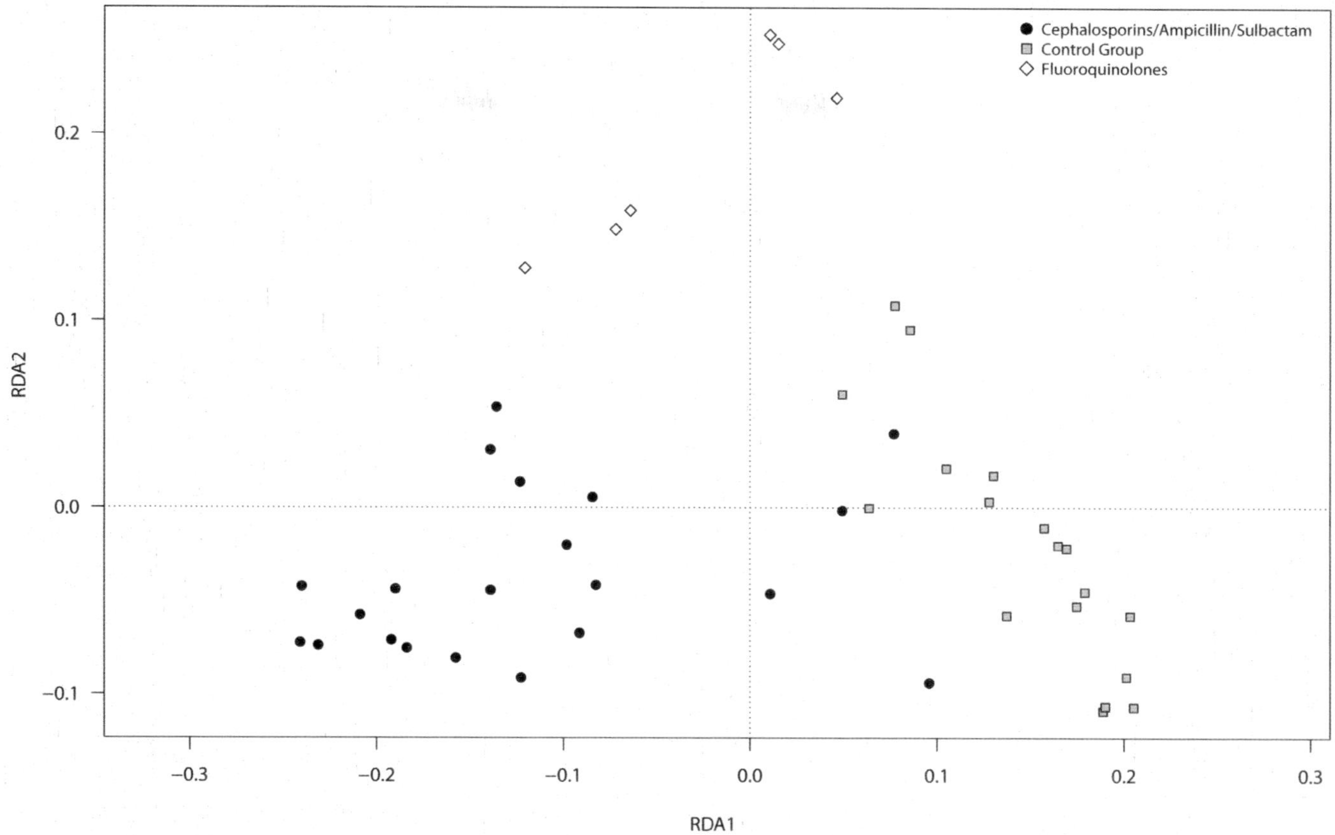

Figure 3. Graphical representation (distance plots) of the redundancy analysis (RDA) model of Hellinger-transformed OTU abundances. The model illustrate the relationship of gut microbes of healthy controls, individuals treated with ß-lactam antibiotic (Cephalosporins/Ampicillin/Sulbactam) and individuals treated with fluoroquinolones at DNA level.

the DNA and RNA levels, respectively. Eight OTUs at RNA level were indicators for healthy controls and showed homology to *Faecalibacterium prausnitzii*, *Coprococcus*, *Eubacterium*, Lachnospiraceae and *Clostridium*. Twelve OTUs were indicators for AB treatment, affiliated with *Blautia*, *Streptococcus parasanguinis*, *Clostridium ramnosum*, *Enterococcus lacti*, *Halomonas*, *Propionibacterium acnes and Staphylococcus epidermidis*. At DNA level six OTUs indicating healthy controls showed homology to *Faecalibacterium prausnitzii*, *Coprococcus* and *Eubacterium*. Ten OTUs indicating fluoroquinolone treatment were associated with *Blautia*, *Subdoligranulum*, *Adlercreutzia*, *Clostridium and Ruminococcus*. Two OTUs (*Enterobacter*, and *Enterococcus lacti*) indicated treatment with ß-lactam antibiotics.

No overall effect on the gut microbial composition was found in case CDAD. Rather an effect was found on single OTUs, as few microbial indicators could be identified as specific for CDAD during AB treatment. Table S1c shows the indicator OTUs found in individuals with and without CDAD at RNA and DNA levels; briefly, four indicator OTUs associated to individuals with CDAD (*Streptococcus*, *Enhydrobacter* and *Granulicatella* at RNA, and, as expected, *Clostridium difficile* at the DNA level) and two in non-CDAD individuals (*Adlercreutzia* and *Collinsella* at DNA level).

Discussion

C. difficile infections can be provoked by intestinal detrimental events caused by AB-induced microbial imbalances and a loss of colonization resistance. As bacterial protein synthesis potential may indicate an important pathophysiological role, we examined additionally to DNA the amounts of 16S rRNA amplicons generated from cDNA in individuals receiving AB treatment. Although a few studies have investigated these imbalances based on AB treatment in the context of CDAD development in humans, we present the first study based on high-throughput sequencing technology that investigates the development of CDAD depending on the gut microbial profiles associated with specific AB therapy. As it was not possible to obtain larger sample sizes for each group we expected to recognize only large effects between the compared groups.

Decreased alpha diversity in CDAD development at the DNA, but not at the RNA level

Alpha diversity expressed as effective OTU richness ^1D (a.k.a. Shannon numbers equivalent) was used to assess differences in cumulative OTU abundance. ^1D was consistently and significantly higher (by factor 2) in individuals without CDAD than in individuals with CDAD at the DNA level but not at the RNA level. Higher ^1D is associated with higher species richness and/or evenness. Our results reveal that lower species richness at the DNA level might be indicative of colonization with *C. difficile*. These results at the DNA level are in agreement with the results of Chang *et al.*, who used bacterial clone libraries and observed that an overall collapse of bacterial alpha diversity (Shannon index) is responsible for *C. difficile* colonization [15]. Alpha diversity was not significantly different at the RNA level, indicating a rather stable potentially active microbiota. As the potentially active gut microbiota is more important to the host, these results may be more relevant. Results at RNA level contradict those at DNA level

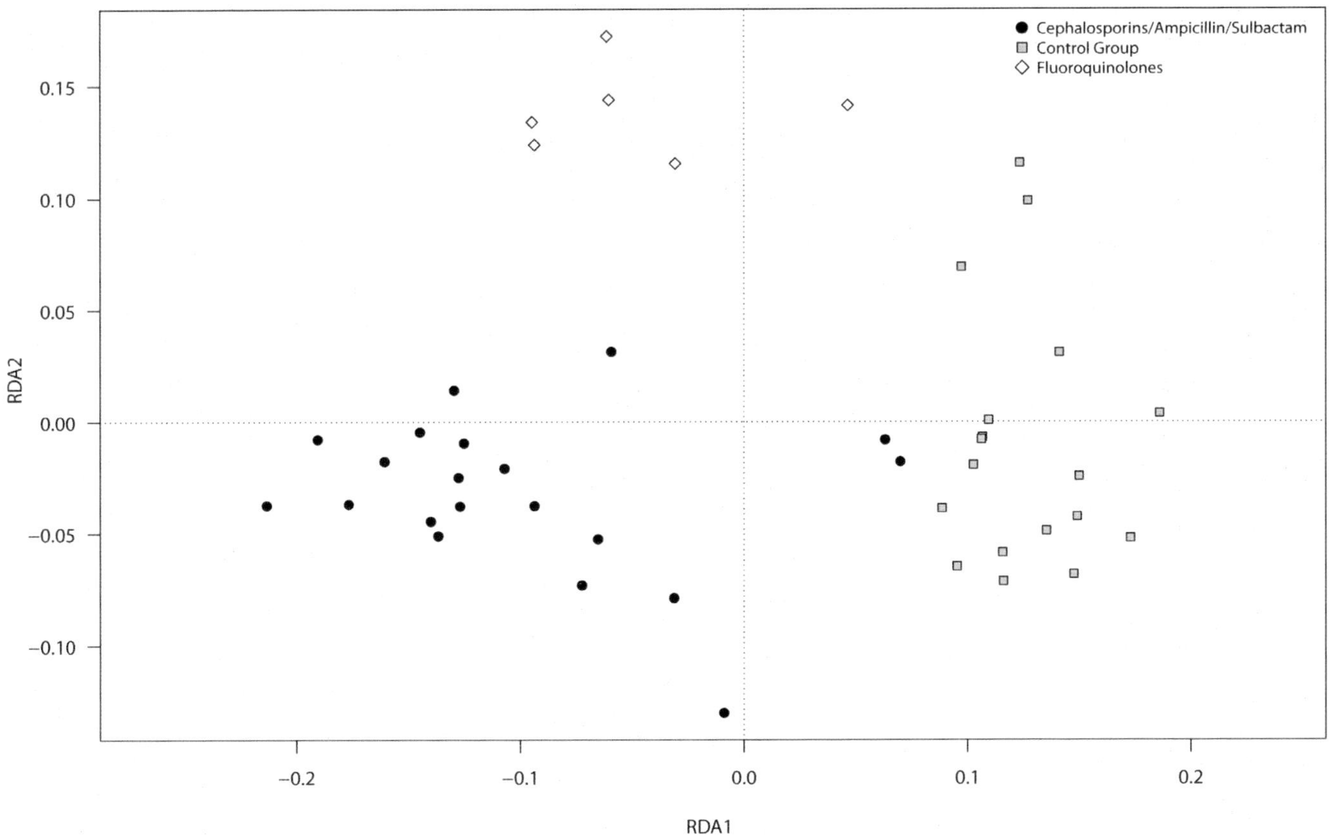

Figure 4. Graphical representation (distance plots) of the redundancy analysis (RDA) model of Hellinger-transformed OTU abundances. The model illustrate the relationship of gut microbes of healthy controls, individuals treated with ß-lactam antibiotic (Cephalosporins/Ampicillin/Sulbactam) and individuals treated with fluoroquinolones at RNA level.

and support the assumption that the development of CDAD is not related to a collapse in alpha diversity of the gut microbiota, although AB therapy has decreased microbial α-diversity. It is possible that a reduction in the amounts of specific potentially active OTUs that may be involved in colonization resistance against *C. difficile* correlates with a loss of their functional role in the gut (i.e. the production of metabolites and antimicrobial substances), which could predispose individuals to *C. difficile* colonization.

Development of CDAD is independent of gut microbial composition

The AB therapy used in this study affected the human gut microbiota and led to compositional shifts. Gut microbial composition showed no connection to CDAD development during AB treatment with ß-lactam antibiotics at DNA or RNA level. Because active gut bacterial diversity did not significantly change with CDAD, the loss of colonization resistance against *C. difficile* does not appear to be related to an overall collapse or overall reduction of the composition of the human gut microbiota during AB treatment. This trend was also shown by Reeves *et al.* in a murine model [20], which suggested that specific changes of single gut microbial members in the course of AB treatment may affect the susceptibility of the host to *C. difficile*. This finding is consistent with the clinical results of Blondeau *et al.* showing that the risk of CDAD development differs with different ABs based on their antimicrobial spectrum [21].

This study showed for the first time that development of CDAD is not dependent on the specific composition of the potentially active gut microbiota. The microbiota with protein synthesis potential are more essential for the host than the inactive microbiota because of factors such as metabolic turnover. Because no specific active gut microbial composition is associated with CDAD, the loss of colonization resistance against *C. difficile* is more likely to depend on the amounts of specific gut microbial members and their functional capacities rather than on the overall compositional level. In cases of CDAD a loss of the functional capacity of single species, possibly involving the production of metabolites such as short chain fatty acids (SCFA) or antimicrobial compounds, could allow the growth of *C. difficile*. Several investigators have reported that low concentrations of SCFA in the gut are associated with the presence of *C. difficile* [22,23]. Reeves *et al.* showed that high levels of Lachnospiraceae contributed to colonization resistance against *C. difficile* or other pathogens in mice [20]. Members of Lachnospiraceae have the ability of ferment complex carbohydrates to SCFA and assist maintaining intestinal homeostasis [24]. In our study the gut microbiota of individuals with CDAD compared to CDAD negative individuals showed lower amounts of Lachnospiraceae as a result of AB treatment. Members of Lachnospiraceae were further identified as an indicator OTU at RNA level belonging to a healthy host. High or low levels of specific gut members such as Lachnospiraceae in relation to their functional role could play a central role in colonization resistance against *C. difficile* in humans. A study involving collection of fecal samples of individuals before and during CDAD development in the course of AB treatment could clarify the role of Lachnospiraceae and other specific gut members in humans with regard to colonization resistance against *C. difficile*.

Different AB classes reduce the same beneficial bacteria and lead to an increase in opportunistic pathogens

We demonstrated that treatment with antibiotics such as Ampicillin/Sulbactam and cephalosporins (both ß-lactam antibiotic) affected the total gut microbiota in a similar manner. Treatment with fluoroquinolones affected the total gut microbiota differently from β-lactam treatment. The effects of Ampicillin/Sulbactam, cephalosporins and fluoroquinolones on the potentially active gut microbiota were indistinguishable. This finding led to the development of identical indicator OTUs at the RNA level for the different AB classes. Indicator OTUs associated with *Faecalibacterium prausnitzii* have been reported to be decreased due to AB treatment [25]. A decrease in *Faecalibacterium prausnitzii* as a result of AB treatment is important because this bacterium exhibits anti-inflammatory capacity and a reduction in the amount of this bacterium was shown to be associated with inflammatory diseases such as Crohn's disease (CD) or ulcerative colitis (UC) [2–27]. A reduction in potentially active *Coprococcus* was induced by both AB classes. This bacterium has been reported to be gut protective and beneficial for human health [28–30]. There was an increase in potentially active bacteria, including *Streptococcus parasanguinis*, *Clostridium rhamosum*, *Enterococcus lacti*, *Eggerthella lenta*, *Halomonas*, *Ralstonia*, and *Propionibacterium acnes* during AB treatment. The presence of *Streptococcus parasanguinis* was shown in previous studies to be associated with healthy oral microflora, and *Eggerthella lenta* has been reported to be a cause of UC [31,32]. *Propionibacterium acnes* is a known opportunistic pathogen that normally does not harm its host. Low host resistance and high amounts of *P. acnes* have been shown to be involved in prostate inflammation, sarcoidosis and SAPHO (synovitis, acne, pustulosis, hyperostosis, osteitis). The increase of these potentially active opportunistic pathogens induced by AB medication may be important, especially in association with decreased host resistance. The observed higher amounts during AB therapy may be caused by AB resistance mechanisms, as it has been reported for *P. acnes* and *E. lenta* [33–35].

The effects of the ABs used in this study were similar at the RNA level. Some ABs target cell wall synthesis (cephalosporins and Ampicillin/Sulbactam), while others interfere with essential bacterial enzymes (fluoroquinolones) [36,37]. This finding suggests that the most important gut microbiota members with protein synthesis potential are affected in similar ways independently of the AB class. The majority of previous studies investigated the gut microbiota during AB treatment at the level of total species (DNA). These studies observed different shifts for different ABs [38–41]. Our results support the previous findings at the DNA level but not at the RNA level. Similar effects of different ABs on the gut microbiota at the RNA level could explain why various ABs are associated with identical intestinal diseases such as AB-associated diarrhea.

Conclusion

Employing high-throughput sequencing we showed that different AB classes (Ampicillin/Sulbactam, cephalosporins and fluoroquinolones) affect the gut microbiota similarly at the RNA level but differently at the DNA level. This finding explains why several different AB classes are associated with similar intestinal problems. CDAD development during AB therapy is not associated with a specific gut microbial composition at the RNA or DNA level. AB treatment affects the microbial composition and decreases the bacterial α-diversity, but no overall diversity collapse caused by AB treatment is responsible for the weak colonization resistance against *C. difficile*. CDAD development is a multifactorial pattern involving the interplay of gut microbial shifts and reduction of specific gut members and diversity caused by AB treatment which can lead to a lack of their functional integrity in colonization resistance against *C. difficile*. Future studies should investigate the development of CDAD and mechanisms of colonization resistance based on functional methods such as metatranscriptomics or metabolomics. Identification of single gut members contributing to colonization resistance may be helpful in determining the process of CDAD development in humans and may allow development of specific probiotics against CDAD. Furthermore, as we could not check for the type of *C.difficile* strains in infected patients, it would be interesting in future studies to characterize the type of *C.difficile* strains from gut samples of CDAD-positive individuals. This has the potential to correlate *C.diffi*cile strain types with specific changes of the gut microbiota as well as severity of clinical symptoms.

Materials and Methods

Study design

Study volunteers provided fecal samples and were divided into three different groups. Feces, collected from eighteen healthy individuals, were used as controls in this study (named "Controls"). Furthermore, fecal samples were obtained from hospitalized individuals five days after starting a therapy with one of the following antibiotic classes classified as fluoroquinolones ($n = 5$), cephalosporins) ($n = 5$) or Ampicillin/Sulbactam (penicillins) ($n = 5$) (named "AB-controls") in the Department for Internal Medicine at the University Hospital Schleswig-Holstein, Campus Kiel (UK-SH). Only samples obtained from individuals who did not develop CDAD during and up to 3 months after the antibiotic therapy were included in the group of AB controls. The third group (named "*C. difficile*") consisted of fecal samples collected from hospitalized individuals immediately after developing CDAD during therapy with cephalosporins or Ampicillin/Sulbactam (each with $n = 5$) (overview of study participants in Table S2). Further criteria for participation in the study were: age 65 years or older; no antibiotic, antimycotic or probiotic therapy in the previous 6 months; no history of hospitalization or diarrhea in the previous 6 months. All study participants gave general written informed consent prior to admission to hospital including molecular analysis of blood, biopsy and stool samples for scientific reasons. An additional ethical vote for intestinal microbiota analysis from stool samples was not deemed necessary by the local ethical board of the Medical Faculty of the Christian-Albrechts-University (CAU) in Kiel. Fecal samples were stored at $-80°C$ until further use.

Tracking of *Clostridium difficile* in fecal samples

Because the production of toxin A and B by *C. difficile* strains is associated with CDAD, all fecal samples were screened for presence of these toxins as well as for *glutamate dehydrogenase* antigen with an enzyme-linked immunosorbent assay (ELISA) at the Institute of Infectious Diseases (UKSH, Campus Kiel). *C. difficile* positivity of stool samples was verified by detection of the specific *C. difficile* toxin A and B, with a membrane immunoassay (TECHLAB; CLOSTRIDIUM DIFFICILE QUIK CHEK COMPLETE KIT, Alere GmbH, Köln, Germany).

Total DNA and RNA extraction

Total DNA extraction was performed with incubation of fecal samples in 200 µl TL-buffer and 25 µl proteinase-K for two hours at 56°C, before using the FastDNASPIN KIT FOR SOIL (Qiagen, Hilden, Germany) as previously described [42]. Total RNA from feces was isolated using the PowerMicrobiome RNA Isolation Kit (MO BIO Laboratories Inc, Carlsbad, CA) following the manufacturer's protocol. Extracted RNA was reverse transcribed into cDNA with the High Capacity cDNA Reverse Transcription Kit (Applied Biosystems, Foster City, USA) according to the manufacturer's instructions.

PCR amplification of variable region V1 to V2

The variable regions V1 and V2 of the 16S rRNA were amplified. Samples preparation and high throughput sequencing were performed according to previous studies [43].

Data cleansing and statistics

Data were preprocessed using MOTHUR version 1.27 [44] as described before [43]. Data analysis and multivariate statistical approaches were done in R v3.0.0 (http://www.R-project.org/). Analyses were separately performed with DNA-and RNA-level data. P-values in multiple testing scenarios were subjected to Benjamini-Hochberg correction ("q-values") [45]. Beta diversity analysis was conducted via redundancy analysis (RDA) [46] as implemented in the R package vegan v2.0-7 [47]. Count data of operational taxonomic units (OTU; defined by 97% sequence similarity) were Hellinger-transformed in order to produce valid results in RDA [48]. Alpha diversity was described by effective OTU richness ^1D (known as the Shannon numbers equivalent) [49,50], taking both the numbers and relative abundances of OTUs into account. The ^1D values were Box-Cox transformed to meet homoscedasticity and normality of residuals in subsequent analysis of variance (ANOVA).

In a first step, the effect of *C. difficile* associated diarrhea development in connection with β-lactam AB classes cephalosporins and Ampicillin/Sulbactam was assessed by a 2×2 factorial ANOVA. A subsequent one-way ANOVA was conducted with only AB as the independent factor, including also quinolones as well as the control group. Data from *C. difficile*-positive individuals were included in the second ANOVA if the *C. difficile* infection effect was non-significant in the first one. With significance of the second ANOVA, pairwise comparisons of factor levels were conducted.

In beta diversity, OTUs most likely to be responsible for differences between the group of AB treated individuals and controls were determined. OTUs were pre-filtered by profile likelihood selection [51] according to their vector lengths calculated from RDA scores (scaling 1). Pre-filtered OTUs significantly correlated with axes in the RDA model were subjected to indicator analysis with the R package indicspecies v1.6.7 [52].

Supporting Information

Figure S1 Distribution of Shannon number equivalents at RNA level in healthy controls and during treatment with Cephalosporins/Ampicillin/Sulbactam and Fluoroquinolones.

Figure S2 Distribution of OTUs at bacterial phylum level in fecal samples of healthy controls and during antibiotic treatment with Ampicillin/Sulbactam, Cephalosporins and Fluoroquinolones in CDAD positive and CDAD negative individuals at DNA and RNA level.

Figure S3 Distribution of OTUs at bacterial family level in fecal samples of healthy controls and during antibiotic treatment with Ampicillin/Sulbactam, Cephalosporins and Fluoroquinolones in CDAD positive and CDAD negative individuals at DNA and RNA level.

Table S1 **a:** Indicator OTUs of controls and AB treatment at the DNA level (Ctrl - controls, Fluoro-quinol - Fluoroquinolones). **b:** Indicator OTUs of controls and AB treatment at the RNA level (Ctrl - controls; AB includes Ampicillin/Sulbactam, Cephalosporins and fluoroquinolone). **c:** Indicator OTUs of individuals with and without CDAD at RNA and DNA level after treatment with Ampicillin/Sulbactam and cephalosporins.

Table S2 Characteristics of study participants.

Acknowledgments

We thank the Institute of Infectious Diseases (UKSH, Campus Kiel), Anita Hellmann, Manuela Kramp, Sanaz Sedghpour Sabet and Katja Cloppenborg-Schmidt for technical assistance and Markus B. Schilhabel as well as Sven Künzel for their expertise in 454 sequencing.

Author Contributions

Conceived and designed the experiments: VMdS SO. Performed the experiments: HK FAH AS AZ MF. Analyzed the data: HK SCN CK RAS VMdS MF AKF SO. Contributed reagents/materials/analysis tools: SCN CK VMdS MF. Wrote the paper: HK FAH RAS VMdS MF PCR SS AKF SO. Wrote application and received funding: SO.

References

1. Kyne L, Hamel MB, Polavaram R, Kelly CP (2002) Health care costs and mortality associated with nosocomial diarrhea due to C. difficile. Clin Infect Dis 23: 653–9.
2. Lawley TD, Walker AW (2013) Intestinal colonization resistance. Immunology 138: 1–11.
3. Thomas V, Rochet V, Boureau H, Ekstrand C, Bulteau S, et al. (2002) Molecular characterization and spatial analysis of a simplified gut microbiota displaying colonization resistance against Clostridium difficile. Microbial ecology in Health and Disease 14: 203–210.
4. Pepin J, Alary ME, Valiquette L, Raiche E, Ruel J, et al. (2005) Increasing risk of relapse after treatment of Clostridium difficile colitis in Quebec, Canada. Clin Infect Dis 40: 1591–7.
5. McDonald LC (2006) Confronting C. difficile in inpatient health care facilities. Clin Infect Dis 45: 1274–6.
6. Cloud J, Kelly CP (2007) Update on C. difficile associated diseases. Curr Opin Gastroenterol 23: 4–9.
7. Bartlett JG (2006) Narrative review: the new epidemic of C. difficile-associated enteric diseases. Ann Intern Med 145:758–64.
8. Loo VG, Poirier L, Miller MA, Oughton M, Libman MD, et al. (2005) A predominant clonal multi-institutional outbreak of C. difficile-associated diarrhea with high morbidity and mortality. N Engl J Med 353: 2442–9.
9. Gerding DN (2004) Clindamycine, cephalosporins, fluoroquinolones, and C. difficile-associated diarrhea: this is an antimicrobial resistance problem. Clin Infect Dis 38: 646–648.
10. Sullivan A, Edlund C, Nord C (2001) Effect of antimicrobial agents on the ecological balance of human microflora. Lancet Infect Dis 1: 101–114.
11. Jernberg C, Löfmark S, Edlund C, Jansson JK (2007) Long-term ecological impacts of antibiotic administration on the human intestinal microbiota. ISME J 1:56–66.
12. Freeman HJ (2008) Recent developments on the role of C. difficile in inflammatory bowel disease. World J Gastroenterol 14: 2794–2796.
13. Wilson K (1993) The microecology of C. difficile. Clin Infect Dis 16:214–218.

14. Manges A, Labbe A, Loo V, Atherton J, Behr M, et al. (2010) Comparative metagenomic study of alterations to the intestinal microbiota and risk of nosocomial C. difficile-associated disease. J Infect Dis 202: 1877–1884.
15. Chang JY, Antonopoulos DA, Kalra A, Tonelli A, Khalife WT, et al. (2008) Decreased diversity of the fecal Microbiome in recurrent C. difficile-associated diarrhea. J Infect Dis 197: 435–8.
16. Barc MC, Bourlioux F, Rigottier-Gois L, Charrin-Sarnel C, Janoir C, et al. (2004) Effect of amoxicillin-clavulanic acid on human fecal flora in gnotobiotic mouse model assessed with fluorescence hybridization using group-specific 16S rRNA probes in combination with flow cytometry. Antimicrob Agents Chemother 48:1365–8.
17. Tvade M, Rask Madsen J (1989) Bacteriotherapy for chronic relapsing C. difficile diarrhea in six patients. Lancet 1: 1156–1160.
18. Rosseau C, Lemee L, Le Monnier A, Poilane I, Pons JL, et al. (2011) Prevalence and diversity of C. difficile strains in infants. J Med Microbiol 60: 1112–8.
19. Blazewicz SJ, Barnard RL, Daly RA, Firestone MK (2013) Evaluating rRNA as an indicator of microbial activity in environmental communities: limitations and uses. ISME 7: 2061–8
20. Reeves AE, Theriot SM, Bergin IL, Huffnagle GB, Schloss PD, et al. (2011) The interplay between microbiome dynamics and pathogen dynamics in a murine model of Clostridium difficile infection. Gut Microbes 2: 145–58.
21. Blondeau JM (2009) What have we learned about antimicrobial use and the risks for Clostridium difficile-associated diarrhea? Journal of Antimicrobial Chemotherapy 63: 238–242.
22. Hove H, Tvede M, Mortensen PB (1996) Antibiotic-associated diarrhea, Clostridium difficile, and short-chain fatty acids. Scand J Gastroenterol 31: 688–93.
23. Rolfe RD (1984) Role of volatile fatty acids in colonization resistance to Clostridium difficile. Infect. Immun 45: 185–191.
24. Cotta M, Forster R (2006) The family Lachnospiraceae, including the genera Butyrivibrio, Lachnospira and Roseburia. Prokaryotes 4: 1002–1021.
25. Hill DA, Hoffmann C, Abt MC, Du Y, Kobuley D, et al. (2010) Metagenomic analysis reveal antibiotic-induced temporal and spatial changes in the intestinal microbiota with associated alterations in immune cell homeostasis. Mucosa Immunology 3; 148–158.
26. Fujimoto T, Imaeda H, Takahashi K, Kasumi E, Bamba S, et al. (2013) Decreased abundance of Faecalibacterium prausnitzii in the gut microbiota of Crohn's disease. J Gastroenterol Hepatol 28: 613–9.
27. Duboc H, Rainteau D, Rajca S, Humbert L, Farabos D, et al. (2012) Increase in fecal primary bile acids and dysbiosis in patients with diarrhea-predominant irritable bowel syndrome. Neurogastroenterol Motil 24:513–20.
28. Bajaj JS, Hylemon PB, Ridlon JM, Heuman DM, Daita K, et al. (2012) Colonic mucosal microbiome differs from stool microiome in cirrhosis and hepatic encephalopathy and is linked to cognition and inflammation. Am J Physiol Gastrointest Liver Physiol 303: G675–85.
29. Chen W, Liu F, Ling Z, Tong X, Xiang C (2012) Human intestinal lumen and mucosa-associated microbiota in patients with colorectal cancer. PloS One 7: e39743.
30. Kassinen A, Krogius-Kurikka L, Mäkivuokko H, Rinttilä T, Paulin L, et al. (2007) The fecal microbiota of irritable bowel syndrome patients differs significantly from that of healthy subjects. Gastroenterology 133: 24–33.
31. Lau S, Woo PC, Fung AM, Chan KM, Woo GK, et al. (2004) Anaerobic, non-sporulating, Gram-positive bacilli bacteraemia characterized by 16S rRNA gene sequencing. J Med Microbiol 53: 1247–1253.
32. Lau S, Woo PC, Woo GK, Fung AM, Wong MK, et al. (2004). Eggerthella hongkongensis sp. nov. and Eggerthella sinensis sp. nov., two novel Eggerthella species, account for half of the cases of Eggerthella bacteremia. Diagn Microbiol Infect Dis 49: 255–263.
33. Rajeshwair DS, Basappa BK (2011) Vancomycin Resistance Genes in Various Organisms- An Insilico Study. IJBB 5(2).
34. Coates P, Vyakrnam S, Eady EA, Jones CE, Cove JH, et al. (2002) Prevalence of antibiotic-resistant propionibacteria on the skin of acne patients: 10-year surveillance data and snapshot distribution study. Br J Dermatol 146: 840–8.
35. Tzellos T, Zampelli V, Makrantonaki E, Zouboulis CC (2011) Treating acne with antibiotic-resistant bacterial colonization. Expert Opin Pharmacother 12: 1233–47.
36. Mutschler E, Geisslinger HK, Kroemer P (2008) Arzneitmittelwirkungen. Lehrbuch der Pharmakologie und Toxikologie p794.
37. Köhler W, Eggers HJ, Fleischer B (2001) Medizinische Mikrobiologie. 8. Auflage, Elsevier, Munick, p.200.
38. Antonopoulos DA, Huse SM, Morrison HG, Schmidt TM, Sogin ML, et al. (2009) Reproducible community dynamics of the gastrointestinal microbiota following antibiotic perturbation. Infect Immun; 77: 2367–75.
39. Croswell A, Amir E, Teggatz P, Barman M, Salzman NH (2009) Prolonged impact of antibiotics on intestinal microbial ecology and susceptibility to enteric Salmonella infection. Infect Immun 77: 2741–2753.
40. De La Cochetiere MF, Durand T, Lepage P, Bourreille A, Galmiche JP (2005) Resilience of the dominant human faecal microbiota upon short-course antibiotic challenge. L Clin Microbiol 43: 5588–92.
41. Dethlefsen L, Huse S, Sogin ML, Relman DA (2008) The pervasive effects of an antibiotic on the human gut microbiota, as revealed by deep 16S rRNA sequencing. PLoS Biol 6:e280.
42. Rehman A, Sina C, Gavrilova O, Häsler R, Ott S, et al. (2011) Nod2 is essentiell for temporal development of intestinal microbial communities. Gut 60: 1354–62.
43. Stratil SB, Neulinger SC, Knecht H, Friedrichs AK, Wahl M (2013) Temperature-driven shifts in the epibiotic bacterial community of the brown macroalgae Fucus vesiculosus. Microbiologyopen 2: 338–49.
44. Schloss PD, Westcott SL, Ryabin T, Hall JR, Hartmann M, et al. (2009) Introducing mothur: open—source, platform-independent, community-supported software for describing and comparing microbial communities. Appl Environ Microbiol 75: 7537–41.
45. Benjamini Y, Hochberg Y (1995) Controlling the false discovery rate: a practical and powerful approach to multiple testing J R Statist Soc B 57: 289–300.
46. Borcard D, Gillet F, Legendre P (2011) Numerical ecology with R. New York : Springer. 319 p.
47. Oksanen J, Blanchet FG, Kindt R, Legendre O, Minchin PR, et al. (2013) Vegan: Community ecology package. R package version 2.0-7 ed.
48. Legendre P, Gallagher ED (2001) Ecologically meaningful transformation for ordination of species data. Oecologia 129: 271–280.
49. Jost L (2006) Entropy and diversity. Oikos 113: 363–375.
50. Jost L (2007) Partitioning diversity into independent alpha and beta components. Ecology 88: 2427–2439.
51. Zhu M, Ghodsi A (2006) Automatic dimensionality selection from the scree plot vial the use of profile likelihood. Computitional Statistics & Data Analysis 51: 918–930.
52. De Caceres M, Legendre P (2009) Association between species and groups of sites: indices and statistical interference. Ecology 90: 3566–3574.

Combination of ^{1}H NMR- and GC-MS-Based Metabonomics to Study on the Toxicity of *Coptidis Rhizome* in Rats

Yuting Zhou[1]❡, Qiongfeng Liao[2]❡, Manna Lin[1,2], Xuejiao Deng[1], Peiting Zhang[1], Meicun Yao[1], Lei Zhang[2], Zhiyong Xie[1]*

1 School of Pharmaceutical Sciences, Sun Yat-sen University, Guangzhou, People's Republic of China, **2** School of Chinese Materia Medica, Guangzhou University of Chinese Medicine, Guangzhou, People's Republic of China

Abstract

Background: *Coptidis Rhizome* (CR), widely applied to treat with heat and toxicity, is one of the most commonly used traditional Chinese medicine (TCM), however, an extensive dosage can induce toxicity. Diarrhea is one of the most frequent side effects of CR treatment.

Methodology/Principal Findings: In this study, metabonomics was combined with the multivariate statistical analysis to discover the endogenous metabolites which related to the diarrheal induced by CR. The male Sprague–Dawley rats were dosed with 4.95 g CR/kg weight. Urine samples were collected at day −1 (before treatment), and days 14 and 21 for NMR analysis. Serum and tissues were collected at day 14 for GC-MS analysis and histopathological examination, respectively. The urine and serum metabolic profiles provided clearer distinction between CR-treated group and control group, which was confirmed by body weight change and diarrhea. Through multivariate statistical analysis, 12 marker metabolites from ^{1}H NMR and 8 ones from GC-MS have been found. Among those metabolites, hippurate, acetate, alanine, glycine and glutamate are likely to break the balance of gut microbiota, whereas, lactate and 2-ketoisovalerate showed association with energy metabolism. Meanwhile, we observed that the CR-induced toxicity will recover when the treatment was stopped.

Conclusions/significance: These results suggest that the main reason for the CR-associated diarrhea might be disturbance in the normal gut microbiota. This metabonomics approach may provide an effective way to study the alteration of gut microbiota, which is expected to find broader application in other drug-induced gastrointestinal reaction assessment.

Editor: Daniel Monleon, Instituto de Investigación Sanitaria INCLIVA, Spain

Funding: This work was supported by Natural Science Foundation of China, number 81274028. The funders had no role in study design, data collection and analysis, decision to publish, or preparation of the manuscript.

Competing Interests: The authors have declared that no competing interests exist.

* E-mail: xiezy2074@yahoo.com

❡ These authors contributed equally to this work.

Introduction

Traditional Chinese Medicine (TCM) has gained increasing worldwide acceptance in recent years and is generally considered natural and harmless [1,2,3]. *Coptidis Rhizome* (CR, Chinese name is Huanglian) is a widely used Chinese herbal medicine and has been used as a heat-clearing and detoxifying agent for two thousand years. Extensive studies showed CR has many pharmacological actions with strong clinical implications, including antibacterial, anti-inflammatory, antihypertensive, antioxidative, antihyperglycemic and cholesterol-lowering effects [4,5,6,7,8,9]. CR is relatively safe in normal dosage, however, it can also cause adverse effects. Diarrhea is one of the most frequent side effects in CR treatment, with a prevalence rate about 19% [10], while the mechanisms of CR-induced diarrhea have not been fully elucidated. In addition, CR has also been reported to cause adverse reactions such as arrhythmia and liver function injury and even lead to death in some patients, in clinic in China [11]. Therefore, it is reasonable to speculate that CR is not safe to some extent. Up to now, most studies about CR toxicity focus on the toxic components of CR and its acute toxicity. There are relatively few studies on the diarrhea associated mechanism by CR treatment.

Diarrhea usually results from increasing amounts of fluid in the intestinal lumen due to osmotically active substances (osmotic diarrhea), impairing absorption or increasing secretion of water and electrolytes (secretory diarrhea) and accelerating intestinal transit [12,13]. Furthermore, persistent diarrhea leads to intestinal malabsorption of nutrients such as fat or bile acids and influences the composition of the microbial community. One universal activity of the intestinal microbiota is breakdown and fermentation of polysaccharides into short chain fatty acids (SCFAs) [14]. SCFAs, the major anion in stool, are synthesized from non-absorbed carbohydrate by the colonic microbiota, interfering with the production of SCFA in the colon may result in diarrhea [15]. Alterations in the diversity of the gut microbiota are believed to

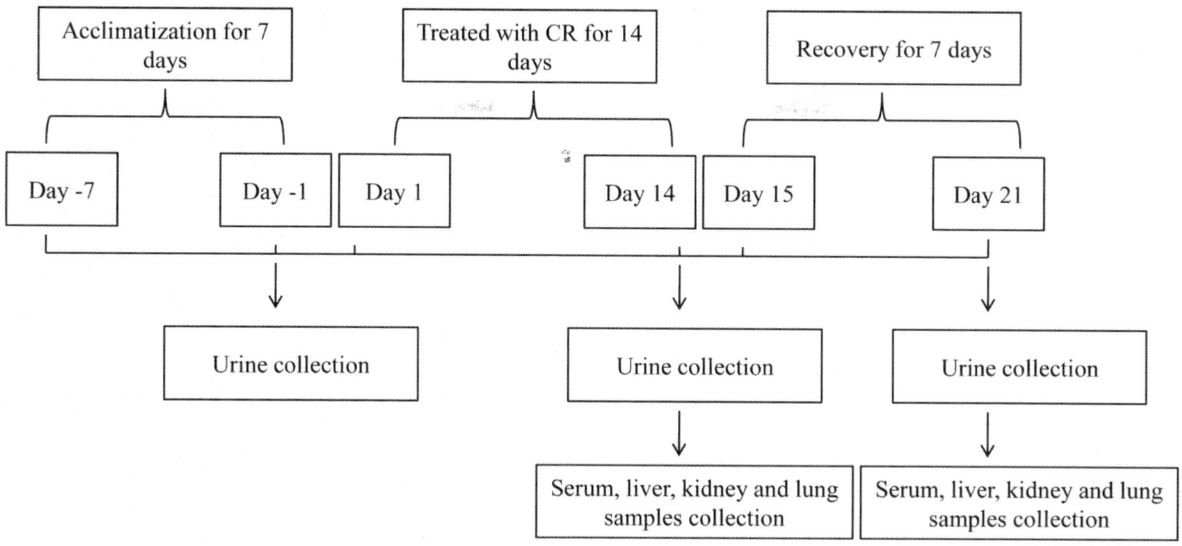

Figure 1. Schematic representation of animal treatment and sample collection. The experiment lasted 21 days, including 14 days of treatment with CR and 7 days of recovery, urine sample, serum sample and tissues were collected after 14 days of treatment and 7 days of recovery.

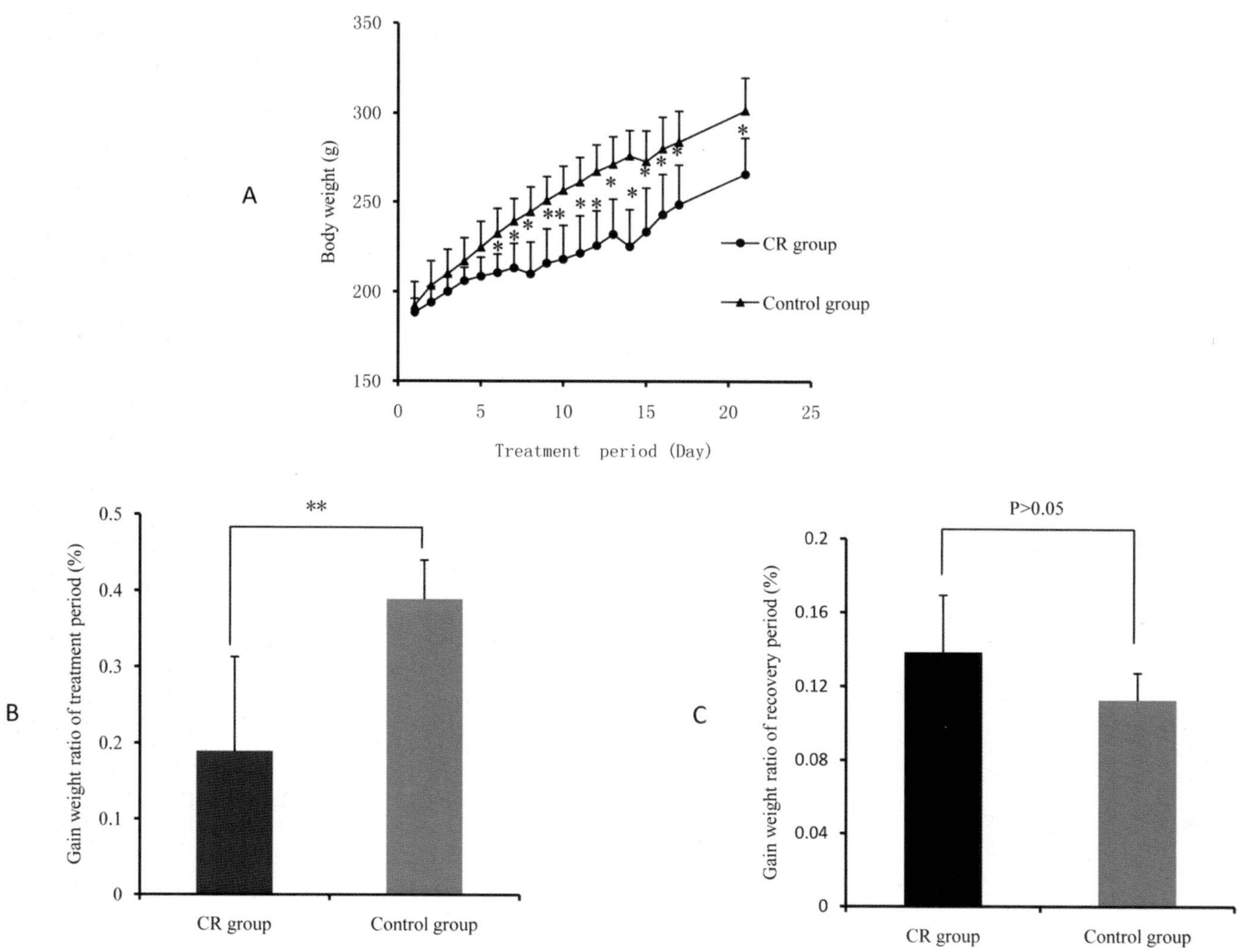

Figure 2. Changes of Body weight and increased body weight ratio of rats in CR-treated group and control group. A, body weight of rats in the whole experimental period; B, increased body weight ratio of treatment period; C, increased body weight ratio of recovery period. The data are expressed as means ± SD (*P<0.05; **P<0.01).

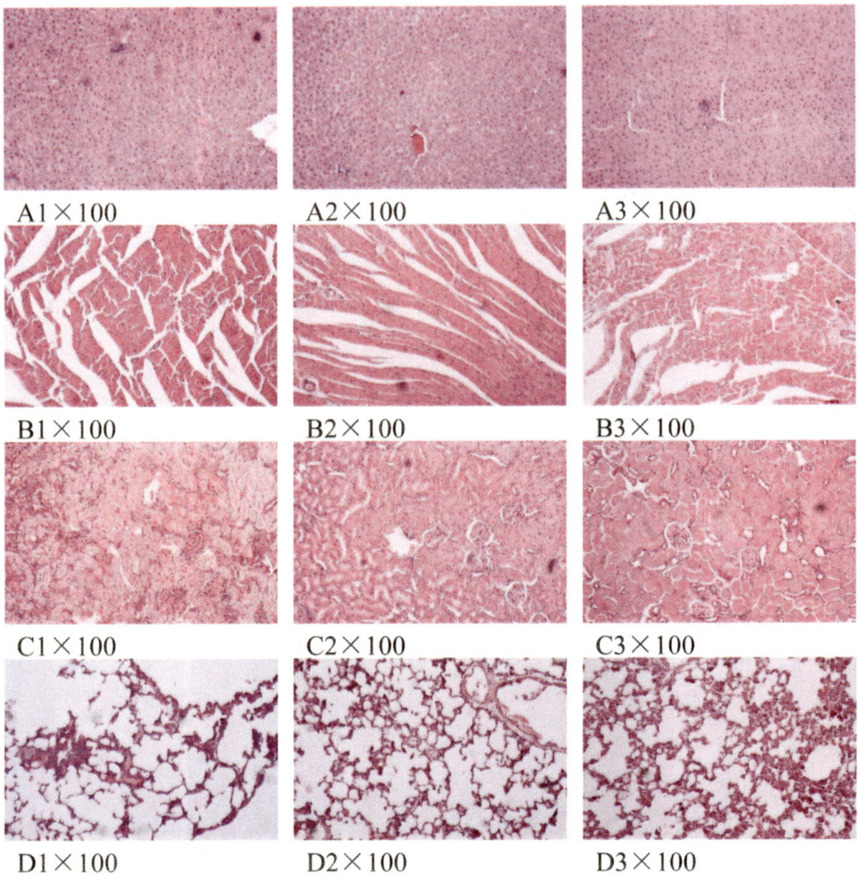

Figure 3. Histopathology of liver (A), heart (B), kidney (C) and lung (D) tissues. The tissues were collected after 14 days of CR treatment and 7 days of recovery. The tissues were fixed in 10% formaldehyde, and then stained using Hematoxylin and Eosin (H&E). Original magnification×100. A1, B1, C1 and D1, controls group of day 14; A2, B2, C2 and D2, CR-treated group of day 14; A3, B3, C3 and D3, CR-treated group after 7 days of recovery.

underlie the development of antibiotic-associated diarrhea (AAD) [16,17]. Therefore, we hypothesized CR-associated diarrhea may be caused by disruption of intestinal microbiota for its antibacterial activity. Hence, in this study we intend to figure out if CR induced diarrhea related to disturbance in gut microbiota and find out the biomarkers associated with gut dysbiosis to elucidate the mechanism of CR induced diarrhea.

Metabolomic investigations attempt to detect and profile changes in metabolites, which reflect changes in metabolic pathways and may provide information indicate the underlying mechanisms induced by a disease or toxic insults [18]. Nowadays, metabonomics is considered as a well-established system approach to characterize the metabolic phenotype, which results from a coordinated physiological response to various intrinsic and extrinsic parameters including environment, drugs, dietary patterns, lifestyle, genetics, and microbiome [19]. Lately, metabonomics had been successfully applied to study the mechanism of the hepatotoxicity induced by hydrazine [20] and toxicity of aconite root and its processed products [21], and to assess the associations between changes in bacterial communities' structure and dynamics of host metabolic patterns in humans [22]. In addition, as a systemic approach, metabolomics has brought enormous opportunities for improving detection of toxicity and biomarker discovery. Metabolomics reflects the function of organisms from terminal symptoms of metabolic networks and demonstrates metabolite changes of a complete system caused by interventions in a holistic context, which perfectly coincides with the holistic thinking of TCM [23,24]. High resolution ^{1}H nuclear magnetic resonance (NMR) spectrometry and gas chromatography–mass spectrometry (GC-MS)-based metabolome analysis study are well-established techniques for detection of the endogenous metabolic changes in biofluids such as serum and urine [25,26]. Because of the fundamental differences in the nature of NMR and GC-MS measurements, the results obtained using each platform contribute supplementary understanding of the complex metabolic response of rats treated with CR [27].

The main objective of this study was to apply the histopathology examination and metabolomics to confirm whether the diarrhea induced by CR treatment results from interference in gut microbiota. ^{1}H NMR and GC-MS were used to analyze the small molecular metabolites in the urine and serum samples. Multivariate data analysis, such as principal components analysis (PCA) and partial least squares-discriminant analysis (OPLS-DA) were utilized to find out related biomarkers, which could indicate the biological response to CR treatment. Our results showed that metabonomics approach may provide an effective way to study the alteration of gut microbiota.

Materials and Methods

Ethics statement

All animal experiments were conducted at the Sun Yat-sen University Animal Experiment Center (Guangzhou, China). The animal experiments were reviewed and approved by the Institu-

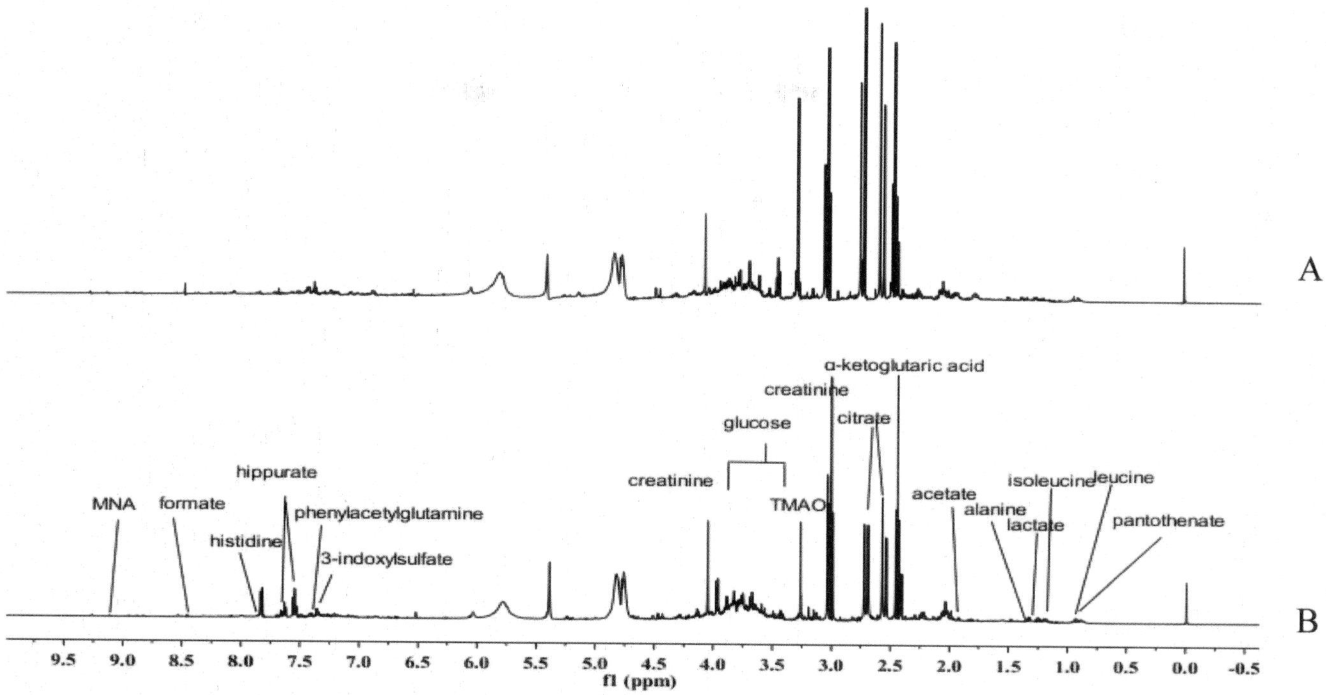

Figure 4. Representative urine ^{1}H NMR spectra from control and CR treated rats after 14 days of treatment: A, CR-treated group; B, control group. Assignments of endogenous metabolites were based on comparing chemical shifts and multiplicities of peaks to the literature as well as the Metabonomics Toolbox (http://www.hmdb.ca). The spectra were taken for urine samples containing 0.2 M Na_2HPO_4/NaH_2PO_4, pH 7.4 and 0.05% TSP as a chemical shift reference.

tional Animal Care and Use Committee of Sun Yat-sen University (SYXK, Licence No. 2011-0112), and conformed to the National Institute of Health guidelines on the ethical use of animals. All surgeries were operated under sodium pentobarbital anesthesia. Because this experiment was aim to investigate the toxicity of Coptidis Rhizome in rats, we did not stop the experiment when we observed the animals were beginning to loss of body weight & diarrhea. However, considering the suffering caused by loss of body weight & diarrhea, we stopped CR treatment after 14 days of CR administration. During the 14-day administration and 7-day recovery, no animal died as a result of CR treatment and all rats were sacrificed by sodium pentobarbital anesthesia. During the period of recovery, we found that the rats began to stop diarrhea gradually after three days of recovery. Besides, the growth of rats also returned to normal level.

Materials and chemicals

Coptidis Rhizome was purchased from Zhixin Medicine Health co., Ltd (Guangzhou, China), and identified by Prof. Ling Jiang (School of Pharmaceutical Sciences, Sun Yat-sen University). D_2O (with 0.05% sodium 3-trimethylsilyl-(2, 2, 3, 3-$^2H_4$)-1-propionate, TSP), Bis (Trimethylsilyl) -Trifluo-roacetamide (BSTFA, with 1% Trimethylchlorosilane, TMCS) and heptadecanoic acid were purchased from Sigma-Aldrich. Pyridine and chloroform were GC grade from China National Pharmaceutical Group Corporation (Shanghai, China).

Preparation of *Coptidis Rhizome* decoction

The dried roots of *Coptidis Rhizome* were ground into powder (about 30 meshes). The powder (200 g) was dipped in 2 liters of water for 1 h and then decocted to boil for 1 h. The decoction was filtered through four layers of gauze. Next, the residues were boiled once again for 1 h with 1.6 liters of water and the decoction was filtrated out with the above method. All filtrates were merged and concentrated to a volume equivalent 0.495 g *Coptidis Rhizome*/ml and stored at 4°C.

Animal treatment and sample collection

Male Sprague-Dawley (SD) rats with specific pathogen free (SPF) (weight: 180–200 g) were purchased from the medical laboratory animal center of Guangdong province (Guangzhou, China) and allowed to acclimate to the new environment for 7 days prior to experiment in a standard experimental room (12 h light/dark cycle, 24°C and 50%–70% humidity). All animals had ad libitum access to food and water. After acclimatization for 7 days, all rats were randomly divided into two groups (control group and CR-treated group). Controls were subjected to oral gavage with distilled water, while the CR-treated group was orally administered CR water solution at a dose of 4.95 g *Coptidis Rhizome*/kg of body weight for 14 days, respectively. The dosage of 4.95 g *Coptidis Rhizome*/kg weight was determined with reference to the Chinese Pharmacopoeia (10 g per human per day) and our pre-study results.

The experiment lasted 21 days, including 14 days of treatment and 7 days of recovery. Body weights were measured every day just before CR administration. The animals were observed daily for abnormalities of general appearance and behavior. Urine samples were collected from the metabolic cages with an ice packed Eppendorf tube on pre-dose day 1 and on days 14 and 21 post-dose. The fresh urine samples were immediately centrifuged at 10,000 g for 10 min, 4°C and the supernatants were collected and stored at −80°C for subsequent analysis. At the end of 14th day, five rats of each group were sacrificed by sodium pentobarbital anesthesia, intraperitoneal injection. Blood was

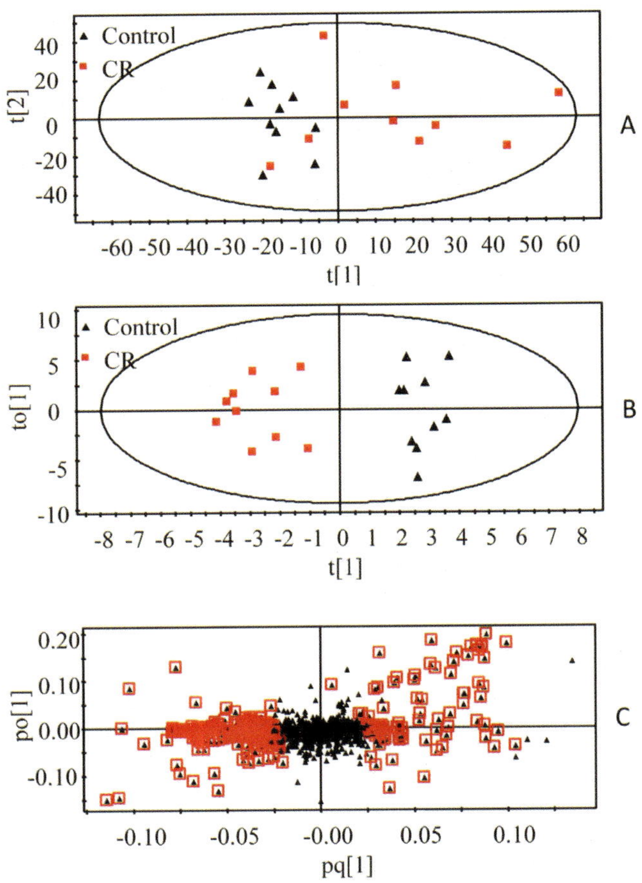

Figure 5. Multivariate analysis of urine samples from CR and control groups. A, PCA score plot, B, OPLS-DA score plot, C, OPLS-DA loadings plot. The urine samples were collected after 14 days of treatment. The model was established using one predictive and one orthogonal component.

Table 1. Endogenous metabolites selected as biomarkers in urine profile and their change trends.

Metabolites	Chemical shift(ppm)	CR vs. control
2-Keto-isovalerate	1.25	↑*
Lactate	1.33	↑*
Alanine	1.46	↑*
Acetate	1.91	↑**
N-acetylglycoprotein	2.03	↑*
Glutamate	2.36	↑**
Trimethylamine	2.82	↑*
Creatine	3.00	↓*
Phenylacetylglulamine	7.41	↑**
Hippurate	7.53,7.62,7.83	↓**
Trigonelline	8.07	↓*
Formate	8.46	↓**

↑, the increase in signal; ↓, the decrease in signal.
*Key: $p<0.05$.
**Key: $p<0.01$.

obtained from the abdominal aorta and collected in tubes without heparin in order to collect the serum. The liver, kidney, lung and heart specimens were removed and immediately fixed in 10% neutral buffered formalin for histopathological studies. The remaining rats were fed for another 7 days to recover and sacrificed at day 21 to collect serum sample and tissue specimens. The serum samples were stored at −80°C until analysis. A schematic presentation of animal treatment and sample collection was shown in Figure 1.

Histological examination

After fixation for 48 hours, all tissues were embedded in paraffin wax according to routine procedures. Five μm thick sections were cut and stained with hematoxylin-eosin (H&E) for histopathological evaluation. Two expert testers at the department of Pathology of Sun-yat-sen University analyzed the tissue slices.

Sample preparation and analysis

For NMR analysis, urine samples were removed from −80°C storage and thawed at room temperature, 500 μL of urine was mixed with 100 μL of phosphate buffer (0.2 M Na_2HPO_4/ NaH_2PO_4, pH 7.4) to minimize chemical shift variations and then centrifuged (14,000×g, 10 min, 4°C) to remove any precipitates. The supernatant was then pipetted into 5 mm NMR tube and 80 μL of D_2O containing 0.05% sodium 3-trimethylsilyl-(2, 2, 3, 3-$^2H_4$)-1-propionate (TSP) was added.

All ^{1}H NMR spectra of urine were collected at 298 K on a Bruker Avance 500 MHz spectrometer equipped with a Bruker inverse probe. The acquisition parameters were essentially refer to those previously reported [28,29]. The NMR spectrum was recorded using the water-presaturated standard one-dimensional Carr–Purcell–Meiboom–Gill (CPMG) pulse sequence, which can eliminate interference by macromolecules. The 90° pulse length, varying from 14.44 to 15.35 μs, was adjusted for each sample individually. 64 transients were collected into 128 k data points using a spectral width of 10 kHz with a relaxation delay of 3 s, and relaxation time (2 nτ) of 100 ms. The free induction decays (FIDs) were multiplied by an exponential function with a line-broadening factor of 0.3 Hz before Fourier transformation. The ^{1}H NMR spectra were corrected for phase and baseline distortion using software MestreNova (http://www.mestrelab.com/software/).

For GC-MS analysis, Serum metabolites were subjected to trimethylsilyl derivatization and analyzed by GC-MS according to Wei Jia [30]. Briefly, internal standard solution (10 μL of L-2-chlorophenylalanine in water, 0.3 mg/mL) was spiked into 100 μL aliquot of serum sample. A mixture of methanol/ chloroform (3:1) (300 μL) was used to extract the metabolites from the serum. After a vortexing period of 30 s and storage at −20°C for 10 min, the samples were centrifuged at 10000 g for 10 min. An aliquot of the 300 μL supernatant was vacuum-dried at room temperature in a glass vial. The residue was derivatized with 80 μL of methoxyamine (15 mg/mL in pyridine) at 30°C for 90 min, and followed by 80 μL of BSTFA (1%TMCS) at 70°C for 60 min, then centrifuged at 12 000 g for 10 min.

Each 1-μL of derivatized solution was injected into a DB-5MS capillary column (30 m×250 μm i.d., 0.25 μm film thickness; Agilent J&W Scientific, Folsom, CA) and conducted on a Finnigan gas chromatograph (Thermo Fisher Scientific Inc., U.S.A.) coupled with a mass spectrometer (TRACEDSQ). Helium was used as the carrier gas at a constant flow rate of 1.0 mL/min. The injection and transfer interface temperatures were both set to 280°C. Electron impact ionization at full scan mode (m/z 50–500) was used. Source temperature, electron energy, and solvent delay

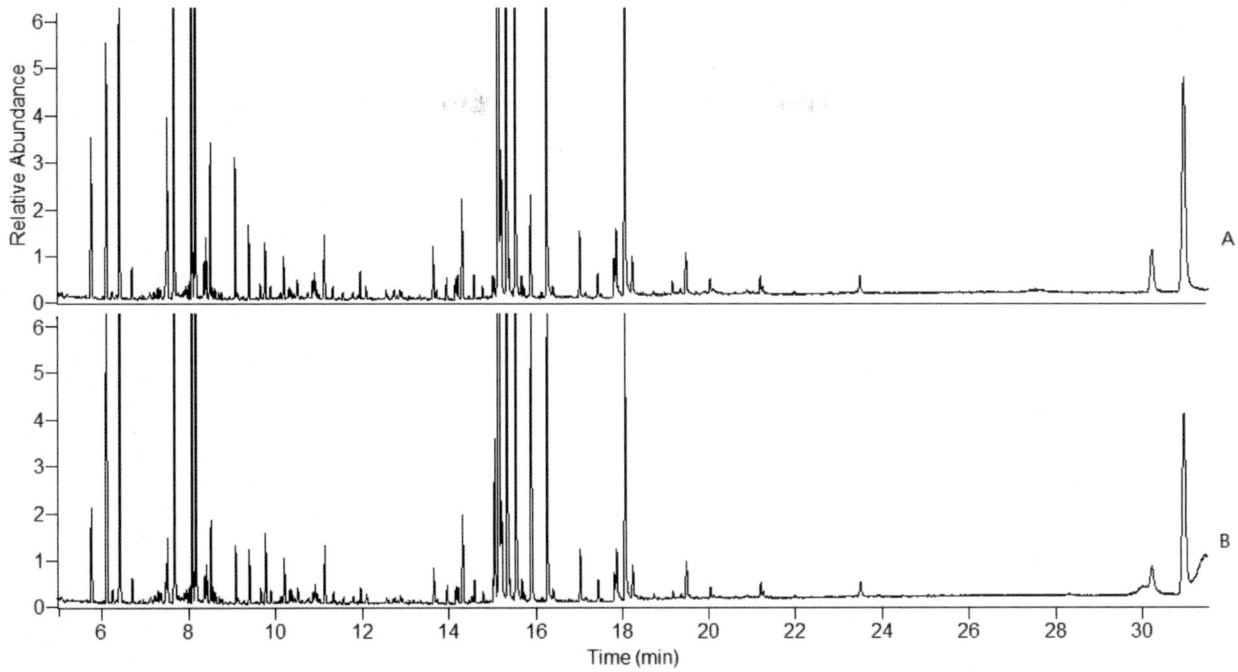

Figure 6. Representative GC-MS total ion chromatograms from the serum samples of control and CR treated rats after 14 days of treatment: A, control group; B, CR-treated group.

were set at 230°C, 70 eV, and 5 min, respectively. The GC oven temperature programming was started at 100°C and maintained for 5 min, followed by 20°C/min ramps to 170°C and maintained at 170°C for 1 min, 10°C/min to 270°C and maintained at 270°C for 1 min, and 2°C/min to 280°C, and a final 6 min maintenance at 280°C.

Data Processing

^{1}H NMR spectra data was analyzed using the established method of spectral binning and the new technique of targeted profiling [31]. Spectral binning was performed using the software MestreNova (http://www.mestrelab.com/software/). The chemical shifts of spectra were referenced to the TSP at δ 0.00. Each NMR spectrum was reduced to 0.04 ppm-wide segments between δ 0.5 and δ 9.5 ppm. The spectral regions of water (δ 4.60–5.20 ppm) and urea (δ 5.52–6.00 ppm) were removed from the analysis for all groups in order to prevent variation in each sample. The resonance from the NMR internal standard and reference (TSP) was also excluded from the dataset prior to analysis. Each NMR variable was normalized to the total area in order to allow a spectrum-to-spectrum comparison. Bins that showed significant differences between CR-treated group and control group were then assigned to the corresponding metabolites by comparing chemical shifts and multiplicities of peaks to the literature or online databases.

Raw GC-MS files were exported into the platform-independent net CDF (*.cdf) and loaded into XCMS software (version 1.6.1) based on R-program version 2.4.0 (R-Foundation for statistical computing, www.Rproject.org), where peak peaking, integration and alignment in the time domain were performed. Integrated intensities of each m/z-retention time pair (MZRT) were obtained for each one of the samples used in the study. NIST mass spectral databases were used for metabolite identification.

Statistical analysis

Both univariate and multivariate statistical analyses were applied using SPSS 17.0 software (SPSS, Chicago, USA) and SIMCA-P+ 12.0 (Umetrics, AB, Umeå, Sweden), respectively. Data of body weight gain and the ratio of body weight (weight gain to weight at week 0) were expressed as the mean ± standard deviation. Student's t-test was used for comparison of gain of body weight and the ratio of body weight. Significant difference was defined at $p<0.05$. In the multivariate statistical analyses, all normalized ^{1}H NMR and GC-MS spectral data were imported to SIMCA-P+ 12.0 for principal components analysis (PCA), and orthogonal partial least-squares discriminant analysis (OPLS-DA). PCA, an unsupervised multivariate statistical approach, was performed to achieve the natural inter-relationship (grouping, clustering, and outlier detection) among samples. To maximize class discrimination, the OPLS-DA results were further analyzed. Criteria of quality of modeling were R^2X, the cumulative modeled variation in metabolite data, R^2Y, the cumulative modeled variation in class values, and Q^2, the cumulative predicted variation in metabolite data according to cross-validation (7-fold cross validation). These parameters range between 0 and 1, where 1 indicates a perfect fit. Metabolites responsible for the separation between classes in supervised models were identified based on the Variable Influence on Projection (VIP) values, which correspond to the importance of the variables for the model. The variables with a VIP value larger than 1.0 were considered significant and used for further analysis and identification of the responsible peak(s) within the spectrum.

Results

Body weight

During the 14-day administration and 7-day recovery, no animal dead, but rats in the CR-treated group began diarrhea after 5 days of treatment. To investigate the toxic effects of CR,

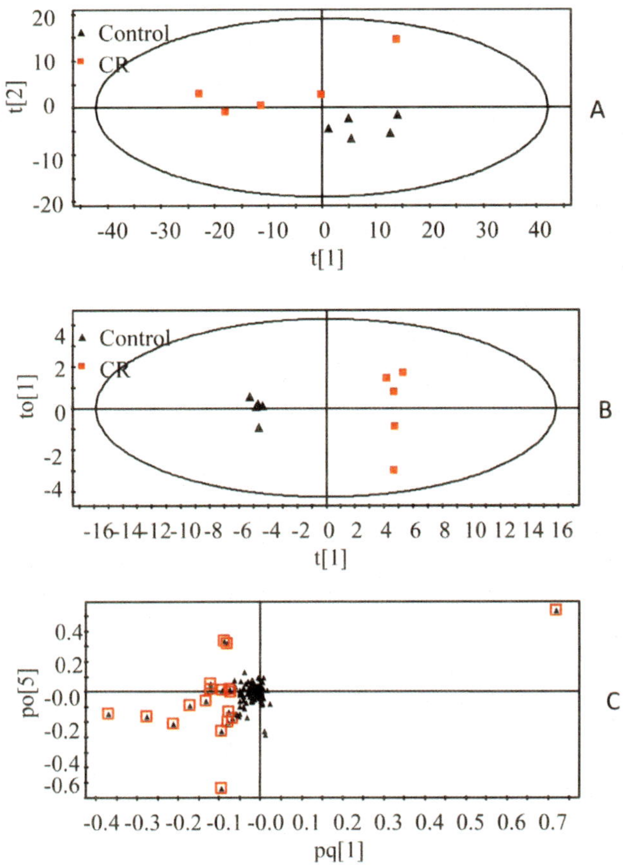

Figure 7. Multivariate analysis of serum samples from CR and control groups. A, PCA score plot, B, OPLS-DA score plot, C, OPLS-DA loadings plot. The urine samples were collected after 14 days of treatment. The model was established using one predictive and one orthogonal component.

growth was firstly examined. The representative change tendency of body weight during the experiment period is showed in Figure 2A. The body weights of rats in CR-treated group were significantly lower than those in control group after 14 days of CR treatment. Furthermore, the ratio of body weight (weight gain to weight at week 0) of CR-treated group is approximately 20% lower than control group (Figure 2A and 2B). However, the ratio of body weight was no significant difference during recovery period (Figure 2C).

Histopathology

To examine the toxicity at the tissue, we analysed the histopathological data on liver, kidney, lung and heart tissues. H&E staining of liver, kidney, lung and heart tissues revealed that there was no apparent toxicity at these tissues by CR treatment. After CR administration of 14 days, three rats in CR-treated group and one in control group had only a slight morphological variation in liver (Figure 3B), in which less than 10% of cells showed infiltration or edema. Therefore, we considered this as the normal organic change in liver. The hepatic lobules in other rats had normal cell shapes. In addition, the hepatic lobular structure and portal tract were not inflammatory or hydropic (Figure 3A). There was no obvious variation in liver tissue after recovery of 7 days compared with controls (Figure 3C).

Table 2. Endogenous metabolites selected as biomarkers in serum profile and their change trends.

Metabolite	RT(min)	CR vs. control
Alanine	5.74	↑*
L-proline	8.4	↑*
Glycine	8.5	↑*
Hisoindol	8.55	↑*
Serine	9.08	↑*
Glutamate	11.95	↑*
L-ornithine	14.16	↑*
D-Glucose	15.14	↓*

↑, the increase in signal; ↓, the decrease in signal.
*Key: $p<0.05$.

NMR Spectroscopy of urine samples

Representative ^{1}H NMR spectra of urine samples collected on the 14th day from different group are shown in Figure 4. Assignments of endogenous metabolites involved in ^{1}H NMR spectra were based on comparing chemical shifts and multiplicities of peaks to the literatures [32,33,34,35] as well as the Metabonomics Toolbox (http://www.hmdb.ca). Due to the high information content and complexity of the spectra, multivariate statistical analyses were applied to reveal the metabolic changes-related CR treatment. Initially, the unsupervised principal component analysis (PCA) was applied to explore correlations between control group and CR-treated group, and a tendency to separate the two classes was detected in the score plot ($R^2X = 0.721$, $Q^2 = 0.526$) (Figure 5A). Since we observed intra-group variation, the supervised method, OPLS-DA, was also used to isolate the variables responsible for the differences observed between the CR and control groups ($R^2X = 0.451$, $R^2Y = 0.921$, $Q^2 = 0.783$) (Figure 5B). The model showed an overall goodness of fit. To high light metabolite differences between the control group and CR-treated group, feature selections were performed using loadings plot, followed by OPLS-DA (Figure 5C). VIP analysis showed the order of metabolites according to their critical influence on clustering. The points marked red in Figure 4C showed the metabolites which VIP value more than 1.00. Some of these segments were found to be from the same metabolite. The key metabolites, which were essential for distinguishing between the CR and control groups were selected from the results of the VIP analysis (VIP>1.00) and Student's t-test ($P<0.05$). After merging the variables from the identical metabolites, 12 metabolites were collected and considered as the urine potential biomarkers (Table 1).

GC-MS spectrometry

Serum samples were analyzed by GC-MS. Figure 6 shows the typical total ion chromatograms (TICs) of serum samples collected on 14th day. The raw GC-MS data from metabolic profiling were pretreated following the procedure in Section 2.7. The XCMS output data containing 536 ion peaks was preprocessed using the Microsoft Excels of software, where the IS (internal standard) peak, and impurity peaks from column bleeds and derivatization procedures were excluded, and the variables presenting in at least 80% of either group were extracted. Then, the remaining ion features were normalized to the internal standard. The most abundant fragment ion with the same retention time (the time bin

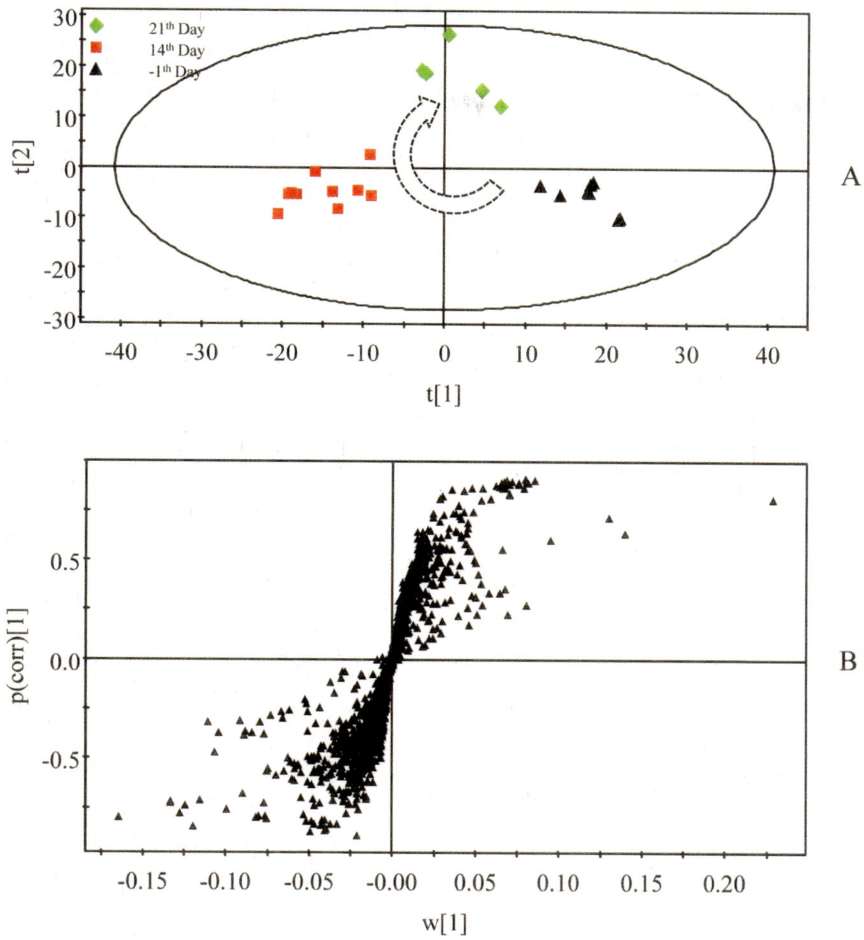

Figure 8. Multivariate analysis of urine samples of pre-treatment, after 14 days of treatment and after 7 days of recovery. A, OPLS-DA score plot, B, OPLS-DA loadings s-plot.

is 0.01 min) was remained and the other ions were excluded. The processed data was further subjected to statistical analysis. In the PCA scores plot (Figure 7A), the CR-treated group and control group can be well distinguished ($R^2 = 0.864$, $Q^2 = 0.687$). As could be observed in the OPLS-DA score plot (Figure 7B), separation between these two groups was also clearly seen ($R^2X = 0.991$, $R^2Y = 0.995$, $Q^2 = 0.888$), indicating that biochemical perturbation significantly happened due to CR treatment. The model showed an overall goodness of fit. According to the loadings plot (Figure 7C) of this OPLS-DA model, and using the above-stated statistically significant threshold, 8 metabolites with VIP-values greater than 1.0 and P values less than 0.05 were finally revealed to be significant in differentiating the CR treated and control groups. Alanine, L-proline, glycine, hisoindol, serine, glutamate and L-ornithine were elevated in CR-treated group, while D-glucose was reduced in this group (Table 2).

Toxic effects of CR based on metabolite profiling

Using the presented ^1H NMR and GC-MS method, the urinary and serum metablic profiles of CR -treated group were obtained. The effects of inhibition of growth on CR-treated rats have been shown in Figure 2. However, after 7 days of recovery, the growth of rats returned to a normal rate. The diarrheal of rats also stopped after days of recovery. As the 12 potential biomarkers from ^1H NMR and 8 ones from GC-MS have been found, it is reasonable to take them as the potential biomarker for further investigating the intervening mechanisms of CR toxicity. Therefore, the metabolic profiling of ^1H NMR on the 21th day was introduced as variables to OPLS-DA. Consequently, the ^1H NMR data of the -1th, 14th and 21th day were analyzed using OPLS-DA. As shown in OPLS-DA scores map derived from ^1H NMR metabolic profile (Figure 8), the 21th day group is closer to the -1th day group, which indicated the CR-induced toxicity tend to recover. To further evaluate the reversed condition of the potential biomarkers when CR treatment was stopped, the normalized integrals of the changes in these endogenous urinary metabolites were investigated. Figure 9 demonstrated the time-related response of these metabolites to CR treatment. Similar to the results of body weight change, the ^1H NMR analysis presented in Figure 9 shows that 11 of the 12 detected metabolites also showed a return toward pretreatment values after 7 days of recovery.

Discussion

CR is relatively safe in normal dosage. However, it reportedly can cause adverse effects such as sicchasia, diarrhea, respiratory failure and extrapyramidal system reactions in some patients, in clinic in China [36]. Our results were similar to those of clinical study in which people treated with CR. During the period of CR treatment, the most obvious toxicity effect of CR treatment was diarrhea. In addition, our results showed there was a significant

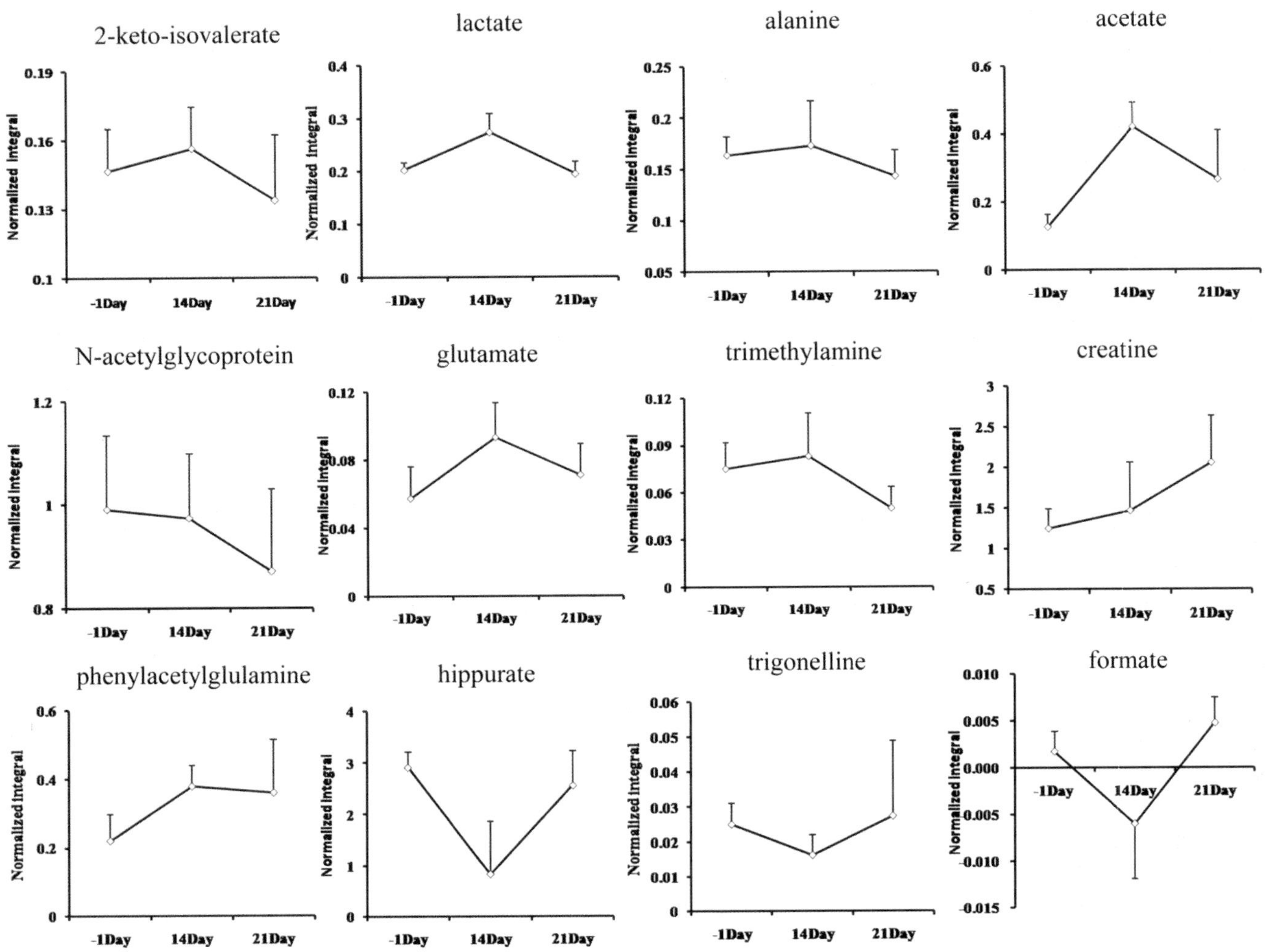

Figure 9. The normalized integral changes of the relevant time-related urinary marked metabolites induced by CR treatment.

decrease in the body weight gain of CR-treated group at during the period of CR treatment compared with the time-matched control. Further, to investigate the mechanisms underlying the toxicity of CR treatment in rats, we compared the urinary and serum metabolic profiles of rats treated with CR decoction and distilled water using ^{1}H NMR and GC-MS based metabonomics.

This is the first study researching the mechanisms of toxicity induced by CR using a holistic approach. The combination of NMR and GC-MS based metabonomics can comprehensively measure the metabolic responses of biological systems. In our study, urine and plasma samples were collected at multiple time points and a set of metabolites were assayed to identify differences in concentration. The results revealed that endogenous metabolites in urine showed time-dependent changes at different period of the experiment. After 14 days of CR administration, by ^{1}H NMR, comparing with controls, we observed that 2-keto-isovalerate, lactate, alanine, N-acetylglycoprotein, glutamate, trimethethylamine and phenylacetylglulamine were markedly increased, while creatine, hippurate, trigonelline and formate were decreased. By GC-MS, alanine, L-proline, glycine, hisoindol, serine, glutamate and L-ornithine were distinctly elevated, while D-glucose and glycerol were decreased. We showed a simplified pathway map based on the metabolite markers identified by NMR and GC-MS (Figure 10). Figure 10 indicated that interference in intestinal microflora and disruption in energy metabolism dominated the altered biochemistry of CR treatment.

Hippurate is an acylglycine formed by the conjugation of benzoic acid with glycine in a reaction (acyl-CoA + glycine→CoA + N-acylglycine) catalyzed by glycine N-acyl trans-ferase [37], which is a metabolite of the amino acid metabolism refer to alanine, glutamate, glycine, serine and phenylalanine (http://www.kegg.jp). It has proved that intestinal microflora play an important role in the excretion of aromatic phenolic compounds. Hippurate, is generated from the conjugation of glycine and benzoic acid that is produced from aromatic amino acids by gut microbes and excreted into the urine [38]. In addition, it was reported that hippurate is a biomarker of breaking the balance of normal microorganisms, and that low levels of hippurate have been found in intestinal flora disturbance induced by GI damage [39]. Therefore, it is possible that CR treatment may correlate with a disturbance in the gut microbiota. The lower level of hippurate in urine at 14 days after CR administration may account for interference in amino acid metabolism. After 7 days of recovery, the level of hipprate was back to the value of pretreatment, which implied the gut microbiota may remold when CR treatment was stopped.

In addition, gut microbiota extensively catabolized protein and aromatic amino acids, including phenylalanine and tyrosine, to

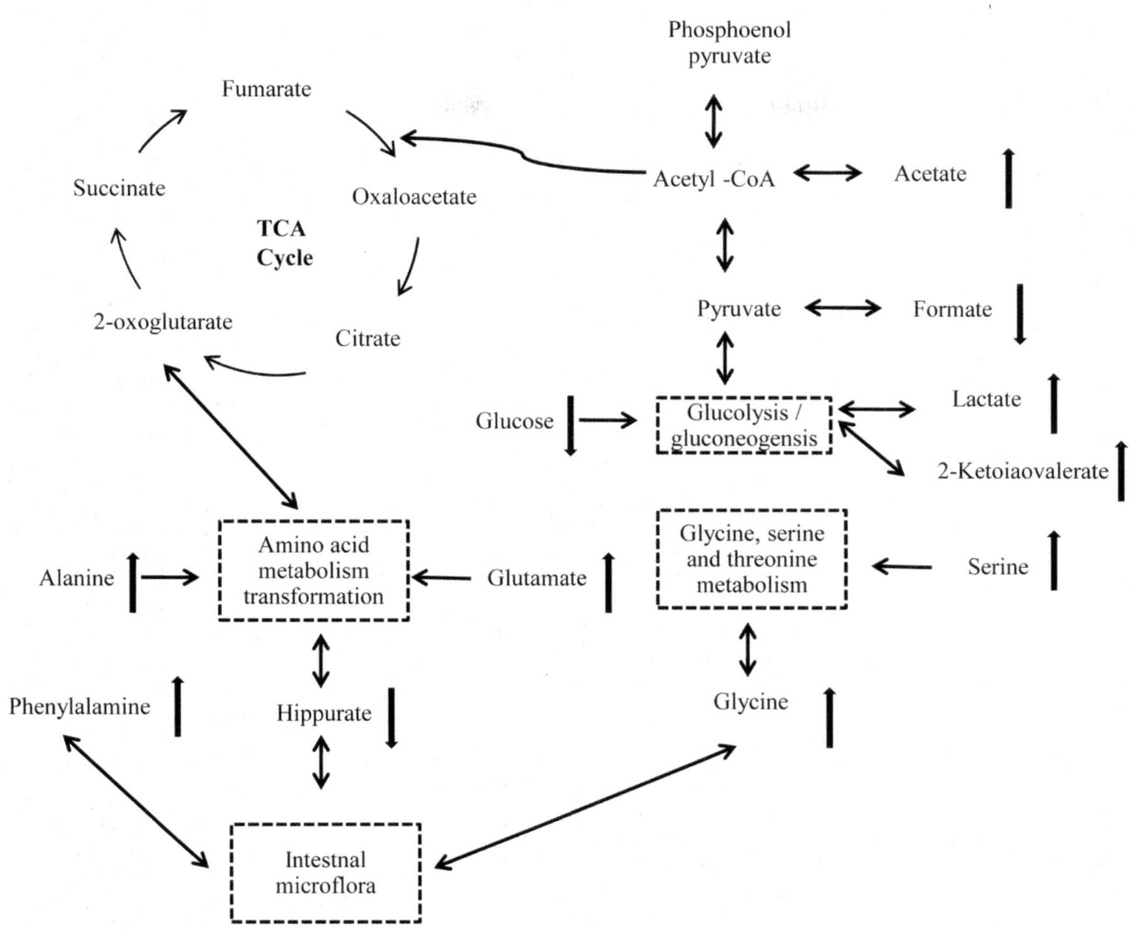

Figure 10. Altered metabolism pathways for the most relevant metabolic differences between rats treat with CR and control group. The network of the potential biomarkers changing according to the KEGG PATHWAY.

form phenylacetylglutamine and p-cresol sulfate [40]. As discussed the relationships between urine metabotypes and microbiota composition, phenylacetylglutamine displays positive correlation with Proteobacteria species, namely *Campylobacter, E. coli, Haemophilus, Pseudomonas, Serratia, Yersinia et rel* [22] . In this study, increased urinary level of phenylacetylglutamine may suggest that CR exposure enhanced the aromatic amino acid metabolism for disturbance in the gut microbiota. After 7 days of recovery, the concentration of Phenylacetylglutamine showed a similar turn back tendency, but it was not so obvious compared with hippurate. The urinary level of trigonelline, which produced via the conversion of S-adenosyl-methionine (SAM) to S-adenosylhomocysteine (SAH) by gut microflora [41], was also significantly decreased in CR treated rats, when compared to controls. This suggested that SAM was consumed and thus depleted in the transsulfuration pathway to produce glutathione that was depleted in CR treated group [41,42]. Figure 9 showed the urinary level of trigonelline increased when stopped CR administration.

We observed a higher urinary level of lactate and 2-ketoisovalerate, and a lower level of serum glucose. These compounds were main metabolites involved in biochemical pathway of glycolysis or gluconeogenesis. Glycolysis is the process of converting glucose into pyruvate and generating small amounts of ATP and NADH. This is a central pathway that produces important precursor metabolites for the citrate cycle. Lactate is typically interpreted as a marker of anaerobic metabolism, and accumulation of it usually accounted for a higher energy demand in the biological system [43]. Under normal circumstances, lactate transform into pyruvic acid by Lactate Oxidase, then pyruvic acid participate in the citrate cycle (TCA cycle). The TCA cycle is an important aerobic pathway for the final steps of the oxidation of carbohydrates and fatty acids, simultaneously, produce ATP. ATP deficiency from mitochondrial dysfunction can be partially offset by increased glycolysis, and the AMP-activated protein kinase (AMPK) will promote glycolysis through phosphorylation and activation of phosphofructokinase-2 (PFK2), leading to increase levels of the glycolytic stimulator, fructose-2, 6-bisphosphate. In this study, increased lactate and 2-keto-isovalerate in combination with decreased glucose suggest that CR exposure may disturb the energy metabolism.

An acetic acid is usually fully ionized to acetate, a derivative of acetic acid [44]. In biochemistry, acetate and acetic acid are equivalent. When bound to coenzyme A, it becomes to acetyl-CoA, another important precursor metabolite, which is produced by oxidative decarboxylation of pyruvate and an important intermediate in the TCA cycle, central to the metabolism of carbohydrates and fats [43]. In this study, elevation of acetate also suggests that the metabolism of fats and carbohydrates was affected. The suppression of body growth in rats treated with CR may attribute to energy metabolism disorder. We supposed that CR-induced diarrhea leads to intestinal malabsorption of carbohydrates or fats, furthermore results in energy deficiency and energy metabolism disorder.

Besides interference in above biochemical pathways, there were significant differences in trimethylamine, ornithine and proline between CR and control groups. Trimethylamine (TMA), a product of choline degradation and an osmolyte that counteracts the effects of increased urine concentrations [45,46]. The concentration of TMA in urine was elevated after 14 days of CR treated, suggesting suppression of the choline degradation pathway. Ornithine is one of products derived from biodegradation alkaloids [47], and increased concentrations of ornithine in serum may because of the primary components of CR are alkaloids [48]. Increased proline concentration in serum might be related to disturbance in arginine and proline metabolism (www.genome.jp/kegg).

Conclusion

This paper integrated NMR and GC-MS metabonomics in combination with the multivariate statistical analysis (SIMCA-P) to discover the marker metabolites which contribute to the toxicity of CR treatment. The results showed the main toxic effect of CR is diarrhea, coupling with resistance of body growth. Through multivariate statistical analysis 12 marker metabolites from NMR and 8 ones from GC/MS have been found. Among those metabolites, hippurate, acetate, alanine, glycine and glutamate showed association to the gut dysbiosis, whereas others, such as lactate and 2-ketoisovalerate are likely to increase anaerobic glycolysis, meanwhile the CR-associated toxicity will recover when treatment was stopped. These results suggest that the main reason for the CR-associated diarrhea might be disturbance in the normal gut microbiota. This metabonomics approach may provide an effective way to study the alteration of gut microbiota, which is expected to find broader application in other drug-induced gastrointestinal reaction assessments.

Author Contributions

Conceived and designed the experiments: YZ QL ZX. Performed the experiments: YZ ML XD PZ. Analyzed the data: YZ ML MY LZ. Contributed reagents/materials/analysis tools: QL ZX. Wrote the paper: YZ ML ZX.

References

1. Normile D (2003) Asian medicine. The new face of traditional Chinese medicine. Science (New York, NY) 299: 188–190.
2. Stone R (2008) Biochemistry. Lifting the veil on traditional Chinese medicine. Science (New York, NY) 319: 709–710.
3. Tan G, Liao W, Dong X, Yang G, Zhu Z, et al. (2012) Metabonomic profiles delineate the effect of traditional Chinese medicine sini decoction on myocardial infarction in rats. PloS one 7: e34157.
4. Lu J, Wang J, Kong L (2011) Anti-inflammatory effects of Huang-Lian-Jie-Du decoction, its two fractions and four typical compounds. Journal of ethnopharmacology 134: 911–918.
5. Choi U, Kim M, Lee N (2007) Optimization of antibacterial activity by Gold-Thread (Coptidis Rhizoma Franch) against Streptococcus mutans using evolutionary operation-factorial design technique. Journal of microbiology and biotechnology 17: 1880–1884.
6. Wang N, Feng Y, Cheung F, Chow O-Y, Wang X, et al. (2012) A comparative study on the hepatoprotective action of bear bile and coptidis rhizoma aqueous extract on experimental liver fibrosis in rats. BMC Complementary and Alternative Medicine 12: 239.
7. Tjong Y, Ip S, Lao L, Fong HH, Sung JJ, et al. (2011) Analgesic Effect of Coptis chinensis rhizomes (Coptidis Rhizoma) Extract on Rat Model of Irritable Bowel Syndrome. Journal of ethnopharmacology 135: 754–761.
8. Tang J, Feng Y, Tsao S, Wang N, Curtain R, et al. (2009) Berberine and Coptidis rhizoma as novel antineoplastic agents: a review of traditional use and biomedical investigations. Journal of ethnopharmacology 126: 5–17.
9. Jung H, Min B, Yokozawa T, Lee J, Kim Y, et al. (2009) Anti-Alzheimer and antioxidant activities of Coptidis Rhizoma alkaloids. Biological & pharmaceutical bulletin 32: 1433–1438.
10. Xigyan Z, Xiaolin T, Linhua Z, Qiang Zhou, Zhiping Peng, et al. (2013) Advances in study on the adverse reaction of coptis razma and its major components, China journal of Chinese Materia Medica 38: 546–547.
11. Yuqin Bao. (1983) The adverse reaction of berberine and coptis razma,Chinese journal of integrated traditional and western medicine 3: 31–33.
12. Guirl M, Högenauer C, Santa Ana C, Porter J, Little K, et al. (2003) Rapid intestinal transit as a primary cause of severe chronic diarrhea in patients with amyloidosis. The American journal of gastroenterology 98: 2219–2225.
13. Read N (1986) Diarrhée motrice. Clinics in gastroenterology 15: 657–686.
14. Bugaut M (1987) Occurrence, absorption and metabolism of short chain fatty acids in the digestive tract of mammals. Comparative biochemistry and physiology B, Comparative biochemistry 86: 439.
15. Clausen M, Bonnen H, Tvede M, Mortensen P (1991) Colonic fermentation to short-chain fatty acids is decreased in antibiotic-associated diarrhea. Gastroenterology 101: 1497.
16. Walker A, Lawley T (2012) Therapeutic modulation of intestinal dysbiosis. Pharmacological research: the official journal of the Italian Pharmacological Society 69: 75–86.
17. Young VB, Schmidt TM (2004) Antibiotic-Associated Diarrhea Accompanied by Large-Scale Alterations in the Composition of the Fecal Microbiota. Journal of Clinical Microbiology 42: 1203–1206.
18. Robertson D, Watkins P, Reily M (2011) Metabolomics in toxicology: preclinical and clinical applications. Toxicological sciences: an official journal of the Society of Toxicology 120: S146–S170.
19. Li M, Wang B, Zhang M, Rantalainen M, Wang S, et al. (2008) Symbiotic gut microbes modulate human metabolic phenotypes. Proceedings of the National Academy of Sciences of the United States of America 105: 2117–2122.
20. Bando K, Kunimatsu T, Sakai J, Kimura J, Funabashi H, et al. (2010) GC-MS-based metabolomics reveals mechanism of action for hydrazine induced hepatotoxicity in rats. Journal of applied toxicology: JAT 31: 524–535.
21. Wang X, Wang H, Zhang A, Lu X, Sun H, et al. (2012) Metabolomics study on the toxicity of aconite root and its processed products using ultraperformance liquid-chromatography/electrospray-ionization synapt high-definition mass spectrometry coupled with pattern recognition approach and ingenuity pathways analysis. Journal of proteome research 11: 1284–1301.
22. Collino S, Montoliu I, Martin F-PJ, Scherer M, Mari D, et al. (2013) Metabolic Signatures of Extreme Longevity in Northern Italian Centenarians Reveal a Complex Remodeling of Lipids, Amino Acids, and Gut Microbiota Metabolism. PloS one 8: e56564.
23. Wang X, Sun H, Zhang A, Sun W, Wang P, et al. (2011) Potential role of metabolomics apporoaches in the area of traditional Chinese medicine: as pillars of the bridge between Chinese and Western medicine. Journal of pharmaceutical and biomedical analysis 55: 859–868.
24. P LI LY, Y GONG (2009) Application of Systems Biology Technology in Research of Traditional Chinese Medicine. Journal of Traditional Chinese Medicine 2: 019–024.
25. Ciborowski M, Lipska A, Godzien J, Ferrarini A, Korsak J, et al. (2012) Combination of LC-MS and GC-MS based metabolomics to study the effect of ozonated autohemotherapy on human blood. Journal of proteome research 11: 6231–6241.
26. Ni Y, Su M, Qiu Y, Chen M, Liu Y, et al. (2007) Metabolic profiling using combined GC-MS and LC-MS provides a systems understanding of aristolochic acid-induced nephrotoxicity in rat. FEBS letters 581: 707–711.
27. Wuolikainen A, Moritz T, Marklund SL, Antti H, Andersen PM (2011) Disease-Related Changes in the Cerebrospinal Fluid Metabolome in Amyotrophic Lateral Sclerosis Detected by GC/TOFMS. PloS one 6: e17947.
28. Yang H-j, Choi M-J, Wen H, Kwon HN, Jung KH, et al. (2011) An Effective Assessment of Simvastatin-Induced Toxicity with NMR-Based Metabonomics Approach. PloS one 6: e16641.
29. Tang B, Ding J, Wu F, Chen L, Yang Y, et al. (2012) 1H NMR-based metabonomics study of the urinary biochemical changes in Kansui treated rat. Journal of ethnopharmacology 141: 134–142.
30. Lu J, Zhou J, Bao Y, Chen T, Zhang Y, et al. (2012) Serum Metabolic Signatures of Fulminant Type 1 Diabetes. Journal of proteome research 11: 4705–4711.
31. Holmes E, Bonner F, Sweatman B, Lindon J, Beddell C, et al. (1992) Nuclear magnetic resonance spectroscopy and pattern recognition analysis of the biochemical processes associated with the progression of and recovery from nephrotoxic lesions in the rat induced by mercury (II) chloride and 2-bromoethanamine. Molecular pharmacology 42: 922–930.
32. Pechlivanis A, Kostidis S, Saraslanidis P, Petridou A, Tsalis G, et al. (2012) 1) H NMR study on the short-and long-term impact of two training programs of sprint running on the metabolic fingerprint of human serum. Journal of proteome research 12: 470–480.
33. O'Sullivan A, Willoughby R, Mishchuk D, Alcarraz B, Cabezas-Sanchez C, et al. (2012) Metabolomics of cerebrospinal fluid from humans treated for rabies. Journal of proteome research 12: 481–490.
34. Hochrein J, Klein M, Zacharias H, Li J, Wijffels G, et al. (2012) Performance Evaluation of Algorithms for the Classification of Metabolic (1) H-NMR Fingerprints. Journal of proteome research 11: 6242–6251.

35. Mackinnon N, Somashekar B, Tripathi P, Ge W, Rajendiran T, et al. (2012) MetaboID: A graphical user interface package for assignment of (1) H NMR spectra of bodyfluids and tissues. Journal of magnetic resonance (San Diego, Calif: 1997) 226: 93–99.
36. Xiyan Z, Xiaolin T, Linhua Z, Qiang Z, Zhiping P, et al. (2013) Advances in study on the adverse reaction of coptis razma and its preparation, China journal of Chinese Materia Medica 38: 292–295.
37. Phipps A, Stewart J, Wright B, Wilson I (1998) Effect of diet on the urinary excretion of hippuric acid and other dietary-derived aromatics in rat. A complex interaction between diet, gut microflora and substrate specificity. Xenobiotica; the fate of foreign compounds in biological systems 28: 527–537.
38. Garaulet M, Pérez-Llamas F, Pérez-Ayala M, Martínez P, de Medina FS, et al. (2001) Site-specific differences in the fatty acid composition of abdominal adipose tissue in an obese population from a Mediterranean area: relation with dietary fatty acids, plasma lipid profile, serum insulin, and central obesity. The American journal of clinical nutrition 74: 585–591.
39. Um S, Park J, Chung M, Kim K, Kim S, et al. (2012) Nuclear magnetic resonance-based metabolomics for prediction of gastric damage induced by indomethacin in rats. Analytica chimica acta 722: 87–94.
40. Smith E, Macfarlane G (1997) Formation of phenolic and indolic compounds by anaerobic bacteria in the human large intestine. Microbial ecology 33: 180–188.
41. Sun J, Schnackenberg LK, Holland RD, Schmitt TC, Cantor GH, et al. (2008) Metabonomics evaluation of urine from rats given acute and chronic doses of acetaminophen using NMR and UPLC/MS. J Chromatogr B Analyt Technol Biomed Life Sci 871: 328–340.
42. Calvani R, Miccheli A, Capuani G, Tomassini Miccheli A, Puccetti C, et al. (2010) Gut microbiome-derived metabolites characterize a peculiar obese urinary metabotype. Int J Obes (Lond) 34: 1095–1098.
43. Kokushi E, Uno S, Harada T, Koyama J (2012) 1) H NMR-based metabolomics approach to assess toxicity of bunker a heavy oil to freshwater carp, Cyprinus carpio. Environmental toxicology 27: 404–414.
44. March J (1992) Advanced organic chemistry: reactions, mechanisms, and structure: John Wiley & Sons.
45. Park J, Hong Y, Kim Y, Yang J, Kim E, et al. (2009) A metabonomic study on the biochemical effects of doxorubicin in rats using (1) H-NMR spectroscopy. Journal of toxicology and environmental health Part A 72: 374–384.
46. Nicholls A, Mortishire-Smith R, Nicholson J (2003) NMR spectroscopic-based metabonomic studies of urinary metabolite variation in acclimatizing germ-free rats. Chemical research in toxicology 16: 1395–1404.
47. Boyd D, Sharma N, O'Dowd C, Carroll J, Loke P, et al. (2005) cis-Dihydrodiol, arene oxide and phenol metabolites of dictamnine: key intermediates in the biodegradation and biosynthesis of furoquinoline alkaloids. Chemical communications (Cambridge, England): 3989–3991.
48. Fan G, Zhang M, Zhou X, Lai X, Yue Q, et al. (2012) Quality evaluation and species differentiation of Rhizoma coptidis by using proton nuclear magnetic resonance spectroscopy. Analytica chimica acta 747: 76–83.

Disgust Sensitivity Is Not Associated with Health in a Rural Bangladeshi Sample

Mícheál de Barra[1]*, M. Sirajul Islam[2], Val Curtis[1]

1 Environmental Health Group, London School of Hygiene and Tropical Medicine, London, United Kingdom, 2 Environmental Microbiology Lab, ICDDR,B, Dhaka, Bangladesh

Abstract

Disgust can be considered a psychological arm of the immune system that acts to prevent exposure to infectious agents. High disgust sensitivity is associated with greater behavioral avoidance of disease vectors and thus may reduce infection risk. A cross-sectional survey in rural Bangladesh provided no strong support for this hypothesis. In many species, the expression of pathogen- and predator-avoidance mechanisms is contingent on early life exposure to predators and pathogens. Using childhood health data collected in the 1990s, we examined if adults with more infectious diseases in childhood showed greater adult disgust sensitivity: no support for this association was found. Explanations for these null finding and possible directions for future research are discussed.

Editor: Christine A Caldwell, University of Stirling, United Kingdom

Funding: This research was supported by a grant from Hindustan Unilever Ltd to Valerie A. Curtis. The funders had no role in study design, data collection and analysis, decision to publish, or preparation of the manuscript.

Competing Interests: This research was supported by a grant from Hindustan Unilever Ltd to Valerie A. Curtis.

* Email: mdebarra@gmail.com

Introduction

The emotion disgust is characterized by behavioral avoidance or rejection. A broad range of stimuli including body wastes, deformity, spoilage and certain immoral and sexual acts elicit the emotion [1]. People vary in the degree to which they experience disgust in response to these things, and this variation is known as disgust sensitivity. Disgust often motivates avoidance of things that carry an infection risk; this overlap between infective substances and disgust elicitors suggests that disgust may play a functional role in preventing infection [2]. Over evolutionary timescales the costs associated with parasitism have been an important selection pressure and have sculpted several host defense mechanisms, including behavioral strategies [3–5]. Functionally speaking, our feeling of revulsion and the associated avoidance behavior can be considered a psychological arm of the broader immune system [6].

One implication of the parasite-avoidance model is that people prone to strong feelings of disgust will be exposed to pathogens less frequently. Disgust sensitivity is associated with unwillingness to approach/touch things that can cause infection [7] and this reduced exposure could translate into fewer bouts of infectious disease. Consistent with this, Stevenson et al. found that people who were both highly sensitive to disgusting stimuli and inclined to make inferences about spreading contamination reported less recent infections [8]. While the health benefits of disgust were modest, these results suggest that disgust sensitivity can influence health in a high-income population where public health infrastructure is well developed and where infectious disease is rare. In this paper, we examine if individual variation in disgust sensitivity influences infection rates in rural Bangladesh. In this environment, people are exposed to diseases uncommon in high-income settings [9]. If disgust does indeed provide a protective effect, the relationship between infection rate and disgust sensitivity should be clear in this population.

Another prediction derived from the parasite-avoidance model is that disgust sensitivity will be higher where the threat of infection is greater. Systems that protect organisms from pathogens or predators often entail trade-offs: the individual benefits from fewer infections or reduced risk of predation but must pay a cost to develop or maintain the system. The costs of disgust may include rejected food and social partners, or an increased risk of psychopathology [10]. In other species, the costs of disease avoidance can be considerable. For example, Hutchings and colleagues found that sheep with conservative foraging behavior also had lower weight because avoiding pathogens also entailed avoiding high quality forage [11]. Finding the right balance of cost and benefit is an important problem, and one solution lies in facultative expression of the protective system. In humans, food disgust sensitivity appears to decline when the costs of rejection increase, i.e., when people are hungry [12]. Conversely, when the immune system is weakened by pregnancy, there is a compensatory increase in disgust sensitivity [13]. In other species, adjustment to local pathogen/predator risk often occurs in during development and is relatively stable over the lifespan; the organism can use early-life cues to estimate the current threat and develop accordingly [14]. In humans, many life history parameters such as age-at-first birth and age-at-marriage appear to be influenced by early life cues indicative of a risky environment [15,16]. Local infection risk depends on factors like immunocompetence, sanitation and water infrastructure, local hygiene practices, animal husbandry, and climate. These factors change relatively slowly (i.e., over decades) and so childhood infection rates should provide a reliable medium-term measure of local infection risk and could

Table 1. Illness among the 284 participants in the year prior to data collection.

Disease	Number of participants experiencing disease
Flu	118 (42%)
Gastric Pain	105 (37%)
Cough	82 (29%)
Vomiting	70 (25%)
Diarrhea	61 (21%)
Eye Infection	33 (12%)
Tooth Ache	28 (10%)
Skin Infection	27 (10%)
Fever	9 (3%)
Ear Ache	8 (3%)
Sinus Infection	8 (2%)
Dysentery	7 (0%)
Tuberculosis	0 (%)

thus be used to benchmark a locally appropriate level of disgust sensitivity. Consistent with this, we previously found that childhood exposure to disease is associated with a greater preference for opposite sex faces with exaggerated sex typical characteristics, a putative health cue [17]. In other words, people sick more often as children prioritize health cues in partner choice as adults. Thus, our second hypothesis was that people with more infections in childhood would show greater disgust sensitivity in adulthood. We tested this hypothesis using disgust sensitivity data collected in 2010 and longitudinal childhood health data collected in the 1990s.

Materials and Methods

The data was collected as part of a broader study on health, hygiene and psychology in rural Bangladesh. Participants, all of whom were 16 years of age or older, saw an information sheet, had the aims and methods explained, and were given the opportunity to ask questions. Participants gave written consent before data collection began. Informed consent from participants' next of kin, caretaker or guardian was not sought. The London School of Hygiene and Tropical Medicine Review Board approved the research, including the information sheets, consent forms, and consent procedure.

Sample

Sample size calculation was based on hypothesis one; that disgust sensitivity will correlate negatively with recent infection frequency. We anticipated that the correlation between disgust and health in the present study would be of small or medium magnitude ($r \approx .2$). A sample size calculation with $r = .2$, significance threshold $= .05$, and power $= .9$ indicated that 258 participants were needed.

Participants were randomly selected from a list of people born between July 1990 and August 1997 and living in one of 13 villages familiar to the field workers (i.e., in regions where they had previously conducted field work). The wording of childhood health questions and the frequency of interview remained constant for

Table 2. Exploratory factor analysis of disgust items: two factor solution.

Back Translated Item	Factor 1	Factor 2	Communality
Picking your nose	.80		.51
Touching the inside of a toilet	.65	.32	.75
Skin with scabies	.59		.35
Eating from dirty plate	.55		.38
Spit on the road	.54		.26
Accidentally using other persons toothbrush	.50		.25
Sour milk	.50		.26
Dead animal	.45		.44
Eating something with left hand	.45		.36
Small acne	.43		.29
Person who never washes himself	.36		.33
Infected eye	.35		.24
Hand without a finger		.79	.64
Deformed body		.67	.56
Perished/decomposed fish		.66	.38
Animal feces in yard		.66	.34
Touching an animal		.53	.52
Eating last nights food		.50	.30
Unkempt beggar		.49	.40
Child with diarrhoea		.38	.23
Very obese man		.31	.22

Note: Items are ordered according to loading on relevant factor. Loadings less than .3 are omitted for clarity.

children born within this period. The sample included 113 men and 171 women and had an average age of 18 years (SD = 1.3). Most participants were unmarried (88%) and Muslim (87%).

Data collection

Participants were interviewed by one of four FWs (field workers). All four FWs had worked as enumerators in two or more previous research projects. Before data collection began, FWs underwent one week of training that included mock interviews and group discussion. During data collection, progress and evaluation meetings were held every third day. Interviews were conducted in Bengali and took place in the participants' homes in the afternoon or evening. Matlab is the site of a long-term health and demographic research project and people are accustomed to visits from field workers and researchers.

Measures

The Disgust Scale [18] (revised in [19]) and the Three Domain Disgust Scale [20] are the most commonly used measures of disgust sensitivity. However, neither has been translated into Bengali, and both contain include items with little relevance to a rural, low-income Bangladeshi sample (e.g., "eating vanilla ice cream with ketchup", "seeing some mold on old leftovers in your refrigerator"). In order to measure disgust sensitivity we designed a simple measure with locally relevant items modeled on these two measures and our previous work on disgust sensitivity in the UK [21]. Consistent with the disease-avoidance model discussed above, these were items related to infectious disease transmission. Hence, this disgust measure focused on what Tybur et al. have termed 'pathogen disgust' [20] and what Haidt et al. have referred to as 'core' or 'contagion' disgust [19]. It is this pathogen related disgust that is most likely to influence participant health and is therefore most relevant to the current analysis. Items were first written in English, then translated into Bengali by a native speaker, and then back translated into English by a second translator who was fluent in both English and Bengali. Minor discrepancies between the versions were resolved through discussion with the translators. Participants were read each item and asked to rate it from 0 ('not at all disgusting') to 4 ('extremely disgusting'). The Bengali and English versions of the questionnaire, as well as the individual-level response data, are available on the Figshare data repository [22].

Participants' current health (i.e. health as adults) was measured using a Benagli- language questionnaire adapted from the 1996 Matlab Health and Socio-Economic Survey [23]. Participants were asked whether or not they had a list of ailments/diseases in the previous twelve months, how many bouts of the illness they experienced, and the recency of the last bout. 73% of participants reported experiencing an infectious disease in the previous 12 months; see Table 1 for more detailed health information. In our analysis *number of infectious diseases* refers to the total number of different infectious diseases experienced in the year before data collection. Following Stevenson et al. [8] we coded the recency of each disease as '4' if the illness was current, '3' if it occurred within the past week, '2' if it occurred in the past month, '1' if it occurred in the past year, and '0' for all other values. By summing the recency score for each disease, an illness recency score was calculated for each participant.

The health of participants during their childhood was estimated using data collected by the ICDDR,B in the early nineties [24]. During this period, all mothers of children under 5 years were visited each month and asked if their children had experienced diarrhea in the past fortnight or pneumonia in the past month. These two diseases are the major causes of child mortality in rural Bangladesh [25]. On average, 6.1 (SD: 4.8) bouts of diarrhea and 1.8 (SD: 1.4) bouts were recorded per child. There was a marginal association between childhood diarrhoea and current number of infectious diseases (Spearman's $\rho = .11$, $p = .06$) and no association between childhood pneumonia and number of infectious diseases (Spearman's $\rho = .06$, $p = .4$). Childhood diarrhea and pneumonia correlate positively (Spearman's $\rho = .22$, $p < .001$).

Results

The raw data and analysis code are available from figshare.com [22]. Disgust responses were first analyzed using exploratory factor analysis. We used the ordinary least squared method to find the solution with minimum residuals. A parallel analysis [26] indicated that the data was best summarized with two factors: The first five

Table 3. A multilevel model of number of infections over past year and disgust sensitivity (two disgust factors).

	Model 1		Model 2		Model 3	
	Estimate	95% CI	Estimate	95% CI	Estimate	95% CI
Fixed effects						
Intercept	2.18	[1.45, 2.91]	3.06	[1.51, 4.63]	2.87	[0.02, 5.75]
disgust1			−0.19	[−0.73, 0.35]	−0.18	[−0.73, 0.36]
disgust2			−0.13	[−0.64, 0.39]	−0.13	[−0.64, 0.40]
sex					0.03	[−0.32, 0.38]
age					0.01	[−0.13, 0.14]
Random effects						
Intercept	0.52		0.39		0.40	
Residual	2.07		2.08		2.10	
Model fit statistics						
Deviance	1023		1022		1022	
Model AIC	1030		1034		1043	
Model AIC – minimum AIC	-		4		13	

Table 4. A multilevel model of illness recency and disgust sensitivity (two disgust factors).

	Model 1		Model 2		Model 3	
	Estimate	95% CI	Estimate	95% CI	Estimate	95% CI
Fixed effects						
Intercept	3.32	[2.50, 4.14]	5.28	[2.77, 7.89]	6.33	[0.93, 11.72]
disgust1			−0.51	[−1.48, 0.45]	−0.49	[−1.46, 0.48]
disgust2			−0.17	[−1.11, 0.78]	−0.15	[−1.10, 0.80]
sex					0.21	[−0.48, 0.90]
age					−0.07	[−0.33, 0.19]
Random effects						
Intercept	0.58		0.32		0.32	
Residual	7.99		8.03		8.06	
Model fit statistics						
Deviance	1402		1400		1399	
Model AIC	1408		1410		1416	
Model AIC – minimum AIC	-		2		8	

eigenvalues were 7.42, 1.76, 1.26, 1.01, and 0.98 while the first three average eigenvalues from 1,000 randomly generated datasets with the same dimensions were 1.59, 1.48, 1.40, 1.33, and 1.29. (95th percentile: 1.68, 1.54, 1.46, 1.38, and 1.31). A scree plot similarly indicated a two-factor solution. For eight of the disgust items, these two latent variables explained less than 20% of the variance and therefore these items were removed and the analysis was repeated [26]. Two items that cross-loaded weakly on both factor 1 and factor 2 were also excluded. To allow for correlation between factors, a direct oblimin rotation was performed. Factor loadings and communality for the surviving items are shown in Table 2. Factor one was primarily associated with unhygienic behavior while several items about people and food loaded on factor two. By averaging the items that loaded most strongly on factor 1 and factor 2 we created two variables, *disgust1* and *disgust2*. These two disgust measures were positively correlated ($r = .67$, $p < .001$). Cronbach's alpha for disgust1 and disgust2 were .85 and .81, respectively.

Men rated disgust1 items ($M = 3.15$ versus 2.96, $t(282) = 2.74$, $p = .007$, Cohen's $d = .33$) and disgust2 items ($M = 2.62$ versus 2.47, $t(282) = 2.18$, $p = .03$, Cohen's $d = .26$) as more disgusting than women did. Disgust sensitivity differed according to which field worker conducted the interview (disgust1 ANOVA: $F(3,280) = 173$, $p < .001$; disgust2: $F(3, 280) = 149$, $p < .001$). These interview effects – i.e., measurement error attributable to characteristics of the interviewer [27] – were accommodated in the analysis using multilevel (mixed) models [28]. Field worker group was modeled as a random effect while disgust, age, and sex were modeled as fixed effects. Using the AIC [29] we compared the fit of different models to the data. In the case of number of infections, a model with no fixed effects (i.e. without disgust, sex or age) fit the data better than a model including disgust, see Table 3. A similar analysis was conducted to investigate the relationship between disgust and recency of infection. As Table 4 indicates, disgust sensitivity had no strong relationship with illness recency.

Childhood health was measured by a different team of FWs and so interviewer effects and the associated correlated error are not

Table 5. Adult disgust sensitivity and childhood health: multiple regression analyses.

	Disgust1		Disgust2		Disgust: Single factor	
	Beta	95% CI	Beta	95% CI	Beta	95% CI
Intercept	2.64***	[2.06, 3.22]	1.17***	[1.55, 2.79]	2.28***	[1.72, 2.85]
Childhood Diarrhea	0.00	[−0.01, 0.01]	0.00	[−0.01, 0.01]	0.00	[−0.00, 0.01]
Childhood Pneumonia	0.02	[−0.01, 0.05]	0.01	[−0.03, 0.04]	0.02	[−0.01, 0.05]
Field Worker 1 (ref)						
2	0.90***	[0.79, 1.01]	0.31***	[0.20, 0.43]	0.87***	[0.76, 0.98]
3	0.78***	[0.68, 0.90]	1.03***	[0.92, 1.15]	1.26***	[1.16, 1.37]
4	−0.27***	[−0.39, −0.14]	−0.16**	[−0.30, −0.03]	−0.13*	[−0.26, −0.01]
Age	0.00	[−0.03, 0.03]	0.00	[−0.03, 0.04]	0.01	[−0.03, 0.03]
Sex (female)	−0.11*	[−0.20, −0.04]	−0.11*	[−0.20, −0.02]	−0.10**	[−0.18, −0.02]

Note: *** indicates $p < .001$, ** indicates $p < .01$ and * indicates $p < .05$.

Table 6. Exploratory factor analysis of disgust items: one factor solution.

Back Translated Item	Factor Loading	Communality
Touching the inside of a toilet	0.83	0.68
A stranger touching your things	0.74	0.55
Eating dropped sweet	0.73	0.53
Touching an animal	0.72	0.52
Deformed body	0.69	0.47
Hand without a finger	0.68	0.46
Dead animal	0.68	0.46
Eating something with left hand	0.62	0.38
Unkempt beggar	0.6	0.36
Person who never washes himself	0.59	0.35
Eating from dirty plate	0.57	0.33
Picking your nose	0.53	0.29
Eating last nights food	0.52	0.27
Sour milk	0.51	0.26

Note: Items ordered according to factor loading

relevant in the analysis of childhood health and disgust sensitivity. The data were analyzed using multiple regression. As Table 5 shows, there was no relationship between disgust1 (adjusted $R^2 = .65$, $F(7,276) = 77.3$, $p < .001$) or disgust2 (adjusted $R^2 = .61$, $F(7,276) = 65.22$, $p < .001$) and childhood diarrhea or pneumonia.

Although the parallel analysis and scree plot indicated that disgust sensitivity is best measured by two variables, disgust1 and disgust2, these two factors do correlate strongly and have some overlap in content (e.g., items that could be considered hygiene related load on both factors). Thus disgust sensitivity might be better measured as a single variable. Following a reviewer's recommendation, we reexamined the relationship between disgust sensitivity and health with a single disgust variable. The factor analysis was repeated, items with a communality <.2 were excluded, and all items with a loading of .5 or higher that factor were averaged to created a general disgust score (Cronbach's alpha = .9; see Table 6). The multivariate analyses results were broadly consistent with those presented above. Number of infectious diseases was best predicted by a simple model excluding disgust (see Table 7). Results displayed in Table 8 indicate that people higher in disgust sensitivity were sick less recently than people lower in disgust. However, this effect was not statistically significant and the AIC statistic indicates that a model excluding disgust provides a better fit. Finally, we found no relationship between disgust and childhood diarrhea or pneumonia (Table 5). To summarize, disgust, when measured as a single construct, is unrelated to the number of infections in childhood or adulthood, or the recency of disease.

Table 7. A multilevel model of number of infections over past year and disgust sensitivity (single disgust factor).

	Model 1		Model 2		Model 3	
	Estimate	**95% CI**	**Estimate**	**95% CI**	**Estimate**	**95% CI**
Fixed effects						
Intercept	2.18	[1.45, 2.91]	2.78	[1.41, 4.16]	2.60	[0.20, 5.40]
disgust			−0.22	[−0.68, 0.23]	−0.21	[−0.68, 0.24]
sex					0.04	[−0.31, 0.40]
age					0.01	[−0.13, 0.14]
Random effects						
Intercept	0.52		0.39		0.37	
Residual	2.07		2.08		2.09	
Model fit statistics						
Deviance	1023		1022		1022	
Model AIC	1030		1032		1040	
Model AIC – minimum AIC	-		2		10	

Table 8. A multilevel model of illness recency and disgust sensitivity (single disgust factor).

	Model 1		Model 2		Model 3	
	Estimate	95% CI	Estimate	95% CI	Estimate	95% CI
Fixed effects						
Intercept	3.32	[2.50, 4.14]	5.00	[3.01, 6.98]	6.14	[0.96, 11.31]
disgust			−0.62	[−1.32, 0.08]	−0.60	[−1.31, 0.11]
sex					0.23	[−0.46, 0.92]
age					−0.07	[−0.33, 0.19]
Random effects						
Intercept	0.58		0.23		0.22	
Residual	7.99		8.00		8.04	
Model fit statistics						
Deviance	1402		1400		1399	
Model AIC	1408		1409		1414	
Model AIC – minimum AIC	-		1		6	

Discussion

Contrary to our hypotheses, we found no relationship between disgust sensitivity and childhood health, or between disgust sensitivity and recent health. Below we discuss theoretical and methodological explanations for these null findings

One possible explanation is that disgust sensitivity is unrelated to infection risk. A number of different processes, enumerated below, may weaken the association between disgust and health. (1) Disease exposure depends on community and family behavior as well as individual behavior. If the role of these other people is relatively strong, we are unlikely to detect and relationship between individual psychology and health. Most of our participants were young adults still living at home and their health may therefore be more dependent on parents' and siblings' precautionary behavior. (2) Removing pathogen risks from the one's environment often involves interaction with disgust elicitors and in some circumstances high disgust sensitivity may inhibit actions that benefit health. (3) There is good evidence that people socially learn what constitutes a disgust elicitor [30]. It may be the case that the overlap of disgust elicitors and disease risks is a more important determinant of health than disgust sensitivity itself. In other words, high disgust sensitivity may prevent infection only in individuals who are disgusted by the locally important disease threats. (4) As the findings of Stevenson *et al.* [8] suggests, the interaction of disgust and the tendency to make strong inferences about the spread of contamination may be more important than disgust sensitivity alone. (5) Stevenson *et al.* also suggest that disease exposure results in an increase in disgust sensitivity. Such an effect may mask the protective effects of disgust in a cross-sectional study. Longitudinal data on both disgust sensitivity and health would help to resolve this question.

Our results do not support the hypothesis that adult disgust sensitivity is calibrated by childhood disease exposure. We estimated childhood health using incidence of diarrhea and pneumonia. Although these are important causes of childhood mortality, they kill relatively few adults. Moreover, data from this sample suggests a weak relationship between diarrhea and adult health, and no relationship between pneumonia and adult health. It may be the case the there are other diseases/pathogens that are better predictors of adult pathogen stress and consequently adult disease avoidance behavior.

A more general point is that in some circumstances, a more risky environment can counter-intuitively favor individuals who invest *less* in precautionary behavior [31]. E.g., consider how a solider likely to die in battle gains little in life expectancy from not smoking compared to a general who can expect to survive the war. Unavoidable risks make precautionary behavior for avoidable risks less worthwhile. We have assumed that disease risk is, by in large, an avoidable risk which can be mitigated through precautionary behavior. If, however, a large proportion of infection risk is unavoidable, then individuals in high-risk environments are unlikely to invest more. More research on the extent to which disease risks are avoidable – and are *perceived* to be avoidable – would be help to clarify this issue.

An alternative explanation for these null results is that the measures of health and/or disgust were lacking in validity or reliability. Measuring psychological constructs like disgust sensitivity in a low-income, non-English speaking population is not straightforward. Although Bengali is the 6th most commonly spoken language, few, if any, psychological measures have been translated and validated in Bengali. Our disgust measure followed the format of some commonly used and well-validated measures and was well understood by participants and field workers. However, there are two causes for concern. Contrary to several published studies [2,32,33], male participants rated the items more disgusting that women. This indicates that either sex differences in pathogen related disgust are not as consistent as previously argued, or that the measure is biased in some way. However, there are some reasons to think that sex differences in disgust play out differently in this population. In Matlab there is an uneven exposure to disgust-relevant stimuli; women do almost all cleaning and cooking, and they care for infants and the infirm. Rozin has argued that repeated interaction with disgust cues reduces sensitivity [34] and thus this may account for the reversal of sex differences. Another point of concern with the disgust measure was that sensitivity appeared to vary according to field worker. Some interviewer effects are inevitable in this kind of study, and the effects were statistically controlled for in the analysis, but nevertheless they may have weakened our ability to detect a real relationship. Future research on disgust sensitivity may benefit from asking participants to rate pre-recorded audio versions of the items or to rate images of disgust stimuli instead. Another possible explanation for this null result is health was not accurately measured. In particular, our measure of recent health was relatively crude; participants may have forgotten disease events or misremembered the exact timing. However, the positive correlation between childhood and adult disease frequency does suggest these measures have some validity.

We argued that high disgust sensitivity would be associated with fewer infections because more sensitive individuals have less contact with infectious matter. However, actual sickness is a relatively poor measure of pathogen exposure. Most exposure events (e.g., eating contaminated food, being coughed upon) do not result in disease because the pathogenic organisms are destroyed by the immune system or because the infection remains 'latent' [35]. Moreover, people differ in the extent to which they can prevent disease occurring, given exposure. A more direct way to study the protective effects of disgust may be to examine immunological markers of disease exposure. By measuring specific antibody levels, researchers may be able to estimate the frequency of pathogen exposure more accurately [36,37]. Such a study should have a more power to detect the relationship between disgust and pathogen exposure, if one does indeed exist.

Acknowledgments

We thank Dr Zahid Hayat, Mr Zakir Hossain and Mr Rashed Zaman for their support during fieldwork.

Author Contributions

Conceived and designed the experiments: MDB VC SI. Performed the experiments: MDB SI. Analyzed the data: MDB. Wrote the paper: MDB VC.

References

1. Curtis V, Biran A (2001) Dirt, disgust, and disease: Is hygiene in our genes? Perspect Biol Med 44: 17–31.
2. Curtis V, Aunger R, Rabie T (2004) Evidence that disgust evolved to protect from risk of disease. Proc Biol Sci 271 Suppl: S131–3. doi:10.1098/rsbl.2003.0144.
3. Curtis V, de Barra M, Aunger R (2011) Disgust as an adaptive system for disease avoidance behaviour. Philos Trans R Soc B 366: 389–401. doi:10.1098/rstb.2010.0117.
4. Wisenden BD, Goater CP, James CT (2003) Behavioral Defenses against Parasites and Pathogens. In: Zaccone C, Perriere A, Mathis A, Kapoor G, editors. Fish Defenses. Vol 2 Enfield, USA. pp. 151–168.
5. Hart BL (2011) Behavioural defences in animals against pathogens and parasites: parallels with the pillars of medicine in humans. Philos Trans R Soc B 366: 3406–3417. doi:10.1098/rstb.2011.0092.
6. Oaten M, Stevenson RJ, Case TI (2009) Disgust as a disease-avoidance mechanism. Psychol Bull 135: 303–321. doi:10.1037/a0014823.
7. Rozin P, Haidt J, McCauley C, Dunlop L, Ashmore M (1999) Individual Differences in Disgust Sensitivity: Comparisons and Evaluations of Paper-and-Pencil versus Behavioral Measures. J Res Pers 33: 330–351.
8. Stevenson RJ, Case TI, Oaten MJ (2009) Frequency and recency of infection and their relationship with disgust and contamination sensitivity. Evol Hum Behav 30: 363–368. doi:10.1016/j.evolhumbehav.2009.02.005.
9. Lozano R, Naghavi M, Foreman K, Lim S, Shibuya K, et al. (2012) Global and regional mortality from 235 causes of death for 20 age groups in 1990 and 2010: a systematic analysis for the Global Burden of Disease Study 2010. Lancet 380: 2095–2128. doi:10.1016/S0140-6736(12)61728-0.
10. Davey GCL, Bond N (2006) Using controlled comparisons in disgust psychopathology research: The case of disgust, hypochondriasis and health anxiety. J Behav Ther Exp Psychiatry 37: 4–15.
11. Hutchings MR, Judge J, Gordan IJ, Athanasiadou S, Kyriazakis I (2006) Use of trade-off theory to advance understanding of herbivore-parasite interactions. Mamm Rev 36: 1–16. doi:10.1111/j.1365-2907.2006.00080.x.
12. Hoefling A, Likowski KU, Deutsch R, Mu A, Weyers P, et al. (2009) When hunger finds no fault with moldy corn: food deprivation reduces food-related disgust. Emotion 9: 50–58. doi:10.1037/a0014449.
13. Fessler DMT, Navarrete CD (2003) Domain-specific variation in disgust sensitivity across the menstrual cycle. Evol Hum Behav 24: 406–417. doi:10.1016/S1090-5138(03)00054-0.
14. Lively C (1986) Predator-induced shell dimorphism in the acorn barnacle Chthamalus anisopoma. Evolution (N Y) 40: 232–242.
15. Nettle D, Coall DA, Dickins TE (2011) Early-life conditions and age at first pregnancy in British women. Proc R Soc B 278: 1721–1727. doi:10.1098/rspb.2010.1726.
16. Waynforth D (2012) Life-history theory, chronic childhood illness and the timing of first reproduction in a British birth cohort. Proc R Soc B 279: 2998–3002. doi:10.1098/rspb.2012.0220.
17. De Barra M, DeBruine LM, Jones BC, Mahmud ZH, Curtis VA (2013) Illness in childhood predicts face preferences in adulthood. Evol Hum Behav 24: 384–389. doi:10.1016/j.evolhumbehav.2013.07.001.
18. Haidt J, McCauley C, Rozin P (1994) Individual differences in sensitivity to disgust: A scale sampling seven domains of disgust elicitors. Pers Individ Dif 16: 701–713. doi:10.1016/0191-8869(94)90212-7.
19. Olatunji BO, Cisler JM, Deacon BJ, Connolly K, Lohr JM (2007) The Disgust Propensity and Sensitivity Scale-Revised: psychometric properties and specificity in relation to anxiety disorder symptoms. J Anxiety Disord 21: 918–930. doi:10.1016/j.janxdis.2006.12.005.
20. Tybur JM, Lieberman D (2009) Microbes, mating, and morality: Individual differences in three functional domains of disgust. J Pers Soc Psychol 97: 103–22.
21. Curtis V (2013) Don't Look, Don't Touch: The Science Behind Revulsion. Chicago: University of Chicago Press.
22. De Barra M (2013) Infectious disease and disgust sensitivity in Bangladesh. Figshare. doi:10.6084/m9.figshare.839646.
23. Rahman O, Menken J, Foster A, Peterson CE, Khan MN, et al. (1999) The 1996 Matlab Health and Socioeconomic Survey. RAND Corporation.
24. Rahman MM, Alam MN, Razzaque A, Streatfield PK (2012) Health and Demographic Surveillance System–Matlab, v. 44. Registration of health and demographic events 2010. Dhaka.
25. Baqui AH, Black RE, Arifeen SE, Hill K, Mitra SN, et al. (1998) Causes of childhood deaths in Bangladesh: results of a nationwide verbal autopsy study. Bull World Health Organ 76: 161–171.
26. Hayton JC, Allen DG, Scarpello V (2004) Factor Retention Decisions in Exploratory Factor Analysis: a Tutorial on Parallel Analysis. Organ Res Methods 7: 191–205. doi:10.1177/1094428104263675.
27. Freeman J, Butler E (1976) Some sources of interviewer variance in surveys. Public Opin Q 40: 79–91.
28. Hox J (1994) Hierarchical regression models for interviewer and respondent effects. Sociol Methods Res 22: 300–318.
29. Akaike H (1974) A new look at the statistical model identification. Autom Control IEEE Trans.
30. Bayliss AP, Frischen A, Fenske MJ, Tipper SP (2006) Affective evaluations of objects are influenced by observed gaze direction and emotional expression. Cognition 104: 644–663. doi:10.1016/j.cognition.2006.07.012.
31. Nettle D (2010) Why are there social gradients in preventative health behavior? A perspective from behavioral ecology. PLoS One 5: e13371. doi:10.1371/journal.pone.0013371.
32. Tybur JM, Bryan AD, Lieberman D, Caldwell Hooper AE, Merriman L a. (2011) Sex differences and sex similarities in disgust sensitivity. Pers Individ Dif 51: 343–348. doi:10.1016/j.paid.2011.04.003.
33. Olatunji BO, Moretz MW, McKay D, Bjorklund F, de Jong PJ, et al. (2009) Confirming the Three-Factor Structure of the Disgust Scale–Revised in Eight Countries. J Cross Cult Psychol 40: 234–255. doi:10.1177/0022022108328918.
34. Rozin P (2008) Hedonic "adaptation": Specific habituation to disgust/death elicitors as a result of dissecting a cadaver. Judgm Decis Mak 3: 191–194.
35. Janeway CA, Travers P, Walport M, Shlomchik MJ (2001) Immunobiology. 5th ed. New York: Garland Science.
36. Albers R, Antoine J-M, Bourdet-Sicard R, Calder PC, Gleeson M, et al. (2007) Markers to measure immunomodulation in human nutrition intervention studies. Br J Nutr 94: 452. doi:10.1079/BJN20051469.
37. Drakeley CJ, Corran PH, Coleman PG, Tongren JE, McDonald SLR, et al. (2005) Estimating medium- and long-term trends in malaria transmission by using serological markers of malaria exposure. Proc Natl Acad Sci U S A 102: 5108–5113. doi:10.1073/pnas.0408725102.

Icotinib Is an Active Treatment of Non-Small-Cell Lung Cancer: A Retrospective Study

Xiaofeng Chen[1]❘, Quan Zhu[2]❘, Yiqian Liu[1], Ping Liu[1], Yongmei Yin[1], Renhua Guo[1], Kaihua Lu[1], Yanhong Gu[1], Lianke Liu[1], Jinghua Wang[3], Zhaoxia Wang[4], Oluf Dimitri Røe[5,6], Yongqian Shu[1]*, Lingjun Zhu[1]*

1 Department of Oncology, the First Affiliated Hospital of Nanjing Medical University, Nanjing, China, **2** Department of Cardiothoracic Surgery, the First Affiliated Hospital of Nanjing Medical University, Nanjing, China, **3** Department of Oncology, Jinling Hospital, Nanjing University School of Medicine, Nanjing, China, **4** Department of Oncology, the Second Affiliated Hospital of Nanjing Medical University, Nanjing, China, **5** Department of Cancer Research and Molecular Medicine, Norwegian University of Science and Technology, Trondheim, Norway, **6** Norwegian University of Science and Technology, Trondheim, Norway, Cancer Clinic, Levanger Hospital, Nord-Trøndelag Health Trust, Levanger, Norway

Abstract

Background: Icotinib hydrochloride is a novel epidermal growth factor receptor (EGFR) tyrosine kinase inhibitor (TKI) with preclinical and clinical activity in non-small cell lung cancer (NSCLC). This retrospective analysis was performed to assess the efficacy of icotinib on patients with non-small-cell lung cancer (NSCLC).

Methods: 82 consecutive patients treated with icotinib as first (n = 24) or second/third line (n = 58) treatment at three hospitals in Nanjing were enrolled into our retrospective research. The Response Evaluation Criteria in Solid Tumors (RECIST) was used to evaluate the tumor responses and the progression-free survival (PFS) and overall survival (OS) was evaluated by the Kaplan-Meier method.

Results: Median PFS was 4.0 months (95% CI 2.311–5.689). Median OS was 11.0 months (95% CI 8.537–13.463) in this cohort. Median PFS for first and second/third line were 7.0 months (95% CI 2.151–11.8) and 3.0 months (95% CI 1.042–4.958), respectively. Median OS for first and second/third line were 13.0 months (95% CI 10.305–15.695) and 10.0 months (95% CI 7.295–12.70), respectively. In patients with EGFR mutation (n = 19), icotinib significantly reduced the risk of progression (HR 0.36, 95% CI 0.18–0.70, $p = 0.003$) and death (HR 0.10, 95% CI 0.02–0.42, $p = 0.002$) compared with those EGFR status unknown (n = 63). The most common adverse events were acne-like rash (39.0%) and diarrhea (20.7%).

Conclusions: Icotinib is active in the treatment of patients with NSCLC both in first or second/third line, especially in those patients harbouring EGFR mutations, with an acceptable adverse event profile.

Editor: Srikumar P. Chellappan, H. Lee Moffitt Cancer Center & Research Institute, United States of America

Funding: This work was partly supported by the Program for Development of Innovative Research Teams, by Jiangsu Province Clinical Science and Technology Projects (Clinical Research Center, BL 2012008), and by the Priority Academic Program Development of Jiangsu Higher Education Institutions (PAPD) and by Provincial Initiative Program for Excellency Disciplines, Jiangsu Province, China. No additional external funding was received for this study. The funders had no role in study design, data collection and analysis, decision to publish, or preparation of the manuscript.

Competing Interests: The authors have declared that no competing interests exist.

* E-mail: yongqianshu@126.com (YS); zhulingjun@njmu.edu.cn (LZ)

❘ These authors contributed equally to this work.

Introduction

The epidermal-growth-factor receptor (EGFR) is part of a signalling pathway that regulates tumor cell proliferation, invasion, angiogenesis, metastasis, and apoptosis [1]. EGFR tyrosine-kinase inhibitors (TKIs) can inhibit tumor cells by blocking the EGFR signaling via binding to ATP binding site on the tyrosine kinase domain of the EGFR. Activating EGFR mutations are found in about 60% of lung adenocarcinomas in the East Asian population and nonsmoker or former light smoker [2]. Numerous phase III studies have shown that EGFR TKIs such as gefitinib or erlotinib have strong anti-tumor activity and increase survival in patients with NSCLC harboring activating EGFR mutation not only in second and third line [3,4,5], but also in first line [2,6,7] and maintenance treatment [8,9,10].

Icotinib hydrochloride is a new type of small molecule EGFR-TKI, developed and patented by Zhejiang BetaPharma Co., Ltd. (Hangzhou, Zhejiang, China, Patent No. WO2003082830). Its chemical name is 4-((3-ethynylphenyl) amino)-6, 7-benzo-12-crown-4- quinazoline hydrochloride. The molecular formula is $C_{22}H_{21}N_3O_4 \cdot HCl$, with a small molecular weight of 427.88. Preclinical studies showed that icotinib is a potent and specific EGFR TKI. *In vitro,* icotinib could significantly inhibit the EGFR tyrosine kinase activity at a concentration of 0.5 μM including the EGFR (91%), EGFR (L858R) (99%), EGFR (L861Q) (96%), EGFR (T790M) (61%) and EGFR (T790M, L858R) (61%) [11].

In EGFR-mutated lung cancer cell lines (PC-9 and HCC827), icotinib showed similar anti-tumor effect compared with gefitinib [12]. *In vivo*, icotinib strongly inhibited the tumor growth in several xenograft models in a dose related manner [11].

Two phase I studies evaluated the safety and tolerability of icotinib in Chinese patients with NSCLC and other solid tumors [13,14]. Generally, icotinib showed favorable safety and tolerability. Mild and reversible rash, diarrhea and nausea were the main adverse events. Notably, positive anti-tumor activities were observed in patients with advanced NSCLC. A dose of 125 mg or 150 mg q8h/day was recommended for phase II/III studies.

A randomized, double-blind phase III study [15] was carried out to compare the efficacy and safety of icotinib with gefitinib in NSCLC patients previously treated with chemotherapy (ICOGEN) [16]. A total of 399 patients with advanced NSCLC who had progressed after one or two lines of chemotherapies were randomized to receive icotinib (n = 200, 125 mg q8h) or gefitinib (n = 199, 250 mg qd). Compared with gefitinib, icotinib provided similar median progression-free survival (PFS, icotinib vs. gefitinib: 4.6 months vs. 3.4 months, HR 0.84, 95% CI 0.67–1.05) and median overall survival benefit (OS, icotinib vs. gefitinib: 13.3 months vs. 13.9 months, HR 0.90, 95% CI 0.79–1.02). As with gefitinib, biomarker analysis revealed that EGFR mutation status was the strongest predictor for icotinib. The PFS in patients treated with icotinib was 7.8 months in EGFR mutant subgroup and 2.3 months in EGFR wild type population.

Based on the encouraging results of ICOGEN reported in ASCO annual meeting in 2011, icotinib was approved for the second or third line treatment of advanced NSCLC by the State Food and Drug Administration of China. Gefitinib and erlotinib have shown good efficacy as first line treatment in clinically selected patients, while icotinib has the similar molecular structure with gefitinib and erlotinib. In addition, icotinib is much cheaper than gefitinib or erlotinib in China. Thus icotinib was also an alternative choice for first line treatment in the clinic. Here, we retrospectively analyzed the efficacy of icotinib on the treatment of advanced NSCLC patients as first line or second/third line treatment in clinical practice.

Patients and Methods

Ethics Statement

This study was approved by the three hospitals Review Boards: the First and Second Affiliated Hospital of Nanjing Medical University, and Jinling Hospital of Nanjing University School of Medicine. Patient records were anonymized and de-identified prior to analysis.

Patients

We conducted a retrospective search of the medical records in the First and Second Affiliated Hospital of Nanjing Medical University, and Jinling Hospital of Nanjing University School of Medicine, from July 2011 to February 2013. Excluding the patients received icotinib as forth or later lines treatment and those whose clinical data were not available, 82 patients who received icotinib as first line (n = 24) or second/third line (n = 58) treatment were enrolled into our retrospective search. All these patients received oral icotinib at a dose of 125 mg q8h/day continuously until either a disease progression (radiographic or obvious clinical) or severe toxicity was observed. No other chemotherapeutic drug was administered concurrently with icotinib treatment.

Assessment of the Efficacy and Adverse Events

The Response Evaluation Criteria in Solid Tumors (RECIST) was used to evaluate the tumor responses [17]. The evaluation was from the patients' original medical records and in some uncertain cases, was re-evalatued by two radiologist (H.L & Y.J, radiology department in the First Affiliated Hospital of Nanjing Medical University). Objective response comprises complete response (CR) and partial response (PR). Disease control was defined as CR, PR or stable disease (SD). Generally, after starting with icotinib, the first evaluation was performed at one month, and then assessed every two months or at overt signs of progression. PFS was defined as the period from the initial administration of icotinib to tumor progression or death of any cause (calculated according to the event occurred firstly). OS was defined as the span between the start of icotinib and the date of death. Adverse events were assessed according to Common Terminology Criteria for Adverse Events of the National Cancer Institute (version 3.0) [18]. Clinical data and outcomes were collected by patient medical records search, consulting the doctors in charge, interview in the clinic and phone calls to the patients or their relatives.

Statistical Analysis

The chi-square ($\chi 2$) test was used for intergroup comparisons of response rate and disease control rate at a significance level of 5% ($\alpha = 0.05$, two-sided). PFS and OS were obtained using the Kaplan-Meier method. Log-rank test was applied to compare the significance between groups. Multivariate Cox-regression model was also used to detect the hazard ratios. SPSS software package (SPSS 17.0 Inc., Chicago, IL, USA) was applied.

Results

Patients Characteristics

A total of 82 patients who received icotinib as first (n = 24) or second/third (n = 58) line treatment were enrolled in this retrospective analysis. The median age of the population was 64 years. All patients were Chinese. Most patients were non-smokers, had adenocarcinoma, stage IV disease and relatively low performance status (Table 1). EGFR sensitive mutation was found in 19 patients (8 in first line and 11 in second/third line) while unknown in the remaining cases. This may due to the lack of proper tissue and some patients were reluctant to receive the gene detection. Five patients had diagnosed brain metastasis before they received icotinib. In the second/third lines subset, the most frequently used chemotherapy regimens for first/second line treatment were pemetrexed+cisplatin/carboplatin, paclitaxel+cisplatin/carboplatin, docetaxel+cisplatin/carboplatin and gemcitabine+cisplatin. Two patients received gefitinib as first line treatment.

Response Rate

The CR, PR and SD of the whole group were 1%, 22% and 41%, respectively, a 65% overall disease control rate. Twelve of 19 patients (63%) bearing EGFR mutation experienced an objective response, which was significantly higher than that in patients with EGFR status unknown (7 out of 63, 11%). Higher response rates were observed in EGFR mutation positive patients in first as well as second/third line, while a higher disease control rate was only seen in the first line subset (Table 2).

Progression-free Survival and Overall Survival

Median progression-free survival for the 82 patients was 4.0 months (95% CI 2.311–5.689). Patients bearing EGFR mutation had a significantly longer PFS (9.0 months, 95% CI 3.661–14.339)

Table 1. Patient characteristics.

	First line N = 24	Second/third line N = 58	Total N = 82 (%)
Median age	64(37–79)	65(30–80)	64
Sex			
Male	9	32	41 (50)
Female	15	26	41 (50)
ECOG			
0–1	7	20	27 (32.9)
2	14	28	42 (51.2)
3	3	10	13 (15.8)
Smoking history			
Non-smoker	14	36	50 (60.9)
Smoker	10	22	32 (39.1)
EGFR mutation			
Del 19	5	7	12 (14.6)
L858R	3	4	7 (8.5)
Not available	16	47	62 (36.9)
Clinical stage			
IIIb	2	7	9 (11)
IV	22	51	73 (89)
Pathological type			
Adeno	23	52	75 (91)
Squamous	1	5	6 (7.3)
Other	0	1	1 (1.7)

than those with EGFR status unknown (3.0 month, 95% CI 2.284–5.151, $p = 0.001$) or the whole population ($p = 0.014$) (Figure 1–1). Median progression-free survival was 7.0 months (95% CI 2.151–11.849; Figure 1–2) in first line subset and 3.0 months (95% CI 1.042–4.958, Figure 1–3) in second/third lines subset. Consistently, patients with EGFR sensitive mutation had longer PFS both in first line ($p = 0.020$) and in second/third line subgroups ($p = 0.034$) compared with those whose EGFR status were unknown. Multivariate analysis using Cox regression model indicated that icotinib significantly decreased the risk of progression in patients with EGFR mutation compared with EGFR status unkown (HR, 0.36, 95% CI 0.18–0.70, $p = 0.003$). In patients with EGFR mutation icotinib showed decreased risk of progression in the first line subset, (HR, 0.21, 95% CI,0.05–0.97, $p = 0.046$), while insignificant/trend of risk reduction in the second/third line subset (HR, 0.51, 95% CI 0.24–1.07, $p = 0.073$).

Median overall survival for all patients was 11.0 months (95% CI 8.537–13.463, Figure 2–1). Consistent with the results in PFS, patients with EGFR mutation had statistically longer OS (not reached) than those with EGFR status unknown (mOS 9.0 months, 95% CI 7.207–10.793, $p = 0.000$) or the whole population ($p = 0.001$). This superiority was consistently observed both in first and second/third line subsets. The median overall survival was 13.0 months (95% CI 10.305–15.695,) in the first line treatment subgroup (Figure 2–2), and 10.0 months (95% CI 7.295–12.70) in the second/third line (Figure 2–3). Multivariate analysis showed that icotinib significantly reduced the risk of death in EGFR mutation patients (HR 0.10, 95% CI 0.02–0.42, $p = 0.002$). This significant reduction were found both in first line (HR 0.27, 95% CI 0.10–0.87, $p = 0.032$) and second/third line subsets (HR 0.18, 95% CI 0.04–0.75, $p = 0.018$).

Adverse Events

Drug related adverse event were registered in 61 of 82 patients (74.3%, Table 3). The most common adverse events were skin-related events and diarrhea. The incidence of acne-like rash and diarrhea were 39.0% and 20.7% respectively. Other common adverse events include dry skin, oral ulcer, nausea, fatigue, elevated ALT/AST, and leukopenia. However, most of the adverse events were grade 1 or 2, and only two grade 3 acne-like rashes were recorded. No possible drug-related interstitial lung disease and drug related death was noted and no patient had dose reduction due to the adverse events. The two patients with grade 3 rash refused to reduce the dose of icotinib, and the symptoms were alleviated through symptomatic treatment.

Discussion

Since the appearance of gefitinib and erlotinib, a novel TKI inhibitor, icotinib, has recently showed effect in NSCLC [16]. This relatively small retrospective study of a novel EGFR inhibitor, icotinib, in unselected NSCLC patients from three hospitals showed an encouraging disease control rate (65%), progression-free survival (4.0 m) and overall survival (11.0 m). We observed that a large proportion of patients who responded to icotinib and longer PFS were observed in patients with EGFR mutation. Although the OS in patients with EGFR mutation was not reached, it was statistically longer than that in patients with EGFR status unknown. These results suggest activity of icotinib in non-

Table 2. Best response according to RECIST 1.0.

	First line n=24			Second/third line n=58			All patients N=82			Total response
	EGFR mut+N=8	EGFR status unknown N=16	P*	EGFR mut+N=11	EGFR status unknown N=47	P**	EGFR mut+N=19	EGFR status unknown N=63	P***	
CR	0 (0%)	0 (0%)	/	1 (9%)	0 (0%)	0.190	1 (5%)	0 (0%)	0.232	1 (1%)
PR	6 (75%)	2 (13%)	0.005	5 (45%)	5 (11%)	0.013	11(58%)	7 (11%)	0.000	18 (22%)
SD	2 (25%)	7 (44%)	0.380	3 (27%)	22 (47%)	0.320	5 (26%)	29 (46%)	0.184	34 (41%)
DC	8 (100%)	9 (57%)	0.034	9 (82%)	27 (53%)	0.178	17 (89%)	36 (57%)	0.013	53 (65%)
PD	0 (0%)	7 (44%)	0.034	2 (18%)	20 (43%)	0.178	2 (11%)	27 (43%)	0.013	29 (35%)

Notes: CR, complete response; PR, partial response; SD, stable disease; DC, disease control; PD, progressive disease.
*EGFR mut vs EGFR unknown in first line icotinib treatment,
**EGFR mut vs EGFR unknown in second/third line icotinib treatment,
***EGFR mut vs EGFR unknown in all patients who received icotinib treatment.

1-1

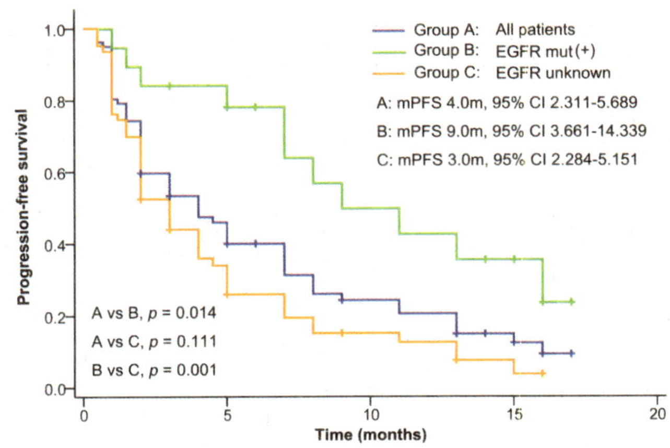

1-2

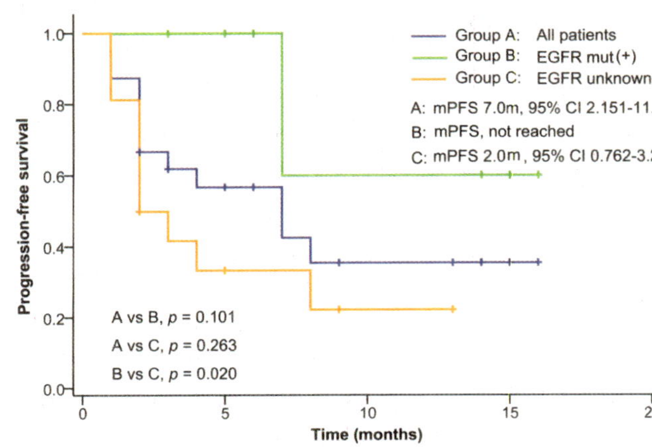

1-3

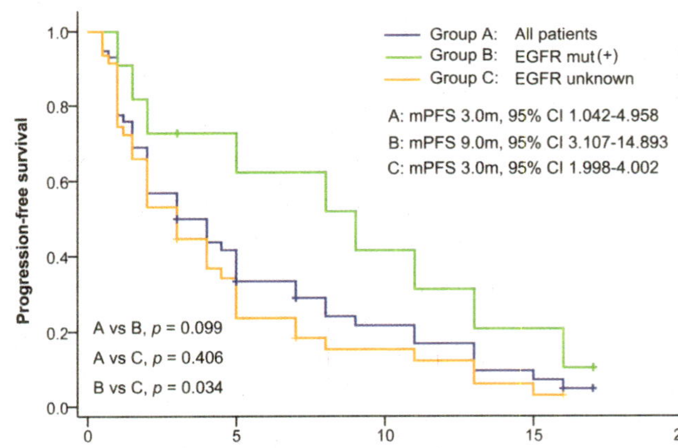

Figure 1. Progression-free survival. 1-1 shows the PFS in all patients in this study, 1-2 shows the PFS in first line subset, 1-3 shows the PFS in second/third line subset.

small cell lung cancer, and robust activity of icotinib in patients with EGFR mutation.

In the second/third line subset (n = 58), the PFS were 3.0 m for all patients, 9.0 m for EGFR mutation patients and 3.0 m for EGFR status unknown patients. The OS was 10.0 for all patients,

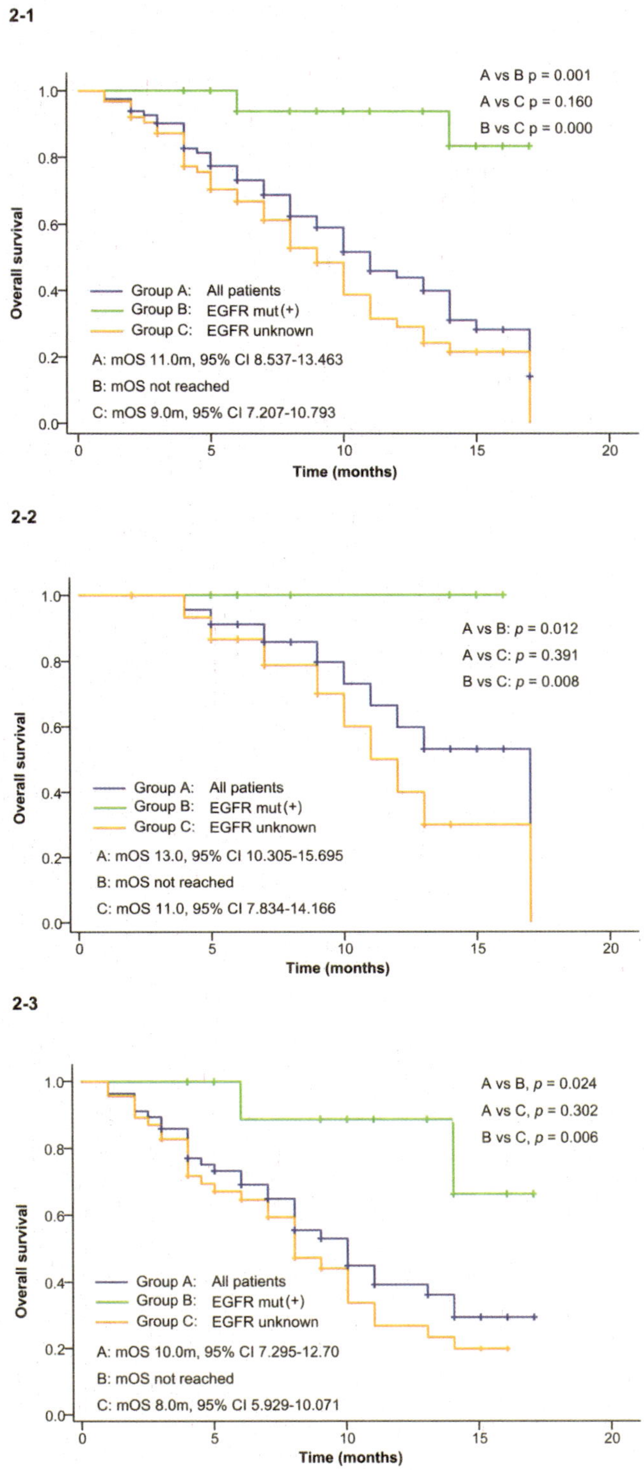

Figure 2. Overall survival. 2–1 shows the OS in all patients in this study, 2–2 shows the OS in first line subset, 2–3 shows the OS in second/third line subset.

while the OS for EGFR mutation patients was not reached. These results were similar with those reported in ICOGEN. In the ICOGEN study, patients with NSCLC that progressed after one or two lines of chemotherapies were randomized to receive icotinib (150 mg tid) or gefitinib (250 mg qd). In the icotinib group, the median PFS were 4.6 m for all patients and 7.8 m in patients with EGFR mutation, and the OS was 13.3 months, comparable with the results of gefitinib group [16,19]. Gefitinib and erlotinib has been widely tested as second/third line treatment for lung cancer in a series of prospective studies, such as INTREST [3], ISEL [5], TITAN [4] and BR.21 study [20]. The PFS of tyrosine kinase inhibitors (TKIs) groups in these studies ranged from 6.3 weeks to 3.3 months, and the OS ranged from 5.3 to 7.6 months. Our retrospective study, based on the real clinical practice, together with results from ICOGEN, showed that icotinib produced a comparable benefit with gefitinib or erlotinib, and indicated that it could be an alternative choice for patients in second/third line treatment.

In first line subset, the PFS and OS were 7.0 m and 13.0 m for all patients, 2.0 m and 11.0 m for EGFR status unknown patients respectively. PFS and OS for EGFR mutation patients were not mature. Currently, no other study reports the efficacy of icotinib as first line treatment. Three ongoing prospective trials will give more information about the activity of icotinib in first line (NCT01646450, NCT01665417, NCT01719536). Patients in our study were all Asian, 96% of them had adenocarcinoma, 63% were female, and 58% were non-smoker. These clinical features indicate that there may be a relative high rate of EGFR mutation. The PFS in this study was very similar with that in patients treated with gefitinib in IPASS study [2], which enrolled patients with clinical enrichment of EGFR mutation, including East Asian, female, non-smoker or light smoker and adenocarcinoma. Compared with those data in gefitinib and erlotinib studies, the PFS and OS in this study were numerically good, considering that there were 55 patients (67.1%) had a PS ≥ 2 in this population. However, one should note that this is a retrospective study and the assessment bias caused by clinical doctors may exist while the abovementioned studies on gefitinib and erlotinib were all prospective randomized controlled trials. In addition, the number of cases in this study was small, thus the results may be heavily influenced by individual cases, especially those with EGFR active mutation.

EGFR mutation is a prognostic factor regardless of the treatment with EGFR TKIs [21] or chemotherapy [22]. Moreover, it is also the strongest predictive factor for the efficacy of EGFR TKIs [2], Similarly, in the current study, significantly better response rates and survival results were noted in patients with EGFR mutation, compared with those with EGFR status unknown, in both first line and second/third lines subsets. Ren Guanjun et al [23] analysed the relationship between EGFR mutations and the efficacy of icotinib in patients enrolled in a phase I study, the results showed that EGFR exon 19 deletions and exon 21 point mutation are predictive biomarkers for response to icotinib hydrochloride as second line or subsequent lines of treatment. In the ICOGEN study, PFS and OS were longer in patients with EGFR mutation (7.8 m and 20.9 m, respectively) than those with EGFR mutation-negative (2.3 m and 7.8 m, respectively). Thus, EGFR mutation status is the strongest predictor in identifying which patients are most likely to benefit from icotinib. Based on these results and previous evidence from gefitinib and erlotinib, EGFR mutation should be detected when considering the use of icotinib.

The adverse events in this study was similar with those observed in ICOGEN study, while numerically less than those with gefitinib [2,24,25] and erlotinib [6,26]. Although skin related events and diarrhea were common, most of the events were grade 1, and no patient needed dose reduction. However, the available data for both the efficacy and safety of icotinib are limited, and more studies are needed to address the role of icotinib in the treatment

Table 3. Summary of the treatment-related adverse events.

Adverse events	Grade 1	Grade 2	Grade 3	Grade 4	Total (%)
Acne-like rash	24 (29.3%)	6 (7.3%)	2 (2.4%)	0	32 (39.0%)
Dry skin	7 (8.5%)	2 (2.4%)	0	0	9 (11.0%)
Oral ulcer	4 (4.9%)	1 (1.2%)	0	0	5 (6.1%)
Diarrhea	12 (14.6%)	5 (6.1%)	0	0	17 (20.7%)
Nausea	5 (6.1%)	0	0	0	5 (6.1%)
Fatigue	3 (3.7%)	2 (2.4%)	0	0	5 (6.1%)
Elevated ALT/AST	6 (7.3%)	2 (2.4%)	0	0	8 (9.8%)
Leucopenia/neutropenia	2 (2.4%)	0	0	0	2 (2.4%)

of non-small cell lung cancer. Besides the ICOGEN study, 13 prospective trials about icotinib are now active.

The key weakness of this report is its retrospective nature. The evaluation of efficacy and toxicity was not predefined. Another weakness is that the sample was small, especially for the first line subset. In addition, only a small portion of patients had EGFR status known both in first and second/third line.

In summary, a novel TKI, icotinib showed clinically meaningful activity in the treatment of patients with lung adenocarcinoma, especially in those patients harbouring EGFR mutations, with an acceptable adverse event profile. The outcomes of the ongoing trials on icotinib will give more evidence for the value of icotinib in the treatment of NSCLC.

Acknowledgments

We thank the patients and their families for their support for this work. We thank colleagues in radiology department for their work on imaging (H.L & Y.J)

Author Contributions

Conceived and designed the experiments: XFC QZ YQS LJZ. Performed the experiments: XFC QZ YQL PL YMY RHG YHG LKL JHW ZXW YQS LJZ KHL. Analyzed the data: XFC YQL ODR LJZ YQS. Contributed reagents/materials/analysis tools: XFC YQS. Wrote the paper: XFC QZ YQL.

References

1. Yarden Y, Shilo BZ (2007) SnapShot: EGFR signaling pathway. Cell 131: 1018.
2. Mok TS, Wu YL, Thongprasert S, Yang CH, Chu DT, et al. (2009) Gefitinib or carboplatin-paclitaxel in pulmonary adenocarcinoma. N Engl J Med 361: 947–957.
3. Kim ES, Hirsh V, Mok T, Socinski MA, Gervais R, et al. (2008) Gefitinib versus docetaxel in previously treated non-small-cell lung cancer (INTEREST): a randomised phase III trial. Lancet 372: 1809–1818.
4. Ciuleanu T, Stelmakh L, Cicenas S, Miliauskas S, Grigorescu AC, et al. (2012) Efficacy and safety of erlotinib versus chemotherapy in second-line treatment of patients with advanced, non-small-cell lung cancer with poor prognosis (TITAN): a randomised multicentre, open-label, phase 3 study. Lancet Oncol 13: 300–308.
5. Thatcher N, Chang A, Parikh P, Rodrigues Pereira J, Ciuleanu T, et al. (2005) Gefitinib plus best supportive care in previously treated patients with refractory advanced non-small-cell lung cancer: results from a randomised, placebo-controlled, multicentre study (Iressa Survival Evaluation in Lung Cancer). Lancet 366: 1527–1537.
6. Zhou C, Wu YL, Chen G, Feng J, Liu XQ, et al. (2011) Erlotinib versus chemotherapy as first-line treatment for patients with advanced EGFR mutation-positive non-small-cell lung cancer (OPTIMAL, CTONG-0802): a multicentre, open-label, randomised, phase 3 study. Lancet Oncol 12: 735–742.
7. Han JY, Park K, Kim SW, Lee DH, Kim HY, et al. (2012) First-SIGNAL: first-line single-agent iressa versus gemcitabine and cisplatin trial in never-smokers with adenocarcinoma of the lung. J Clin Oncol 30: 1122–1128.
8. Zhang L, Ma S, Song X, Han B, Cheng Y, et al. (2012) Gefitinib versus placebo as maintenance therapy in patients with locally advanced or metastatic non-small-cell lung cancer (INFORM; C-TONG 0804): a multicentre, double-blind randomised phase 3 trial. Lancet Oncol 13: 466–475.
9. Cappuzzo F, Ciuleanu T, Stelmakh L, Cicenas S, Szczesna A, et al. (2010) Erlotinib as maintenance treatment in advanced non-small-cell lung cancer: a multicentre, randomised, placebo-controlled phase 3 study. Lancet Oncol 11: 521–529.
10. Chen X, Liu Y, Roe OD, Qian Y, Guo R, et al. (2013) Gefitinib or erlotinib as maintenance therapy in patients with advanced stage non-small cell lung cancer: a systematic review. PLoS One 8: e59314.
11. Tan F, Shen X, Wang D, Xie G, Zhang X, et al. (2012) Icotinib (BPI-2009H), a novel EGFR tyrosine kinase inhibitor, displays potent efficacy in preclinical studies. Lung Cancer 76: 177–182.
12. Yang G, Yao Y, Zhou J, Zhao Q (2012) Effects of icotinib, a novel epidermal growth factor receptor tyrosine kinase inhibitor, in EGFR-mutated non-small cell lung cancer. Oncol Rep 27: 2066–2072.
13. Wang HP, Zhang L, Wang YX, Tan FL, Xia Y, et al. (2011) Phase I trial of icotinib, a novel epidermal growth factor receptor tyrosine kinase inhibitor, in Chinese patients with non-small cell lung cancer. Chin Med J (Engl) 124: 1933.
14. Zhao Q, Shentu J, Xu N, Zhou J, Yang G, et al. (2011) Phase I study of icotinib hydrochloride (BPI-2009H), an oral EGFR tyrosine kinase inhibitor, in patients with advanced NSCLC and other solid tumors. Lung Cancer 73: 195–202.
15. Shi Y, Zhang L, Liu X, Zhou C, Zhang S, et al. (2013) Icotinib versus gefitinib in previously treated advanced non-small-cell lung cancer (ICOGEN): a randomised, double-blind phase 3 non-inferiority trial. Lancet Oncol.
16. Y Sun YS, Zhang L, Liu X, Zhou C, Zhang L, et al. (2011) A randomized, double-blind phase III study of icotinib versus gefitinib in patients with advanced non-small cell lung cancer (NSCLC) previously treated with chemotherapy (ICOGEN). J Clin Oncol 29: (suppl; abstr 7522).
17. Therasse P, Arbuck SG, Eisenhauer EA, Wanders J, Kaplan RS, et al. (2000) New guidelines to evaluate the response to treatment in solid tumors. European Organization for Research and Treatment of Cancer, National Cancer Institute of the United States, National Cancer Institute of Canada. J Natl Cancer Inst 92: 205–216.
18. Trotti A, Colevas AD, Setser A, Rusch V, Jaques D, et al. (2003) CTCAE v3.0: development of a comprehensive grading system for the adverse effects of cancer treatment. Semin Radiat Oncol 13: 176–181.
19. Yan Sun YS, Zhang L, Liu X, Zhou C, Zhang L, et al. (2012) Final overall survival and updated biomarker analysis results from the randomized phase III ICOGEN trial. J Clin Oncol 30: (suppl; abstr 7559).
20. Shepherd FA, Rodrigues Pereira J, Ciuleanu T, Tan EH, Hirsh V, et al. (2005) Erlotinib in previously treated non-small-cell lung cancer. N Engl J Med 353: 123–132.
21. Han SW, Kim TY, Hwang PG, Jeong S, Kim J, et al. (2005) Predictive and prognostic impact of epidermal growth factor receptor mutation in non-small-cell lung cancer patients treated with gefitinib. J Clin Oncol 23: 2493–2501.
22. Wu M, Zhao J, Song SW, Zhuo M, Wang X, et al. (2010) EGFR mutations are associated with prognosis but not with the response to front-line chemotherapy in the Chinese patients with advanced non-small cell lung cancer. Lung Cancer 67: 343–347.
23. Ren GJ, Zhao YY, Zhu YJ, Xiao Y, Xu JS, et al. (2011) Tumor gene mutations and messenger RNA expression: correlation with clinical response to icotinib hydrochloride in non-small cell lung cancer. Chin Med J (Engl) 124: 19–25.
24. Maemondo M, Inoue A, Kobayashi K, Sugawara S, Oizumi S, et al. (2010) Gefitinib or chemotherapy for non-small-cell lung cancer with mutated EGFR. N Engl J Med 362: 2380–2388.

25. Mitsudomi T, Morita S, Yatabe Y, Negoro S, Okamoto I, et al. (2010) Gefitinib versus cisplatin plus docetaxel in patients with non-small-cell lung cancer harbouring mutations of the epidermal growth factor receptor (WJTOG3405): an open label, randomised phase 3 trial. Lancet Oncol 11: 121–128.

26. Rosell R, Carcereny E, Gervais R, Vergnenegre A, Massuti B, et al. (2012) Erlotinib versus standard chemotherapy as first-line treatment for European patients with advanced EGFR mutation-positive non-small-cell lung cancer (EURTAC): a multicentre, open-label, randomised phase 3 trial. Lancet Oncol 13: 239–246.

27

Socio-Economic Gradients in Maternal and Child Health-Seeking Behaviours in Egypt: Systematic Literature Review and Evidence Synthesis

Lenka Benova[1]*, Oona M. R. Campbell[2], George B. Ploubidis[1]

1 Department of Population Health, Faculty of Epidemiology and Population Health, London School of Hygiene and Tropical Medicine, London, United Kingdom, **2** Department of Infectious Disease Epidemiology, Faculty of Epidemiology and Population Health, London School of Hygiene and Tropical Medicine, London, United Kingdom

Abstract

Background: Health-seeking behaviour lies on the direct pathway between socio-economic position (SEP) and health outcomes. The objective of this systematic review is to identify and synthesise evidence of socio-economic gradients in health-seeking behaviours related to maternal and child health in Egypt.

Methods: Four databases (Medline, Embase, Global Health and Web of Science) were searched in September 2013 for material published in English from 1992 to 2013 for a combination of terms describing health-seeking behaviours, indicators of socio-economic position and geographical limitation to Egypt. Findings of studies were described and synthesised in a narrative format as meta-analysis was not possible.

Findings: Among the 786 references identified, 10 articles met the inclusion criteria. Six studies examined maternal and five studies child health-seeking behaviours (one study examined both). For maternal health, three dimensions of health-seeking behaviour (receipt of any care, type of care and intensity of care) were covered by studies of ante-natal and one dimension (type of care) by analyses of delivery care. For child health, two dimensions of preventive care (coverage of and intensity of immunisation) and three dimensions of curative care (receipt of any care, type and cost of care) were analysed.

Conclusions: Based on two studies of time trends in nationally-representative surveys, socio-economic inequalities in seeking care for basic preventive and curative interventions in maternal and child health appear to have narrowed. Limited evidence of gradients in intensity of maternal preventive and provider selection in child curative care showed that inequalities may have widened. In studies of more geographically and socially homogeneous samples, fewer gradients were identified. Current body of evidence contains numerous limitations and gaps and is insufficient to draw a conclusive summary of such gradients. Improved understanding of SEP gradients is crucial in designing and prioritising interventions to equitably improve maternal and child health outcomes.

Editor: Zulfiqar A. Bhutta, Aga Khan University, Pakistan

Funding: This work was supported by the Economic and Social Research Council (ESRC) 1+3 Studentship grant award (ES/I903224/1); and Medical Research Council (MRC) Population Health Science fellowship (G0802442). The funders had no role in study design, data collection and analysis, decision to publish, or preparation of the manuscript.

Competing Interests: The authors have declared that no competing interests exist.

* E-mail: lenka.benova@lshtm.ac.uk

Introduction

In virtually every context where they have been studied, inequalities in health outcomes based on living standards or on social hierarchy (as observed through various measures of socio-economic position, SEP) have been identified.[1] This association is hypothesised to arise mainly on the basis of causal pathways, encompassing healthcare access and utilisation, psychosocial determinants, health knowledge and behaviours, as well as environmental hazards.[2–5] As one of these pathways, health-seeking behaviour comprises several sequential decisions and actions through which individuals proceed in their contact with the healthcare system; including experiencing and reporting symptoms, seeking care, choosing a provider, paying for care, adhering to treatment, as well as timing and intensity of follow-up visits. Health-seeking behaviour includes preventive (immunisation or screening) and curative care (after the onset of symptoms).

A review of socio-economic determinants of health-seeking behaviour in low and middle income countries indicated that a variety of individual and households-level indicators have been used to reflect socio-economic position, including education, occupation, absolute or relative poverty level, and access to material, financial and productive resources (income, landholding, assets).[6] Rigorously evaluated interventions, such as conditional cash transfer (CCT) programs, showed that provision of cash transfers to female heads of households can lead to an increase in healthcare utilization patterns.[7] Socio-economic status is hypothesised to influence health-seeking behaviour through several mechanisms, such as material and intellectual resources and access to health facilities.[8,9] However, individuals rarely make health-related decisions in a social vacuum and their socio-economic position is not solely an individual-level characteristic. Therefore, the association between SEP and health-seeking behaviour can be examined on various levels, spanning from the individual and familial environment, to the wider community and country.

Objectives

The objective of this systematic review is to identify and synthesise evidence published in the previous two decades about the existence, magnitude and trends in socio-economic gradients in health-seeking behaviours related to maternal and child health in Egypt. Firstly, a summary of the types and dimensions of health-seeking behaviour analysed by included studies is presented. Secondly, we synthesise the evidence regarding the extent of gradients identified, and lastly, limitations of current evidence and recommendations for future research are outlined. Maternal health-seeking behaviour for the purposes of this review refers to the timing and intensity of care, as well as provider choice and cost incurred during pregnancy, childbirth and in the immediate post-partum period. Child health-seeking behaviour is defined as actions taken in relation to healthcare for children under five years of age. Preventive and curative health-seeking behaviours are included.

Methods

Data sources and search strategy

Four databases (Medline, Embase, Global Health and Web of Science) were searched in September 2013 for material published in English from 1992 to 2013. Where available, MeSH terms were combined with free-text terms capturing components of health-seeking behaviour (access, utilization, provider selection, and cost of care), a wide range of indicators of socio-economic position (education, literacy, employment, wealth, income, consumption, expenditure, assets, poverty, indebtedness) and geographic limitation to Egypt. The reference lists of included articles were also screened. The complete search strategy is presented in Table 1. The review is reported according to the Preferred Reporting Items for Systematic Reviews and Meta-Analyses (PRISMA) guideline (Table S1).[10] The review protocol was not registered.

Study selection and data extraction

Abstracts of all references identified in searches were screened and discarded if they did not contain data from Egypt or maternal or child health-seeking behaviour as an outcome measure. Cognizant of the fact that SEP indicators may be included in analyses as confounders and may thus not be identified as exposures in the abstracts, full-text versions of remaining references were screened. At this stage, we eliminated studies without SEP as an exposure or confounder, those in which the SEP variable used was not clearly defined, and those not presenting any statistical test (p value, confidence interval or standard error) of the association between SEP and health-seeking behaviour. Descriptive information abstracted from studies included study design, study objective, study population and data sources, type of health-seeking behaviour examined and measures of SEP used. We classified each study according to its main objective into one of the following three groups: SEP was the main determinant examined by the study, SEP was one of the several risk factors examined by the study or SEP was one of the confounders used in the study. Abstracted information on study findings included type of statistical analysis and tests used, crude and adjusted parameters that quantified the association between SEP measure(s) and health-seeking behaviour outcomes and confounders included in adjusted analyses, if any. No data were obtained from investigators, but results were confirmed with authors of Stephenson et al (2012). For the results of Gwatkin et al (2007), binary significance levels of the concentration indices (<0.05, >0.05) were calculated by using the standard errors by this study.

Analysis

No meta-analysis was performed due to insufficient number of comparable estimates for any single health-seeking behaviour. Findings of studies were described and synthesised in a narrative format. The results of analyses are presented separately for each dimension of health-seeking behaviour: 1) Seeking any care, 2) Type of care sought/received, 3) Intensity of care received, and 4) Cost of care incurred, based on a conceptual approach used by

Table 1. MeSH and text search terms used in databases searched according to algorithm (1 AND 2 AND 3).

Search Concept	Text search terms	MeSH terms
Database	(Medline, Embase, Global Health and Web of Science)	(Medline, Embase and Global Health)
1. Health-seeking behaviour	((health OR health-care OR healthcare OR health-related OR provider OR help OR care OR therap* OR treatment) AND (seeking OR behavio?r OR decision OR choice* OR utili?ation OR narrative OR network)) OR ((illness OR sick*) AND (perception OR narrative)) OR ((out?of?pocket OR private OR health) AND (expen* OR cost* OR payment OR fee OR charge)) OR pathways to doctor OR pathways to the doctor OR health-seeking OR help-seeking OR care-seeking	**Medline:** Attitude to Health, Health Behavior, Illness Behavior, Direct Service Costs, Cost of Illness, Fees, Medical. **Embase:** health related behavior, patient attitude, health care utilization, health care access. **Global Health:** health care utilization, social barriers, Health care costs.
2. Socio-economic determinants	socio-economic OR socioeconomic OR social status OR social class OR social position OR economic position OR poverty OR inequalit* OR gradient* OR deprivation OR SES OR SEP OR employment OR occupation OR unemployment OR education* OR school* OR graduat* OR literacy OR numeracy OR income OR wage OR pension OR salary OR wealth OR asset* OR loan OR debt OR borrow* OR consumption OR expenditure OR spend* OR housing OR crowding OR determinant* OR sociodemographic	**Medline:** Socioeconomic Factors, Sociometric Techniques, Social Class. **Embase:** Social status. **Global Health:** Socioeconomic status.
3. Egypt	Egypt*	**Medline, Embase, Global Health:** Egypt.

* Truncation symbol.

Pokhrel and colleagues.[11] A risk of bias assessment was developed based on the Newcastle-Ottawa quality assessment scale.[12] This tool was used in consideration of the strengths and limitations of the available evidence.

Results

A total of 786 unique references were identified and screened. The majority (83%) of excluded references did not examine any component of health-seeking behaviour. From 64 references reviewed in full-text, 10 articles met the inclusion criteria (Figure 1). Six studies examined maternal health-seeking behaviours and five studies child health-seeking behaviours (Tables 2 and 3, respectively, studies listed in chronological order by year of publication); one study included both behaviours. Among the ten included studies, nine set out to examine the association between socio-economic position and health-seeking behaviour, either as the main exposure or one of several main exposures.

Maternal health-seeking behaviours

Three of the six studies analysing maternal health-seeking behaviours were based on the nationally representative population-level Demographic and Health surveys (DHS) collected between 1995 and 2008.[13–15] The remaining three studies analysed small samples of (<250) women in specific geographic locations; the city of Alexandria,[16] six villages in Beni Sueif governorate [17] and a Giza village.[18] All six studies were based on cross-sectional data.

Four studies analysed whether women received any ante-natal care (ANC) or ANC from a medical professional during pregnancy (Figure 2, Table 2). The proportion of women receiving any ANC in the samples used by the studies ranged from 33.8% to 71.4% for any ANC and 42.5% to 73.2% for any ANC with a medical professional. Four studies examined ANC regularity (number of ANC visits during pregnancy) and one study each looked at the timing of the first ANC visit and at the pattern of ANC use (combining regularity and timing into one indicator). In regard to delivery care, four studies assessed various characteristics of the health provider (skilled or traditional birth attendant) or facility (any, public, private, home) where women sought care.

Four studies of maternal health-seeking behaviour used women's individual-level SEP measures; education or literacy appeared in four studies and employment-related SEP measurement reflected in occupation status and cash income earnings were used by one study each. Two studies evaluated individual-level SEP measures (education and occupation) of the spouse. All studies that analysed DHS surveys relied partly or solely on quintiles of the wealth index, a household-level measure.[19] Other household-level measures of SEP included family socio-economic status (SES) based on a score suggested in 1983 by Fahmy and Sherbini [20] and binary variables indicating ownership of various assets (land, house, cattle), access to potable water, and monthly meat consumption. One study examined the association between health-seeking behaviour and community-level economic prosperity, which was constructed as mean of the DHS household-level wealth scores within each survey primary sampling unit (PSU). Two of the six studies showed the absolute levels of health-seeking behaviours under investigation for each SEP category. To assess the existence and magnitude of the association between SEP and maternal health-seeking behaviours, four studies used odds ratio measure of effect and two studies presented the value of the concentration index, both relative effect measures.

Ante-natal care. The two studies which analysed more than one DHS survey both reported only a crude measure of association between SEP and health-seeking behaviours (Gwatkin 2007, Khadr 2009), shown in Table 4. However, their use of concentration index, a method which quantifies the extent of a SEP gradient, allowed for comparison of time trends. Concentration index is formally expressed as twice the area under the Lorenz curve of inequality, showing the cumulative distribution of an outcome according to cumulative distribution of wealth. Concentration index values range between -1, indicating absolute inequality of the outcome concentrated among the poorest and +1, showing absolute inequality concentrated among the wealthiest, with 0 signifying perfect equality. The definitions of health-seeking behaviours reported were similar (except for a difference in receiving 'regular' ANC, where definition varied between Gwatkin ≥3 and Khadr ≥4 visits). Both studies showed that women from lower wealth quintiles were significantly less likely to have received any ANC and regular ANC than women from richer wealth quintiles. Concentration index values for 1995 and 2000 differed between the two studies for the four indicators they both evaluated. Wealth score and quintile became available to users of the DHS starting with the 2005 survey, and authors calculated their own wealth index for the two prior surveys, possibly using different component variables, which may be the main reason for this difference. For both indicators of ante-natal care, the concentration index value decreased between the 1995 and 2005 surveys, but remained higher for regular ANC than for any ANC use. Khadr found that while the concentration index value for these two ANC behaviours based on education level remained significant and concentrated among women with higher SEP; the

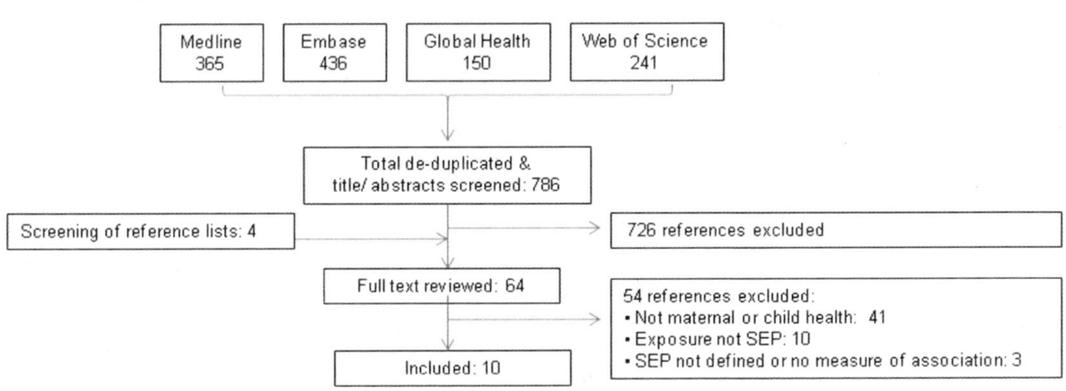

Figure 1. Systematic review search and inclusion flowchart.

Table 2. Descriptive characteristics of included maternal health-seeking behaviour studies.

#	Author, Year	Study design	Study sample and objective	Exposure: SEP definition	Outcome: Health-seeking behaviour(s) – type, definition and level in sample
1	Abdel Houssein, 1997[16]	Cross-sectional	Pregnant women in third trimester attending 6 randomly selected MCH centers in Alexandria, all pregnant women in third trimester interviewed (no date of study provided), n = 240. SEP: One of risk factors.	**IS: Education level** (no information on number or types of categories). **HH: Family SES score** based on education (woman and husband), monthly per capita income (no further information), crowding and household sanitation.	**Pattern of attendance of ANC clinics:** based on timing of initial visit (1st ANC visit during 1st trimester) and total number of ANC visits for current pregnancy; classified (no further information) into adequate and inadequate. Level: 28.8% adequate.
2	Yassin et al., 2003[17]	Cross-sectional	6 villages in Beni Sueif, all mothers of children less than one year old living in an area around a sentinel site (no date of study provided), n = 231. SEP: One of risk factors.	**IS: Literacy** (binary), **occupation** (binary). **IO: Spouse literacy** (binary), **spouse occupation** (binary). **HH: Land ownership** (binary), **house ownership** (binary), **cattle ownership** (binary), **access to potable water** (binary), **meat consumed <4 times in previous month** (binary).	**Receipt of any ANC** at local primary center during most recent pregnancy (with child <1 year old). Level: 33.8% received any ANC.
3	Gwatkin et al., 2007[13]	Cross-sectional	EDHS 1995, 2000. Population representative sample of ever-married women. Last birth among women with at least one birth in the five years preceding the survey, n: 1995 = 7797, 2000 = 7953. SEP: Main determinant.	**HH: DHS Wealth index quintile.**	**Any ANC by a medically-trained person** (at least one consultation from a doctor, nurse or trained midwife). Level: 1995: 42.5%, 2000: 55.7%. **Multiple (3+) ANC visits with medically-trained person.** Level: 1995: 34.9%, 2000: 43.7%. **Delivery with skilled attendance** (doctor, nurse or midwife). Level: 1995: 46.2%, 2000: 60.9%. **Delivery location: Public facility.** Level: 1995: 17.9%, 2000: 22.2%. **Delivery location: Private facility.** Level: 1995: 14.6%, 2000: 26.0%. **Delivery location: Home (woman's or another home).** Level: 1995: 67.0%, 2000: 51.7%.
4	Khadr, 2009[14]	Cross-sectional	EDHS 1995, 2000, 2005 Population representative sample of ever-married women. Last birth among currently married women with at least one birth in the 5-years preceding survey; n: 1995 = 7828, 2000 = 7823, 2005 = 9744. SEP: Main determinant.	**IS: Education level** (no education, some primary, primary to secondary, completed secondary and higher). **HH: DHS Wealth index quintile.**	**Any ANC received** (no further definition). Level: 1995: 42.4%, 2000: 54.1%, 2005: 71.4%. **Regular ANC received** (4+ visits during pregnancy). Level: 1995: 31.0%, 2000: 40.7%, 2005: 61.3%. **Delivery with skilled attendance** (no further definition). Level: 1995: 41.7%, 2000: 55.8%, 2005: 70.5%. **Home delivery.** Level: 1995: 64.5%, 2000: 49.1%, 2005: 33.6%.
5	Chiang et al., 2012[18]	Cross-sectional	2007 survey of married women <50 years from a Giza village, n = 189. SEP: One of risk factors.	**IS: Woman's education** (no primary, completed primary or higher), **existence of cash income** (binary). **IO: Husband's education** (primary school or lower, higher than primary).	**Regular ANC (4+ visits) during most recent pregnancy. Level: 48.7%. Delivery with skilled medical professional at most recent delivery.** Level: 79.4%. **Delivery in a health facility at most recent delivery.** Level: 61.4%.
6	Stephenson et al., 2012[15]	Cross-sectional	EDHS 2008. Population representative sample of ever-married women. Last birth among women with at least one birth in the five years preceding the survey, n = 7813. SEP: One of risk factors.	**C: Community-level economic prosperity** - mean score of household wealth (DHS wealth score) per PSU (primary sampling unit), continuous variable.	**Any ANC received** (from a medically trained person). Level: 73.23%. **Regular ANC received** (4+ visits). Level: 65.75%. **First ANC visit received in 1st trimester.** Level: 59.48%. **Delivery in a health facility.** Level: 71.25%.

EDHS – Egypt Demographic and Health Survey. Measures of SEP: **IS**: Individual – self, **IO:** Individual– other (spouse, mother, etc), **HH:** Household-level, **C**: Community-level.

Table 3. Descriptive characteristics of included child health-seeking behaviour studies.

#	Author, Year	Study design	Study sample and objective	Exposure: SEP – type, definition, level in sample	Outcome: Health-seeking behaviour(s) – type, definition and level in sample
1	Reichler et al., 1998[26]	Cross-sectional	Nationally-representative survey of children under 48 months of age surveyed one month after second National Immunisation Day (NID, polio) round in 1995, n = 4188 children from 3216 households. SEP: One of risk factors.	**HH: Radio in household** (binary), **TV in household** (binary).	**Number of doses of OPV (oral poliomyelitis vaccine) received.** Level: 0 doses: 9% (CI95%: 7.1%–9.9%). Level: 1 dose: 17% (CI95%: 14.6%–19.7%). Level: 2 doses: 74% (CI95%: 71.4%–77.3%).
2	Yount, 2003[27]	Cross-sectional.	Two Governorates Linkages Survey 1995–1997, children <5 years with diarrhoea in past 2 weeks in 12 rural villages of Minya governorate, n = 129 children, 152 episodes of care-seeking. SEP: Confounder in analysis of gender.	**IO: Maternal education** (binary). **HH: Major asset ownership** (binary).	If reported symptoms of diarrhoea: **Type of provider sought** (episodes, n = 152). Other:15%, Lay:16%, Pharmacist: 40%, Doctor: 29%. **Location of care** (episodes, n = 152). Other: 28%, Public:12%, Private: 21%, Pharmacy: 39%. **Cost of care** (children, n = 129). Free, ≤ 1 EPG, > 1 EGP (Proportions by category not provided, but median expenditure for boys 0.5 EGP, girls 0.2 EPG).
3	Yount, 2004[28]	Cross-sectional	Two Governorates Linkages Survey 1995–1997, Minya governorate, children <5 years of age of currently married women who were sick in 2 weeks before interview, n = 1579. SEP: One of risk factors.	**IO: Mother's education level** (none, primary, preparatory, secondary and higher, **mother's ever-employment for cash** (binary), **mother's ownership of assets** (none, one, two or more), **father's years education** (none, 1–11, 12+). **HH: Number of assets/durables owned:** (none, low [1 asset/0–2 durables], medium [≤1 asset, 3+ durables], high [2+ assets]. (Assets include 6 items of means of transportation, land and building ownership; Durables are 10 household assets such as TV, fridge etc.)	If reported symptoms of illness (with diarrhoea, fever, cough or rash): **Utilized private treatment (private doctor).** Level: 18.8%.
4	Fadel, et al. 2007[29]	Pros-pective cohort	257 healthy infants (0–9 months) followed for 12 months (October 1999–October 2000) in Assiut university primary health center catchment area, n = 631 diarrhoeal episodes. SEP: One of risk factors.	**IO: Mother's education, father's education** (illiterate, literate/primary, preparatory, secondary, university/higher), **mother's employment status** (binary). **HH: TV ownership** (binary), **Radio ownership** (binary).	If reported symptoms of diarrhoea in preceding 2 weeks: **Sought any treatment** (caretakers of children sought medical care outside the home). Level: 53.1% of diarrhoeal episodes (335 of 631). **Utilized private treatment** (medical care not under government control). Level: 37.3% of diarrhoeal episodes for which care was sought (210 of 335).
5	Gwatkin,et al, 2007[13]	Cross-sectional	EDHS 1995, 2000 (children under 5 years), n immunization: 1995 = 2085, 2000 = 2170; treatment for ARI: 1995 = 2479, 2000 = 1032; treatment for fever: 1995 = 4295, 2000 = 1923; treatment for diarrhoea: 1995 = 1701, 2000 = 771. SEP: Main determinant.	**HH: DHS Wealth index quintile**	**Coverage of immunisations:** BCG: 1995: 94.7%, 2000: 99.3%. Measles: 1995: 89.2%, 2000: 96.9%. DPT(3 doses): 1995: 83.0%, 2000: 94.0%. Hepatitis B: 1995: 57.0%, 2000 not reported. Full basic: 1995: 79.1%, 2000: 92.2%. No basic (not received full basic): 1995: 2.5%, 2000: 0.2%. **Sought any medical treatment.** Fever: 1995: 47.6%, 2000: 35.1%. ARI: 1995: 61.7%, 2000: 66.0%. Diarrhoea: 1995: 47.5%, 2000: 46.3%. **Utilized private treatment.** Fever: 1995: 34.8%, 2000: 21.7%. ARI: 1995: 43.5%, 2000: 41.5%. Diarrhoea: 1995: 33.2%, 2000: 30.0%. **Utilized public treatment.** Fever: 1995:12.0%, 2000: 12.6%. ARI: 1995: 17.1%, 2000: 23.1%. Diarrhoea: 1995: 13.7%, 2000: 15.6%.

EDHS – Egypt Demographic and Health Survey EGP – Egyptian pound BCG – Bacillus Calmette–Guérin (TB) DPT- Diphtheria, pertussis (whooping cough) and tetanus. Measures of SEP: **IO:** Individual – other (spouse, mother, etc), **HH:** Household-level.

values were closer to equality than the concentration index values based on wealth quintile.

In order to approximate the level of community affluence, Stevenson et al (2012) constructed a community level wealth index based on the household wealth index of respondents in the same primary sampling units. This study concluded that community-level economic prosperity was not associated with any ANC, regular ANC or timely ANC (first visit in first trimester of

Domain	Dimension	Health-seeking behaviour	Study #
Maternal health			
Ante-natal care	1. Any care received	Any ANC received	2, 4
	2. Type of care (provider, facility)	Any ANC with medical professional	3, 6
	3. Intensity (frequency, timing)	Regularity of ANC (> or ≥3 visits)	3, 4, 5, 6
		Timing of ANC (start in 1st trimester)	6
		Pattern of ANC (adequate timing and regularity)	1
Delivery care	2. Type of care (provider, facility)	Delivery with skilled attendance	3, 4, 5
		Delivery at any health facility	5, 6
		Delivery at public facility	3
		Delivery at private facility	3
		Delivery at home	3, 4
Child health			
Immunisation	1. Any care received	Immunisation received (various types)	1,5
	3. Intensity (coverage)	Full basic immunisation	5
Childhood illness	1. Any care received	Any medical assistance received	4, 5
	2. Type of care (provider, facility)	Type of healthcare provider	2
		Type of facility	2
		Private care (binary)	3, 4, 5
		Public care (binary)	5
	4. Cost of care	Amount spent	2

- - - Preventive care ——— Curative care

Figure 2. Maternal and child health-seeking behaviours analysed in included studies.

pregnancy) use. Receiving regular ANC in a Giza village was associated with primary or higher education level - both woman's as well as her husband's, but not with woman's cash income, in crude analysis (Chiang 2012). Crude analysis of a sample from villages in Beni Sueif showed a significant positive association between maternal and paternal literacy (individual-level) and land ownership (household-level) with the likelihood of receiving any ANC (Yassin 2003). A study in Alexandria reported that neither education nor family SES score were significantly associated with adequate pattern of ANC clinic attendance among women attending an ANC clinic, when adjusted for woman's age group, parity, knowledge of ANC use, level of medical risk, and health belief model score (Abdel Houssein 1997).

Delivery care. The concentration index values for obtaining skilled delivery care appeared to have decreased between 1995 and 2005, yet the values remained significant, and higher based on wealth quintile than on education level (Gwatkin 2007, Khadr 2009). Gwatkin and colleagues reported that women from lower household wealth quintiles were significantly less likely to deliver in private facilities and in public facilities, compared to women from higher quintile households, in both 1995 and 2000, but the concentration index value had decreased over this timeframe. Both Gwatkin and Khadr concluded that women from lower wealth quintiles were significantly more likely to deliver at home in all surveys analysed. However, whereas Gwatkin reported that the concentration index value increased between 1995 and 2000, Khadr noted a decrease between 1995 and 2005. Khadr's analysis showed that the concentration index value for home delivery was smaller when SEP was measured by education level rather than household wealth quintile, but remained significant, favouring women with higher SEP. Using the 2008 DHS, Stephenson et al reported no significant difference, in adjusted analysis, in the odds of delivery in any health facility compared to at home based on community-level wealth. Lastly, crude analysis of health-seeking behaviour in a Giza village revealed that higher level woman's and husband's education were significantly positively associated with the odds of delivery with a skilled medical professional and delivery in any health facility. However, woman's cash income was not associated with either delivery-related health-seeking behaviour (Chiang 2012).

Child health-seeking behaviours

Five studies analysing SEP determinants of health-seeking behaviour for children were identified; two included assessment of immunisation coverage and four examined aspects of curative health-seeking for common childhood illnesses (Figure 2, Table 3).

Table 4. Summary of results from included maternal health-seeking studies.

#	Author, Year	Statistical method, type of analysis, effect estimate	Results and confounders (if applicable)
1	Abdel Houssein, 1997[16]	**Crude analysis:** Not reported. **Adjusted analysis:** Logistic regression. **Effect estimate:** Odds ratio.	**Pattern of attendance of ANC clinics:** Education (number of categories not reported): OR 1.42 (0.64–3.13), p = 0.387. SEP (ref category not specified) OR 1.38 (0.75–2.56), p = 0.302. **Confounders:** age group (<20, 21–29, 30+), parity (0, 1–4, 5+), knowledge about adequate ANC use, level of risk, and health belief model score.
2	Yassin et al., 2003[17]	**Crude analysis:** Logistic regression. **Effect estimate:** Odds ratio.	**Any ANC:** Maternal literacy (ref: literate) OR 3.3 (1.6–6.7), p<0.001. Maternal occupation (ref: unskilled worker) OR 0.8 (0.3–1.8), p>0.05. Paternal literacy (ref: literate) OR 3.1 (1.4–6.9), p<0.01. Paternal occupation (ref: unskilled worker) OR 1.8 (0.7–4.5), p>0.05. Land ownership (ref: yes) OR 3.6 (1.4–9.3), p<0.01. House ownership (ref: yes) OR 1.0 (0.3–3.5), p>0.05. Cattle ownership (ref: yes) OR 0.5 (0.3–1.1), p>0.05. Access to safe water OR 1.1 (0.6–2.2), p>0.05. Meat consumption (ref: <4 times/month) OR 0.9 (0.4–2.1), p>0.05.
3	Gwatkin et al., 2007[13]	**Crude analysis:** Concentration index (CoI)*. **Effect estimate:** Concentration index value.	**Any ANC by a medically trained person:** Women from households in lower quintiles were less likely to receive but CoI decreased from 0.2703 (p<0.05) in 1995 to 0.2028 (p<0.05) in 2000. **Multiple (3+) ANC visits:** Women from households in lower quintiles were less likely to receive multiple ANC visits, but CoI decreased from 0.3580 (p<0.05) in 1995 to 0.2614 (p<0.05) in 2000. **Delivery with skilled attendance:** Women from households in lower quintiles were less likely to deliver with skilled medical assistance, but CoI decreased from 0.2911 (p<0.05) in 1995 to 0.2189 (p<0.05) in 2000. **Delivery location:** Public or Private facility: Women from households in lower quintiles were less likely to deliver in private facilities (CoI1995: 0.4379, p<0.05; CoI2000: 0.3422, p<0.05) and in public facilities (CoI1995: 0.2472, p<0.05; CoI2000: 0.1708, p<0.05), both indexes decreased between 1995 and 2000. **Delivery location: Home:** Women from households in lower quintiles were more likely to deliver at home and gradient increased over time (CoI1995: −0.1630, p<0.05; CoI2000: −0.2457, p<0.05).
4	Khadr, 2009[14]	**Crude analysis:** Concentration index (CoI). **Effect estimate:** Concentration index value.	**Any ANC received:** Education: CoI value has remained the same (0.41) between 1995 and 2005 (p<0.001). Wealth: Decreased inequality from 0.50 (1995) to 0.45 (2005) but significant (p<0.001). **Regular ANC received:** Education: Decreased inequality from 0.49 (1995) to 0.39 (2005) but significant (p<0.001). Wealth: Decrease in inequality from 0.60 (1995) to 0.49 (2005) but significant (p<0.001). **Delivery with skilled attendance:** Education: Decrease in inequality from 0.41 (1995) to 0.37 (2005) but significant (p<0.001). Wealth Decrease in inequality from 0.55 (1995) to 0.47 (2005) but significant (p<0.001). **Home delivery:** Education: Decrease in inequality from −0.42 (1995) to −0.35 (2005) but significant (p<0.001). Wealth: Decrease in inequality from −0.53 (1995) to −0.47 (2005) but significant (p<0.001).
5	Chiang et al., 2012[18]	**Crude analysis:** Logistic regression. **Effect estimate:** Odds ratio.	**Regular ANC:** Maternal education (ref: no primary education) OR 5.59 (2.98–10.47), p<0.01. Cash income (ref: no) OR 0.52 (0.25–1.09), p>0.05. Husband education (ref: ≤primary) OR 2.31 (1.26–4.23), p<0.01. **Delivery with skilled medical professional:** Maternal education (ref: no primary education) OR 2.98 (1.36–6.54), p<0.01. Cash income (ref: no) OR 0.79 (0.34–1.85), p>0.05. Husband education (ref: ≤primary) OR 2.38 (1.05–5.36), p<0.05. **Delivery in a health facility:** Maternal education (ref: no primary education) OR 5.42 (2.78–10.57), p<0.01. Cash income (ref: no) OR 0.51 (0.25–1.04), p>0.05. Husband education (ref: ≤primary) OR 2.82 (1.46–5.42), p<0.01.
6	Stephenson et al., 2012[15]	**Crude analysis:** Not reported. **Adjusted analysis:** Multi-level logistic regression. **Effect estimate:** Odds ratio.	**Any ANC received:** OR 1.0 (1.0–1.0), p>0.05. **Regular ANC received:** OR 1.0 (1.0–1.0), p>0.05. **First ANC in 1st trimester:** OR 1.0 (1.0–1.0), p>0.05. Delivery in a health facility: OR 1.0 (1.0–1.0), p>0.05. **Confounders:** Woman's age, marriage duration, partner age difference, death of a child, number of living children, sex ratio of children, education (woman and partner), employment status (woman and partner), household wealth, reproductive health knowledge, media exposure, violence justification, and decision-making autonomy.

* Only values of standard error (SE) were provided by this study. Binary significance levels (<0.05, >0.05) were calculated by multiplying the SE by 1.96 to obtain the upper and lower confidence intervals.

Two studies analysed nationally-representative samples; one by following up on National Immunisation Days (Reichler 1998) and the other examined two rounds of EDHS (Gwatkin 2007). Two papers reported findings from samples in Minia governorate based on the Two Governorates Linkages Survey (Yount 2003 and Yount 2004), and the remaining study assessed health-seeking behaviours for infants in a primary health centre catchment area in Assiut (Fadel 2007). Although this study included prospective cohort data collection method, all findings were based on cross-sectional analyses.

Between the two studies examining receipt of immunisations, socio-economic determinants of both disease-specific coverage (BCG, measles, DPT, Hepatitis B, polio), as well as overall immunisation status based on national guidelines (full basic immunisation, no basic immunisation) were assessed. In regard to curative care, health-seeking behaviours following reported childhood illnesses (any illness, diarrhoea, acute respiratory infection-ARI, or fever) were examined, specifically whether any medical care was sought, the type of medical provider and health facility approached, and cost incurred. Three of the five studies used measures of parental SEP, namely maternal and paternal education level and employment status, and maternal asset ownership. All three studies using individual-level variables also used household-level measures of SEP, the remaining two studies analysed solely household-level measures. The household-level SEP measures included DHS wealth quintiles, binary TV and radio ownership, and major asset ownership. Four of the five studies showed the absolute levels of health-seeking behaviours under investigation for each SEP category. The assessment of the association between SEP and maternal health-seeking behaviours was conducted using relative effect measures in four studies (three used odds ratios and one concentration index value) and absolute measure in one study (risk difference).

Immunisation coverage. Both studies examining the association between SEP and receipt of immunisations presented only crude effect estimates (Table 5). In their analysis of polio vaccine

Table 5. Summary of results from included child health-seeking studies.

#	Author, Year	Statistical method, type of analysis, effect estimate	Results and confounders (if applicable)
1	Reichler et al., 1998[26]	**Crude analysis:** T-test. **Effect estimate:** Risk difference.	Children in households with a radio were more likely to have received 2 doses (77%) than one (69%) or no doses of OPV (72%), p<0.01. Children in households with a TV were more likely to have received 2 doses (94%) than one (86%) or no doses of OPV (84%), p<0.001.
2	Yount, 2003[27]	**Crude analysis:** Not reported. **Adjusted analysis:** Logistic regression. **Effect estimate:** Odds ratio.	**Type of provider**: Household assets (ref: none) Any: Pharmacist OR 1.78 (p>0.05), Doctor OR 2.46 (p>0.05). Maternal education (ref: none) Any: Pharmacist OR 2.10 (p>0.05), Doctor OR 0.75 (p>0.05). **Location of care**: Household assets (ref: none) Any: Public OR 3.65 (p>0.05), Pharmacy OR 2.01 (p>0.05), Private OR 2.20 (p>0.05). Maternal education (ref: none) Any: Public OR 0.66 (p>0.05), Pharmacy OR 2.09 (p>0.05), Private OR 0.72 (p>0.05). **Cost of care** (categorical variable, 3 levels): Household assets (ref: none) Any: OR 0.76 (p>0.05). Maternal education: not reported. **Confounders**: child gender and age; severity, cause and duration of diarrhoea; presence and gender of siblings; and family members' involvement in decision-making.
3	Yount, 2004[28]	**Crude analysis:** Not reported. **Adjusted analysis:** Logistic regression. **Effect estimate:** Odds ratio.	**Odds of utilizing private treatment:** Father's education (ref: 0 years): 1–11 years OR 0.84 (p>0.05); 12+ years OR 1.10 (p>0.05). Maternal ever-employment (ref: no): Yes: OR 0.79 (p>0.05). Maternal education (ref: none): Primary/preparatory: OR 0.81 (p>0.05), secondary or more: OR 0.92 (p>0.05). Maternal assets (ref: none): One OR 0.74(p<0.05), Two or more: OR 0.79 (p>0.05). Household assets/durables (ref: none): Low: OR 1.84 (p<0.01), Medium: OR 2.55 (p<0.001), High: OR 3.62 (p<0.001). **Confounders**: child gender and age; severity, cause and duration of illness; presence and gender of siblings; religion; urban/rural residence; maternal social resources and social constraints; and proximity of health services.
4	Fadel, et al. 2007[29]	**Crude analysis:** X^2 test. **Adjusted analysis:** Logistic regression. **Effect estimate:** Odds ratio.	**Crude analysis - Utilized treatment:** Mother's education p = 0.285, Father's education p = 0.339, Mother's employment status p = 0.486, TV ownership p = 0.042 (diarrhoeal episodes where households have TV more likely to utilize care), Radio ownership p = 0.196. **Utilized private providers, if utilized treatment:** Mother's education p<0.001 (higher levels of education are more likely to utilize private providers), Father's education p = 0.020 (higher levels of education are more likely to utilize private providers), Mother's employment status p<0.001 (working mothers are more likely to utilize private providers), TV ownership, Radio ownership: not reported. **Adjusted analysis - Utilized treatment:** Mother's education, Father's education, Mother's employment status, Radio ownership: not reported. TV ownership (ref: not clear) OR 0.63, p = 0.418. **Confounders**: Perception of severe attack, vomiting, bloody stool, fever, duration of episode, age of infant, frequency of stool, presence of cough, associated any symptoms with diarrhoea, watery stool, history of child death, presence of preschool children, using self-prescribed drugs. **Utilized public versus private providers:** Mother's education (ref: illiterate): reads/writes/primary: OR 0.04 (p<0.001), preparatory: OR 0.02 (p<0.001), secondary: OR 0.04 (p<0.01), university/higher: OR 0.07 (p<0.01). Father's education (ref: illiterate): reads/writes/primary: OR 2.04 (p = 0.212), preparatory: OR 1.27 (p = 0.726), secondary: OR 0.82 (p = 0.785), university/higher: OR 1.93 (p = 0.209). Mother's employment status (ref: not working): working: OR 0.61 (p = 0.278). TV ownership, radio ownership: not reported. **Confounders**: age and sex of infant, mother's age and mother's perception of diarrhoeal episode severity.
5	Gwatkin, et al, 2007[13]	**Crude analysis:** Concentration index (CoI)*. **Effect estimate:** Concentration index value.	**Coverage of immunisation:** BCG: Children from lower quintiles less likely covered, CoI decreased from 0.0317 (p<0.05) in 1995 to 0.004 (p<0.05) in 2000. Measles: Children from lower quintiles less likely covered, CoI decreased from 0.058 (p<0.05) in 1995 to 0.009 (p<0.05) in 2000. DPT: Children from lower quintiles less likely covered, CoI decreased from 0.0691 (p<0.05) in 1995 to 0.0022 (p>0.05) in 2000. HepB: Children from lower quintiles less likely covered, 0.0984 (p<0.05) in 1995, no 2000 estimate. Full basic: Children from lower quintiles less likely covered, CoI decreased from 0.0819 (p<0.05) in 1995 to 0.0052 (p>0.05) in 2000. No basic: Children from lower quintiles more likely to have no coverage, CoI decreased from −0.7434 (p<0.05) in 1995 to −0.7212 (p>0.05) in 2000. **Sought any treatment**: Fever: Children from lower quintiles less likely to receive, CoI decreased from 0.1076 (p<0.05) in 1995 to 0.077 (p<0.05) in 2000. ARI: Children from lower quintiles less likely to receive, CoI decreased from 0.0965 (p<0.05) in 1995 to 0.0897 (p<0.05) in 2000. Diarrhoea: Children from lower quintiles less likely to receive, CoI increased from 0.0357 (p<0.05) in 1995 to 0.0688 (p<0.05) in 2000. **Utilized private provider:** Fever: Children from lower quintiles less likely to receive, CoI increased from 0.1609 (p<0.05) in 1995 to 0.1928 (p<0.05) in 2000. ARI: Children from lower quintiles less likely to receive, CoI increased from 0.1543 (p<0.05) in 1995 to 0.1932 (p<0.05) in 2000. Diarrhoea: Children from lower quintiles less likely to receive, CoI increased from 0.1095 (p<0.05) in 1995 to 0.1713 (p<0.05) in 2000. **Utilized public treatment**: Fever: Children from lower quintiles more likely to receive, CoI increased from −0.0411 (p>0.05) in 1995 to −0.1240 (p<0.05) in 2000. ARI: Children from lower quintiles more likely to receive, CoI increased from −0.0469 (p<0.05) in 1995 to −0.0892 (p<0.05) in 2000. Diarrhoea: Children from lower quintiles more likely to receive, CoI decreased from −0.1446 (p<0.05) in 1995 to −0.1180 (p<0.05) in 2000.

* Only values of standard error (SE) were provided by this study. Binary significance levels (<0.05, >0.05) were calculated by multiplying the SE by 1.96 to obtain the upper and lower confidence intervals.

coverage during the 1995 National Immunisation Days, Reichler et al concluded that children living in households with a radio or a TV were significantly more likely to have received two oral polio virus vaccine doses than one or zero doses. Using concentration index based on household wealth quintile, Gwatkin et al reported that children from lower quintile households were less likely to be immunised against BCG, measles, and DPT (3 doses) than those from higher quintiles, although the concentration index value had decreased between 1995 and 2000. The concentration index value for Hepatitis B immunisation was only available for 1995 and showed the highest level (higher coverage among children from wealthier quintile households) among the various vaccines. Children from lowest wealth quintile households were significantly more likely to have received no basic immunisation coverage, and the concentration index value declined only marginally in the five-year period between surveys.

Curative care. In terms of the first dimension of curative health-seeking, seeking advice from a medical provider, Gwatkin's crude analysis showed that children from lower quintiles were less likely to receive care with symptoms of fever, acute respiratory infection (ARI) and diarrhoea compared to children from higher quintile households. However, whereas the concentration index value decreased between 1995 and 2000 for symptoms of fever and ARI, these values increased with respect to diarrhoea. The highest concentration index value in 2000 for this dimension was seen in health-seeking for symptoms of ARI. In a small sample of infants in Assiut, Fadel examined the association between SEP and seeking medical advice following symptoms of diarrhoea. In crude analysis, only household TV ownership was marginally positively associated with seeking care, but ceased to be significant in adjusted analysis.

Four studies examined the association between SEP and type of care chosen for childhood illness among the subsamples of children for whom any medical care was sought. In the nationally-representative DHS surveys, Gwatkin reported results of a crude association, finding that children from lower quintile households were less likely to have received care from a private provider. Whereas the concentration index value was smaller for symptoms of diarrhoea compared to ARI or fever in both surveys, the value had increased for all three illnesses between 1995 and 2000. Among infants in Assiut for whom medical care was sought for diarrhoea, utilisation of private care was associated with higher levels of both mother's and father's education, as well as mother's employment status in crude analysis (Fadel 2007). Among these three SEP indicators, only mother's education remained significantly positively associated with private care utilisation in adjusted analysis. In a sample of children taken for care for diarrhoea, fever, cough or rash in Minia, adjusted odds of seeking a private doctor were significantly higher for those with higher number of maternal as well as household assets, but not associated with maternal or paternal education or maternal ever-employment (Yount 2004). Analysing a smaller sample of children with diarrhoea in Minia, Yount (2003) found that neither the type of medical provider (doctor, pharmacist, other, lay) nor the type of facility (public, private, pharmacy) sought was associated with maternal education or household assets in adjusted analysis. This study also found no association, after adjustment for various confounders, between household asset ownership and cost of care incurred.

Discussion

Studies using nationally representative datasets found evidence of an association between SEP and maternal health-seeking behaviours. Women living in lower wealth quintile households were less likely than those from wealthier households to receive any and regular ANC, to deliver with skilled attendance and in health facilities. The magnitude of this association appeared smaller when women's SEP position was measured by education level compared to household wealth. However, no association was found between community-level affluence and maternal health-seeking behaviours. These differences in the existence and extent of SEP gradients raise the question whether material/financial resources may be a more important determinant of utilisation (potentially via direct and indirect costs of care) than women's knowledge of the need for care or its availability. On the other hand, the only adjusted analysis of a small sample found that women's education or household-level SES score did not predict the pattern of ANC attendance among women attending ANC clinics, potentially suggesting that once women access ANC care, determinants other than SEP contribute to the intensity of care they receive.

Children from wealthier households were significantly more likely to have been immunised, for separate illnesses and for a combination of basic immunisations, compared to children from poorer households. Analysis of time trends revealed that this gradient had decreased between 1995 and 2000, potentially as a result of high overall immunisation coverage. Crude analysis of a nationally representative sample showed that the gradient in care-seeking for symptoms of childhood illnesses favoured children from higher wealth quintile households, but while remaining significant, decreased over time. A significant and increasing inequality in private provider use based on household wealth was identified for all three childhood illnesses examined. This may be a result of the fact that the cost of private care is higher than of public care.[21,22] However, in smaller samples from Upper Egypt, conflicting results about the existence of an association between SEP and utilisation of any curative care and private provider selection for child illnesses were reported. This may be due to real differences between the populations from which samples were drawn, or be partially or fully explained by the difference in analysis methods (crude versus adjusted) or definition of illness (diarrhoea and any illness). The evidence on existence of an association between SEP and the cost of care-seeking was limited to one study (not adjusted for provider type) of a small sample, and therefore carried limited generalizability.

Limitations of available evidence

We considered selection bias, information bias (related to exposure or outcome) and analysis methods in assessing data quality of each study (Table 6).

Five studies used nationally representative survey data. Whereas the remaining smaller surveys considered selection bias (by including, for example, all women attending ANC, all mothers living in villages, or utilising simple random sampling in a community), they often neglected to describe the specifics of the population their samples represent. It was unclear whether sample sizes were calculated based on sufficient power to detect gradients in health-seeking behaviours, or whether previously collected data was used in analysis of health-seeking. Therefore, the findings of several such studies have limited generalizability not only on the general population level, but also for the understanding of local-level determinants of health-seeking. All included studies relied on cross-sectional analysis, and no analysis of individual-level time patterns of health-seeking behaviours was presented.

Two of the included studies specifically analysed socio-economic determinants of health-seeking behaviours. Seven studies attempted to identify determinants of health-seeking behaviours and one paper included SEP as a confounder in analysis of gender. Studies using separate variables, such as education level or binary asset ownership described the definition and categorisation of exposure categories better than those using component variables (SES score, household wealth quintile). Potential bias may stem from data collection methods – studies failed to report on and examine which member of the household reported on the various indicators of SEP (own, other members' or household-level) and whether this person could do so reliably.

Limitations in the definitions of health-seeking behaviours in included studies relate mainly to type of provider or facility. The method of categorising health providers into skilled or unskilled and health facilities into public or private was not always made explicit and may have relied of respondents' self-report. This concern is particularly pertinent to the use of pharmacies without previous medical consultation, a common practice in Egypt. The

Table 6. Risk of bias in included studies.

	Health-seeking behaviour	Maternal						Child				
Risk of bias category	**Study**	**Abdel Houssein, 1997**	**Yassin, 2003**	**Gwatkin, 2007**	**Khadr, 2009**	**Chiang 2012**	**Stephenson, 2012**	**Reichler, 1998**	**Yount, 2003**	**Yount, 2004**	**Fadel,2007**	**Gwatkin, 2007**
Selection	Representativeness (consecutive or obviously representative)	–	?	+	+	?	+	+	?	?	?	+
	Missing data or loss to follow up minimal	?	?	+	+	?	+	?	?	?	?	+
Exposure (SEP)	Clear definition of exposure	–	+	?	+	+	?	+	+	+	+	?
	Ascertainment of exposure	?	+	+	+	+	+	+	+	+	?	+
Outcome (HSB)	Clear definition of outcome	–	+	+	+	+	+	+	?	?	+	+
	Ascertainment of outcome	–	+	?	?	+	+	?	+	+	+	?
Analysis	Statistical test used to analyze the data is clearly described* and appropriate	+	+	+	+	+	?	+	+	+	+	+
	Minimal adjustment for age (maternal, child), parity (maternal) and gender (child)	+	–	–	–	–	+	–	+	+	+	–
	Correctly adjusting for several indicators of SEP	–	NA	NA	NA	NA	–	NA	–	–	–	NA

SEP – socio-economic position, HSB – health-seeking behaviour.
* Presenting a test of statistical significance was one of the inclusion criteria.
NA – not applicable (no adjusted analysis was conducted).
Key: + Low risk of bias, ? Potential/unclear risk of bias, - High risk of bias.

existence and extent of an SEP gradient by provider type may change as a result of the inclusion and categorization of pharmacies. Misclassification may have occurred in regard to type of provider, because many public sector medical professionals also practice privately. In addition, respondents may not know, correctly recall, or be willing to report the level of medical qualification of the provider used. The recall period used by studies for reporting of health-seeking behaviours seemed appropriate – longer for maternal care where information surrounding a birth is more likely to be remembered, and shorter (two weeks preceding survey or prospective data collection) for events related to child health. Child curative care relies heavily on the perception and reporting of child ill health. However, only Yount 2004 and Fadel 2007 used perceived severity of illness in their adjusted analyses of health-seeking determinants. On the conceptual level, the use of such an approach also challenges the underlying assumption that all perceived childhood illness symptoms ought to be attended to by a health provider.

Several important gaps in the body of evidence are present. In regard to maternal health-seeking, no study analysed SEP determinants of the type of facility (public or private) chosen by users of ante-natal care. Further, no study modelled the intensity of ANC care as a continuous variable, which would enable detailed analysis of the dose-response effects of SEP. No analysis of post-natal care, a crucial component of the maternal health package, was identified. Neither the determinants of facility level (health centre, hospital) nor of a combination of provider qualification and facility characteristics were examined for delivery care health-seeking. Lastly, expenditures related to maternal health-seeking and their association with SEP were not examined by any study. In comparison with maternal care, available evidence for child health-seeking included more dimensions of behaviours related to curative, but less for preventive care. No studies analysed types of providers and facilities approached or costs encountered in obtaining childhood immunisations. No evidence examining gradients in intensity of care (number of visits made and types of providers approached, if more than one) received for childhood illnesses was identified. Lastly, the type of symptoms for which curative health-seeking was analysed is limited to three; no evidence examining other important issues, such as childhood injuries or mental health was identified.

The use of a statistical test to assess the existence and extent of SEP gradients was an inclusion criterion in this review. However, included studies suffered from several other limitations in their analyses. Six studies only presented results of crude analyses and this was a major limitation of the usefulness of studies that employed nationally-representative data. The usefulness of analyses to policy is also limited by the number of following dimensions of health-seeking behaviour assessed in any given study. A gradient in intensity of care (dimension 3) may not only be a result of inequalities experienced at that point, but also a consequence of accumulated inequalities in seeking care (dimension 1) and the type of provider used (dimension 2). For example, in the only analysis of cost of care identified by this review (Yount, 2003), adjusted analysis did not include provider type and cannot therefore elucidate the SEP gradient in expenditures based on provider choice. Further, all five studies presenting adjusted analyses used various SEP indicators in one adjusted model, thereby controlling for (eliminating) the pathways of association from one SEP indicator through those remaining.

Strengths and limitations of systematic review

In addition to limitations of the studies included in this review and the gaps in the body of evidence, limitations of this systematic review were also assessed. The search strategy targeted global and regional databases, but only English sources were searched. Complete retrieval of studies identified for full-text review was achieved. Health-seeking behaviour is not a new concept, although it is a recent term, and care was taken to identify and use as many synonyms and components as possible in the text and MeSH terms used. Likewise, a wide range of potential SEP indicators was compiled and used in searches. However, the search strategy may have missed studies which used socio-economic indicators as confounders, but did not list them in the title, abstract or keywords. One author was responsible for study selection and data extraction. Most studies looked at a range of factors associated with health-seeking behaviours, not solely SEP. Therefore, while no formal assessment of publication bias was conducted, it is possible that studies which failed to find an association between health-seeking behaviour and SEP did not report the estimates. Such studies may also not have been submitted or accepted for publication. Despite the fact that only quantitative studies assessing the existence and extent of SEP gradient were included in the review, it was not possible to produce a summary measure of association due to the variability of definitions, effect estimates and analysis methods in individual studies.

Conclusion

Following large improvements in coverage of maternal and child health interventions in Egypt, socio-economic inequalities, and in particular the rural concentration of poverty, have been identified as the primary determinants of remaining disparities.[23,24] As one of the pathways in this association, health-seeking behaviours could contribute to such gradient in health outcomes. While the body of evidence presented in this study contains several limitations, we have attempted to synthesise the available evidence related to inequalities in dimensions of maternal and child health-seeking behaviour.

On the national level, socio-economically patterned inequalities in seeking any care for basic preventive and curative interventions in maternal and child health appear to have narrowed, potentially as a result of increased overall coverage. However, the extent of this gradient seems larger measured by wealth compared to education, and further exploration to determine whether and how knowledge and affordability of care drive these inequalities is necessary. On the other hand, the limited evidence of gradients in intensity of preventive care in maternal, and provider type in child curative care, showed that inequalities may have widened. In studies of more geographically and socially homogenous samples, fewer gradients were identified, signifying that in areas with comparable health service supply, future research will need to examine determinants of health-seeking beyond the traditionally used SEP indicators.

Overall, although ten studies examining socio-economic inequalities in health-seeking behaviours were identified, the body of research contains numerous gaps and the quality of available evidence is insufficient to draw a conclusive summary of the extent of gradients in Egypt. Future research needs to address gaps in the assessment of the various dimensions of maternal and child health-seeking behaviours, while carefully defining constructs underlying SEP indicators and correctly modelling this association in statistical analyses. This understanding will be crucial in designing and prioritising interventions to equitably improve maternal and child health outcomes in Egypt.[25]

Author Contributions

Conceived and designed the experiments: LB OMRC GBP. Analyzed the data: LB OMRC GBP. Wrote the paper: LB OMRC GBP.

References

1. Marmot M (2005) Social determinants of health inequalities. Lancet 365: 1099–1104.
2. Marmot M, Bobak M, Davey Smith G (1995) Explanations for social inequalities in health. In: Amick BC, Levine S, Tarlov A, Walsh DC, editors. Society and Health. Oxford: Oxford University Press. pp. 172–210.
3. Palloni A, Milesi C, White R, Turner A (2009) Early childhood health, reproduction of economic inequalities and the persistence of health and mortality differentials. Social Science & Medicine 68: 1574–1582.
4. Adda J, Chandola T, Marmot M (2002) Socio-Economic Status and Health: Causality and Pathways. Journal of Econometrics 112: 57–63.
5. Stowasser T, Heiss F, McFadden D, Winter J (2011) "Health, wealthy and wise?" Revisited: An analysis of the causal pathways from socio-economic status to health. Cambridge, MA: National Bureau of Economic Research.
6. Tipping G, Segall M (1995) Health care seeking behaviour in developing countries: an annotated bibliography and literature review. Brighton: Institute of Development Studies at the University of Sussex.
7. Lagarde M, Haines A, Palmer N (2007) Conditional Cash Transfers for Improving Uptake of Health Interventions in Low- and Middle-Income Countries. Journal of the American Medical Association 298: 1900–1910.
8. Mechanic D (2002) Disadvantage, Inequality, And Social Policy. Health Affairs 21: 48–59.
9. Andersen R (2008) National Health Surveys and the Behavioral Model of Health Services Use. Medical Care 46: 647–653.
10. Moher D, Liberati A, Tetzlaff J, Altman DG, Group P (2009) Preferred reporting items for systematic reviews and meta-analyses: the PRISMA statement. PLoS Med 6: e1000097.
11. Pokhrel S, Sauerborn R (2004) Household decision-making on child health care in developing countries: the case of Nepal. Health Policy and Planning 19: 218–233.
12. Wells G, Shea B, O'Connell D, Peterson J, Welch V, et al. The Newcastle-Ottawa Scale (NOS) for assessing the quality of nonrandomised studies in meta-analyses.
13. Gwatkin DR, Rutstein S, Johnson K, Suliman E, Wagstaff A, et al. (2007) Socio-Economic Differences in Health, Nutrition, and Population: Egypt. The World Bank.
14. Khadr Z (2009) Monitoring socioeconomic inequity in maternal health indicators in Egypt: 1995-2005. International Journal for Equity in Health 8.
15. Stephenson R, Elfstrom KM (2012) Community Influences On Antenatal And Delivery Care In Bangladesh, Egypt, And Rwanda. Public Health Reports 127: 96–106.
16. Abdel Houssein NA (1997) To what extent women's knowledge, beliefs, and health status influence their pattern of attendance for antenatal care? Bull High Inst Public Health 27: 269–277.
17. Yassin K, Laaser U, Kraemer A (2003) Maternal morbidity in rural upper Egypt: levels, determinants, and care seeking. Health Care for Women International 24: 452–467.
18. Chiang C, Elshair IHH, Kawaguchi L, Fouad NAM, Abdou NM, et al. (2012) Improvements In The Status Of Women And Increased Use Of Maternal Health Services In Rural Egypt. Nagoya Journal of Medical Science 74: 233–240.
19. Rutstein S, Johnson K (2004) The DHS Wealth Index. DHS Comparative Reports No. 6. Calverton, Maryland USA: ORC Macro.
20. Fahmy S, El-Sherbini AF (1983) Determining simple parameters for social classification for health research. The Bulletin of the High Institute of Public Health 13: 95–107.
21. Yip W, Berman P (2001) Targeted health insurance in a low income country and its impact on access and equity in access: Egypt's school health insurance. Health Economics 10: 207–220.
22. Rashad A (2012) Catastrophic health expenditure and poverty in Egypt: an analysis of household survey data. Cairo, Egypt: American University in Cairo.
23. El Deeb B (2005) Social Determinants of Health and Health Inequity in Egypt. Cairo: World Health Organization.
24. Gipson R, El MA, Campbell O, Issa AH, Matta N, et al. (2005) The trend of maternal mortality in Egypt from 1992–2000: an emphasis on regional differences. Maternal & Child Health Journal 9: 71–82.
25. Barros AJ, Victora CG (2013) Measuring coverage in MNCH: determining and interpreting inequalities in coverage of maternal, newborn, and child health interventions. PLoS Med 10: e1001390.
26. Reichler MR, Darwish A, Stroh G, Stevenson J, Abu Al Nasr M, et al. (1998) Cluster survey evaluation of coverage and risk factors for failure to be immunized during the 1995 National Immunization Days in Egypt. Int J Epidemiol 27: 1083–1089.
27. Yount KM (2003) Gender bias in the allocation of curative health care in Minia, Egypt. Population Research and Policy Review 22: 267–295.
28. Yount KM (2004) Maternal resources, proximity of services, and curative care of boys and girls in Minya, Egypt 1995–97. Population Studies 58: 345–355.
29. Fadel KAM, Moftah FM, Hilmy OEGM, Monazea EMM (2007) Health advice seeking behavior during childhood diarrhoea in a semi-urban area in Assiut. Assiut Med J 31: 73–90.

Permissions

All chapters in this book were first published in PLOS ONE, by The Public Library of Science; hereby published with permission under the Creative Commons Attribution License or equivalent. Every chapter published in this book has been scrutinized by our experts. Their significance has been extensively debated. The topics covered herein carry significant findings which will fuel the growth of the discipline. They may even be implemented as practical applications or may be referred to as a beginning point for another development.

The contributors of this book come from diverse backgrounds, making this book a truly international effort. This book will bring forth new frontiers with its revolutionizing research information and detailed analysis of the nascent developments around the world.

We would like to thank all the contributing authors for lending their expertise to make the book truly unique. They have played a crucial role in the development of this book. Without their invaluable contributions this book wouldn't have been possible. They have made vital efforts to compile up to date information on the varied aspects of this subject to make this book a valuable addition to the collection of many professionals and students.

This book was conceptualized with the vision of imparting up-to-date information and advanced data in this field. To ensure the same, a matchless editorial board was set up. Every individual on the board went through rigorous rounds of assessment to prove their worth. After which they invested a large part of their time researching and compiling the most relevant data for our readers.

The editorial board has been involved in producing this book since its inception. They have spent rigorous hours researching and exploring the diverse topics which have resulted in the successful publishing of this book. They have passed on their knowledge of decades through this book. To expedite this challenging task, the publisher supported the team at every step. A small team of assistant editors was also appointed to further simplify the editing procedure and attain best results for the readers.

Apart from the editorial board, the designing team has also invested a significant amount of their time in understanding the subject and creating the most relevant covers. They scrutinized every image to scout for the most suitable representation of the subject and create an appropriate cover for the book.

The publishing team has been an ardent support to the editorial, designing and production team. Their endless efforts to recruit the best for this project, has resulted in the accomplishment of this book. They are a veteran in the field of academics and their pool of knowledge is as vast as their experience in printing. Their expertise and guidance has proved useful at every step. Their uncompromising quality standards have made this book an exceptional effort. Their encouragement from time to time has been an inspiration for everyone.

The publisher and the editorial board hope that this book will prove to be a valuable piece of knowledge for researchers, students, practitioners and scholars across the globe.

List of Contributors

Daniel R. Feikin and Robert F. Breiman
International Emerging Infections Program, Centers for Disease Control and Prevention Kisumu, Kenya

Godfrey Bigogo, Allan Audi and George Aol
International Emerging Infections Program, Centers for Disease Control and Prevention Kisumu, Kenya
Kenya Medical Research Institute, Nairobi, Kenya

Sherri L. Pals
Division of Global HIV/AIDS, United States Centers for Disease Control and Prevention, Atlanta, Georgia, United States of America

John Williamson
Center for Global Health, United States Centers for Disease Control and Prevention, Atlanta, Georgia, United States of America

Charles Mbakaya
Kenya Medical Research Institute, Nairobi, Kenya

Charles P. Larson
International Centre for Diarrhoeal Disease Research, Bangladesh, Dhaka, Bangladesh
Department of Pediatrics, University of British Columbia, Vancouver, Canada

Mícheál de Barra and Val Curtis
Environmental Health Group, London School of Hygiene and Tropical Medicine, London, United Kingdom

M. Sirajul Islam
Environmental Microbiology Lab, ICDDR,B, Dhaka, Bangladesh

Naomi J. Launders
Gastrointestinal, Emerging and Zoonotic Infections Department, Public Health England, London, United Kingdom
EU Shipsan Trainet Project, Public Health Program, European Agency for Health and Consumers, Luxembourg, Luxembourg

Gordon L. Nichols
Gastrointestinal, Emerging and Zoonotic Infections Department, Public Health England, London, United Kingdom
EU Shipsan Trainet Project, Public Health Program, European Agency for Health and Consumers, Luxembourg, Luxembourg
Department of Hygiene and epidemiology, Medical Faculty, University of Thessaly, Larissa, Greece
Norwich Medical School, University of East Anglia, Norwich, United Kingdom

Rodney Cartwright
Federation of Tour Operators, London, United Kingdom

Joanne Lawrence and Jane Jones
Travel and Migrant Health Section

Christos Hadjichristodoulou
Public Health England, London, United Kingdom
Department of Hygiene and epidemiology, Medical Faculty, University of Thessaly, Larissa, Greece

Yue Li, Shan-Shan Zhen, Ying Chen and Xuan-Yi Wang
Key Laboratory Medical Molecular Virology, MoE/MoH, and the Institutes of Biomedical Sciences, Shanghai Medical College, Fudan University, Shanghai, People's Republic of China

Song-Mei Wang
Training Center of Medical Experiments, Shanghai Medical College, Fudan University, Shanghai, People's Republic of China

Wei Deng
Department of Health Statistics and Social Medicine, School of Public Health, Shanghai Medical College, Fudan University, Shanghai, People's Republic of China

Paul E. Kilgore
Eugene Applebaum College of Pharmacy and Health Sciences, Wayne State University, Detroit, United States of America

Mia Catharine Mattioli, Alexandria B. Boehm and Angela R. Harris
Environmental and Water Studies, Department of Civil and Environmental Engineering, Stanford University, Stanford, California, United States of America

Jennifer Davis and Amy J. Pickering
Environmental and Water Studies, Department of Civil and Environmental Engineering, Stanford University, Stanford, California, United States of America
Woods Institute for the Environment, Stanford University, Stanford, California, United States of America

Mwifadhi Mrisho
Ifakara Health Institute, Bagamoyo Research and Training Unit, Bagamoyo, Tanzania

Musthafa Chalikandy Peedikayil and Fahad Ibrahim AlSohaibani
Department of Medicine, King Faisal Specialist Hospital and Research Center, Riyadh, Kingdom of Saudi Arabia

Abdullah Hamad Alkhenizan
Department of Family Medicine and Polyclinics, King Faisal
Specialist Hospital and Research Center, Riyadh, Kingdom of Saudi Arabia

Takeshi Yamamoto, Toshihisa Kodama, Jaemin Lee, Naho Utsunomiya, Shusaku Hayashi and Makoto Kadowaki
Division of Gastrointestinal Pathophysiology, Institute of Natural Medicine, University of Toyama, Toyama, Toyama, Japan

Hiroshi Sakamoto
Department of Physical Therapy, Health Science University, Fujikawaguchiko, Yamanashi, Japan

Hirofumi Kuramoto
Department of Applied Biology, Kyoto Institute of Technology, Kyoto, Kyoto, Japan

Xiaofeng Chen, Yiqian Liu, Ping Liu, Yongmei Yin, Renhua Guo, Kaihua Lu, Lingjun Zhu Yanhong Gu, Lianke Liu, Yongqian Shu and Lingjun Zhu
Department of Oncology, the First Affiliated Hospital of Nanjing Medical University, Nanjing, China

Quan Zhu
Department of Cardiothoracic Surgery, the First Affiliated Hospital of Nanjing Medical University, Nanjing, China

Jinghua Wang
Department of Oncology, Jinling Hospital, Nanjing University School of Medicine, Nanjing, China

Zhaoxia Wang
Department of Oncology, the Second Affiliated Hospital of Nanjing Medical University, Nanjing, China

Oluf Dimitri Røe
Department of Cancer Research and Molecular Medicine, Norwegian University of Science and Technology, Trondheim, Norway
Norwegian University of Science and Technology, Trondheim, Norway, Cancer Clinic, Levanger Hospital, Nord- Trøndelag Health Trust, Levanger, Norway

Timothy J. Dallman, Marie A. Chattaway, Lauren A. Cowley, Kathie A. Grant and Claire Jenkins
Gastrointestinial Bacteria Reference Unit, Public Health England, London, United Kingdom

Michel Doumith
Antimicrobial Resistance and Healthcare Associated Infections Reference Unit, Public Health England, London, United Kingdom

Rediat Tewolde and Anthony Underwood
Applied Laboratory and Bio- Informatics Unit, Public Health England, London, United Kingdom

David J. Wooldridge
Department for Bio-analysis and Horizon Technologies, Next Generation Sequencing, Public Health England, London, United Kingdom

Derren Read
Public Health Laboratory London, Barts and The London Hospital Trust, London, United Kingdom

John Wain
Innovation Centre, University of East Anglia, Norwich, United Kingdom

Kirsty Foster
North East Public Health England Centre, Newcastle upon Tyne, United Kingdom

Filemón Bucardo and Yaoska Reyes
Department of Microbiology, University of León (UNAN-León), León, Nicaragua,

Lennart Svensson and Johan Nordgren
Division of Molecular Virology, Department of Clinical and Experimental Medicine, Linköping University, Linköping, Sweden

Saskia Luttikholt, Renévan den Brom, Lammert Moll, Karianne Lievaart-Peterson and Piet Vellema
Department of Small Ruminant Health, GD Animal Health, Deventer, The Netherlands

Anouk Veldhuis and Gerdien van Schaik
Department of Epidemiology, GD Animal Health, Deventer, The Netherlands

Klaas Peperkamp
Department of Pathology, GD Animal Health, Deventer, The Netherlands

Sabrina J. Moyo
Department of Clinical Science, University of Bergen, Bergen, Norway
Department of Microbiology and Immunology, Muhimbili University of Health and Allied Sciences, Dar es Salaam, Tanzania

Samuel Y. Maselle
Department of Microbiology and Immunology, Muhimbili University of Health and Allied Sciences, Dar es Salaam, Tanzania

Bjørn Blomberg and Kurt Hanevik
Department of Clinical Science, University of Bergen, Bergen, Norway
Department of Microbiology, Haukeland University Hospital, Bergen, Norway

Oyvind Kommedal
Centre for Tropical Infectious Diseases, Haukeland University Hospital, Bergen, Norway

Kirsti Vainio
Division of Infectious Disease Control, Norwegian Institute of Public Health, Oslo, Norway

Nina Langeland
Department of Clinical Science, University of Bergen, Bergen, Norway
Department of Medicine, Haukeland University Hospital, Bergen, Norway

Beatrice Olack, Kennedy O. Odero and George O. Okoth
Kenya Medical Research Institute and Centers for Disease Control and Prevention Collaboration (KEMRI-CDC), Nairobi, Kenya

Daniel R. Feikin, Leonard O. Cosmas, Joel M. Montgomery and Robert F. Breiman
Global Disease Detection Division, Kenya Office of the US Centers for Disease Control and Prevention, Nairobi, Kenya

Nicolas Faller, Ivan Gautschi and Laurent Schild
Department of Pharmacology and Toxicology, University of Lausanne, Lausanne, Switzerland

Ke Wen, Christine Tin, Haifeng Wang, Xingdong Yang, Guohua Li, Ernawati Giri-Rachman, Lijuan Yuan, Jacob Kocher and Tammy Bui
Department of Biomedical Sciences and Pathobiology, Virginia-Maryland Regional College of Veterinary Medicine, Virginia Polytechnic Institute and State University, Blacksburg, Viginia, United States of America

Sherrie Clark-Deener
Department of Large Animal Clinical Sciences, Virginia-Maryland Regional College of Veterinary Medicine, Virginia Polytechnic Institute and State University, Blacksburg, Viginia, United States of America

Rita Prager, Christina Lang, Philipp Aurass, Angelika Fruth, Erhard Tietze and Antje Flieger
Divison of Enteropathogenic Bacteria and Legionella, National Reference Centre for Salmonella and other Bacterial Enteric Pathogens, Robert Koch-Institut, Wernigerode, Germany

Joshua S. Gruber, Ayse Ercumen and John M. Colford, Jr.
Division of Epidemiology, University of California, Berkeley, California, United States of America

Zhang Fangbin, Hao Weiwei, Zheng Cong, Chu Yanjun and Xu Feng
Department of Gastroenterology, The First Affiliated Hospital of Zhengzhou University, Zhengzhou, People's Republic of China

Zhao Wugan
Department of Pathology, The First Affiliated Hospital of Zhengzhou University, Zhengzhou, People's Republic of China

Patricia Rarau, Mary Salib, Doris Manong and Peter Siba
Vector Born Unit, PNG Institute of Medical Research, Madang (MAD), Papua New Guinea

Stephen Rogerson
Department of Medicine, University of Melbourne, Melbourne, Australia

Ivo Mueller
Vector Born Unit, PNG Institute of Medical Research, Madang (MAD), Papua New Guinea
Dept. of Infections and Immunity Walter and Eliza Hall Institute of Medical Research, Melbourne, Australia
Centre de Recerca en Salut Internacional de Barcelona (CRESIB), Barcelona, Spain

Blaise Genton
Health Intervention Unit, Swiss Tropical and Public Health Institute, Basel (BS), Switzerland
University of Basel, Basel (BS), Switzerland

Nicolas Senn
Vector Born Unit, PNG Institute of Medical Research, Madang (MAD), Papua New Guinea
Health Intervention Unit, Swiss Tropical and Public Health Institute, Basel (BS), Switzerland

University of Basel, Basel (BS), Switzerland
Department of Medicine, University of Melbourne, Melbourne, Australia

Phimpha Paboriboune
Centre d'Infectiologie Christophe Mérieux du Laos, Ministry of Health, Vientiane, Lao Peoplés Democratic Republic
UMI 233, Institut de Recherche pour le Développement-UniversitéMontpellier 1, Montpellier, France

Eric Delaporte and Jean- Franc¸ois Etard
UMI 233, Institut de Recherche pour le Développement-UniversitéMontpellier 1, Montpellier, France

Niranh Phoumindr, Bouachanh Sengphilom and Yathmany Vansilalom
Department of Parasitology, University of Health Sciences, Vientiane, Lao People's Democratic Republic

Elisabeth Borel
Facultéde Médecine Lyon-Sud Charles Mérieux, UniversitéLyon 1, Lyon, France

Khamphang Sourinphoumy
Department of Infectious Diseases, Provincial Hospital, Savannakhet, Lao People's Democratic Republic

Saykham Phaxayaseng
Department of Infectious Diseases, Setthatirath Hospital, Vientiane, Lao People's Democratic Republic

Elodie Luangkhot
Service de Parasitologie, Hospices Civils de Lyon, Lyon, France

Peter Odermatt
Department of Epidemiology and Public Health, Swiss Tropical and Public Health Institute, Basel, Switzerland

Meja Rabodonirina
Facultéde Médecine Lyon-Sud Charles Mérieux, UniversitéLyon 1, Lyon, France
Service de Parasitologie, Hospices Civils de Lyon, Lyon, France

Lenka Benova and George B. Ploubidis
Department of Population Health, Faculty of Epidemiology and Population Health, London School of Hygiene and Tropical Medicine, London, United Kingdom

Oona M. R. Campbell
Department of Infectious Disease Epidemiology, Faculty of Epidemiology and Population Health, London School of Hygiene and Tropical Medicine, London, United Kingdom

Marieke Heijnen, Oliver Cumming, Rachel Peletz and Gabrielle Ka-Seen Chan
Faculty of Infectious and Tropical Diseases, London School of Hygiene and Tropical Medicine, London, United Kingdom

Kelly Baker
Department of Environmental Health, Rollins School of Public Health, Emory University, Atlanta, Georgia, United States of America

Joe Brown
School of Civil and Environmental Engineering, Georgia Institute of Technology, Atlanta, Georgia, United States of America

Thomas Clasen
Faculty of Infectious and Tropical Diseases, London School of Hygiene and Tropical Medicine, London, United Kingdom
Department of Environmental Health, Rollins School of Public Health, Emory University, Atlanta, Georgia, United States of America

Pascal Geldsetzer
Department of Global Health and Population, Harvard School of Public Health, Boston, Massachusetts, United States of America

Thomas Christie Williams, Amir Kirolos, Sarah Mitchell, Louise Alison Ratcliffe, Maya Kate Kohli-Lynch, Esther Jill Laura Bischoff, Sophie Cameron and Harry Campbell
Public Health Sciences Section, Division of Community Health Sciences, University of Edinburgh, Edinburgh, United Kingdom

Yeon Joo Lee and Eric R. Littmann
Infectious Diseases Service, Memorial Sloan Kettering Cancer Center, New York, New York, United States of America

Robert R. Jenq
Adult Bone Marrow Transplant Service, Memorial Sloan Kettering Cancer Center, New York, New York, United States of America

Lauren Lipuma, Asia Gobourne and Daniel No
Lucille Castori Center for Microbes, Inflammation, and Cancer, Memorial Sloan Kettering Cancer Center, New York, New York, United States of America

Marcel van den Brink
Adult Bone Marrow Transplant Service, Memorial Sloan Kettering Cancer Center, New York, New York, United States of America

Lucille Castori Center for Microbes, Inflammation, and Cancer, Memorial Sloan Kettering Cancer Center, New York, New York, United States of America
Immunology Program, Sloan-Kettering Institute, New York, New York, United States of America
Weill Cornell Medical College, New York, New York, United States of America

Eric G. Pamer
Infectious Diseases Service, Memorial Sloan Kettering Cancer Center, New York, New York, United States of America
Lucille Castori Center for Microbes, Inflammation, and Cancer, Memorial Sloan Kettering Cancer Center, New York, New York, United States of America
Immunology Program, Sloan-Kettering Institute, New York, New York, United States of America
Weill Cornell Medical College, New York, New York, United States of America

Ying Taur
Infectious Diseases Service, Memorial Sloan Kettering Cancer Center, New York, New York, United States of America
Lucille Castori Center for Microbes, Inflammation, and Cancer, Memorial Sloan Kettering Cancer Center, New York, New York, United States of America
Weill Cornell Medical College, New York, New York, United States of America

Melissa A. Kinnebrew
Immunology Program, Sloan-Kettering Institute, New York, New York, United States of America
Weill Cornell Medical College, New York, New York, United States of America

Halvor Sommerfelt
Centre for International Health, University of Bergen, Norway

Manjeswori Ulak
Centre for International Health, University of Bergen, Norway
Department of Child Health, Institute of Medicine, Kathmandu, Nepal

Ramesh K. Adhikari and Pushpa R. Sharma
Department of Pediatrics, Kathmandu Medical College, Nepal

Ram K. Chandyo
Centre for International Health, University of Bergen, Norway
Community Medicine, Kathmandu Medical College, Nepal

Helga Refsum
Department of Nutrition, Institute of Basic Medical Sciences, University of Oslo, Norway

Tor A. Strand
Centre for International Health, University of Bergen, Norway
Medical Microbiology, Innlandet Hospital Trust, Lillehammer, Norway

Xiaohui Zeng and Yunhua Wang
PET-CT Center, the Second Xiangya Hospital of Central South University, Changsha, Hunan, People's Republic of China

Jianhe Li, Xiaomin Wan and Chongqing Tan
Department of Pharmacy, the Second Xiangya Hospital of Central South University, Changsha, Hunan, People's Republic of China
School of Pharmaceutical Sciences, Central South University, Changsha, Hunan, People's Republic of China

Liubao Peng, Qiong Lu and Lidan Yi
Department of Pharmacy, the Second Xiangya Hospital of Central South University, Changsha, Hunan, People's Republic of China

Gannong Chen
Department of Surgery, the Second Xiangya Hospital of Central South University, Changsha, Hunan, People's Republic of China

Henrik Knecht, Femke Anouska Heinsen, Alexandra Zimmermann and Philip C. Rosenstiel
Institute of Clinical Molecular Biology (IKMB), Christian-Albrechts-University (CAU), Kiel, Germany

Sven C. Neulinger, Anke Schilhabel and Ruth A. Schmitz
Institute for General Microbiology (IFAM), Christian-Albrechts- University (CAU), Kiel, Germany

Carolin Knecht
Institute of Medical Informatics and Statistics (IMIS), Christian-Albrechts-University (CAU), Kiel, Germany

Vitor Martins dos Santos
Systems and SyntheticBiology, Wageningen University, Wageningen, The Netherlands LifeGlimmer GmbH, Berlin, Germany

Manuel Ferrer
Laboratory of Enzyme Discovery, CSIC - Institute of Catalysis,Madrid, Spain

Stefan Schreiber, Anette K. Friedrichs and Stephan J. Ott
Institute of Clinical Molecular Biology (IKMB), Christian-Albrechts-University (CAU), Kiel, Germany
Department of Internal Medicine I, University Hospital Schleswig-Holstein (UKSH), Kiel, Germany

Yuting Zhou, Xuejiao Deng, Peiting Zhang, Meicun Yao and Zhiyong Xie
School of Pharmaceutical Sciences, Sun Yat-sen University, Guangzhou, People's Republic of China

Qiongfeng Liao and Lei Zhang
School of Chinese Materia Medica, Guangzhou University of Chinese Medicine, Guangzhou, People's Republic of China

Manna Lin
School of Pharmaceutical Sciences, Sun Yat-sen University, Guangzhou, People's Republic of China
School of Chinese Materia Medica, Guangzhou University of Chinese Medicine, Guangzhou, People's Republic of China

George B. Ploubidis
Department of Population Health, Faculty of Epidemiology and Population Health, London School of Hygiene and Tropical Medicine, London, United Kingdom

Index